ONCOLOGY

ONCOLOGY

A multidisciplinary textbook

Edited by

Alan Horwich

Head of the Academic Unit
Department of Radiotherapy and Oncology
The Royal Marsden Hospital
Surrey, UK

CHAPMAN & HALL MEDICAL

London · Glasgow · Weinheim · New York · Tokyo · Melbourne · Madras

Published by Chapman & Hall, 2–6 Boundary Row, London SE1 8HN, UK

Chapman & Hall, 2–6 Boundary Row, London SE1 8HN, UK

Blackie Academic & Professional, Wester Cleddens Road, Bishopbriggs, Glasgow G64 2NZ, UK

Chapman & Hall GmbH, Pappelallee 3, 69469 Weinheim, Germany

Chapman & Hall USA, One Penn Plaza, 41st Floor, New York NY 10119, USA

Chapman & Hall Japan, ITP-Japan, Kyowa Building, 3F, 2-2-1 Hirakawacho Chiyoda-ku, Tokyo 102, Japan

Chapman & Hall Australia, Thomas Nelson Australia, 102 Dodds Street, South Melbourne, Victoria 3205, Australia

Chapman & Hall India, R. Seshadri, 32 Second Main Road, CIT East, Madras 600 035, India

First edition 1995

© 1995 Chapman & Hall except Chapter 16
© 1995 Chapter 16 William F. Hendry

Typeset in 10/12pt Palatino by EXPO Holdings, Malaysia.

Printed in Great Britain at the University Press, Cambridge

ISBN 0 412 55250 7

A catalogue record for this book is available from the British Library

Library of Congress Catalog Card Number: 94-71825

CONTENTS

CONTRIBUTORS

SIMON M. ALLAN FRCS
Clinical Research Fellow and Surgical
  Registrar,
Department of Surgery
The Royal Marsden Hospital,
Downs Road,
Sutton, Surrey, SM2 5PT, UK

T.G. ALLEN-MERSH MD, FRCS
Consultant Surgeon and Senior Lecturer in
  Surgery,
Department of Surgery,
Chelsea & Westminster Hospital,
Fulham Road,
London SW10 9NH, UK

S. BAL MS, FRCS
Senior Registrar Surgery and Assistant
  Professor of Surgery,
All India Institute of Medical Sciences,
New Delhi, India

RACHAEL BARTON MA, MRCP
Department of Radiotherapy and
  Oncology,
The Royal Marsden Hospital,
Sutton, Surrey, SM2 5PT, UK

PETER R. BLAKE MD, FRCR
Head of Unit,
Consultant Radiotherapist/Oncologist,
Gynaecology Unit,
The Royal Marsden Hospital,
Fulham Road,
London SW10 9NH, UK

MICHAEL BRADA BSc, MB, ChB, MRCP,
  FRCR
Senior Lecturer and Consultant in
  Radiotherapy and Oncology,
Head of Neuro-oncology Unit,
The Royal Marsden Hospital,
Downs Road,
Sutton, Surrey SM2 5PT, UK

DERMOT BURKE MB, ChB, FRCS
Department of Surgery,
Chelsea & Westminster Hospital,
369 Fulham Road,
London SW10 9NH, UK

RICHARD L. CARTER MA, DM, DSc,
FRCPath
Reader in Pathology,
The Institute of Cancer Research and
  Consultant Histopathologist,
The Royal Marsden Hospital,
Downs Road,
Sutton, Surrey SM2 5PT, UK

DANIEL CATOVSKY DSc(Med), FRCPath,
  FRCP
Academic Department of Haematology and
  Cytogenetics,
The Royal Marsden Hospital and Institute of
  Cancer Research,
Fullham Road,
London SW3 6JJ, UK

MICHEL P. COLEMAN BA, BM, BCh, MSc,
  MFPHM
Medical Director,
Thames Cancer Registry,
15 Cotswold Road,
Sutton, Surrey SM2 5PY, UK

JESSICA CORNER PhD, BSc, RGN
Senior Macmillan Lecturer,
Chairman, Section of Nursing,
The Royal Marsden Hospital, and Institute of
  Cancer Research,
Fulham Road,
London, SW3 6JJ UK

DAVID CUNNINGHAM MD, MRCP
Consultant Medical Oncologist and Head GI
  and Lymphoma Units,
Section of Medicine,
Institute of Cancer Research, and
The Royal Marsden Hospital,
Downs Road,
Sutton, Surrey SM2 5PT, UK

TIM DAVIDSON ChM, MRCP, FRCS
Senior Lecturer and Honorary Consultant
  Surgeon,
Department of Surgery,
University College London Medical
  School,
Riding House Street,
London WIP 7LD, UK

DAVID P. DEARNALEY MA, MD, FRCP,
  FRCR
Bob Champion Senior Lecturer and
  Honorary Consultant,
Academic Unit of Radiotherapy and
  Oncology,
The Royal Marsden Hospital,
Downs Road,
Sutton, Surrey SM2 5PT, UK

MARTIN J.S. DYER MA, DPhil, MRCP
Leukaemia Research Fund Senior Lecturer
  and Honorary Consultant Physician,
Academic Department of Haematology and
  Cytogenetics,
Institute of Cancer Research,
The Royal Marsden Hospital,
Downs Road,
Sutton, Surrey SM2 5PT, UK

SUZANNE A. ECCLES PhD
Section of Immunology,
The Institute of Cancer Research,
Haddow Laboratories,
Sutton, Surrey, SM2 5PT, UK

PAUL A. ELLIS MB, ChB, FRACP
Lung Unit,
The Royal Marsden Hospital,
Downs Road,
Sutton, Surrey SM2 5PT, UK

MICHAEL FINDLAY FRACP
Staff Specialist in Medical Oncology,
Royal Prince Alfred Hospital,
Missenden Road,
Camperdown 2050,
Sydney, New South Wales, Australia

J-C. GAZET MS, MB, BS FRCS
Consultant Surgeon,
The Royal Marsden Hospital,
Downs Road,
Sutton, Surrey SM2 5PT, UK

PETER GOLDSTRAW FRCS
Consultant Thoracic Surgeon,
Department of Thoracic Surgery,
The Royal Brompton National Heart and
  Lung Hospital, London, UK

MARTIN GORE PhD, FRCP
Consultant Medical Oncologist,
The Royal Marsden Hospital, and the
  Institute of Cancer Research,
Sutton, Surrey, SM2 5PT, UK

STEVEN GREER MD, FRCPsych
Cancer Research Campaign,
Psychological Medicine Group,
The Royal Marsden Hospital,
Sutton, Surrey, SM2 5PT, UK

ROSIE GUY MB, BS, MRCP, FRCR
Consultant Radiologist,
Conquest Hospital
St Leonards on Sea
East Sussex

CHRIS C. HARLAND MA, MB, MRCP
Consultant Dermatologist,
St. Helier Hospital, Wrythe Lane, Carshalton,
Surrey SM5 1AA, UK

CLIVE HARMER MB, FRCP, FRCR
Chief of Radiotherapy Services,
Department of Radiotherapy and
   Oncology,
The Royal Marsden Hospital,
Fulham Road,
London SW3 6JJ, UK

SUE E. HEIGHT BSc, MRCP
Academic Department of Haematology
   and Cytogenetics,
Institute of Cancer Research and The Royal
   Marsden Hospital,
Downs Road,
Sutton, Surrey SM2, 5PT, UK

WILLIAM F. HENDRY MD, ChM, FRCS
Consultant Urologist,
Department of Urology,
The Royal Marsden and St Bartholomew's
   Hospital,
London, UK

J. MICHAEL HENK MA, MBBCh, DMRT,
   FRCR
Consultant Radiotherapist, Head and Neck
   Unit,
The Royal Marsden Hospital
Downs Road,
Sutton, Surrey SM2 5PT, UK

TAMAS HICKISH MA, BM, MRCP
Department of Medicine,
The Royal Marsden Hospital,
Downs Road,
Sutton, Surrey SM2 5PT, UK

ALAN HORWICH MBBS, PhD, FRCP,
   FRCR
Professor and Consultant,
Academic Department of Radiotherapy and
   Oncology,
The Royal Marsden Hospital and Institute of
   Cancer Research,
Downs Road,
Sutton, Surrey SM2 5PT, UK

MARJAN JAHANGIRI FRCS
Department of Cardiothoracic Surgery,
The Royal Brompton National Heart and
   Lung Hospital,
London, UK

BERYL JAMESON MB, ChB, FRCPath
Consultant in Medical Microbiology,
The Royal Marsden Hospital,
Fulham Road,
London SW3 6JJ, UK

ALISON L. JONES MD, MRCP
Consultant Medical Oncologist,
Royal Free Hospital,
Pond Street,
London NW3 2QG, UK

IAN R. JUDSON MA, MD, MRCP
The Institute of Cancer Research Drug
   Development Section,
Clinical Pharmacology Team
Cotswold Road, Belmont,
Sutton, Surrey SM2 5NG, UK

ESTELLA MATUTES MD, PhD, MRCPath
Academic Department of Haematology and
   Cytogenetics,
The Royal Marsden Hospital and Institute of
   Cancer Research,
Fulham Road,
London SW3 6JJ, UK

JAYESH MEHTA MD
Leukaemia Unit,
The Royal Marsden Hospital,
Sutton, Surrey, SM2 5PT, UK

JANE MERCIECA MRCP, MRCPath,
Academic Department of Haematology and
   Cytogenetics,
The Royal Marsden Hospital
Fulham Road,
London SW3 6JJ, UK

BARBARA C. MILLAR BSc, PhD
The Institute of Cancer Research,
McElwain Laboratories,
Cotswold Road,
Sutton, Surrey SM2 5NG, UK

PETER S. MORTIMER MD, FRCP
Consultant Skin Physician,
The Royal Marsden Hospital,
Downs Road
Sutton, Surrey SM2 5PT, UK

ANTHONY G. NASH FRCS
Consultant Surgeon,
The Royal Marsden Hospital,
Downs Road,
Sutton, Surrey SM2 5PT, UK

ROBERT J. OTT PhD, FInstP
Head of Department,
Joint Department of Physics,
The Royal Marsden Hospital and Institute
   of Cancer Research,
Downs Road,
Sutton, Surrey SM2 5PT, UK

HELEN PATTERSON PhD
Academic Unit of Radiotherapy,
The Royal Marsden Hospital,
Fulham Road,
London SW3 6JJ, UK

ROSS PINKERTON MD, DCH, FRCPI
Consultant Paediatric Oncologist,
Children's Department,
The Royal Marsden Hospital,
Downs Road,
Sutton, Surrey SM2 5PT, UK

MERON E. PITCHER MB, BS, FRACS
The Royal Marsden Hospital,
Downs Road,
Sutton, Surrey SM2 5PT, UK

RAY POWLES BSc, MD, FRCP, FRCPath
Head and Physician-in-Charge, Leukaemia
   and Myeloma Units,
The Royal Marsden Hospital,
Downs Road,
Sutton, Surrey SM2 5PT, UK

TREVOR J. POWLES PhD, FRCP
Consultant Medical Oncologist,
Department of Medicine,
The Royal Marsden Hospital,
Downs Road,
Sutton, Surrey SM2 5PT, UK

PETER RHYS EVANS MB, BS, FRCS
Consultant Surgeon, Head and Neck Unit,
The Royal Marsden Hospital,
Fulham Road,
London SW3 6JJ, UK

GORDON J.S. RUSTIN MD, MSc, FRCP
Senior Lecturer in Medical Oncology,
Charing Cross and Westminster School,
Honorary Consultant Physician,
Charing Cross Hospital and Consultant
   Physician,
Mount Vernon Hospital,
Northwood, UK

NIGEL P.M. SACKS MS, FRACS, FRCS
Director, Surgical Oncology Unit,
St George's Hospital,
London SWI7 0QT, UK

AN E. SMITH MD, FRCPE, FRCP
Lung Unit,
The Royal Marsden Hospital,
Downs Road,
Sutton, Surrey SM2 5PT, UK

DIANA TAIT MB, ChB, MRCP, FRCR, MD
Clinical Oncologist,
The Royal Marsden Hospital,
Downs Road,
Sutton, Surrey SM2 5PT, UK

ANNE TAYLOR MB, BS, FRACP
Department of Medicine,
The Royal Marsden Hospital,
Fulham Road,
London SW3 6JJ, UK

J. MEIRION THOMAS MS, MRCP, FRCS
Consultant Surgeon, Sarcoma and Melanoma
   Unit,
The Royal Marsden Hospital,
Fulham Road,
London SW3 6JJ, UK

JENNIFER G. TRELEAVEN MD, MRCP,
   MRCPath
Consultant Haematologist,
The Royal Marsden Hospital,
Leukaemia Unit,
Downs Road,
Sutton, Surrey SM2 5PT, UK

ROSE TURNER MBs, MRCP
Consultant in Palliative Medicine
South Downs Health NHS Trust
The Community Palliative Care Team
The PortaKabin
Hazel Cottage
Warren Road
Woodingdean
Brighton BN2 6DA, UK

GERALD WESTBURY OBE, MB, FRCP, FRCS
Professor of Surgery (Emeritus),
Institute of Cancer Research,
Fulham Road,
London SW3 6JJ

EVE WILTSHAW OBE, MD, FRCP, FRCOG
The Royal Marsden Hospital,
Fulham Road,
London SW3 6JJ, UK

CHRISTOPHER R.J. WOODHOUSE MB,
   FRCS
Consultant Urologist,
Department of Urology,
The Royal Marsden Hospital and St George's
   Hospital and Senior Lecturer in Urology,
   The Institute of Urology, London, UK

JOHN YARNOLD MBBS, MRCP, FRCR
Academic Unit of Radiotherapy,
The Royal Marsden Hospital,
Downs Road,
Sutton, Surrey SM2 5PT, UK

PREFACE

In considering the wealth of oncological expertise to be found in many parts of the world, it may seem something of an arrogance to present an oncology textbook largely deriving from a single institution, the Royal Marsden Hospital and Institute of Cancer Research. The explanation is embodied in the subtitle of the book, stimulated by the development within the institution of a postgraduate multidisciplinary course in clinical oncology for a London University diploma.

For academic and administrative purposes the Royal Marsden Hospital is structured on a tumour unit basis: each clinical unit comprises specialized surgeons, clinical and medical oncologists. Protocols for assessment and management – as well as frequently the individual patient care plans – are defined within multidisciplinary discussion. Thus, the purpose underlying the structure and authorship of this book is to present a perspective on this multidisciplinary approach to the cancer patient and certainly not to suggest that this institution has a monopoly on authoritative teachers of oncology. A secondary fact has been that each unit and many of the institute's research departments have contributed directly to teaching students on the oncology course, and in essence, this textbook represents the didactic component of this course refined by presentations to, and feedback from, our previous students.

The book is intended as an introduction to oncology for those embarking on careers in surgical, radiation or medical oncology, it also provides a general management context for those in allied subjects such as pathology, diagnostic oncology, nursing and radiography. The inclusion of references with each chapter serves to emphasize that cancer therapy is a discipline in evolution; no textbook, however comprehensive, can substitute for the careful appraisal of original studies to obtain a true understanding of current practice.

In as much as the book may prove useful, full credit must go to the individual chapter authors, recognizing their willingness to sacrifice the indulgence of a personal hobbyhorse for the sake of clarity, balance and brevity. Christine Evans and Christine Martin organized respectively the book chapters and my timetable, and I will dedicate the book to Phyllis Cunningham, Chief Executive of the Royal Marsden Hospital in recognition of her zealous support for the concept and actuality of a multidisciplinary cancer centre.

Alan Horwich

PART ONE

THE PRINCIPLES OF ONCOLOGY

EPIDEMIOLOGY OF CANCER 1

Michel P. Coleman

Cancer will afflict up to one in three persons before their seventy-fifth birthday in developed countries, and one in four persons will die from it. In the UK, almost a quarter of a million new cancers are diagnosed each year, and there are some 160 000 deaths (OPCS, 1993). The frequency and lethality of cancer underlie the persistent public concern about this group of diseases, and the great interest in any news of progress in cancer treatment. The figures also give some idea of the magnitude of the public health challenge which cancer now represents in industrialized societies.

This chapter will provide a brief introduction to some of the information available about cancer from epidemiological research, and to the ways in which this research is carried out; an explanation will also be given of some key terms which may not be familiar to clinicians. Statistical methods for epidemiology will not be covered here.

Epidemiology is the study of the distribution and causes of disease in human populations. It is the basic science of public health. Epidemiology has been extremely informative about the patterns and the causes of cancer. We now have a clear description of the burden of disease and death caused by cancer in many populations around the world, and of the way cancer risk is evolving with time. Many of the causes of cancer have also been identified (Tomatis *et al.*, 1990). There is controversy over whether recent trends in mortality can be regarded as satisfactory progress towards the control of cancer

(Bailar and Smith, 1987; Doll, 1989), but there is widespread agreement that research into discovering avoidable causes of cancer is now of paramount importance (Breslow and Cumberland, 1988): 'Understanding biological mechanisms can be useful but is not essential for important progress in disease control... Hence, research aimed directly at cancer prevention and promoting use of available knowledge for cancer prevention is highly desirable in the present state of cancer control.'

1.1 EPIDEMIOLOGY

The epidemiological approach aims to provide an accurate and representative picture of the pattern of cancer in the population as a whole, and to help uncover the causes of cancer. Such information provides a factual basis for the development of rational public health policies for cancer control. The policies may relate to primary prevention, screening (secondary prevention) or treatment. Primary prevention policies require knowledge of the cause(s) of cancer, but not necessarily of the precise mechanism by which they operate. It may be enough simply to break the causal sequence of events, for example, by avoidance of excessive exposure to ultraviolet rays in sunlight (melanoma, other skin cancers) or by avoidance of exposure to cigarette smoke and tobacco products (cancers of lung, oral cavity, larynx, pancreas, bladder). Screening programmes are designed to diagnose cancers early, before the development of clinical symptoms and signs (preclinical detectable phase), when treatment at an earlier stage of disease may be expected to confer better survival. There is reliable evidence from randomized controlled trials that mammographic screening for breast cancer in women aged 50–69 can reduce mortality by 25%, and there is adequate evidence from observational studies of the efficacy of regular Pap smear screening in reducing incidence and mortality from invasive cancer of the uterine cervix. In the development of cancer treatment policies, epidemiological methods can be applied to describe the patterns of treatment or the extent of adherence to standard protocols, and the efficacy of treatment strategies in the population as a whole, including their costs. In this context, there is some overlap with the recent development of clinical audit.

The basis of the epidemiological approach is simple. Information is collected in a rigorously standardized manner for every individual (or a representative sample of individuals) diagnosed with or dying from cancer in a defined population, and the resulting data set is analysed with suitable statistical techniques. For a cohort study of cancer risk in an occupational group, the population might be defined as all persons who have worked in the industry or factory for more than some minimum time during a given calendar period. For a case-control study of cancer risk in relation to dietary habits, information obtained from a defined group of patients diagnosed with the cancer of interest (cases) would be compared with equivalent information obtained from a comparable group of persons who do not have cancer (controls). For a descriptive study of cancer in the general population, the population would be defined as all persons normally resident in a defined geographical area, such as that of a health authority or other administrative unit, and all cases of cancer diagnosed in members of that population would be recorded, either by an occasional survey or, more usually, by a population-based cancer registry conducting continuous surveillance of cancer in its territory.

Statistics may remain unfamiliar to some clinicians, but there has certainly been great progress since the last century, when one critic of an early trial of bloodletting to cure pneumonia felt able to write (Cairns, 1985): 'By invoking the inflexibility of arithmetic in order to escape the encroachment of the imagination, one commits an outrage upon good sense!' Randomized controlled clinical trials and the statistical rigour they impose are now accepted as the gold standard for evaluating the efficacy of new treatments, and basic epidemiological study designs such as surveys, cohort studies and case-control studies are widely used to describe the patterns of disease, to investigate its causes and to assess the side-effects of its treatment.

1.2 DESCRIPTIVE EPIDEMIOLOGY

Variation in cancer risk is usually described in relation to characteristics of person, place and time, the three classical epidemiological descriptors. Cancer risk is known to vary greatly with age and between the sexes, but also by other personal characteristics such as racial or ethnic group, and with occupation, dietary habits and other known or presumed surrogates for exposure to carcinogens, such as tobacco smoking and chewing, alcohol consumption and sexual behaviour. There is substantial geographical variation in cancer risk, both on a global scale and, for some cancers, over quite small distances. The incidence of colon cancer, for example, varies more than 10-fold around the world in both sexes (Table 1.1), while the range is several hundred-fold for cancer of the oesophagus, for which small areas of very high incidence can be found within short distances of low-incidence area, both in parts of Iran and Kazakhstan on the Caspian littoral, and in Brittany (France). Many atlases of geographical variation in cancer risk have now been published. Geographical variations offer

Table 1.1 Age-standardized[a] incidence rates per 100 000 for selected major cancers and selected populations, 1983–87

Country	Lung	Stomach	Colon	Melanoma	Prostate	Hodgkin's disease	Non-Hodgkin lymphoma	Naso-pharynx	All sites
Males									
Denmark	58.5	12.5	20.3	7.7	29.9	2.5	8.0	0.7	278.9
UK – South Thames	66.1	14.9	16.5	3.5	24.8	2.7	8.2	0.4	242.9
UK – Scotland	88.1	19.2	21.8	4.4	7.8	2.7	8.8	0.5	297.7
Japan – Osaka	41.5	73.6	14.8	0.2	6.6	0.5	6.1	0.6	265.4
India – Bombay	14.0	7.3	3.2	0.2	6.9	1.2	3.7	0.7	124.1
China – Shanghai	53.0	51.7	9.2	0.4	1.7	0.4	3.9	4.0	227.2
New Zealand (Maori)	119.1	25.3	11.4	2.0	37.3	1.8	7.1	1.2	350.0
Cuba	44.3	9.8	9.4	1.2	27.3	1.5	3.3	0.7	184.0
USA – Connecticut (whites)	62.5	9.0	35.9	10.5	47.2	4.4	12.6	0.5	320.1
USA – Connecticut (blacks)	87.2	15.0	30.2	1.9	65.0	2.8	8.3	1.0	351.8

Country	Lung	Stomach	Colon	Breast	Cervix	Hodgkin's disease	Non-Hodgkin lymphoma	Naso-pharynx	All sites
Females									
Denmark	23.1	5.7	19.3	68.6	15.9	1.5	5.6	0.3	258.0
UK – South Thames	21.4	5.7	15.0	60.3	9.8	1.7	5.2	0.2	205.4
UK – Scotland	30.5	9.3	18.6	62.6	13.2	2.1	6.3	0.1	238.9
Japan – Osaka	11.7	32.7	10.1	21.9	13.2	0.2	3.4	0.2	155.2
India – Bombay	3.0	4.3	2.6	24.6	19.3	0.6	2.3	0.3	115.3
China – Shanghai	18.1	21.9	8.7	21.2	4.3	0.3	2.2	1.9	146.4
New Zealand (Maori)	62.2	20.4	13.7	64.0	29.9	0.7	5.2	0.0	317.5
Cuba	15.7	5.0	10.2	35.0	20.0	2.8	3.9	0.3	163.6
USA – Connecticut (whites)	29.9	3.9	25.4	88.9	6.9	3.0	9.4	0.2	278.2
USA – Connecticut (blacks)	26.4	4.1	22.8	64.7	13.0	0.3	4.5	0.1	226.8

Source: Parkin *et al.*, 1993.
[a] Standardized to world population

valuable insights into the causes of cancer, and they suggest the extent to which cancer risk may be avoidable if the causes of the variation in risk are amenable to intervention. Changes in cancer risk over time can also provide clues as to the cause of cancer, and information on time trends is essential for evaluating progress towards control of cancer in the community. Cancer is a chronic disease with a long and variable latency between causal exposure and clinical diagnosis, and changes in the recent past are likely to be a fair guide to what will happen in the near future (Coleman *et al.*, 1993). Recent cancer trends can therefore be used as the basis for projecting the future burden of cancer, in order to guide policy-makers in determining priorities for prevention and research, and to assist health care planners in estimating the staff and other resources that will be needed to treat cancer patients.

The frequency of occurrence of new (incident) cases of cancer is usually expressed in the form of an incidence rate – the number of new cases per 100 000 persons per year. Cancer registries are designed to provide this kind of information by recording a standard data set for each new case of cancer diagnosed among usual residents of their territory. Note that the incidence rate refers both to the population, defined geographically in this way, and to a defined period of time; it is expressed per 100 000 persons per year to facilitate comparisons. The incidence rate may refer either to the whole population or to a group defined by age or sex (sex-specific or age-specific rates); separate rates may also be calculated for ethnic or racial groups, to identify variations in risk between them.

1.3 VARIATION WITH AGE

Data for south-east England can be used to examine variation in cancer risk with age for all cancers combined in a predominantly Caucasian population. The data are taken from the Thames Cancer Registry, which covers about a quarter of the population of England and Wales. There is an early peak in risk during childhood, particularly around age 3–5 years, followed by a trough in adolescence, then a rapid increase in risk from the age of 20 years onward (Figure 1.1(a)). This is a typical pattern for developed countries, but it is of course a composite picture, and the age incidence for different cancers varies widely. Lung cancer is rare below the age of 30, but increases continuously with increasing age in both sexes (Figure 1.1(b)). Prostate cancer is rare before the age of 45, but the incidence increases with age more quickly than for lung cancer (Figure 1.1(c)). In both cases, the risk at ages 75 and older is two to three orders of magnitude (100- to 1000-fold) greater than around the age of 30. Cancer of the testis has a quite different pattern; it is one of the most frequent malignancies in young men, but the different morphological types have distinct age-incidence curves, the peak incidence for seminoma occurring some 5 years later than for non-seminoma, itself a mixed group comprising embryonal tumours, arising mainly in young boys, teratoma in young men and an increasing proportion of lymphoma at older ages. Hodgkin's disease, an uncommon lymphoma, has a similar bimodal distribution, with a peak in early adulthood, and a further rise at older ages (Figure 1.1(d)).

Cancer is predominantly a disease of the elderly, and age is the most important determinant of cancer risk for both males and females. Cancers in children generally account for around 1 in 200 of all cancers, while most cancers arise after 65 years of age, and an increasing proportion at age 85 and over. The progressive increase in life expectancy at older ages in developed countries and the resultant rapid increase in the elderly population can therefore be expected to have a disproportionate effect on the numbers of new cancer patients requiring treatment in old age. This will have major implications for the future in the approach to the investigation

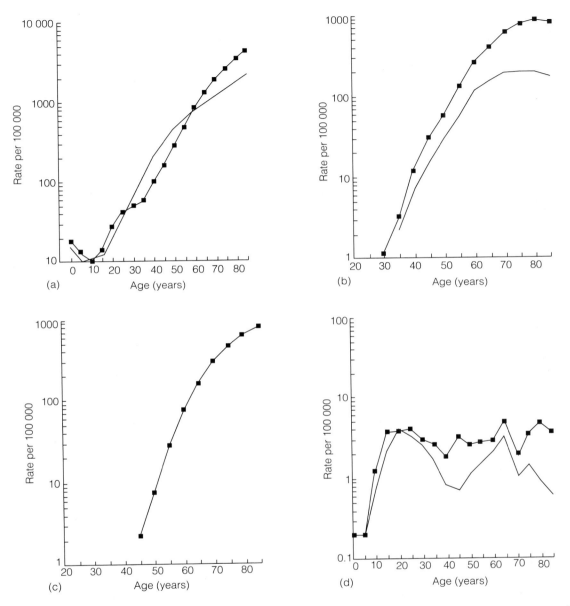

Figure 1.1 (a) Cancer incidence by age, all cancers combined (excluding non-melanoma skin cancer), males and females, south-east England, 1990. (b) Lung cancer incidence by age, south-east England, 1987–89. (c) Prostate cancer incidence by age, south-east England, 1987–89. (d) Hodgkin's disease incidence by age, south-east England, 1987–89. ■, Males; +, females.

and treatment of elderly patients with cancer. The biology of recovery in older patients may be favourably affected by general improve-ments in nutrition and fitness at the point of admission, but it is unlikely that the duration of hospital stay for cancer treatment in the elderly will be substantially reduced by these factors toward the average for younger patients. The overall cost of treating cancer patients may therefore be expected to increase out of proportion to the increase in the actual number or cases.

1.4   VARIATION OVER TIME

Demographic influences on the proportion of elderly persons in the population are only part of the equation, however. The number of cases of cancer arising each year in a population of given size will clearly increase as that population ages, even if the risk of developing cancer at any given age remains the same. But age-specific cancer risks *are* changing, and these changes need to be evaluated alongside the effects of demographic change. Figure 1.2 shows the recent trends in the risk of developing cancer of the stomach, non-Hodgkin's lymphoma and melanoma of the skin in south-east England, shown as the percentage change every 5 years in the age-specific rates for 5 broad age-groups. The decline in stomach cancer is part of a world-wide phenomenon that is still poorly understood, but is presumed to relate to improved quality of food resulting from better storage, reduction in salting and smoking as methods of preserving food, and the increase in consumption of fresh vegetables containing vitamins A, C and E (Coleman *et al.*, 1993). By contrast, the rates of increase in the age-specific risks of non-Hodgkin's lymphoma, testicular cancer and melanoma of the skin are quite substantial, and the causes of these malignancies are also poorly understood. Thus the impact of AIDS and immunosuppression for transplant recipients is unlikely to account for more than a small fraction of the increase in non-Hodgkin lymphoma, particularly in old age. Cryptorchidism is the main risk factor for testicular cancer identified so far, and it appears to be increasingly common, but it is unlikely to be solely responsible for the widespread and rapid increase in inci-

dence of testicular cancer. Recreational exposure to solar ultraviolet radiation certainly plays a part in the increase in melanoma risk, but again, the pattern of international trends by race, geography and sex does not suggest it provides a full explanation. These trends provide a major challenge for research into the causes and prevention of cancer.

1.5   FUTURE TRENDS

When demographic change and underlying trends in cancer risk at each age are taken into account, it is possible to make simple projections of the likely future burden of cancer (Figure 1.3). Such analyses for south-east England suggest that a 10% increase in the number of cases arising each year can be expected in the last decade of the twentieth century, with a further increase up to the year 2010, the increase affecting predominantly the oldest ages. The overall pattern of increase is obviously a weighted average of widely divergent trends in the different cancers, and the detailed patterns of change will need to be taken into account in planning for the future of health care delivery.

1.6   GEOGRAPHICAL VARIATION

There is wide variation in cancer incidence around the world. Each type of cancer has a distinct geographical pattern, and the recorded range in incidence also varies with tumour type. There is a several hundred-fold range of cancers of the oesophagus and liver, but only a ten-fold range or less for cancers of the colon or lung. The true range of incidence is likely to be wider than that shown in Table 1.1, however, because adequate data are not available from many parts of the world, particularly the African continent and developing countries in other areas. The international variation in cancer risk for different types of cancer has considerable implications for the overall cancer patterns within each country. As a simple example, the incidence

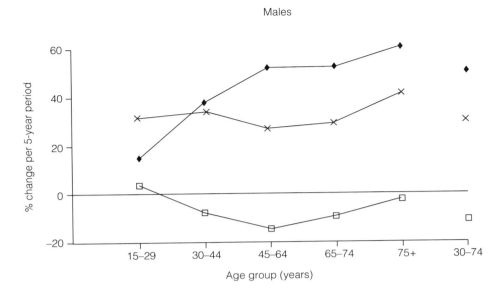

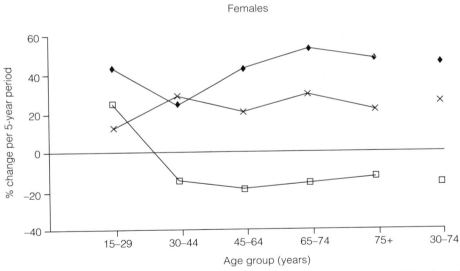

Figure 1.2   Recent trends in the risk of stomach cancer (—□—), non-Hodgkin lymphoma (—♦—) and melanoma of the skin (x), south-east England, 1973–87, by age and sex: percentage change in the age-specific rates per 5-year period.

of lung cancer in Denmark is four to five times greater than that of stomach cancer in both sexes, but the converse is true in Japan: stomach cancer is two to three times as common as lung cancer, and it is the most frequent cancer in both sexes (Table 1.1).

The information on variation in cancer risk around the world comes largely from

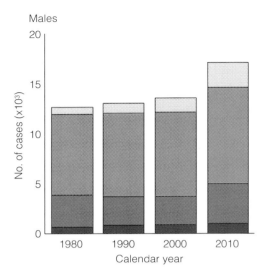

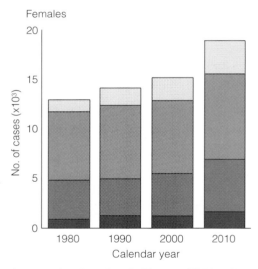

Figure 1.3 Projection of cancer burden, South Thames RHA, 1990–2010, by sex, for selected cancers. Age group (years): ☐, 85 +; ▨, 65–84; ▓, 45–64; ▧, 0–44.

population-based cancer registries. There are more than 250 cancer registries, some covering an entire country, others a region or city; the populations they cover vary in size from less than 100 000 to over 15 million. Some registries have been in continuous operation for more than 40 years, and data from more than 100 registries have been compiled in the quinquennial series *Cancer Incidence in Five Continents* (Smith, 1987). The data in Table 1.1 are taken from the sixth volume in the series, covering the period 1983–87 (Parkin *et al.*, 1993), and they show some of the wide variation in cancer occurrence by geographical area, race and sex for some of the major cancers. The incidence rates have been age-standardized (Smith, 1987), in order to enable direct comparison of rates after eliminating the effect of differences in age structure between the populations being compared. In direct age standardization, the cancer incidence rates observed at each age in the various populations of interest are applied to a common standard population to determine the number of cancers that would have been observed if each population had the same age structure as that of the standard population. The most widely used standard is the hypothetical 'world' population, with an age structure midway between the 'old' populations of the developed countries and the 'young' populations of developing countries.

Table 1.2 shows the most common cancers in south-east England in 1990, as an example of the typical distribution in a Caucasian population. Note that the rank order for the different cancers varies considerably with age, as well as between the sexes. These variations account for the different overall patterns of cancer incidence by age seen for males and females in Figure 1.1(a) which shows that cancer risk is higher in women between the ages of 30 and 60, but higher in men at older ages. Cancers of the breast and female genital tract account for the higher risk among women in middle age, while the rapid increases in cancers of the prostate, bladder and lung in men account for the reversal after the age of 60.

1.7 SEX DIFFERENCES IN CANCER RISK

A striking feature in almost all epithelial cancers is that overall incidence rates are higher in men than in women. The male-to-female ratio of incidence rates is shown in Figure 1.4 for the most common cancers, excluding those restricted to one sex. Apart from breast cancer, the chief exceptions to the male excess are cancers of the gallbladder and thyroid, while the incidence of cancer of the colon is similar in both sexes. The differences in the risk of different cancers between the sexes are not easily explained by different patterns of exposure to known carcinogens, and they must be presumed to represent sex-related differences in susceptibility to cancer development.

1.8 ETHNIC AND RACIAL DIFFERENCES

There are substantial differences in cancer risk between the various ethnic and racial groups, both within and between countries. In the USA, for example, cancers of the oesophagus and prostate are several-fold more common among blacks than among whites, while melanoma of the skin and cancers of the uterus and testis are less common. Nasopharyngeal carcinoma is common in many Chinese populations, particularly those originating from south-east China, and to a lesser extent among North African muslims, but is very uncommon among most Caucasian groups. Again, primary carcinoma of the liver is extremely common in parts of sub-Saharan Africa and in Taiwan, where persistent hepatitis B infection in infancy is widespread, but rare in most parts of Europe and North America. These and other examples do not necessarily imply a major genetic or racial component to the world-wide variation in cancer patterns, since many can be linked to ethnic differences in lifestyle and exposures to risk. Both increases and decreases in cancer risk have been observed among various migrant populations following migration to host countries with different cultural and dietary practices, such as the increase in breast cancer risk among second-generation Japanese women in the USA. Such changes strongly suggest a major environmental component to cancer risk patterns, since no population genetic change would be expected within just one or two generations. This in turn implies a substantial potential for the primary prevention of cancer.

1.9 SCREENING

Screening (secondary prevention) for cancer may be described as the mass application of a

Table 1.2 The 10 most common cancers[a], south-east England, 1990, by sex and broad age group (15 years and over): number of cases and incidence rate per 100 000 per year

		15–34 years		35–64 years			65 and over			All ages 15 and over		
Rank	Site	Cases	Rate	Site	Cases	Rate	Site	Cases	Rate	Site	Cases	Rate
Males												
1	Testis	221	10.1	Lung	1520	63.6	Lung	4933	577.1	Lung	6460	118.9
2	Hodgkin's disease	81	3.7	Colon	525	22.0	Prostate	2950	345.1	Prostate	3337	61.4
3	Melanoma	51	2.3	Bladder	504	21.1	Bladder	1544	180.6	Bladder	2053	37.8
4	Non-Hodgkin	47	2.1	Rectum	390	16.3	Colon	1430	167.3	Colon	1969	36.2
5	Brain	45	2.1	Prostate	385	16.1	Stomach	1209	141.4	Stomach	1549	28.5
6	Bone	24	1.1	Stomach	329	13.8	Rectum	872	102.0	Rectum	1272	23.4
7	Myeloid leukaemia	23	1.1	Kidney	266	11.1	Pancreas	580	67.9	Pancreas	835	15.4
8	Connective tissue	16	0.7	Pancreas	253	10.6	Oesophagus	525	61.4	Oesophagus	751	13.8
9	Lymphoid leukaemia	16	0.7	Brain	247	10.3	Kidney	377	44.1	Kidney	649	11.9
10	Colon	14	0.6	Non-Hodgkin	247	10.3	Non-Hodgkin	353	41.3	Non-Hodgkin	645	11.8
	All sites	706	32.2		6817	285.3		18 213	2130.7		25 736	473.6
Females												
1	Breast	143	6.6	Breast	3916	160.9	Breast	3659	280.5	Breast	7718	131.0
2	Cervix	107	5.0	Lung	738	30.3	Lung	2372	181.8	Lung	3121	53.0
3	Melanoma	75	3.5	Ovary	597	24.5	Colon	1857	142.4	Colon	2313	39.2
4	Hodgkin's disease	67	3.1	Colon	449	18.4	Stomach	841	64.5	Ovary	1365	23.2
5	Ovary	50	2.3	Cervix	446	18.3	Rectum	832	63.8	Rectum	1065	18.1
6	Thyroid	32	1.5	Uterus	432	17.7	Pancreas	768	58.9	Uterus	1012	17.2
7	Brain	30	1.4	Rectum	227	9.3	Ovary	718	55.0	Stomach	979	16.6
8	Myeloid leukaemia	25	1.2	Melanoma	224	9.2	Bladder	675	51.7	Pancreas	926	15.7
9	Bone	21	1.0	Brain	163	6.7	Uterus	573	43.9	Bladder	820	13.9
10	Non-Hodgkin	18	0.8	Pancreas	158	6.5	Oesophagus	488	37.4	Cervix	816	13.8
	All sites	703	32.6		9099	373.8		17 202	1318.8		27 004	458.2

[a] Excluding non-melanoma skin cancer.
Source: Thames Cancer Registry, 1993.

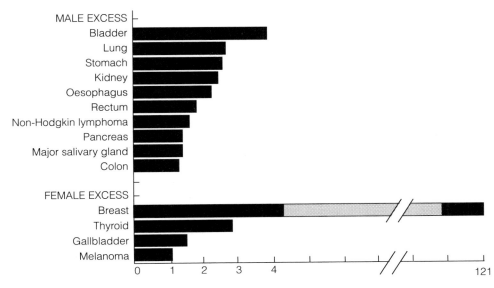

Figure 1.4 Sex differences in cancer risk: ratio of sex-specific age-standardized rates, south-east England, 1990, selected cancer sites.

simple test to detect preclinical cancer in asymptomatic individuals in the general population, in order to provide earlier and more effective treatment. Such organized programmes are thus distinct from the clinical or opportunistic screening done by clinicians in general or hospital practice, or as part of occupational health schemes.

One essential component of a cancer screening programme is that the preclinical phase during which the cancer can be detected must be sufficiently long in most individuals to make regular screening practicable: if metastases often occur before diagnosis is possible, as in lung cancer, screening is likely to be of little value. The test or battery of tests used for early diagnosis must also meet demanding criteria. It must be simple, robust and acceptable to the patient. In other words, it must be extremely reliable as used in the population at large, not just in experimental settings, when the prevalence of the condition to be detected is usually higher than in the general population. It must reliably detect 90–95% of preclinical tumours (sensitivity)

and exclude 98% or more of healthy individual from the need for further investigation (specificity).

On these criteria, screening has so far been unequivocally shown to be effective only for cancers of the female breast and the uterine cervix (Miller *et al.*, 1990). Even for breast cancer, clear evidence of effectiveness from randomized trials is only available for women aged 50–64 years, although further trials are in progress to assess mammography in younger women. A randomized trial of radiology and sputum cytology for lung cancer failed to show any reduction in mortality. Neonatal screening for neuroblastoma has proved difficult to evaluate, because the condition is very rare and the diagnostic test broadens the spectrum of cases to include some which would almost certainly not have developed into clinical disease, while even with a low false-positive rate, the number of healthy individuals requiring further investigation approaches that of those with disease. Colon cancer is potentially an important cancer for screening, since it is extremely common and survival is strongly related to the clinical stage at diagnosis. The nature of the preliminary screening test, detection of occult blood in the faeces, has so far been associated with only limited compliance, even in randomized controlled trials, and there is as yet no conclusive evidence that it will reduce mortality, although a number of trials are in progress.

1.10   CONCLUSIONS

It is perhaps worth stressing for the reader with an essentially clinical background or career plan that, from the broader perspective of cancer control in the whole population, the epidemiological approach is an indispensable part of the overall strategy, alongside basic research into the mechanisms of carcinogenesis and the clinical approach to diagnosis, treatment and management of individuals with cancer – the patients. Important clues to the causes of cancer have come from studies of the distribution of cancer in human populations, from its current patterns, geographical and ethnic differences, and from time trends in cancer incidence and mortality. Evaluation of progress in cancer control, of the current burden of cancer and, especially, assessment of the priorities for cancer control in the future – whether primary prevention, screening or treatment – will all require epidemiological information. Participation in the development of cancer control strategies will also require an ability to interpret such information wisely.

REFERENCES

Bailar, J.C. and Smith, E.M. (1987) Have we reduced the risk of getting cancer or of dying from cancer? An update. *Medical Oncology and Tumor Pharmacotherapy*, **4**, 193–8.

Breslow, L. and Cumberland, W.G. (1988) Progress and objectives in cancer control. *Journal of the American Medical Association*, **259**, 1690–4.

Cairns, J. (1985) The treatment of diseases and the war against cancer. *Scientific American*, **253**, 31–9.

Coleman, M.P., Estève, J., Damiecki, P. *et al.* (1993) *Trends in Cancer Incidence and Mortality (IARC Scientific Publications No. 121)*, IARC, Lyon.

Doll, R. (1989) Progress against cancer: are we winning the war? *Acta Oncologica*, **28**, 611–21.

Miller, A.B., Chamberlain, J., Day, N.E. *et al.* (1990) Report on a workshop of the UICC project on evaluation of screening for cancer. *International Journal of Cancer*, **46**, 761–9.

OPCS (1993) *Cancer Statistics, Registrations: England and Wales, 1987. Series MB1 no. 20*, HMSO, London.

Parkin, D.M., Muir, C.S., Whelan, S. *et al.* (eds) (1993) *Cancer Incidence in Five Continents, Vol. VI (IARC Scientific Publications No. 120)*, IARC, Lyon.

Smith, P. (1987) *Comparison between registries: age-standardised rates*, in *Cancer Incidence in Five Continents, Vol. V (IARC Scientific Publications No. 88)*, (eds C.S. Muir, J.A.H. Waterhouse, T. Mack *et al.*), IARC, Lyon, pp. 790–5.

Thames Cancer Registry (1993) *Cancer in South East England, 1990–1992*, Thames Cancer Registry, Sutton.

Tomatis, L., Aitio, A., Day, N.E. *et al.* (eds) (1990) *Cancer: Causes, Occurrence and Control (IARC Scientific Publications No. 100)*, IARC, Lyon.

CELL BIOLOGY OF CANCER 2

Barbara C. Millar

Nobel laureate, Richard Feynman, once compared understanding nature with trying to decipher the rules of chess when only a corner of the chess board is visible. These sentiments apply equally to understanding the development and nature of malignancy. The principal question that concerns cell biologists in relation to cancer is why certain cells have escaped from the normal homeostatic behaviour in multicellular organisms. This raises the question of what regulates normal multicellular behaviour.

Given the diversity of biochemical processes occurring in mammalian cells which arises because of the development of tissues with specific functions, it is likely that the regulation of cell proliferation and transformation to malignancy is determined by both external events, related to soluble factors and intercellular contact, and by intrinsic events, determined by the nature of specific cell types. Consequently, malignant transformation may result from many routes and involve a wide variety of different chemicals. Furthermore, because transforming gene products may be normal cellular components, differences in the behaviour of malignant and normal cells may result from quantitative behavioural anomalies rather than novel or unusual biochemical events. As a paradigm, the discussion will concern haematological disorders, as these represent malignant transformations in a heterogeneous tissue in which proliferation and differentiation are required to produce functionally mature cells. Also, repeated biopsy samples are available which

obviate the need to rely on cell lines which may have undergone further genetic changes *in vitro*.

When normal solid tissue or haemopoietic cells are cultured *in vitro* most have a finite capacity for growth. Occasionally, spontaneous mutations occur resulting in the expansion of subpopulations of cells which have infinite capacity to proliferate (secondary cell lines). Chemicals and viruses can accelerate this phenomenon *in vitro*. In each instance the resultant transformed cells may be tumorigenic in immune-suppressed recipients whereas the parental cells are not. Similarly, the autonomous proliferation of growth factor dependent malignant cells can be achieved following a single translocation event with viral DNA or cDNA for specific molecules, e.g. growth factors or cytokines. In considering the development of cancer it is important to remember that it may take years to evolve *in vivo* whereas transformation *in vitro* can occur in relatively short time periods.

2.1 NORMAL HOMEOSTASIS AND THE DEVELOPMENT OF MALIGNANCY

The control of homeostasis *in vivo* is dependent on the constant replenishment of old and damaged cells in the absence of immunological stimuli. In solid tissue such as gut epithelium, goblet cells in the crypts proliferate and differentiate as they progress up the villi to replace mature cells which are sloughed off into the lumen. In other tissue, e.g. bladder and skin, proliferation may occur in the absence of differentiation. In the haemopoietic system some blood elements have half-lives as short as 7 hours (neutrophils) or as long as 120 days (erythrocytes) or several years (some T cells). Thus, the differentiation pathways which regulate each lineage must be controlled accordingly. The majority of blood cells necessary for this 'constitutive' haematopoiesis in the mature animal are produced in the bone marrow microenvironment from a population of pluripotent stem cells which have the capacity for self renewal as well as differentiation (Till and McCulloch, 1961) (Figure 2.1). In general most stem cells are in a nonproliferative state. Since a percentage of these cells are retained throughout life it is likely that initial commitment to differentiation occurs concomitantly with self renewal. This may occur by asymmetric mitosis in which one daughter cell retains the properties of the stem cell whilst the other becomes committed to differentiation. Following commitment, there is rapid proliferation which can be demonstrated *in vitro* (Bradley and Metcalf, 1966), resulting in differentiation and maturation. In man the earliest recognizable haemopoietic progenitor cell has a surface epitope designated CD34, which is lost during differentiation.

In contrast, stress-induced haemopoiesis consists of a network of host cells comprising the immune system which are activated into proliferation and terminal differentiation in acute situations such as infections or bleeding (Figure 2.2). The hallmark of the immune system is specificity, which lies in the specific cellular recognition of numerous foreign antigens. This specificity is a property of T and B lymphocytes, which originate in the bone marrow but mature at distinct locations. In addition bone marrow derived macrophages, which do not recognize antigen, play a crucial

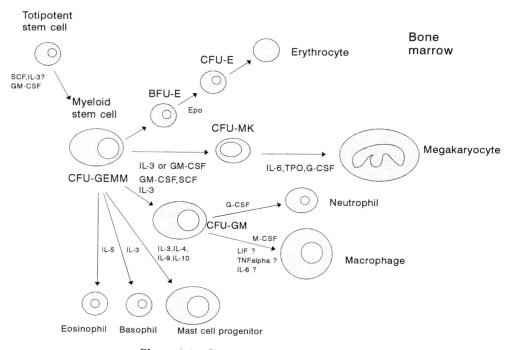

Figure 2.1 Constitutive haemopoiesis.

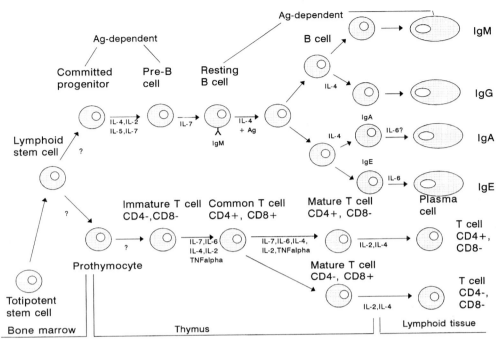

Figure 2.2 Inducible haemopoiesis.

role by presenting antigen to T cells and by providing both T and B cells with the extracellular signals required for functional activation. Interaction among these cell types is driven by antigenic stimuli to enable the recognition of self versus nonself, elimination of foreign pathogens, neutralization of toxins and even tumour cell killing (natural killer cells (NK) and lymphocyte activated killer cells (LAK)).

In considering the evolution of haematological malignancies, the aberrant expression of an oncoprotein(s) which results in malignant transformation must occur in cells which are capable of division. Thus, the target cells are either stem cells or committed progenitors that can proliferate as well as differentiate. Transformation could occur by two independent processes; either by enhancing the ability of self renewal, resulting in a clonal

advantage, e.g. chronic myeloid leukaemia (CML), or by arresting differentiation, resulting in the inhibition of maturation, e.g. acute myeloid leukaemia (AML). Despite the prevalence of immature cells, many acute leukaemias have similar phenotypes to their normal counterparts, suggesting that both mechanisms may be operable. In contrast, in multiple myeloma, which is characterized by the presence of excess abnormal but mature plasma cells in the bone marrow, it appears that mutations have resulted in clonal advantage in the absence of inhibition of maturation. Because myeloma cells produce an idiotypic paraprotein with concomitant light chain isotype suppression (LCIS), the consensus is that the major proliferative compartment occurs because of clonal expansion at an early stage of B-cell development, after gene rearrangement.

Additionally, it is likely that in accelerated disease in leukaemia and at relapse in drug-resistant multiple myeloma either additional mutations may have occurred or tumour control mechanisms have been subverted since progression often takes place in parallel with a further left-shift in the cells' stage of differentiation. Whether these changes in phenotype result from changes in the tumour cells themselves or because of changes in the control mechanisms mediated by other cells is unclear *in vivo*. From studies *in vitro* there is evidence that genetic changes in stromal cells, which are components of the bone marrow microenvironment, can affect the proliferation of bone marrow haemopoietic progenitor cells. When normal mouse progenitor cells were cultured *in vitro* with stroma which had been transfected with the v-*src* oncogene, the number of mature cells decreased whereas there was an increase in early progenitors compared with numbers seen in cultures exposed to non-transfected stroma. This change was mediated by the inappropriate signal from the viral oncogene since the same cells were able to reconstitute potentially lethally irradiated mice who lived a normal life span and did not develop leukaemia. However, one fundamental change had occurred because spleen colony forming units (CFU-S) from *src* transfected cultures had increased ability for self renewal in situations unfavourable for normal stem cells (Boettinger, Anderson and Dexter, 1984).

2.2 GENETIC CHANGES AND MALIGNANT TRANSFORMATION

It has been recognized for 25 years that gross changes in genetic material, particularly non-random chromosomal abnormalities such as translocations, characterize many human tumours. Approximately 90% of patients with CML have the Philadelphia (PH[1]) chromosome (Nowell and Hungerford, 1960) which results from the reciprocal translocation of DNA between chromosome 9 and 22. More recently, characteristic chromosomal rearrangements have been shown to be a feature of Burkitt's lymphoma (Manolov and Manolova, 1972).

Although changes in karyotype are not necessarily indicative of cancer, for example trisomy of chromosome 21 in Down's syndrome, evidence that they can contribute to malignant transformation has been provided from experimental systems. Seminal work by Harris *et al.* (1969) showed that fusion of malignant mouse cells with normal mouse fibroblasts often produced hybrids with a non-malignant phenotype, suggesting that 'normality' is dominant to 'malignancy'. However, subsequent chromosomal loss resulted in further hybrids which had reverted to the malignant phenotype. This was shown to be due to a specific loss of chromosome 4 in the mouse (Jonasson *et al.*, 1977) and chromosome 1 in man (Stoler and Bouck, 1985). These early experiments initiated studies into tumour suppressor genes for which the retinoblastoma (rb) gene is a paradigm (Lee *et al.*, 1987). In patients with hereditary retinoblastoma, karyotypic examination has demonstrated the frequent and specific loss of a polymorphic genetic marker enzyme, esterase D, from the long arm of chromosome 13 in tumour cells compared with normal cells from the same patients (Godbout *et al.*, 1983).

In other studies, Revell (1974) showed that malignant transformation can occur spontaneously *in vitro* from normal diploid hamster fibroblasts following chromosomal loss from a subpopulation of tetraploid cells. The resultant aneuploid cells develop during culture. Neither diploid nor tetraploid cells were tumorigenic whereas aneuploid cells formed tumours in immune suppressed animals. These and other karyotypic findings laid the foundation for the molecular genetics of malignancy and were antecedents to the more subtle genetic changes that have been detected in malignant cells.

The understanding of events which may contribute to abnormal cellular behaviour has been assisted by advances in the study of acute or rapidly transforming RNA tumour viruses which induce neoplastic change within weeks of infection of the host. The presence of oncogenes (v-*onc*) in these retroviruses and the identification of cellular homologues (proto-oncogenes) (Stehelin *et al.*, 1976) which code for growth factors (v-*sis* (β-chain PDGF)), their receptors (c-*src*, c-*erbB*, c-*fms*) or components of signal transduction pathways (*ras*), provided the first evidence for the existence of cellular genes with oncogenic potential. At least 35 such proto-oncogenes have now been identified which, as suggested by their names, require modification (mutation) to change them from their normal configuration and activate their oncogenic potential. These developments would not have been possible without concomitant advances in molecular techniques together with the availability of monoclonal antibodies which have permitted cell biologists to take advantage of recombinant protein technology to study relatively complex molecules and processes that are involved in cell proliferation and differentiation. There is general agreement that many, if not all, of the lesions in the genome of malignant cells result in the disruption of the recognition of, or response to, interactive signals that should regulate homeostasis. These signals which are provided by soluble factors combine with specific cell-surface receptors and result in the elaboration of a series of chemical events which lead to activation and transcription of specific gene products. Thus, mutation in any gene which codes for mediators of these events and may lead to the continuous message 'proliferate', is potentially oncogenic. Conversely, genes which in normal cells inhibit the production, receipt or implementation of signals are designated anti-oncogenes or tumour suppressor genes. Mutation of these genes or genes which regulate their function in cells which have undergone mutation in one or more other proto-oncogene can also lead to deregulated proliferation.

Based on these considerations, there are at least four mechanisms which might become disordered in malignant cells and result in aberrant proliferation:

1. Abnormalities in growth factor production
2. Abnormalities in growth factor receptors
3. Disturbances of post-receptor signalling
4. The reduced production of or sensitivity to growth inhibiting factors.

In general, these disturbances may be recognized at the behavioural level *in vitro* by loss of anchorage dependent proliferation, lack of density dependent growth inhibition and the secretion of excess or abnormal proteins. In haematological malignancies, the failure to produce mature functional cells is characteristic of the leukaemias and the accumulation of abnormal end cells and an idiotypic paraprotein that of multiple myeloma.

2.3 GROWTH FACTORS AND CYTOKINES

It has been known for years that serum is essential for the proliferation of mammalian cells *in vitro* and cannot be replaced by cell-free plasma, because of the presence of a factor, platelet derived growth factor (PDGF), released from platelets which behaves as a mitogen (Ross *et al.*, 1974). In fact, the proliferation and differentiation of all mammalian cells is generally controlled by extracellular signals which are referred to as peptide regulatory factors (PRFs). They include PDGF, epidermal growth factor (EGF), nerve growth factor (NGF) and fibroblast growth factor (FGF). More recently, glycoproteins produced by activated T cells (lymphokines), monocytes and macrophages (monokines) have been added to this list, including the interleukins (IL-) *viz.* IL-1, IL-2, IL-3, IL-4, IL-5, IL-6, IL-10, granulocyte macrophage colony stimulating factor (GM–CSF), granulocyte colony stimulating factor (G–CSF), the interferons (INFs) α and γ, tumour necrosis factor (TNFα) and lymphotoxin. These molecules may mediate both the immune and inflammatory responses as well as constitutive haematopoiesis. In addition, other factors produced by stromal cells, e.g. M-CSF (CSF-1), IL-7, leukaemia inhibitory factor (LIF) and stem cell factor (SCF; c-*kit* ligand) form a group of molecules collectively called cytokines. Unlike the response to hormones and neurotransmitters, which act within minutes to evoke a response, several hours may elapse between the binding of a growth factor or cytokine to its receptor and the induction of DNA synthesis. Thus PRFs must be capable of activating signal pathways for protracted periods. This may be important in determining some of the interactions which occur when cells are exposed to mixtures of cytokines *in vitro.*

Most cytokines are pleiotropic and have multiple biological activities. They may stimulate or inhibit or in some instances do both, depending on the dose and the target cell. In most cases they act synergistically or additively and may induce paracrine, autocrine or endocrine loops, thereby further evolving a wider range of cytokines. At least 40 cytokines are known to act on the haemopoietic system and it has been calculated that the number of possible combinations (with their order of administration being important) is at the minimum 2.1×10^{48} (Queensenberry, 1993).

Many cytokines are produced *in vivo* in response to immunological stimuli, e.g. IL-1, IL-6, INF, or following cytotoxic chemotherapy, for example G-CSF. During immunomodulatory events *in vivo*, the activation of cytokine genes in T cells and macrophages is temporal and may be restricted to the site of cytokine production to involve the appropriate inflammatory response or wound healing. Whilst there is considerable information concerning which cytokines are involved in these stress-inducible processes, very little is known about the cytokine requirement for constitutive haemopoiesis *in vivo.*

Although IL-3 is a suitable candidate for this regulatory role because it stimulates the growth and differentiation of pluripotent haemopoietic stem cells *in vitro* leading to the production of macrophages, monocytes, eosinophils, megakaryocytes and mast cells, its production from T cells requires their activation (i.e. stress). Furthermore, the mRNA and protein for IL-3 has only been detected in man following cytotoxic chemotherapy (Adshead *et al.*, 1992). Also, despite the isolation of IL-3 from culture supernatants of the murine cell line WEHI-3 cells, this is unlikely to represent a normal cellular byproduct and probably occurs because of aberrant rearrangement of DNA in the region of the IL-3 gene (Ymer *et al.*, 1985). Recently, SCF (McNiece *et al.*, 1992), which stimulates the proliferation and differentiation of early myeloid and erythroid progenitor cells via its interaction with the c-*kit* proto-oncogene, has been identified as a major regulator of basal haematopoiesis. SCF is produced constitutively in soluble and membrane bound forms from stomal cells and vascular endothelium. Although it has no direct effect on cell proliferation, SCF significantly increases the proliferative response in combination with all later CSFs including IL-3, GM–CSF, G–CSF and erythropoietin (EPO). Stromal cells which produce SCF do not express c-*kit*, whereas normal bone marrow progenitors express c-*kit* but not the ligand (Aye *et al.*, 1992). Based on qualitative differences between the effects of soluble and membrane associated SCF, current evidence suggests that the membrane bound form may be important in the cell–cell interaction between stromal and haemopoietic cells *in vivo* and *in vitro.* Similarly, microvascular endothelia and pulmonary arterial and venous cells produce GM–CSF constitutively (Malone *et al.*, 1989). Since GM–CSF can support the growth of multipotent progenitor cells in a later stage than IL-3 and can be associated with stromal cells by binding to the extracellular matrix, it also may be a key regulator of constitutive haematopoiesis possibly via an interaction with SCF. However, this should not preclude the existence of other IL-3-like molecules or the possibility that other mechanism(s) may fulfil the function of IL-3.

2.4   GROWTH FACTORS AND CYTOKINES IN CANCER AND *IN VITRO* TRANSFORMATION

One of the earliest hypotheses for the autonomous growth of transformed cells was attributed to autostimulation by an endogenous factor(s), which was thought to be one of the causes of unrestrained cell growth (Temin, 1967; Sporn and Todaro, 1980). Although many cell types have been shown to produce growth promoting activity, less have been shown to co-express the corresponding receptor and even fewer have been shown to be mitogenically stimulated in an autocrine way. For example, the bladder carcinoma cell line 5637 produces substantial amounts of IL-6; however proliferation is not inhibited by antibody to the cytokine (Millar B.C. and Bell J.B.G., unpublished observation). In contrast, cells transformed with simian sarcoma virus (v-*sis*) *in vitro* produce a homologue of the B chain of PDGF (v-*cis*). The v-*sis* oncogene only transforms cells which are responsive to PDGF and transformation can be blocked by antibody to the growth factor. Several glioma, sarcoma and osteosarcoma cell lines which are presumably derived from PDGF responsive tissue produce PDGF-like activity (Heldin *et al.*, 1980; Betsholtz *et al.*, 1983). In other cell types, TNFα which has 40% homology with EGF is produced in some retrovirally transformed cells (Twardzik *et al.*, 1982, Lee *et al.*, 1985); however its control by the retroviral oncogene product indicates that it is not itself an oncogene. An autocrine function has been described for the proliferation of small cell lung cancer by bombesin-like peptides (Cuttita *et al.*, 1985) and by insulin-like growth factor 1 (Macaulay *et al.*, 1990).

In most instances, constitutive growth factor synthesis in tumour cells occurs without any noticeable changes in gene structure or gene dosage. In such cases it may be impossible to determine whether growth factor production is different from that of normal progenitor cells perhaps by subtle changes in gene structure or control. For example, studies on the production of PDGF-like activity have shown that there is no evidence for rearrangement or amplification of the PDGF/c-*sis* or A chain gene (Nister *et al.*, 1988). Furthermore, genes in normal cells can be constitutively or inducibly expressed. In the case of PDGF this may either stimulate cell growth by an autocrine mechanism (e.g. placental cytotrophoblasts) or a paracrine mechanism (e.g. endothelial cells and macrophages). It is clear that more information is needed about the involvement of growth factors in the autocrine stimulation of normal growth, its developmental control and the molecular mechanisms of gene expression in order to fully understand its relevance in tumour cell proliferation.

In leukaemogenesis, autocrine stimulation occurs rarely in cells taken from biopsy samples and in general their proliferation is dependent on the addition of the same cytokines as those required for the proliferation of normal progenitor cells *in vitro*. The finding of an autocrine response to GM–CSF in acute myeloblastic leukaemia may thus be regarded as an exception to the rule (Young and Griffin, 1986). Also, the expression of SCF mRNA in some leukaemia blast cell lines (Pietsch *et al.*, 1992) is not necessarily indicative of autonomous proliferation *in vitro* since SCF is not a growth factor but augments the proliferative response to other cytokines. Even cells derived from Ph[1] CML patients, where there is known oncogene activation of the *bcr-abl* fusion gene, are usually dependent on the provision of cytokines to elicit proliferation. Nevertheless, it is arguable that when these phenotypic changes occur *in vivo* leukaemia cells may have a proliferative advantage because of their proximity to the haemopoietic microenvironment. Although immortalized myeloid leukaemia cell lines have been rendered factor independent following transfection with GM–CSF c-DNA, the failure to inhibit cell proliferation with antibody to GM–CSF suggested that other mutations had occurred which abolished growth factor dependency (Lang *et al.*, 1985). This has been shown to occur in a two-step process in which autonomy precedes a second mutational event (Laker *et al.*, 1987).

In B-cells transformed by Epstein–Barr virus (EBV) growth factors are not required for proliferation *in vitro* unless the cells are cultured in dilute solutions and B-cell stimulatory factors can be harvested from these cultures (Blazar *et al.*, 1983). However, lymphocytic tumour-derived cell lines differ from EBV-transformed lymphoblastoid cells in their total or partial lack of the requirement for their own growth factor (Gordon *et al.*, 1985). In some leukaemia cell lines derived from human T-cell leukaemias transformed by human T-cell lymphotrophic virus-1 (HTLV-1), the cells may progress in culture from IL-2 dependence to factor independence because of the autocrine expression of IL-2. However, some IL-2 independent HTLV-1 transformed cell lines do not require or express IL-2, suggesting that ligand binding to an appropriate receptor is no longer required to generate the proliferation signal.

In multiple myeloma there is considerable controversy concerning the role of cytokines, particularly IL-6, in the proliferation of malignant cells. In normal B-cell development IL-6 stimulates the secretion of immunoglobulin from mature human plasma cells and induces the proliferation of murine plasmacytomas (van Snick *et al.*, 1987) and hybridomas (Astaldi *et al.*, 1980). Experiments using clonogenic assays have failed to demonstrate any proliferative stimulus by IL-6 in cultures of plasma cells taken from bone marrow aspirates (Montes-Borinaga *et al.*, 1990), even

though it may stimulate the incorporation of tritiated thymidine in some cultures enriched for plasma cells (Kawano *et al.*, 1988). Similarly, in cell lines derived from human multiple myeloma there is no consistent requirement for IL-6 to induce proliferation. Since malignant plasma cells are often multinucleate this discrepancy may arise because DNA synthesis does not necessarily represent proliferation. In most instances, the proliferation of multiple myeloma cells *in vitro* does not show any specific cytokine requirement. Furthermore, the cells which proliferate *in vitro* usually have lymphoplasmacytoid morphology, rather than that of mature plasma cells, providing further support for the proposition that the proliferative compartment precedes the mature plasma cell.

2.5 GROWTH FACTOR AND CYTOKINE RECEPTOR

In most processes which involve the receipt of an extracellular signal, its translation and amplification in the cell involve protein phosphorylation. The first step in this pathway involves the association of ligand with the appropriate receptor which initiates the activation of protein kinase in the cytoplasm and results in the phosphorylation of target proteins (the nature of which are largely unknown). Events which follow ligand binding may be coupled with the activation of guanidine binding proteins (G-proteins), phospholipid hydrolysis and/or activation of adenylate cyclase. Generally PRFs constitute a group of structurally unrelated peptides whereas their receptors have conserved elements suggesting evolutionary diversity (Figure 2.3). Growth factor receptors have been identified by their intrinsic tyrosine kinase activity, e.g. the receptors for PDGF, EGF, FGF, T-cell, SCF and M-CSF (CSF-1). At least a third of the known proto-oncogenes code for growth factor receptors. Receptors for growth factors share a conserved core of 260 amino acids, indicating a common mechan-

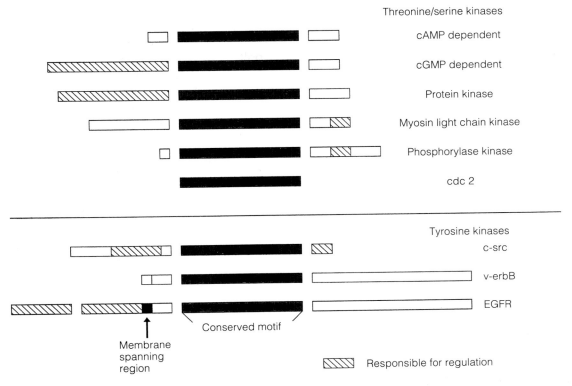

Figure 2.3 Growth factor receptor diversity.

ism of catalysis. In fact the residue required for both catalysis and Mg^{++} ATP binding are often conserved throughout the protein kinase family. Diversity in this group of receptors can occur because of substrate specificity as well as the number of subunits which contribute to the active enzyme and the distribution of peptide motifs either side of the conserved domain (Figure 2.3). Activation of growth factor receptors is mediated by dimerization and conformational changes induced by ligand binding, resulting in autophosphorylation of the internal domain of the receptor.

Overexpression of EGF receptors and amplification of the EGF receptor gene have been implicated in the growth of human tumours, e.g. glioblastomas (Libermann *et al.*, 1985). Truncated forms of growth factor receptors like v-*erb*-B and v-*fms*, which correspond to the EGF and M-CSF (CSF-1) receptors respectively, lack their external ligand binding domain but express tyrosine kinase activity constitutively. Transfection studies have shown that both v-*erb*-B and v-*fms* can render cells growth factor independent, by providing stimulatory signals in the absence of ligand (Wheeler *et al.*, 1986). The *neu* oncogene, which arises because of a point mutation and is structurally related to EGF, has been identified in mammary cell lines and salivary gland adenocarcinomas where it is thought that over-expression of the putative growth factor receptor can lead to unregulated proliferation. Similarly, amplification and enhanced expression of the c-*met* gene has been ascribed to the spontaneous transformation of NIH 3T3 cells following trans-

Table 2.1   Oncogenes and their cellular homologues

Oncogenes	Source	Cellular homologue	Function of homologues	Mechanism of oncogene activation
v-*src*	Rous sarcoma virus	c-*src*	Tyrosine kinase pp60^{src}	
v-*erb-B*	Avian erythroblastosis virus	EGF(R) c-*erb-B*	Tyrosine kinase	Truncation of EGF(R) amplification insertional mutagenesis
v-*sis*	Simian sarcoma virus	B chain of PDGF		
neu	Carcinogen induced rat neuroglioblastoma	EGF(R) c-*neu*	Tyrosine kinase	Point mutation in EGF(R)
v-*erb-A*	Avian erythroblastosis virus	c-*erb-A*	Nuclear receptor for thyroid hormone	
v-*fms*	Friend murine leukaemia virus	M-CSF(CSF-1)(R)	Tyrosine kinase	Truncation of M-CSF(R)
v-*abl*	Abelson murine virus	c-*abl*	Tyrosine kinase	
met	Carcinogen induced human osteosarcoma cells	c-*met*	Tyrosine kinase	Amplification and over expression

fection with normal cellular DNA (Cooper *et al.*, 1986) (Table 2.1).

Although inappropriate activation of growth factor receptors by an autocrine mechanism or by qualitative or quantitative changes in the receptor protein may illicit proliferation it may be insufficient to cause malignancy. In haematopoiesis such an event may also require a differentiation block. For example, the transformation of erythroid cells by v-*erb*-B necessitates the cooperation with v-*erb*-A which may act as the inhibitor of differentiation.

Unlike growth factor receptors, those for cytokines do not have integral tyrosine kinase activity in their cytoplasmic domain, e.g. receptors for IL-1, IL-2, IL-3, IL-4, IL-5, IL-6, GM–CSF, G-CSF, INFα, β and γ, suggesting that effecter subunits may be required for signal transduction, as has been suggested for the IL-6 receptor (IL-6R) (Taga *et al.*, 1989). Cytokine receptors are classified into distinct families based on their extracellular amino

acid sequences (Figure 2.4). The simplest type of receptor, e.g. IL-2β chain, IL-3, IL-4, IL-5, IL-6, GM–CSF, G–CSF and EPO, has conversed cysteine and tryptophan-serine-x-tryptophan-serine (x is any amino acid) motifs; however more complex receptors have evolved in which additional Ig-like motifs (IL-6R) or fibronectin-like as well as Ig-like motifs (G-CSFR) (Figure 2.4) are present extracellularly. The receptor for IL-1 differs in that it has only Ig-like motifs in the extracellular domain, thereby resembling the tyrosine kinase receptor family. Additional receptor diversity occurs because some cytokine receptors require at least two distinct subunits to form a high affinity receptor whereas others have high affinity ligand binding on their own or as a homodimer (Figure 2.5). The IL-6R consists of a soluble 80 kDa binding protein which associates with a 130 kDa membrane glycoprotein (gp130). Transfection of an IL-3 dependent cell line with the cDNA for human gp130 conferred

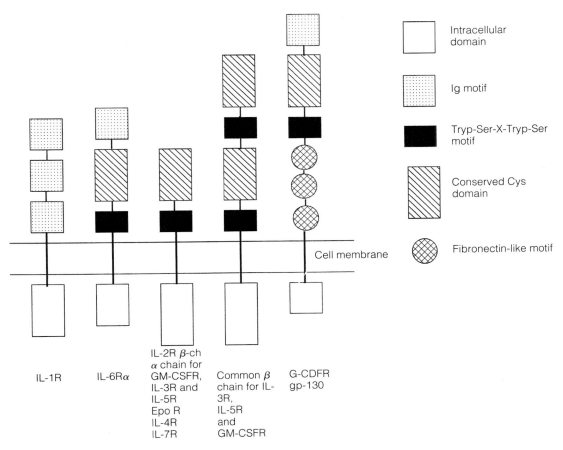

		IL-2R β-ch α chain for GM-CSFR, IL-3R and IL-5R Epo R IL-4R IL-7R	Common β chain for IL-3R, IL-5R and GM-CSFR	G-CDFR gp-130
IL-1R	IL-6Rα			

Figure 2.4 Cytokine receptor diversity.

Legend:
- Intracellular domain
- Ig motif
- Tryp-Ser-X-Tryp-Ser motif
- Conserved Cys domain
- Fibronectin-like motif
- Cell membrane

proliferative potential in the presence of IL-6 and the 80 kDa protein, thereby suggesting that gp130 is necessary for signal transduction (Taga *et al.*, 1989). Similarly, both mouse and human erythropoietin receptors (EPOR) expressed in an IL-3 dependent cell line transmit signals in response to EPO and a single point mutation in the extracellular domain of EPOR induced ligand independent growth of IL-3 dependent cells and tumorogenicity (Yoshimuro *et al.*, 1990). Elaboration of abnormal yet functional forms of the IL-6R have also been implicated in the development of mouse plasmacytomas.

Some viruses appear to modulate signal pathways at the receptor level. For example, myeloproliferative leukaemia virus (MPLV) carries a novel oncogene v-*mpl* which shares homology with the cytokine receptor family (Souyri *et al.*, 1990). Transfection of cell lines with MPLV yields factor independent cell lines of different lineages. However, in factor dependent cell lines transfected with the viral oncogenes v-*src* and v-*abl*, proliferation occurred independently of growth factors via a non-autocrine mechanism (Cook *et al.*, 1985). It is likely that v-*mpl* interacts with a component(s) of signal transduction pathways

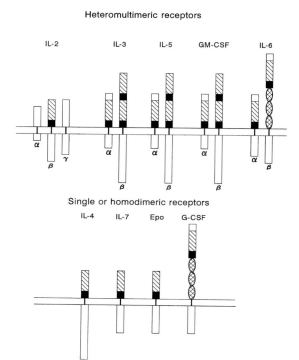

Figure 2.5 High affinity cytokine receptors.

and activates a cascade of events downstream from the cytokine. Because a single haematopoietic cell can respond to a variety of factors, e.g. IL-3, GM–CSF, G–CSF, EPO, which may share common biological activities and evoke similar events such as tyrosine phosphorylation and induction of DNA synthesis, it is possible that these cytokines are linked to a common signal pathway for cell proliferation.

Other oncogene products which may form part of signal transduction pathways have tyrosine kinase activity but are not growth factors since their normal counterparts are not transmembrane proteins. These include *fgr*, *hck*, *lyn*, *abl*, *fes/fps* and *src*. The distribution of the *c-src* family of proteins in non-proliferative cells such as neurones and platelets suggests that they are involved in differentiation rather than proliferation in normal development.

Furthermore, inhibition of tyrosine phosphatase with vanadate, which enhances tyrosine phosphorylation in response to GM–CSF or IL-3 in a factor dependent cell line, also enhanced the proliferative response to these cytokines, thereby implicating tyrosine phosphorylation in signal transduction (Kanakura *et al.*, 1990).

The concept that phosphorylation plays a key role in malignant transformation *in vivo* may be an oversimplification, since it takes little account of concomitant effects which may include the induction of protein phosphatases, of which there are in excess of 1000. Clearly, an understanding of intracellular phosphorylation and its role in the development of cancer should encompass both enzyme systems, since protein phosphatases are potentially powerful tumour suppressors. Nevertheless, the events following receptor–

ligand binding provide numerous sites at which mutation or transformation might result in the inappropriate formation of second messengers, resulting in uncontrolled cell proliferation as well as the expression and/or secretion of aberrant or excess proteins. These effects will be dealt with in a subsequent chapter.

2.6 NEGATIVE REGULATORS

By the time cancer is diagnosed, numerous cellular and molecular events are likely to have occurred from the potential initiating event, which may have happened 20 years earlier. Thus, cancer evolves as a series of genetic changes rather than a single one-off event. Whilst patients with premalignant lesions do not have treatable cancer, they nevertheless represent a population of individuals in the early stages of carcinogenesis which has a probability of progressing to a malignant phenotype. For example, approximately 15% of patients with monoclonal gammopathy of undetermined significance (MGUS) may progress to florid multiple myeloma (Kyle and Lust, 1989). The fact that not all patients with premalignant lesions progress to overt disease indicates that some lesions can be stabilized, arrested or disappear. Additionally, after therapy cancer patients often enter remission which may be sustained for several months or years. This suggests that in mammals there are effective control mechanisms which suppress the development of cancer in some tissues and which can temporarily inhibit tumour regrowth after cytoreduction. Such effects may be mediated by the immune system or by regulators of cell growth which function to inhibit proliferation and differentiation rather than stimulate it. An understanding of these mechanisms may prove as important as understanding the mechanisms that have occurred in aggressive disease, since it may permit their exploitation so that invasive malignancy can be prevented or at least temporarily arrested.

TGFβ is unique among the cytokines because it is synthesized in a biologically inactive form, non-covalently complexed with sequences of its own precursor and with α_2-macroglobulin. Most cells express TGFβ and have specific high affinity receptors for the cytokine. The mechanism for activation *in vivo* is unknown, but the involvement of proteases has been suggested. The most characterized form of TGFβ is TGFβ1, which has been shown to inhibit the proliferation of essentially all epithelial cells *in vitro*, including liver, intestine, pancreas, lung, trachea, bronchus, breast, ovary, prostate and spleen. In the haemopoietic system TGFβ1 inhibits the IL-3 and GM–CSF dependent proliferation of normal and malignant progenitor cells but not of normal progenitors which respond to G–CSF. In contrast, the proliferation of CML cells in response to G–CSF is inhibited by TGFβ1 (Sing *et al.*, 1988), as is the potentiation of G–CSF induced proliferation by IL-4, suggesting a regulatory difference between progenitor cells from normal individuals compared with CML patients. Because the mechanism of activation of TGFβ is unclear it is not known whether any of the cells that can respond to TGFβ *in vitro* can activate and thus respond to the TGFβ they secrete. Recent evidence suggests that an autocrine mechanism may operate in CD34 positive bone marrow cells, since exposure of these cells to antisense oligonucleotides to TGFβ1 resulted in an enhanced proliferation response to cytokines (Hatzfeld *et al.*, 1991). In most instances it is more likely that the action of TGFβ occurs by a paracrine mechanism, which will allow cells to communicate with other cell types and thus regulate tissue homeostasis as a functional unit. In support of this there is evidence that when pericytes and capillary endothelial cells are cultured separately they secrete latent TGFβ1; however, when cultured together, TGFβ1 is secreted in the active form and the growth of the endothelial cells is inhibited (Antonelli-Orlidge *et al.*, 1989). This requirement for cooperation may allow an organ to regulate its growth. It also emphasizes the dangers of relying on simplistic single component culture systems as models of complex biological responses.

Whilst there is no evidence for the direct involvement of INFs in carcinogenesis, they are potentially useful for the arrest and stabilization of malignant disease. INFs are usually induced *in vivo* by bacteria and viruses and *in vitro* by double stranded RNA; α-interferon is produced by bone marrow mononuclear cells, β-interferon by fibroblasts and epithelial cells and γ-interferon by lymphocytes following antigen or mitogen stimulation. *In vitro* cytokines, e.g. IL-1, IL-2, TNFα and β and colony stimulating factors, induce interferon, which inhibits the proliferation of normal and malignant cells. This antiproliferative effect is mediated by the induction of a novel oligonucleotide polymerase, $2'5'$ adenosine synthetase ($2'5'$ A synthetase), which catalyses the synthesis of oligonucleotides from ATP. These oligonucleotides are necessary for the activity and stability of endoribonuclease L (RNAase L) which cleaves single stranded RNA (mRNA and rRNA). Catabolism of RNA ultimately inhibits protein synthesis and cell proliferation. Differentiated and non-growing cells have higher endogenous levels of $2'5'$ A synthetase than do rapidly growing progenitor cells. In cells resistant to INF there is no increase in the enzyme which occurs in sensitive cells. Some myeloid cell lines produce INFβ as their growth rate slows following stimulation to differentiation, whereas resistant lines continue to proliferate. *In vivo* INFα inhibits the growth of virally and chemically induced tumours and evokes regression of human tumour xenografts (Balkwill, 1989). IFNα has been used successfully as primary treatment for hairy cell leukaemia and following minimal treatment for CML. In multiple myeloma INFα has had limited success in primary treatment; however there appears to be a significant increase in the duration of remission among patients given the cytokine as maintenance therapy after intensive chemotherapy (D. Cunningham, personal communication). The cytostatic nature of INFα is evident from studies in which bone marrow aspirates have been cultured during maintenance therapy with INFα (Millar B.C. and Bell J.B.G., unpublished observation). Despite the absence of disease clonogenic myeloma cells have been recovered and grown as colonies *in vitro* up to 10 months from the start of therapy. Thus far INF has had little impact in solid tumours which may reflect differences in the degrees of differentiation which may occur in specific tissues, as well as endogenous levels of $2'5'$ A synthetase.

2.7   IMMUNE RECOGNITION OF MALIGNANT DISEASE

At the cellular level certain T lymphocytes in peripheral blood (NK cells) display natural cytotoxicity towards tumour cells *in vitro* independently of the major histocompatibility complex (MHC). This occurs *in vitro* in the absence of stimulation with IL-2, whereas a subset of NK cells requires activation to evoke a cytotoxic response (LAK). In animal models selective inhibition of NK cells resulted in appreciably more metastases from an experimental tumour (Barlozzari *et al.*, 1985). Furthermore, selective breeding of mice with low NK activity resulted in a greater incidence of lymphomas and breast carcinomas compared with that in animals with high NK activity (Helletier *et al.*, 1988). In man there is a wide range of NK and LAK activity in normal individuals, however there is substantial evidence that individuals with persistently low NK activity have an increased risk of developing cancer. In leukaemia a significant and sudden decrease in NK activity has been associated with relapse (Lotzova *et al.*, 1987), whereas breast cancer patients with high NK activity at diagnosis and before treatment had significantly less lymph node involvement (Levy *et al.*, 1987). Thus, transfer of large numbers of NK cells after expansion *in vitro* may be useful in tumour therapy.

Although the majority of human tumours do not elicit an immune response the presence of tumour associated antigen(s) (TAA) suggest that this lack of immunogenicity could be due to poor antigen presentation. Attempts to augment a T-effector cell response have been undertaken *in vivo* by injecting IL-2 at the tumour challenge site or around tumour draining lymph nodes in mice. In patients with head and neck carcinoma administration of IL-2 to the lymph nodes draining primary and recurrent sites has induced substantial numbers of complete or partial responses (Forni *et al.*, 1987). In other studies murine tumour cells transfected with G–CSF, IL-4, IL-2 or IFN-γ have been shown to be non-tumourigenic *in vivo* and to induce an immune response against the parental cells. The possibility that transfection of human tumour cells with cytokine genes may produce an immunogenic vaccine against human cancer may be of considerable importance for future treatment strategies.

2.8 CONCLUDING REMARKS

Although cell biology can provide a basis for understanding disturbances in cell behaviour that may result in the development of cancer, certain caveats should be remembered because of the nature of the methods employed. The excision of solid tissue or removal of bone marrow or blood from the body and establishment in cell culture puts considerable stress onto cells be they normal or malignant. Conditions *in vitro* are non-physiological, e.g. tissue architecture and spatial association with other tissues is absent, there is no circadian rhythm, no hormonal control (other than that which may result from the cells themselves), an increase in oxygen tension, no removal of catabolic metabolites and the concentration of cells per unit volume is usually profoundly less than that found *in vivo*. In studies involving bone marrow or blood, experimental conditions are usually designed to favour the elaboration of progenitor cells from a specific lineage, thereby ignoring potential interactions from other components of this heterogeneous tissue. In addition, fundamental changes in metabolism occur within days of explant from the host, e.g. the requirement for additional amino acids (arginine, cysteine, glutamine, tryptophan and histidine), the greater reliance on glycolysis as a source of ATP and the consequent accumulation of lactate. Since the removal of physiological control and changes in basic metabolism occur within the cells *in vitro*, it is not surprising that cells in culture have requirements for more complex molecules which may be synthesized *in vivo* by the cells themselves (autocrine) or provided by other cells (paracrine and endocrine).

The maintenance of cells in culture can result in further genetic changes which elicit changes in proliferation or differentiation compared with the parental cells. Additionally, the reliance on cell lines which may have transformed spontaneously *in vitro* or have been transfected with viral oncogenes or the cDNA for specific cellular genes may provide inappropriate models for events that occur in the evolution of cancer in man. In tumour cells taken from patients specific mutations have occurred at specific chromosomal sites in the DNA, whereas in transfection studies there is no evidence that transfected genes are associated at those same sites. Thus, a reductionist approach implying that the addition of a gene to a cell's genetic complement is sufficient to account for the behavioural changes in cancer cells (as opposed *in vitro* transformed cells) may be too simplistic. Ultimately, the validity of concepts concerning the regulation of cellular proliferation in normal and tumour cells must be assessed in animal models; *in vivo* veritas!

ACKNOWLEDGEMENTS

I would like to thank Dr J.B.G. Bell and Dr J.L. Millar for their helpful and constructive criticism and Miss R. Couch for the preparation of the manuscript.

REFERENCES

Adshead, F.J., Hickish, T., Bell, J.B.G. *et al* (1992) Evidence for interleukin-3 expression *in vivo* in human bone marrow. *International Journal of Experimental Pathology*, **73**, A1–13.

Antonelli-Orlidge, A., Saunders, K., Smith, S. and d'Amore, P. (1989) An activated form of TGFβ is produced by co-cultures of endothelial cells and pericytes. *Proceedings of the National Academy of Sciences* USA, **86**, 4544–8.

Astaldi, G.C.B., Janssen, M.C., Lansdorf, P. *et al.* (1980) Human endothelial culture supernatants (HECS): a growth factor for hybridomas. *Journal of Immunology*, **125**, 1411–14.

Aye, M.T., Hashami, S., Leclair, B. *et al.* (1992) Expression of stem cell factor and *ckit* mRNA in cultured endothelial cells, monocytes and cloned human bone marrow stromal cells. *Blood* **79**, 2497–9.

Balkwill, F.R. (1989) Interferons, in *Cytokines in Cancer Therapy*, Oxford University Press, Oxford, pp.8–53.

Barlozzari, T. Leonhard, T.J., Wiltrout, R.H. *et al.* (1985) Direct evidence for the role of LGL on the inhibition of experimental tumour metastasis. *Journal of Immunology*, **134**, 2783–9.

Betsholtz, C., Heldin, C.H., Nister, M. *et al.* (1983) Synthesis of a PDGF-like growth factor in human glioma and sarcoma cells suggests the expression of the cellular homologue of the transforming protein of simian sarcoma virus. *Biochemical and Biophysical Research Communications*, **117**, 176–82.

Blazar, B.A., Sutton, L.M. and Strome, M. (1983) Self-stimulating growth factor production by B-cell lines derived from Burkitt's lymphoma and other cell lines transformed *in vitro* by Epstein–Barr virus. *Cancer Research*, **43**, 4562–9.

Boettinger, D.B., Anderson, S. and Dexter, T.M. (1984) Effect of *src* infection on long term marrow cultures increased self-renewal of haemopoietic progenitor cells without leukaemia. *Cell*, **36**, 767–73.

Bradley, T.R. and Metcalf, D. (1966) The growth of mouse bone marrow cells *in vitro*. *Australian Journal of Experimental Biology and Medical Sciences*, **44**, 287.

Cook, W.D., Metcalf, D., Nicola, N.A. *et al.* (1985) Malignant transformation of a growth factor-dependent cell line by Abelson virus without evidence of an autocrine mechanism. *Cell*, **41**, 677–83.

Cooper, C.S., Tempest, P.R., Beckman, M.P. *et al.* (1986) Amplification and over expression of the *met* gene in spontaneously transformed NIH 3T3 mouse fibroblasts. *EMBO Journal*, **5**, 2623–8.

Cuttita, F., Carney, D.N., Mulshine, J. *et al.* (1985) Bombesin-like peptides can function as autocrine growth factors in human small cell lung cancer. *Nature*, **316**, 823–6.

Forni, G., Giovarelli, M., Santini, A. *et al.* (1987) Interleukin 2 activated tumour inhibition *in vivo* depends on the systemic involvement of host immunoreactivity. *Journal of Immunology*, **138**, 4033–41.

Godbout, R., Dryja, T., Squire, J. *et al.* (1983) Somatic inactivation of genes on chromosone 13 is a common event in both hereditary and non-hereditary retinoblastoma tumours. *Nature* **304**, 451–3.

Gordon, J., Aman, P., Rosen, A. *et al.* (1985) Capacity of B-lymphocytic lines of diverse tumour origin to produce and respond to B-cell growth factors. A progression model for B-cell lymphomagenesis. *International Journal of Cancer*, **35**, 251–6.

Harris, H., Miller, O.J., Klein, G. *et al.* (1969) Suppression of malignancy by cell fusion. *Nature*, **223**, 363–8.

Hatzfeld, J., Li, M-L., Brown, E.L. *et al.* (1991) Release of early human haemopoietic progenitors from quiescence by antisense transforming growth factor β₁ or Rb oligonucleotides. *Journal of Experimental Medicines*, **174**, 925–9.

Heldin, C.H., Westermark, B. and Wasteson, A. (1980) Chemical and biological properties of a growth factor for human cultured osteosarcoma cells: resemblance with platelet derived growth factor. *Journal of Cell Physiology*, **105**, 235–46.

Helletier, H., Olsson, N-L., Faely, C. *et al.* (1988) Differential sensitivity to natural cell mediated cytotoxicity of two rat colony adenocarcinoma variants differing in their tumourigenicity. *Cancer Immunology and Immunotherapy*, **26**, 263–8.

Jonasson, J., Povey, S. and Harris, H. (1977) The analysis of malignancy by cell fusion VII. Cytogenetic analysis of hybrids between malignant and diploid cells and tumours derived from them. *Journal of Cell Science*, **24**, 217–54.

Kanakura, Y., Druker, B., Cannistra, S.A. *et al.* (1990) Signal transduction of the human granulocyte–macrophage colony stimulating factor and interleukin-3 receptors involves tyrosine phosphorylation of a common set of cytoplasmic protein. *Blood*, **76**, 706–15.

Kawano, M., Hirano, T., Matsuda, T. *et al.* (1988) Autocrine generation and essential requirement of BSF-2/16-6 for human multiple myeloma. *Nature*, **332**, 83–5.

Kyle, R.A. and Lust, J.A. (1989) Monoclonal gammopathies of undetermined significance. *Seminars in Hematology*, **26**, 176–200.

Laker, C., Stocking, C., Bergholz, U. *et al.* (1987) Autocrine growth stimulation after viral transfer of the granulocyte–macrophage colony stimulating factor gene and genuine factor independent growth are two distinct but interdependent steps in the oncogenic pathway. *Proceedings of the National Academy of Sciences* USA, **84**, 8458–62.

Lang, R., Metcalf, D., Gough, N.H. *et al.* (1985) Expression of a haemopoietic growth factor cDNA in a factor dependent cell line results in autosomal growth and tumourigenicity. *Cell*, **3**, 531–42.

Lee, D.C., Rochford, R., Todaro, G.J. *et al.* (1985) Development expression of transforming growth factor-like α mRNA. *Molecular and Cellular Biology*, **5**, 3644–6.

Lee, W.-H., Shew, J.-Y., Hong, F. *et al.* (1987) The retinoblastoma gene product is a nuclear phospho protein associated with DNA binding activity. *Nature*, **329**, 642–5.

Levy, S., Heberman, R.B., Lippman, M. *et al.* (1987) Correlation of stress factors with sustained depression of natural killer activity and predicted prognosis in patients with breast cancer. *Journal of Clinical Oncology*, **5**, 348–53.

Libermann, T.A., Nusbaum, H.R., Rozen, N. *et al.* (1985) Amplification, enhanced expression and possible rearrangement of EGF receptor gene in brain tumours of gliol origin. *Nature*, **313**, 144–7.

Lotzova, E., Savary, C.A. and Heberman, R.B. (1987) Impaired NK cell profile in leukaemia patients, in *Immunology of Natural Killer Cells*, vol. 2, (eds E. Lotzova and R.B. Heberman), CRC Press, Boca Ratan, pp. 29–53.

Macaulay, V.M., Everard, M.J., Teale, J.D. *et al.* (1990) Autocrine function for insulin-like growth factor I in human small cell lung cancer cell lines and fresh tumour cells. *Cancer Research*, **50**, 2511–17.

Malone, D.G., Pierce, J.H., Falko, J. *et al.* (1989) Production of granulocyte–macrophage colony stimulating factor by primary cultures of unstimulated rat microvascular endothelial cells. *Blood*, **71**, 684–9.

Manolov, G. and Manolova, Y. (1972) Marker band is one chromosome 14 from Burkitt lymphomas. *Nature*, **237**, 33–4.

McNiece, I., Andrews, R., Williams, D. *et al.* (1992) Biological characteristics of recombinant rat and human stem cell factor. *Bone Marrow Transplantation*, **10**(suppl.2), 2.

Montes-Borinaga, A., Millar, B.C., Bell, J.B.G. *et al.* (1990) Interleukin-6 is a cofactor for the growth of myeloid cells from human bone marrow aspirates but does not affect the clonogenicity of myeloma cells *in vitro*. *British Journal of Haematology*, **76**, 476–83.

Nister, M., Libermann, T., Betsholtz, C. *et al.* (1988) Expression of messenger RNAs for platelet derived growth factor and transforming growth factor-α and their receptors in human malignant glioma cells. *Cancer Research*, **48**, 3910–18.

Nowell, P.C. and Hungerford, D.A. (1960) A minute chromosome in chronic granulocyte leukaemia. *Science*, **132**, 1497.

Pietsch, T., Kyas, S., Steffens, U. *et al.* (1992) Effects of human stem cell factor (c-*kit* ligand) on proliferation of myeloid leukaemia cells. *Blood*, **80**, 1199–206.

Queensenberry, P. (1993) Too much of a good thing "Reductionism Run Amok". *Experimental Haematology*, **21**, editorial.

Revell, S. (1974). The breakage-and-reunion theory and the exchange theory for chromosomal aberrations induced by ionizing radiations. A short history. *Advances in Radiation Biology*, **4**, 367–416.

Ross, R., Glomset, J.A., Kariya, B. *et al.* (1974) A platelet dependent serum factor that stimulates the proliferation of arterial smooth muscle *in vitro*. *Proceedings of the National Academy of Sciences* USA, **72**, 1207–10.

Sing, G.K., Keller, J.R., Ellingsworth, L.R. *et al.* (1988) Transforming growth factor β1 selectively inhibits normal and leukaemic human bone marrow cell growth *in vitro*. *Blood*, **72**, 1504–11.

Souyri, M., Vigon, I., Penciolelli, J.F. *et al.* (1990) A putative truncated cytokine receptor gene transduced by the myeloproliferative leukaemia virus immortalizes haemopoietic progenitors. *Cell*, **63**, 1137–47.

Sporn, M.B. and Todaro, G. (1980) Autocrine secretion and malignant transformation of cells. *New England Journal of Medicine*, **303**, 878–80.

Stehelin, D., Varmus, H.E., Bishop, J.M. *et al.* (1976) DNA related to the transforming gene of avian sarcoma virus is present in normal avian DNA. *Nature*, **260**, 170–3.

Stoler, A. and Bouck, N. (1985) Identification of a single chromosome in the normal human genome essential for suppression of hamster cell transformation. *Proceedings of the National Academy of Sciences USA*, **82**, 570–4.

Taga, T., Hibi, M., Hirata, Y. *et al.* (1989) Interleukin 6 triggers the association of its receptor with a possible signal transducer, gp. 130. *Cell*, **58**, 573–81.

Temin, H.M. (1967) Control by factors in serum of multiplication of uninfected cells and cells infected converted with avian sarcoma viruses, in *Growth Regulating Substances for Animal Cells in Culture*, (ed. V. Defendi), The Wistar Symposium Monograph No. 7, Wistar Institute Press, Philadelphia, pp. 103–116.

Till, J.E. and McCulloch, E.A. (1961) A direct measurement of the radiation sensitivity of normal mouse bone marrow cells. *Radiation Research*, **14**, 213–22.

Twardzik, D.R., Todaro, G.J., Marquerdt, H. *et al.* (1982) Transformation induced by Abelson murine leukaemia virus involves production of a polypeptide growth factor. *Science*, **216**, 894–6.

Van Snick, J., Vink, A., Cayphas, S. *et al.* (1987) Interleukin-HP1, a T-cell derived hybridoma growth factor that supports the *in vitro* growth of murine plasmacytomas. *Journal of Experimental Medicine*, **165**, 641–9.

Wheeler, E.F., Roussel, M.F., Hampe, A. *et al.* (1986) The aminoterminal domain of the v-*fms* oncogene includes a functional signal peptide that directs synthesis of a transferring glycoprotein in the absence of FeLV gag sequence. *Journal of Virology*, **59**, 224–33.

Ymer, S., Tucker, W.Q.J., Sanderson, C.J. *et al.* (1985) Constitutive synthesis of interleukin 3 by leukaemia cell line WEH1-3B is due to retroviral insertion near the gene. *Nature*, **317**, 255–8.

Yoshimuro, A., Longmore, G. and Lodish, H. (1990) Point mutation in the exoplasmic domain of the erythropoietin receptor resulting in hormone independent activation and tumorigenicity. *Nature*, **348**, 647–9.

Young, D. and Griffin, J.D. (1986) Autocrine secretion of GM–CSF in acute myeloblastic leukaemia. *Blood*, **68**, 1178–81.

AN INTRODUCTION TO THE MOLECULAR BIOLOGY OF CANCER

3

Helen Patterson and John Yarnold

3.1 INTRODUCTION

Several lines of evidence have combined to develop the concept of cancer as a genetic disease at the cellular level. Foremost amongst these has been the recognition of heritable cancer syndromes such as familial retinoblastoma and familial polyposis coli, the observation of chromosomal abnormalities in neoplastic cells, and the demonstration that the ability of a chemical to act as a carcinogen is directly related to its ability to bind and to mutate DNA. More recently, the development of the concept of oncogenes and tumour suppressor genes, accompanied by the development and refinement of a number of laboratory techniques such as mammalian cell culture and the ability to recognize, manipulate and amplify DNA sequences of interest, has resulted in a revolution in the field of molecular biology and a concomitant revolution in our understanding of tumorigenesis at the molecular level.

It has recently become apparent that human tumours arise as a result of the accumulation of mutations in two classes of cellular genes – proto-oncogenes, sometimes referred to as dominantly transforming oncogenes, and tumour suppressor genes, also referred to as recessive oncogenes. The nomenclature can be somewhat confusing. Proto-oncogenes are normal cellular genes which when activated by mutation or overexpressed act to promote tumour formation. The phenotypic effect of the activated allele is 'dominant' at the cellular level because the mutation acts to upregulate the activity of the gene. Tumour suppressor genes are normal cellular genes that promote differentiation and regulate proliferation. Loss of function is pertinent to tumorigenesis. Inactivating mutations or deletion of both alleles of a tumour suppressor gene is required before gene function is completely lost. Because mutations in single alleles of tumour suppressor genes are relatively silent at the cellular level they have been termed recessive oncogenes.

Although the demonstration in tumour cells of rearrangement, amplification or point mutation in a gene sequence is often taken as evidence that this sequence is acting as an oncogene, unequivocal proof can only be obtained by demonstrating transforming effects following expression of the cloned gene in appropriate non-transformed cells. Conversely, proof that a gene has suppressor function can only be obtained from experiments in which tumour cells are reverted to a non-tumorigenic phenotype following introduction and expression of the normal gene.

3.2 GENOTYPE, PHENOTYPE AND THE REGULATION OF GENE EXPRESSION

Every somatic cell possesses a diploid genome of 6×10^9 nucleotides encoding an estimated 100 000 genes. In a given individual the genotype of almost every differentiated cell type remains unchanged, and there are important cellular mechanisms involving DNA repair and proof reading of replicated DNA prior to mitosis to ensure that this remains the case throughout the life of the organism. The important exceptions are the T and B lymphocyte lineages which physically rearrange the DNA of their T-cell receptor and immunoglobulin genes as a way of generating diversity of antigenic recognition. In general, however, variation in cellular function, differentiation and behaviour – the cellular phenotype – must be generated by the differential expression of a uniform set of cellular genes.

Gene expression appears to be switched off in some cells because the genes are packed in dense chromatin and are unavailable to the transcription apparatus. Modification of DNA by the methylation of cytosine residues also appears to play a role in switching off gene transcription. More subtle regulatory mechanisms begin at the level of RNA transcription.

The initial step in gene expression involves the transcription of DNA by a cellular enzyme called RNA polymerase II which uses DNA as a template to produce a complementary RNA strand. This is then spliced to remove the intervening intronic sequence, a polyadenylic acid tail is added and the resulting messenger RNA translated into polypeptides which are then modified to produce mature proteins. The process is outlined in Figure 3.1.

The activity of RNA polymerase II is highly regulated. Approximately 100 bp or so upstream of the transcriptional start site exist short conserved nucleotide sequences called promoters which are recognized by proteins called transcription factors. Promoters must be bound by appropriate transcription factors before RNA polymerase II can transcribe the gene at appreciable levels. Enhancers are additional nucleotide sequences, lying at variable distances from the transcriptional start site (and occasionally in downstream regions

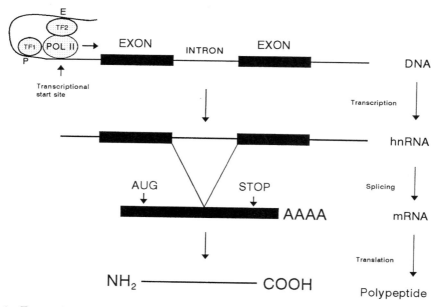

Figure 3.1   Transcription is initiated when RNA polymerase II (Pol II) binds the transcriptional start site. The activity of Pol II is regulated by interaction with transcription factors (TF) which bind the promoter (P) and enhancer (E) sequences illustrated upstream of the transcriptional start site. RNA is initially transcribed as heteronuclear RNA (hnRNA) and this is then spliced and a polyadenylic acid tail (AAAA) is added to produce messenger RNA (mRNA). Polypeptide translation is initiated at an AUG (adenine, uracil, guanine) codon, and terminated at any subsequent codon which fails to encode for an amino acid.

or in intronic sequence), which also bind transcription factors and regulate gene transcription. Some transcription factors are non-specific and are generally required for the efficient functioning of the transcription apparatus, but others act in a promoter specific fashion. The activity of transcription factors themselves appears to be regulated by additional factors. It is easy to see that in this system with its multiple levels of modulation, it is possible to both finely tune gene expression and to activate complicated patterns of expression which then dictate cellular behaviour.

RNA molecules can be spliced in alternative ways. Splicing usually involves the removal of intronic sequences, but many genes can be spliced in ways which variably remove some exonic sequence as well. Thus, a single gene can encode several proteins whose functional activity may vary greatly. In addition, the rate at which RNA molecules are degraded by cytoplasmic RNases, the half-life of the encoded protein and structural modifications to that protein all combine to modulate gene expression in specific cells.

3.3 ONCOGENES

It was not until the late 1970s that two approaches both involving the bioassay and subsequent tracing of tumorigenic genetic elements led to the cloning of the first genes which could be shown to be specifically involved in the process of neoplastic transformation. The study of avian and mammalian transforming retroviruses led to the cloning of a diverse array of viral oncogenes. The recognition that these viral oncogenes were transduced cellular genes (Figures 3.2(a) and (b)) led to the search for cellular genes which were altered and hence activated in primary human tumours and cell lines. The DNA-mediated transfection–transformation assay using NIH3T3 cells proved to be the most useful tool in this respect, but several oncogenes

were subsequently cloned by the analysis of structural alterations in tumour DNA.

3.3.1 ACUTELY TRANSFORMING RETROVIRUSES CARRY MUTATED COPIES OF CELLULAR GENES

Retroviruses possess a diploid genome of single-stranded RNA which replicates via a double-stranded DNA intermediate integrated into the host cell genome – the provirus (Varmus, 1988). Retroviruses are implicated in a variety of disease processes, and in the genesis of naturally occurring leukaemias and tumours in many avian and mammalian species. However, the acutely transforming retroviruses which rapidly induce tumours in experimental animals and efficiently transform cells in culture, produce tumours only in experimental situations. These retroviruses are derived in the laboratory from weakly or non-oncogenic retroviruses by repeated passage in susceptible birds or mammals.

The first tumour-inducing retrovirus was isolated by Peyton Rous as long ago as 1911. He demonstrated that a filtrable agent, derived from a serially passaged spontaneous sarcoma, could induce sarcomas in young chickens and thereby implicated a viral aetiology. Several decades later dissection of the Rous sarcoma virus (RSV) genome ascribed its transforming ability to a distinct portion of the viral genome not involved in viral replication. A close homologue of this sequence appeared to be present as a single copy in the haploid genome of all vertebral species studied, establishing a cellular rather than a viral origin for the transforming sequence of RSV, v-*src*.

Subsequent analysis of a variety of acutely transforming retroviruses capable of producing a variety of tumours in birds and mammals under laboratory conditions, led to the characterization of over 20 distinct oncogenic sequences (Bishop and Varmus, 1982). The paradigm of RSV has held true. In each case the viral oncogene (designated v-*onc*)

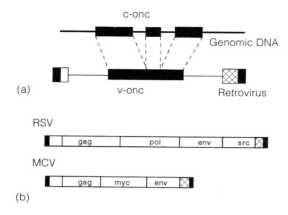

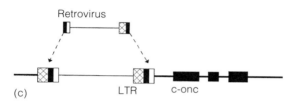

Figure 3.2 **(a)** Retroviral transduction of a cellular gene, c-*onc*. The viral oncogene, v-*onc*, is derived from the exons of a cellular proto-oncogene. **(b)** Schematic representation of the genomes of the Rous sarcoma virus (RSV) and the avian myelocytomatosis virus (MCV). Transduction of the *src* gene in RSV does not disrupt the viral genome leaving the retrovirus competent for replication. In MCV, which is typical of other acutely transforming retroviruses, transduction of the *myc* gene results in disruption of the retroviral genome rendering the virus defective. These defective viruses require co-infection with a competent retrovirus to produce mature acutely transforming viral particles. **(c)** Schematic representation of oncogene activation by proviral insertion. The retrovirus has inserted immediately upstream of a cellular proto-oncogene c-*onc*, and transcription of the proto-oncogene becomes driven by the viral LTR (long terminal repeat) promoter. (Reproduced from Patterson, 1993, with permission.)

was derived by transduction (Figure 3.2(a), (b)) from a cellular proto-oncogene, given the abbreviation c-*onc*. Sequences originally identified as viral oncogenes include the *myc*, H-

ras, K-*ras* and *abl* genes. The cellular genes transduced by transforming retroviruses are usually transcribed at very high levels in retrovirally induced tumours because they are under the control of powerful retroviral promoters. In addition, retroviral oncogenes were frequently shown to be truncated or contain point mutations when compared to their cellular counterparts.

3.3.2   CHRONICALLY TRANSFORMING RETROVIRUSES ACT BY PROVIRAL INSERTION

Chronically transforming retroviruses, so called because they induce tumours in animals with long latency, lack oncogenes but act via proviral integration in the host genome (Figure 3.2(c)). Chance integration of a provirus within the vicinity of an important regulatory gene will bring that gene under proviral transcriptional control, upregulating gene transcription and hence oncogene activity. By cloning retroviral integration sites in tumour DNA several more novel oncogenes were cloned.

3.3.3   THE DNA TRANSFECTION– TRANSFORMATION ASSAY DETECTS ACTIVATED ONCOGENES IN TUMOUR DNA

DNA mediated gene transfer or 'transfection' depends upon the application of DNA to non-tumorigenic cells, usually NIH3T3 cells, as a co-precipitate with calcium phosphate. This allows the uptake (the precipitate is endocytosed) and stable incorporation of exogenous DNA into the recipient cell genome. Using this type of analysis, DNA from cell lines and primary human tumours has been shown to induce cellular transformation, identified by the appearance of foci of morphologically transformed cells on a background of non-transformed cells and the ability of cells from these foci to produce tumours in nude mice. Transformation by transfection does not represent one-step tumorigenesis. NIH3T3 cells are

not primary cultures, they are immortal aneuploid cells which appear to have undergone
many of the changes required for tumorigenesis. They nevertheless retain contact inhibition in culture and do not produce tumours
in nude mice. Primary cultures, for example,
human fibroblasts, are not transformed by
DNA transfection experiments.

In most cases the genes detected by this
method are activated *ras* genes; K-*ras* and H-
ras previously detected as viral oncogenes,
and a third closely related gene N-*ras* first
identified in this assay. Several other genes
including *neu, met, ret, raf, mas, hst, trk* and
dbl have been identified by this route. Several
of these genes carry abnormalities which can
be traced back to the original tumour, but
others appear to be activated by chance
rearrangement during the transfection procedure itself. The spectrum of genes cloned
by transfection may only reflect the category
of genes to which NIH3T3 cells are sensitive.
In addition, genes spanning large regions of
genomic DNA are unlikely to be transfected
intact and for this reason may not be active in
this assay.

3.3.4 ONCOGENES CAN BE CLONED BY THE ANALYSIS OF STRUCTURAL ALTERATIONS IN TUMOUR DNA

(a) Chromosomal translocations

Cytogenetic analyses have identified
numerous specific chromosomal translocations in several classes of human malignancy and many of these translocations have
been shown to result in oncogene activation
by rearrangement. The genes involved in
these translocations have been identified
using two types of approach.

The first reciprocal translocations were
characterized at the molecular level by virtue
of the fact that one of the genes involved in
each translocation had previously been
cloned as a viral oncogene. For example, the
search for the genes involved in the translocation t(9;22) in chronic granulocytic
leukaemia (Heisterkamp *et al.*, 1983) focused
on the c-*abl* proto-oncogene, originally cloned
as v-*abl*, the transforming gene of the Abelson
murine leukaemia virus and subsequently
mapped to chromosome 9. The *abl* gene was
then used as a probe to clone DNA at the c-*abl*
locus in tumour DNA. Analysis of these
clones confirmed that the c-*abl* gene was disrupted by sequences from the *bcr* gene on
chromosome 22. The translocation results in
the production of a chimeric *bcr-abl* fusion
protein which has elevated tyrosine kinase
activity. In Burkitt's lymphomas, translocations involve breakpoints at 8q24 which
becomes transposed to one of the immunoglobulin gene loci at 14q32, 2p13 or 22q11.
Analysis of tumour DNA using a candidate
chromosome 8 proto-oncogene c-*myc* as a
probe confirmed its role in these translocations.

When neither gene involved in a reciprocal translocation is known, the efforts
required to clone the breakpoint are considerably greater. For example, during the
analysis of the translocation t(11,22) in
Ewing's sarcoma, the analysis of candidate
proto-oncogenes was unhelpful. In such
cases the successful approach to the characterization of the breakpoint typically
involves the construction of long-range
physical maps of the breakpoint region, the
cloning of extensive segments of DNA in the
vicinity of the breakpoint and the analysis of
this cloned DNA for the presence of a gene
disrupted by the translocation.

(b) Gene amplification

Genes whose copy number is amplified in
human tumours usually overexpress the same
gene. Hence, amplification provides a mechanism by which oncogenes may be activated.
Southern analysis of tumour DNA using oncogene probes has been used to show amplification of the c-*myc* gene in a number of tumour
types, of the c-*erb*B gene in glioblastomas and

of a *myc*-like gene N-*myc* in neuroblastomas. However, the putative proto-oncogene *gli* and the transforming oncogene *mdm2* were first cloned by manipulating tumour DNA carrying the amplified genes.

3.3.5   STRUCTURAL HOMOLOGY TO KNOWN ONCOGENES HAS BEEN USED TO CLONE NOVEL PROTO-ONCOGENES

Under stringent conditions single-stranded DNA (or RNA) probes will only hybridize to other copies of single-stranded DNA to which they are exactly complementary. However, if the stringency of hybridization is reduced (by reducing the temperature or increasing the salt concentration in which hybridization takes place), then DNA or RNA probes will hybridize to DNA species to which they have only partial homology. Using the premise that genes which share nucleotide sequence homology, and hence amino acid homology, appear to perform similar cellular functions, genes identified as oncogenes by the methods outlined above have been used as probes to clone related genes with sequence homology from DNA libraries. These genes are then examined for transforming activity or alteration in human tumours. *myc* gene probes have been used to isolate three related genes, N-*myc* amplified in neuroblastomas, L-*myc* amplified in small cell lung cancer, and a third gene, R-*myc*. c-*erb*B was used to isolate c-*erb*B2, which is amplified and over-expressed in 30% of breast cancers. *Ras* related genes such as *rho*, *ral* and R-*ras* have been cloned, but these have not yet been implicated in human malignancy.

3.3.6   BIOCHEMICAL FUNCTIONS OF PROTO-ONCOGENES

In excess of 60 proto-oncogenes have been identified and in general they all appear to act in biochemical pathways by which growth factors stimulate cellular proliferation. Bio-chemically three main mechanisms of action have been identified.

(a)   Protein phosphorylation

Phosphorylation of serine, threonine and tyrosine residues is one of the main mechanisms of activating intracellular signal transduction pathways. Several proto-oncogenes with kinase (phosphorylase) activity have been identified: for example, the growth factor receptor *met* and the cytoplasmic signal transduction factors *src* and *raf*. Mutations of these genes appear to up-regulate their kinase activity and hence the proliferative signal to the cell.

(b)   GTP-binding proteins

ras GTP-binding proteins are a large superfamily of signal transduction factors (Downward, 1990). The most important in tumorigenesis are undoubtedly H-*ras*, K-*ras* and N-*ras* genes mutated in approximately 30% of all tumours (Bos, 1989). For example, 95% of pancreatic cancers, 60% of thyroid cancers, 50% of colon carcinomas, 40% of adenocarcinomas of the lung and 30% of acute myeloid leukaemias possess *ras* gene mutations. These genes appear to act as molecular switches in signal transduction pathways. They bind and hydrolyse GTP, are active in the GTP bound form and inactive in the GDP bound form. Their intrinsic GTPase activity is upregulated by GTPase activating proteins (GAP). *ras* genes are almost invariably activated by point mutations at codons 12, 13 and 61, within the GTP binding domain. Such mutations lock ras proteins in the active GTP bound state by inhibiting GAP mediated GTP hydrolysis. Interestingly, the product of the NF1 tumour suppressor gene has activity as a *ras* GTPase activating protein and the *bcr* gene is a GTPase activating protein for a *ras*-related protein called rac.

(c) Transcription factors

Regulation of gene expression as a result of growth factor stimulation and intracellular signal transduction plays a vital role in the control of cellular proliferation. It is of little surprise then that several oncogenes, for example c-*myc*, N-*myc*, *fos* and *jun*, have been shown to function as transcription factors.

3.4 TUMOUR SUPPRESSOR GENES

3.4.1 MALIGNANT SUPPRESSION WAS FIRST DEMONSTRATED IN SOMATIC CELL HYBRIDS

The earliest indication that malignant transformation might involve loss of normal gene function was provided by evidence of malignant suppression in somatic cell hybrids. The basic methodology is to fuse pairs of cells, one normal and one tumorigenic. Hybrid clones are selected by screening for genetic markers from both parents and examined for their ability to form tumours in immunologically appropriate hosts, usually nude mice. Early cultures of hybrid clones continued to grow in culture but were frequently non-tumorigenic when injected into nude mice, indicating that tumorigenicity had been suppressed. However, after continued growth in culture suppressed clones showed a tendency to re-express tumorigenicity. Subsequent cytogenetic analysis of non-tumorigenic hybrids and tumorigenic revertants showed that reversion correlated with loss of specific chromosomes which could be traced back to the normal parent cell (Stanbridge, 1988). The technique was then refined by the development of micro-cell transfer in which single intact chromosomes are transferred to tumorigenic cells as interphase micronuclei and are retained in subsequent generations. Using this method, tumorigenicity has been suppressed in HeLa cells by the introduction of human chromosome 11, in a renal cell carcinoma cell line by chromosome 3p, and in melanoma cell lines by chromosome 6. The main problem with these studies is how to proceed from chromosomal location to the molecular cloning of the suppressor genes. Although some genes cloned by other approaches may be active in this assay, none have been directly isolated through this route.

3.5 THE STUDY OF INHERITED CANCER

3.5.1 RETINOBLASTOMA

Retinoblastoma is a rare tumour of infancy and early childhood. Following the development of effective surgical and radiotherapeutic treatment, two forms of the disease have been recognized. Approximately 30% of these tumours occur in a familial setting where multiple tumours, frequently bilateral, occur at a very early age. Seventy per cent of tumours appear to be sporadic, occurring as single tumours in older children. Following mathematical analysis of age-incidence data for both the familial and sporadic forms of retinoblastoma, Knudson proposed his two-hit hypothesis of retinoblastoma formation (Knudson, 1971). He suggested that whereas sporadic tumours required two hits in the same cell to initiate tumour formation, hereditary tumours required only one hit, the first being inherited from the parent and carried in the germline of every cell in the body. It was not within the scope of the original paper to define the nature of these two hits. However, rare cytogenetic observations of constitutional deletions of the long arm of chromosome 13 in hereditary retinoblastoma patients provided evidence that the first or inherited mutation might involve loss of a region of chromosome 13. Similar interstitial deletions in tumours from patients with normal constitutional karyotypes were observed, implying the second mutation might involve loss of the same region of chromosome 13. Subsequent studies of loss of heterozygosity (LOH) for polymorphic loci on chromosome 13 in tumour DNA from patients with familial retinoblastoma (Cavanee *et al.*, 1983) demonstrated that frequently one copy of chromosome 13 was lost. Furthermore, pedigree analysis (Cavanee *et al.*, 1985) showed that the retained copy of chromosome 13 could always be traced back to the affected parent. Taken together these observations led to the conclusion that retinoblastomas arose as a result of inactivating mutations in both alleles of the same gene on chromosome 13q. The gene, RB1, was subsequently cloned. It is expressed in all normal retinoblasts but its expression is absent in retinoblastomas. When RB1 gene expression is restored in tumorigenic retinoblastoma cells, the cells demonstrate profound inhibition of tumorigenicity *in vivo* (Huang *et al.*, 1988), thus providing proof that RB1 is a tumour suppressor gene.

The study of other familial tumours using a combination of linkage and cytogenetic analyses and molecular cloning has so far been most productive in isolating tumour suppressor genes, for example WT1 (Wilms' tumour), NF1 (neurofibromatosis type 1) and APC (familial polyposis).

3.5.2   GENETIC LOSS IS THE HALLMARK OF TUMOUR SUPPRESSOR GENES

The first hit in tumour suppressor gene inactivation is usually a small deletion or point mutation. However, the loss of the second copy of the gene in tumour cells often involves loss of a large segment or all of the remaining normal chromosome. Such losses can be revealed by cytogenetic analysis, but also as loss of heterozygosity (LOH) for adjacent polymorphic alleles in blot-hybridization experiments of tumour DNA compared to normal DNA (Figure 3.3). Because the second hit can involve the loss of quite extensive regions of DNA from the remaining normal chromosome, polymorphic markers need not be closely linked to the tumour suppressor gene to provide valuable information in LOH analyses. The first polymorphic alleles were represented by proteins with different electrophoretic mobilities. DNA sequence

polymorphisms are usually more highly polymorphic than the protein polymorphisms which they have superceded. They are represented as fragment length polymorphisms separated by electrophoresis in agarose gels following digestion with restriction enzymes which cleave DNA in a sequence-specific manner. Individuals tend to be heterozygous for fragment length polymorphisms at numerous loci throughout their genomes.

Only a handful of tumour suppressor genes have been cloned but the existence of many other suppressor genes has been inferred by the consistent finding of LOH at particular loci in many different tumour types (Table 3.1). Using this approach, early studies mapped the inherited cancer syndrome multiple endocrine neoplasia 1 (MEN1) to chromosome 11q, the Von–Hippel Lindau syndrome to 3p and neurofibromatosis type 2 (NF-2) to chromosome 22. In addition, using one or more highly polymorphic probes for every chromosome arm, allelotypes in which the incidence of LOH for each chromosome arm is recorded have been developed for many types of neoplasm. It has become apparent from these analyses that for most tumour types several loci exhibit LOH, implicating the loss of several tumour suppressor genes in the development of these tumours. The cloning of the genes alluded to by these studies will have a considerable impact on our understanding of molecular tumorigenesis over the next decade.

3.5.3   LINKAGE ANALYSIS IN CANCER FAMILIES

Linkage analysis of affected families (King, 1990) can be used to pinpoint genetic loci associated with familial malignancy. Briefly, linkage analysis exploits the fact that loci which lie closely together on the same chromosome are rarely segregated by homologous recombination at meiosis. In large pedigrees the co-inheritance of the same allele of a specific polymorphic locus with a genetic trait provides evidence that the poly-

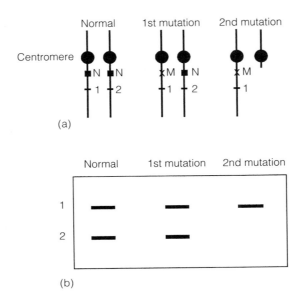

Figure 3.3 **(a)** The diagram represents a pair of homologous chromosomes, and N a normal copy of a tumour suppressor gene. The first mutation (M) is usually a very small deletion or point mutation in one allele of the gene. In inherited malignancies this first mutation will be carried in the germline, and in sporadic malignancies will be an acquired somatic mutation. Loss of the second copy of the gene frequently involves loss of a large part or all of the remaining normal chromosome. In this example, a polymorphic genetic locus in the vicinity of the tumour suppressor gene is represented by alleles 1 and 2, and it can readily be appreciated that the second mutation will not only remove the remaining normal copy of the tumour suppressor gene but also one allele of the polymorphic locus located on the same chromosome. **(b)** Schematic representation of Southern blot analysis of loss of hetrozygosity using a probe which detects the polymorphic locus with alleles 1 and 2. The expected band patterns for normal DNA and after the first and second mutations in the tumour suppressor gene are shown.

morphic locus and the disease locus are linked. In this way neurofibromatosis was mapped to chromosome 17q11.2, MEN II to chromosome 10 and familial adenomatous polyposis (FAP) to chromosome 5q21–q22 (Bodmer *et al.*, 1987). The genes have subsequently been cloned.

The majority of common malignancies arise as a result of spontaneous or environmentally induced somatic mutations. However, a key to identifying the targets for these mutations may lie in the study of families at very high risk of developing a common cancer, e.g. familial breast cancer and non-FAP colon cancer. Familial cancer although epidemiologically distinct is histologically and pathologically identical to cancer in the general population and therefore the identification of genetic alterations which predispose to these familial tumours may have very important implications for related but much more common sporadic tumours. For example, extensive linkage analysis has recently mapped early onset familial breast cancer to chromosome 17q21 (Hall *et al.*, 1990), and a more recently published consortium study provides evidence that up to 100% of familial breast/ovarian cancer and 45% of familial breast cancer is linked to the 17q gene (Easton *et al.*, 1993). Hereditary non-polyposis colorectal cancer, thought to account for up to 13% of all colorectal cancers, has been linked to chromosome 2 (Pelomaki *et al.*, 1993), and the predisposition gene, *msh* 2, identified.

Table 3.1 Examples of tumour suppressor gene loci defined in allele loss studies

Tumour	Chromosome	Tumour suppressor gene
Colorectal cancer	5q, 17p, 18q	APC/MCC, p53, DCC
Breast cancer	11p, 17p, 18q	–, p53, –
Small cell lung cancer	3p, 13q, 17p	–, RB1, p53
Retinoblastoma	13q	RB1
Osteosarcoma	13q	RB1
Renal cell carcinoma	3p	–
Rhabdomyosarcoma	11p	–
Meningioma	22	–

3.5.4 DNA TUMOUR VIRUSES – TRANSFORMATION AT THE LEVEL OF PROTEIN–PROTEIN INTERACTION

The DNA tumour viruses are a large and varied superfamily, the best characterized of which is SV40 (simian virus 40). These viruses have evolved mechanisms which enable them to express and replicate their genomes within host cells free of the restrictions that normally regulate host DNA synthesis. Like the acutely transforming retroviruses they can transform cells in culture, but unlike retroviral oncogenes those of DNA tumour viruses are viral not cellular in origin, and are an important cause of cancer in humans. For example the human papilloma virus (HPV) has been implicated in the development of cervical carcinoma and the Epstein–Barr virus (EBV) in Burkitt's lymphoma and nasopharyngeal carcinoma.

The products of the oncogenes of some of the DNA tumour viruses appear to activate quiescent cells into a pseudo S-phase of the cell cycle. In this state infected cells are permissive to viral replication. Their oncogene products have been shown to interact with host proteins, and it has become apparent that the principle mechanism by which SV40, adenoviruses and human papilloma viruses (types 16 and 18) induce tumour formation is by binding to and presumably inactivating the products of two of the best characterized tumour suppressor genes, RB1 and p53 (Table 3.2). SV40 produces a complex transforming protein

called the large T antigen required for viral DNA synthesis and capable of binding both the RB1 and the p53 genes. The E6 and E7 transforming proteins of HPV types 16 and 18 are both required for the efficient immortalization of primary human keratinocytes. E7 appears to act by binding and inactivating the RB1 protein. The E6 protein acts by binding and targeting the p53 protein for degradation by the ubiquitin–protease pathway. The majority of human cervical and anal carcinomas are associated with HPV infection and in HPV negative tumours the p53 gene appears to be somatically mutated (Crook *et al.*, 1992). In some other types of primary tumour the coincident somatic mutation of both the p53 and the RB1 tumour suppressor genes has been demonstrated. A fascinating parallel can be drawn. Some DNA tumour viruses appear to induce tumours by mimicking genetic mutations seen in some primary human tumours at the level of protein–protein interaction.

3.5.5 THE p53 GENE

Mutations of the p53 gene have emerged as the most commonly recognized alteration in malignant human tumours, occurring in up to 50% of the common adult malignancies (Hollstein *et al.*, 1991). The p53 protein was first identified in association with the large T antigen in cells transformed by SV40. Putative DNA sequence derived from the analysis of

Table 3.2 Interaction of viral oncoproteins with host proteins

Virus	Viral oncoprotein	Associated cellular protein
SV40	Large T antigen	RB1, p53
Adenovirus	E1a	RB1
	E1b	p53
Human papillomavirus (Type 16 and 18)	E6	p53
	E7	RB1

p53 amino acid sequence allowed the cloning of the p53 gene.

Upon transfection, p53 clones were found to be able to immortalize primary cells in culture and if transfected with an activated *ras* gene could contribute to the transformation of primary cells. The p53 gene was thus considered to be a dominantly transforming oncogene. Several observations then emerged which were in conflict with this:

1. Both copies of the p53 gene appeared to be deleted in some cell lines, a feature normally associated with tumour suppressor genes.
2. The p53 gene was localized to the short arm of human chromosome 17, 17p, a region showing allele loss in several types of human tumour.
3. p53 clones derived from normal cells could not immortalize cells and had no transforming potential.
4. Transforming clones of the p53 gene were shown to be mutated copies of the normal gene.
5. Transfection of wild type p53 clones rendered tumorigenic cells lacking p53 expression non-tumorigenic.

These observations established the normal p53 gene as a tumour suppressor gene. Germline mutations of the p53 gene have been associated with the Li–Fraumeni familial cancer syndrome, an observation in keeping with other tumour suppressor genes. Nevertheless the product of the point mutated p53 gene appears to have transforming effects in its own right. One explanation for this derives from the observation that p53 appears to function in the form of protein oligomers. Oligomers formed exclusively from wild type p53 are active, oligomers of wild type and mutant p53 inactive. Hence, mutated p53 can inhibit the action of the wild type protein and in so doing appears to offer a proliferative advantage to the cell.

The majority of p53 mutations are single missense point mutations resulting in an amino acid substitution in the p53 protein. These point mutations are mainly confined to the regions of the p53 gene conserved during evolution. Within this region there are four codons which appear to be mutational hotspots and together account for over 30% of all observed p53 mutations (Hollstein *et al.*, 1991). Comparison has demonstrated that patterns of mutation vary between tumour types and it is thought this may reflect the mechanisms of action of environmental carcinogens which play a role in the aetiology of these tumours (Soussi and Caron de Fromental, 1992). For example, the high rate of G→T nucleotide substitution in the p53 gene in smoking related lung cancers (Takahashi *et al.*, 1991) correlates well with the known mechanisms of action of tobacco related mutagens.

Normal p53 functions as a transcription factor regulating the expression of a number of other genes. Mutant p53 proteins, the SV40 large T antigen and the product of the *mdm*2 gene, a dominantly transforming gene frequently amplified in sarcomas, all inhibit p53 mediated gene transcription. But what exactly does p53 do which makes abrogation of its function so important in tumour development. A number of very recent observations have brought the answer much closer. It has been demonstrated that ultraviolet light, gamma irradiation and DNA-damaging drugs all induce the accumulation of the normal p53 protein. It has also been shown that high levels of normal p53 appear to mediate arrest of the cell cycle in G1 and can also induce apoptosis (programmed cell death). It is proposed that G1 arrest following a genotoxic insult to the cell might allow time for adequate cellular repair of the induced DNA damage. Alternatively, if the cell is sufficiently damaged high p53 levels would induce apoptosis (Lane, 1992). Recent work on apoptosis in thymocytes from p53 'knock-out' mice (mice which lack both p53 genes) has demonstrated that these cells apoptose normally in response to physiological stimuli such as glucocorticoids, but are highly resistant to radiation induced apoptosis (Lane, 1993; Lowe *et al.*, 1993). Hence, it is proposed that cells which lack p53 or possess a mutant p53 gene are highly resistant to DNA damage induced apoptosis. Such cells may be genetically less stable than normal cells, may accumulate mutations unchecked, leading to the rapid selection of increasingly malignant clones.

3.5.6   THE COLORECTAL MODEL OF TUMORIGENESIS

Epidemiological studies of age-dependent tumour incidence in humans indicate kinetics dependent on the fifth or sixth power of elapsed time. In simple terms this suggests a succession of five or six independent rate limiting steps in the development of adult human

malignancies. Unique histological features of colorectal tumours and the extensive work of Vogelstein and his colleagues has meant that the molecular events underpinning the progression to a malignant carcinoma are best understood for colorectal tumorigenesis.

Vogelstein *et al.* (1988) examined a very large series of primary colorectal tumours, representing large numbers of very early to late adenomas and carcinomas, for a series of genetic abnormalities including *ras* gene mutations and LOH on the long arm of chromosomes 5 and 18 (subsequently shown to be the site of tumour suppressor genes mutated in colorectal tumours) and the short arm of chromosome 17 – the p53 locus. In addition he examined tumours for variation in patterns of DNA methylation. By examining the frequency of each type of mutation in early, intermediate and late adenomas and in carcinomas he was able to build up a model of accumulating genetic mutations leading to carcinoma formation (Fearon and Vogelstein, 1990). This model is outlined in Figure 3.4. Identical patterns of mutation are not seen in every tumour and it is the accumulation of mutations, not the absolute order of acquiring those mutations, which appears to be important in the progression to a malignant phenotype. Although the colorectal model is incomplete it represents a sizeable step in understanding colorectal tumorigenesis at the molecular level.

3.6   ONCOGENES AND TUMOUR SUPPRESSOR GENES IN CLINICAL PRACTICE

3.6.1   ONCOGENES AS PROGNOSTIC INDICATORS

The intimate association between molecular pathology and tumour biology has generated widespread interest in the use of molecular markers of oncogene activation or tumour suppressor gene inactivation as prognostic indicators. Numerous studies have generated

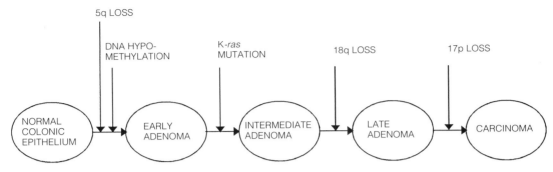

Figure 3.4 Following analysis of numerous adenomas of increasing size, dysplasia and villous content in addition to invasive carcinomas, Fearon and Vogelstein (1990) developed a genetic model for colorectal tumour formation shown in this figure. Although the order of accumulation of mutations was variable, in general 5q loss and hypomethylation were seen in early adenomas followed by K-*ras* mutation, 18q loss and then 17p loss (p53 mutation).

data correlating molecular pathology with clinical stage, histopathological grade and prognosis in univariate analyses, but relatively few have demonstrated that markers of molecular pathology can provide independent prognostic information in multivariate analyses. Particular interest has been directed towards N-*myc* amplification in childhood neuroblastomas, and c-*erb*B2 overexpression and p53 mutation in breast cancer.

Using the Evan's staging system, stage I and II neuroblastomas have a 75–90% overall 2 year survival, whereas stage III and IV tumours have a 10–30% overall 2 year survival. Seeger *et al.* (1985) demonstrated N-*myc* amplification was associated with an advanced tumour stage and a poor prognosis. Moreover, 2/16 stage II tumours analysed demonstrated N-*myc* amplification and both of these tumours metastasized compared to 1/14 stage II tumours which did not possess N-*myc* amplification (P=0.03). In some centres N-*myc* amplification is used to designate an aggressive therapeutic approach in tumours which by other criteria would be deemed to have a favourable prognosis.

In breast cancer, c-*erb*B2 overexpression appears to correlate with reduced disease free and overall survival in both node-positive and node-negative disease. In addition, over-

expression appears to correlate with a poorer therapeutic outcome following endocrine therapy or chemotherapy in both ER-positive and ER-negative breast cancer (Gusterson *et al.*, 1992). Allred *et al.* (1993) analysed 700 node-negative primary breast tumours for p53 mutation and demonstrated p53 mutation was an independent prognostic variable in node-negative disease in multivariate analyses. p53 mutation may therefore represent a clinically useful marker with which to distinguish node-negative patients who may benefit from aggressive postsurgical therapy.

3.6.2 FAMILIAL PREDISPOSITION TO CANCER – USING PREDISPOSITION GENES TO SCREEN FAMILIES AT RISK

Familial clustering of cancer is well documented, and for some familial cancer syndromes genetic predisposition has been demonstrated to be due to a germline mutation in a single tumour suppressor gene; the RB1 gene in familial retinoblastoma, the APC gene in familial polyposis coli and the p53 gene in the Li–Fraumeni syndrome. These are recent developments in rare cancer predisposition syndromes whose burden in clinical practice is not great. However, cloning of a breast cancer gene which appears to account for up to 45% of all familial breast cancer is imminent and the mapping of a locus for hereditary non-polyposis colon cancer, predicted to account for 13% of all colorectal tumours (Pelomaki *et al.*, 1993), heralds the cloning of this gene in the near future. These syndromes both provide a significant cancer burden in clinical practice. The selection, counselling, testing and surveillance of patients and their relatives suspected of carrying a mutation in either of these cancer predisposition genes is likely to become an important part of oncological clinical practice in the very near future.

3.6.3   GENE THERAPY

A precise understanding of the biochemical abnormalities in tumour cells holds promise for the development of effective, non-toxic, tumour-specific therapies by exploiting differences between tumour and normal cellular biology. Gene therapy is yet in its infancy, but a number of therapeutic approaches are being explored, and are reviewed by Harris and Sikora (1993).

One avenue being followed by Rosenberg and his colleagues at the National Institute of Cancer in the USA is to genetically engineer tumour invasive lymphocytes (TILs) from patients with metastatic melanoma by infecting them with retroviruses carrying the gene for tumour necrosis factor (TNF). TNF is then expressed in these cells at very high levels because it is under the influence of strong retroviral promoters. Genetically engineered TILs are transferred back into the patients from whom they were obtained and the lymphocytes home in on tumour cells delivering very high concentrations of TNF locally. Clinical trials are currently in progress in the USA involving 50 patients with metastatic melanoma.

Virally directed enzyme prodrug therapy (VDEPT) proposes to use a similar approach to specifically deliver a toxic drug to tumour cells. A retroviral vector is engineered to carry a foreign gene under the influence of a promoter sequence recognized specifically in tumour cells. The gene encodes an enzyme which can convert a harmless compound into a toxic drug. For example, the conversion of 5-flurocytosine (5-FC) to 5-flurouracil (5-FU) by the enzyme cytosine deaminase. If transcription of the enzyme is driven by a tumour specific promoter sequence, e.g. the αFP promoter in hepatocellular carcinoma or the c-*erb*B2 promoter in breast tumours, then it is predicted that toxic levels of the prodrug metabolite would only be achieved in tumour cells, giving potentially effective chemotherapy with a wide therapeutic ratio. *In vitro* studies are presently underway.

A third approach showing promise involves the use of antisense oligonucleotides. These are short synthetic single-stranded DNA molecules complementary to specific DNA or RNA sequences. When antisense molecules bind complementary DNA or RNA sequences within the cell they can selectively inhibit the transcription or translation of their target genes. A number of specific antisense oligonucleotides have been shown to have antiproliferative activity *in vitro*; for example antisense oligonucleotides to c-*myc* in lymphoma cell lines, to N-*myc* in neuroectodermal cell lines and to *bcr-abl* in chronic myeloid leukaemia cell lines. Their antitumour potential has yet to be tested *in vivo*.

REFERENCES

Allred, D.C., Clark, G.M., Elledge, R. *et al.* (1993) Association of p53 protein expression with tumour cell proliferation rate and clinical outcome in node-negative breast cancer. *Proceedings of the American Society of Clinical Oncology*, **85**, 200–6.

Bishop, J.M. and Varmus, H. (1982) Functions and origins of retroviral transforming genes, in *RNA Tumour Viruses*, 2nd edn, (eds R. Weiss, N. Teich, H. Varmus and J. Coffin), Cold Spring Harbor Laboratory, New York, pp. 999–1108.

Bodmer, W.F., Bailey, C.J., Bodmer, J. *et al.* (1987) Localization of the gene for familial adenomatous polyposis on chromosome 5. *Nature*, **328**, 614–16.

Bos, J.L. (1989) *ras* oncogenes in human cancer: a review. *Cancer Research*, **49**, 4682–9.

Cavanee, W.K., Dryja, T.P., Phillips, R.A. *et al.* (1983) Expression of recessive alleles by chromosomal mechanisms in retinoblastoma. *Nature*, **305**, 779–84.

Cavanee, W.K., Hansen, M.F., Nordenskjold, M. *et al.* (1985) Genetic origin of mutations predisposing to retinoblastoma. *Science*, **228**, 501–3.

Crook, T., Wrede, D., Tidy, J.A. *et al.* (1992) Clonal p53 mutation in primary cervical cancer: association with human-papillomavirus-negative tumours. *Lancet*, **339**, 1070–3.

Downward, J. (1990) The ras superfamily of small GTP-binding proteins. *Trends in Biochemical Science*, **15**, 469–72.

Easton, D.F., Bishop, D.T., Ford, D. *et al.* (1993) Genetic linkage analysis in familial breast and ovarian cancer – results from 214 families. *American Journal of Human Genetics*, **52**, 678–701.

Fearon, E.R. and Vogelstein, B. (1990) A genetic model for colorectal tumourigenesis. *Cell*, **61**, 759–67.

Gusterson, B.A., Gelber, R.D., Goldkirsch, K.N. *et al.* (1992) Prognostic importance of c-erbB2 expression in breast cancer. *Journal of Clinical Oncology*, **10**, 1049–56.

Hall, J.M., Lee, M.K., Newman, B. *et al.* (1990) Linkage of early-onset familial breast cancer to chromosome 17q21. *Science*, **250**, 1648–9.

Harris, J.D. and Sikora, K. (1993) Gene therapy of cancer, in *Molecular Biology for Oncologists*, 1st edn, (eds. J. Yarnold, M. Stratton, T. McMillan), Elsevier Science, Amsterdam, pp. 263–73.

Heisterkamp, N., Stephenson, J.R., Groffen, J. *et al.* (1983) Localization of the c-*abl* oncogene adjacent to a translocation breakpoint in chronic myelocytic leukaemia. *Nature*, **306**, 239–42.

Hollstein, M., Sidransky, D., Vogelstein, B. *et al.* (1991) p53 mutations in human cancers. *Science*, **253**, 49–53.

Huang, H-J. S., Yee, J-K., Shew, J-Y. *et al.* (1988) Suppression of the neoplastic phenotype by replacement of the Rb gene in human cancer cells. *Science*, **242**, 1563–6.

King, M-C. (1990) Genetic analysis of cancer in families. *Cancer Surveys*, **9**, 417–35.

Knudson, A.G. (1971) Mutations and cancer: statistical study of retinoblastoma. *Proceedings of the National Academy of Science USA*, **68**, 820–3.

Lane, D.P. (1992) p53, guardian of the genome. *Nature*, **358**, 15–16.

Lane, D.P. (1993) A death in the life of p53. *Nature*, **362**, 786–7.

Lowe, S.W., Schmitt, E.M., Smith, S.W. *et al.* (1993) p53 is required for radiation-induced apoptosis in mouse thymocytes. *Nature*, **362**, 847–9.

Patterson, H. (1993) Approaches to proto-oncogenes and tumour suppressor gene identification, 1st edn, (eds J. Yarnold, M. Stratton, T. McMillan), Elsevier Science, Amsterdam, p. 28.

Pelomaki, P., Aaltonen, L.A., Sistonen, P. *et al.* (1993) Genetic mapping of a locus predisposing to human colorectal cancer. *Science*, **260**, 810–12.

Seeger, R.C., Brodeur, G.M., Sather, H. *et al.* (1985) Association of multiple copies of the N-*myc* oncogene with rapid progression of neuroblastomas. *New England Journal of Medicine*, **313**, 1111–16.

Soussi, T. and Caron de Fromental, C. (1992) TP53 tumour suppressor gene: a model for investigating human mutagenesis. *Genes, Chromosomes and Cancer*, **4**, 1–15.

Stanbridge, E.J. (1988) Genetic analysis of human malignancy using somatic cell hybrids and monochromosome transfer. *Cancer Surveys*, **9**, 317–24.

Takahashi, T., Takahashi, T., Suzuki, H. *et al.* (1991) The p53 gene is very frequently mutated in small-cell lung cancer with a distinct nucleotide substitution pattern. *Oncogene*, **6**, 1775–8.

Varmus H. (1988) Retroviruses. *Science*, **240**, 1427–35.

Vogelstein, B., Fearon, E.R., Hamilton, S.R. *et al.* (1988) Genetic alterations during colorectal-tumour development. *New England Journal of Medicine*, **319**, 525–32.

IMMUNOLOGICAL APPROACHES TO THE DIAGNOSIS AND TREATMENT OF CANCER

4

Suzanne A. Eccles

Improvements in public awareness and the development of more sophisticated screening techniques are resulting in the earlier diagnosis of cancers. Unfortunately in many cases the disease has already disseminated, and conventional treatments may fail to eradicate it. Clearly there is a need to develop new approaches further to improve detection and control of metastatic disease.

Recent years have seen enormous advances in biotechnology and molecular engineering, and new generations of monoclonal antibodies are already making an impact in clinical medicine (Winter and Milstein, 1991; Adair, 1992). In addition, our increasing understanding of the complexities of immune responses, for example, the importance of correct antigen presentation in association with HLA (human leucocyte antigen) class 1 determinants, and the orchestrated interactions between humoral and cellular effectors, is allowing us to design more rational approaches to immunotherapeutic intervention.

This chapter will focus mainly on the diagnostic and therapeutic applications of monoclonal antibodies in oncology, and briefly on the potential of recruiting host cells to discriminate and destroy neoplastic cells. Cytokines, which provide a pivotal role in the transmission of intercellular messages and amplification of immune responses, and can lead to the direct or indirect killing of tumour cells, are dealt with in Chapter 12.

4.1 POTENTIAL TARGETS FOR HUMAN TUMOUR DIAGNOSIS AND THERAPHY

4.1.1 EVIDENCE FOR HUMAN TUMOUR ANTIGENS AND PATIENT IMMUNOREACTIVITY

The exquisite specificity of immune responses – whether exercised by antibodies or T cells – can only be exploited in the management of cancer if qualitative or quantitative differences can be reliably demonstrated between normal and malignant cells. In early studies of experimental tumour immunology, great excitement was generated by the discovery of 'transplantation-type' antigens on rodent tumours, particularly those induced by acute exposure to chemical carcinogens or oncogenic viruses. This was inevitably followed by disillusionment when evidence for such strong immunogens in human cancers, even those known or suspected to have a similar aetiology, was not immediately forthcoming.

Recently, however, developments in molecular biology and immunology have yielded important insights into the mechanisms of malignant transformation, the nature of oncogene and tumour suppressor gene products, and the requirements for effective host recognition of subtle phenotypic cellular changes. Although it is clear that by the time a patient is suffering from disseminated disease any immune response has failed, this does not necessarily mean that surveillance mechanisms are ineffective in eliminating early clones that have undergone malignant change; we would simply be unaware of the successes. Similarly, if bulky disease can be eliminated by conventional therapies, it is possible that the immune response can be reactivated to eradicate residual micrometastases. In order to do this, however, it is necessary fully to understand the spectrum of changes that cancer cells may exhibit, and devise ways to overcome, supplement or replace ineffective host responses.

4.1.2   HUMAN TUMOUR MARKERS

The earliest tumour markers discovered were named 'carcinoembryonic' antigens because of their expression in fetal, rather than adult, normal tissues; other examples appeared to be differentiation antigens whose tertiary structure or tissue distribution was altered in malignant epithelia. Some of the most venerable of these (e.g. carcinoembryonic antigen (CEA), epithelial membrane antigen (EMA)) have enjoyed useful careers as targets for diagnosis and therapy in spite of their less than perfect profiles in terms of tumour selectivity (Table 4.1). Virally associated antigens may be expressed in tumours where Epstein–Barr virus (EBV), human T-lymphotropic virus 1 (HTLV-1) or certain subtypes of human papilloma virus (HPV) are cofactors in the oncogenic process (McMichael and Bodmer, 1992).

Few antigens are entirely tumour specific, and generally some normal tissues also express the same or cross-reactive epitopes. Exceptions are immunoglobulin idiotypes on B-cell lymphomas (which are clonal in nature), mutated EGFR which have been described in glioblastoma (Humphrey *et al.*, 1990), and fusion proteins produced by DNA translocations, e.g. BCR-ABL gene products. In addition, certain neogangliosides with limited normal tissue distribution have been described in melanoma and neuroblastoma, and from the former a gene encoding a melanoma specific antigen (MZE-2) has

recently been cloned (van der Bruggen *et al.*, 1991).

A further important category of potential cancer targets comprises molecules which are overexpressed on the tumour cell surface compared with normal cells. Significantly, in many cases these molecules are encoded by proto-oncogenes, function as growth factor receptors/intercellular communication devices and appear to confer a selective growth advantage on cells which overexpress them. Prime examples include the EGF receptor, and related proto-oncogenes of the c-*erb*B family (Gusterson, 1992; Lemoine and Epenetos, 1993; Plowman *et al.*, 1993).

Finally, and more speculatively, it has been suggested that neovascularization (on which tumour growth and metastasis critically depends) may provide a target for anti-angiogenic therapy if proliferating capillaries are shown to express unique antigens (Bicknell and Harris, 1991). In a similar vein (no pun intended) molecules thought to be associated with metastatic invasion of extracellular matrix or endothelia (e.g. metalloproteinases) or settling of disseminated cells at secondary sites (e.g. CD44 splice variants) may provide targets for prevention of metastasis (Reber *et al.*, 1990), although cells already lodged in the parenchyma of distant organs would not be susceptible.

Antigens capable of eliciting immune responses in the host (i.e. immunogens) have been demonstrated in experimental tumours by their ability to protect syngeneic (genetically identical) animals from rechallenge with the same malignant cells. Clearly such a direct approach is not feasible in man, and indirect evidence for immune responses to tumours has been adduced. Spontaneous regressions which occur in a few tumour types have sometimes been ascribed to host defence mechanisms, but other mechanisms including induction of differentiation or apoptosis may also be operative. Host lymphocytic or monocytic infiltration of primary tumours and regional lymph nodes,

Table 4.1 Examples of human tumour associated antigens exploitable for diagnosis or therapy

Category	Examples	Distribution	Comments
Onco-fetal antigens	Carcinoembryonic antigen – CEA	Colon, breast and other carcinomas	Often shed; cross-reactive with normal antigen NCA
	Alphafetoprotein – AFP	Hepatocellular carcinoma	Shed; used as serum marker
Differentiation antigens	Epithelial mucins, EMA, PEM	Breast and other carcinomas	Often shed; differential glycosylation may expose immunogenic core peptides
	Gangliosides GM2, GD2	Melanoma, neuroblastoma	Overexpressed normal gangliosides or new structures can be immunogenic
	Cluster 1 (N-CAM) Cluster W4, 5a	Small cell lung cancer (SCLC)	Also on normal (non-lung) tissues
Neo-antigens	Immunoglobulin idiotypes	B-cell lymphomas	Tumour specific
	Mutated EGF-R	Glioblastomas	Tumour specific
	Fusion proteins from DNA translocations (eg BCR-ABL)	CML	Tumour specific
	MAGE gene family (eg MZE-2)	Melanoma, SCLC, breast and other cancers	Some genes present, but not expressed in normal tissues
Virally-associated antigens	Epstein–Barr virus (EBV) Human papilloma virus subtypes (e.g. 16 and 18) HTLV-1	Burkitt's lymphoma, NPC Cervical cancer and other UG malignancies Some T-cell malignancies	Potential cytotoxic T-cell responses inert
Overexpressed growth factor receptors/oncogene products	EGF-R	Squamous cancer of lung, stomach, bladder, pancreas	Present on normal tissues, but tumour cells more dependent on expression for growth
	C-erbB-2, B3, B4	Breast cancer and other adenocarcinomas	Limited expression on normal tissues
	BCL2	B-cell lymphoma	Translocation causes overexpression
Metastasis-associated molecules	CD44 splice variants	Various human tumours	May provide unique target
	metalloproteinases	Various human tumours	Same as in normal tissues – may be overexpressed
Antigens on tumour neovasculature?	Proliferating endothelium may express unique antigens	Theoretically all cancers; histogenic differences may exist	Potential opportunity to inhibit neoangiogenesis by mabs/ADEPT

and in some cases their cytotoxic response to autologous tumours *in vitro* is more direct evidence of immunoreactivity, and in some cases (but not all) carries prognostic significance (McMichael and Bodmer, 1992). In some instances humoral antibodies have been detected, with a frequency which seems to increase following immunotherapeutic interventions and which in some cases is associated with improved survival (Portoukalian *et al.*, 1991). Recently, cytotoxic T lymphocyte (CTL) clones have been derived from a melanoma patient, each capable of responding to one of at least four individual antigenic determinants on the tumour; the gene for one of these (MAGE-1) was cloned, and although present in the patient's normal cells its product was not expressed. It has since been demonstrated on 30% of melanomas, and 15% of breast and lung tumours, although its function is as yet unknown. For a readable account of the research leading up to this important discovery, see Boon (1993).

One of the most important advances in our understanding has come from the realization that an *antigen* will not function as an *immunogen* unless correctly presented in association with class 1 molecules of the major histocompatibility complex (MHC). Thus failure of an effective host response may be due to lack of tumour neoantigens, down-regulation of MHC expression, or insufficient helper factors such as interleukin 2. Clearly it is critically important to identify any deficit in each of these parameters in order effectively to boost the patient's response.

4.2   STRUCTURE AND FUNCTION OF ANTIBODY MOLECULES

The immunoglobulin (Ig) molecule comprises four polypeptide chains (two light chains and two heavy chains) linked by disulphide bonds (Figure 4.1(a)). Each chain has constant and variable regions. The structure of the heavy chain constant region distinguishes the five main classes (isotypes) of antibody (IgG,

IgM, IgA, IgD and IgE), and the terminal Fc portion and adjacent domains determine important functions such as binding to cellular receptors, activation of complement, etc. The Fab (antigen binding fragment) is composed of the variable regions of both light and heavy chains (V_H and V_L). Each chain contains three hypervariable loops or 'complementarity determining regions' (CDR) – which together define the binding specificity – within a framework of flanking peptide domains.

4.2.1   MONOCLONAL ANTIBODIES

Monoclonal antibodies have traditionally been generated by the immunization of rodents with tumour cells, extracts, or purifed peptides of antigens of interest, followed by fusion of their B cells with an immortal myeloma cell line to generate hybridomas. Those secreting antibodies of the desired specificity, affinity and isotype are then cloned and selected by various screening procedures. The production of high affinity monoclonal antibodies using human cells has so far proved more elusive.

Although this approach has generated a number of useful monoclonal antibodies and chemically derived Fab and $F(ab')_2$ fragments, scientists are increasingly attempting to produce second generation recombinant molecules whose behavioural profiles are rationally designed to address specific problems. Immunoglobulin genes have been cloned from a variety of sources, and such libraries can provide a blueprint to generate new therapeutic strategies. For example, chimaeric or 'humanized' composite antibodies in which either the Fab portion or the CDRs of an effective rodent mab are chemically linked or genetically grafted onto a human antibody backbone have been produced to minimize immunogenicity in patients, with some success. If of the appropriate human isotype (e.g. IgG1 or IgG3) such reshaped mabs may also more effectively acti-

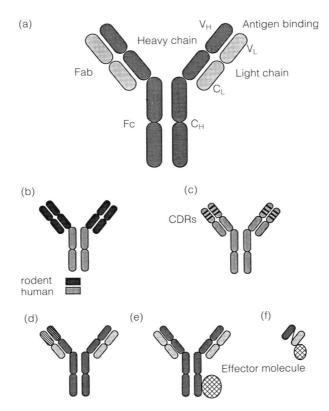

Figure 4.1 Schematic illustration of a basic immunoglobulin molecule **(a)** and various chemically or genetically engineered constructs. **(b)** Chimaeric antibody constructed either by chemical coupling of rodent F(ab')$_2$ onto human Fc, or by grafting rodent genes coding for variable regions (V$_H$ and V$_L$) onto human constant region genes (C$_H$ and C$_L$). **(c)** 'Humanized' antibody produced by grafting rodent hypervariable region genes (CDRs) onto human framework region genes. **(d)** Bifunctional antibody produced either from heterohybridomas (i.e. B-cell hybridomas secreting mabs of two different specificities fused, then recombinant mabs with dual specificity selected), or by genetic engineering. **(e)** Hybrid proteins generated by chemically coupling mabs to molecules with effector function (e.g. toxin, enzyme) or by splicing appropriate genes. This is more practical with smaller molecules, i.e. Fusion proteins **(f)**, e.g. single chain Fv (V$_H$ + V$_L$) plus small toxin molecule (RIP) or hapten.

vate host effector cells and/or complement to destroy target tumour cells (Figure 4.1(b), (c)).

4.2.2 BISPECIFIC ANTIBODIES

Bispecific antibodies in which each Fab arm has a different specificity provide a variety of opportunities (Figure 4.1(d)). Those which bind to tumour antigens and appropriate CD determinants on T lymphocytes (e.g. CD3 molecules associated with the T-cell receptor) can theoretically redirect the specificity of these cells towards the tumour, and activate their cytotoxic potential – this is known as 'effector cell retargeting' (Clark *et al.*, 1988). Antibodies with dual specificity for tumour antigens and suitable haptens would allow delivery of enzymes, isotopes, drugs, toxins or cytokines. Bispecific antibodies recognizing two different epitopes on the same cancer cell should minimize cross-reactivity with normal tissues and increase immunoselectivity. Some such constructs are in early clinical trial, most are still undergoing further refinement (Bolhuis *et al.*, 1991; Fanger *et al.*, 1991). Hybrid molecules or fusion proteins can also be generated, where a portion of the mab with a desired binding specificity is linked to another peptide – perhaps with an effector function. For example, genes for either Fc or single chain Fv (linked variable regions of the light and heavy chains) could be spliced to the gene coding for a small ribosome-inactivating protein and expressed in bacterial or mammalian cells to generate a mini-immunotoxin (Figure 4.1(e), (f)) (Wels *et al.*, 1992).

4.3   DIAGNOSIS

4.3.1   IMMUNOASSAYS, TUMOUR MARKERS, ASSESSMENT OF TUMOUR LOAD

Sensitive *in vitro* immunoassays have revolutionized many areas of medicine, including oncology, and the reader will no doubt be familiar with (and probably take for granted) many of these. Recent developments include the increased specificity afforded by monoclonal (versus polyclonal) antibodies, and advances in the design of more sophisticated assay systems including immunosensors, immunoprobes and various immunoaffinity separation techniques (Herberman and Mercer, 1990).

Only a minority of patients have disease whose response to therapy can be assessed by physical examination or diagnostic radiology, and lesions of less than 1 cm^3 can infrequently be detected. Some tumours release products into the circulation which can be used as markers of residual disease. Examples include human chorionic ganadotrophin (HCG) (choriocarcinoma and teratoma), CEA (some GI tract tumours), alphafetoprotein (hepatoma and teratoma), epithelial mucins (breast carcinoma), monoclonal immunoglobulin (myeloma), and prostate specific antigen. Immunoassays of such products can

give quantitative estimations of tumour load in some cases down to about 10^8 cells, and may give useful 'early warning' of non-responsiveness to treatment and tumour recurrence. Recently it has been shown that a soluble form of the c-*erb*B2 gene product is detectable by ELISA (with certain mabs) in the serum of patients with breast cancer (Leitzel *et al.*, 1992), adding to the list of potential tumour markers which in this case may also carry prognostic significance. Soluble or shed forms of other cell surface transmembrane receptors are also known, for example, the receptors for epidermal growth factor (EGF), tumour necrosis factor (TNF), insulin and IL-2. The latter has been shown to reflect tumour burden and response to therapy in certain forms of T-cell and hairy cell leukaemias.

In addition, mabs specifically recognizing DNA adducts formed by various anti-cancer drugs can precisely determine the relative exposure of normal (e.g. haematopoietic) cells and biopsied tumour cells. Such information could be used to identify individuals (or tumours) hypersensitive to a particular agent, and hopefully to aid in the design of drugs with improved selectivity (Tilby *et al.*, 1993).

4.3.2   IMMUNOHISTOCHEMISTRY

Mabs directed against human oestrogen and progesterone receptors have allowed the development of quantitative and histochemical assays for these proteins in breast cancer, yielding important prognostic information more readily and from smaller samples than is possible using ligand binding assays. The unique specificity of mabs has allowed great improvements to be made in identifying cell lineages in the haematopoietic system, and in immunophenotyping malignancies derived from them. In addition, it is often possible to determine the origin of anaplastic primary tumours (or of tumour cells in lymph node biopsies where no primary tumour has been found) by their expression of surface markers, and hence to select the most appropriate therapy.

Increasingly, it is becoming clear that the presence of oncogenes (e.g. c-*erb*B-2) or gene rearrangements (e.g. *bcr-abl*), or the absence of misregulation of 'suppressor' genes (e.g. p53), may carry important prognostic implications. In some cases, mabs raised against the protein product of these aberrant genes can be used to screen primary tumours to yield valuable information. For example, in breast cancer, the number of tumour-positive lymph nodes is still the most potent prognostic marker for patients with operable disease; however, a significant proportion of node-negative patients suffer tumour recurrence and death. Recent studies have suggested that in patients with otherwise good prognostic markers, overexpression of c-*erb*B2 or the related epidermal growth factor receptor (EGFR) predicted for earlier and more widespread metastases, failure to respond to chemotherapy or tamoxifen, and shorter survival times. Combined expression of both of these receptor tyrosine kinases indicated the worst prognosis (Harris *et al.*, 1992). Such patients may therefore be candidates for immunotherapeutic intervention based on the presence of these cell surface receptors (Allan *et al.*, 1993).

4.4 RADIOIMMUNODETECTION (RAID)

4.4.1 IMMUNOSCINTIGRAPHY

Radiolabelled monoclonal antibodies have been used in attempts to localize tumour deposits by immunoscintigraphy for several years, but in most cases the results have not been appreciably superior to those obtained by imaging techniques such as magnetic resonance spectroscopy or computerized tomography. The problems are caused by the lack of specificity or shedding of many of the commonly employed antigenic targets (e.g. CEA, mucins), the low levels of mab localization in solid tumours, and physical limitations of the isotopes and scanning techniques generally available.

It is likely that some of the recently identified tumour antigens will provide targets with more restricted normal tissue distribution, but probably at the expense of ubiquitous expression on cancers of a particular type; for example, c-*erb*B2 is not present in significant amounts in normal tissues, but is overexpressed in only 20–30% of breast cancers. However, the negative tumours may demonstrate other abnormalities, and it is possible that a relatively small panel of antibodies could be selected to cover all phenotypes while minimizing background. In addition, genetically engineered mabs, designed for improved pharmacokinetics (in terms of serum half-life, affinity, etc.) should also provide better resolution.

The choice of isotopes available, and means of stably conjugating them to mabs, is improving rapidly; the smaller mab fragments are better matched to the short half-life isotopes such as technetium-99m, and the problem of its renal uptake has been reduced by new conjugation chemistry. Radiometals such as yttrium and indium can now be stably coupled using macrocyclic chelators such as DOTA and its descendants. SPECT and PET imaging systems provide enhanced spatial resolution and sensitivity compared with planar gamma scintigraphy, and also enable quantification of the radioisotope distribution *in vivo* (Bakir *et al.*, 1992).

4.4.2 RADIOIMMUNOGUIDED SURGERY (RIS)

Some of the problems associated with detecting radiolabelled mabs in tumours against a high blood or normal tissue background can be avoided by the use of intraoperative probes. In this approach, isotopically labelled mabs are injected into the patient several days before surgery, and lesions in the abdomen detected with a hand-held gamma detecting probe. In one study (Martin *et al.*, 1988), using the anti-mucin antibody B72.3, 79–83% of colorectal tumours scored positive, and lymph node involvement was correctly identified in 17/20 cases. In approximately one-third of patients RIS yielded additional information about subclinical tumour deposits which altered the surgical approach.

4.5 MONOCLONAL ANTIBODY-BASED THERAPEUTIC APPROACHES

4.5.1 DIRECT EFFECTS

Antibodies of the appropriate isotype (which varies between species) can activate complement to lyse target cells (complement-dependent cytotoxicity, CDC) or interact with cells expressing Fc receptors to mediate antibody-dependent cellular cytotoxicity (ADCC) (Dyer, 1992). In some cases mabs directed against growth factor receptors which may be overexpressed on cancer cells (e.g. epidermal growth factor, EGFR) can exert direct growth inhibitory effects by competing with the growth factor(s) on which sustained proliferation of the cells depends (Modjtahedi *et al.*, 1993) (Figure 4.2(a)–(c)).

The use of complement-activating mabs has some limitations. The large size of the first component of complement (C1, 800 kDa) limits its extravascular penetration and hence access to target cells. Also, the haematopoietic system (and perhaps malignancies derived therefrom) is well protected from killing by species restricted membrane activities (such as CD59) which block the activity of autologous complement. Clinical trials using this approach have therefore been restricted to *ex vivo* treatment of bone marrow using heterologous complement, and to a few haematological malignancies *in vivo*. The most notable effects have been obtained with the rat IgG2b mab CAMPATH 1 directed against a human lymphoid cell antigen (CDw52) in non-Hodgkin's lymphoma (Dyer, 1992), and mabs against CD14 and CD15 antigens which are expressed on cells from about 95% of patients with acute myeloid leukaemia (AML) (Ball *et al.*, 1990).

The induction of ADCC by mabs of the correct isotype is an attractive proposition since the cellular effectors readily extravasate, and may gain access to tumours at any site. ADCC is generally inducible at 10–100 fold lower mab concentrations than required to

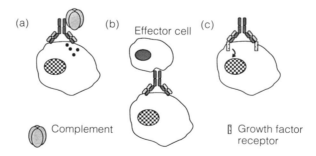

Figure 4.2 Direct mechanisms by which mabs can kill tumour cells. **(a)** Complement-dependent cytotoxicity (CDC). Mabs of certain isotypes can bind and activate complement leading to cytolysis by the formation of perforations in the cell membrane. **(b)** Antibody-dependent cellular cytotoxicity (ADCC). Mabs of certain isotypes can bind to effector cells via their Fc receptors, and direct their cytotoxic potential towards the tumour. Various mechanisms operate (including cytostasis, cytolysis, apoptosis) depending on the nature of the effector cell, the antibody isotype, and the antigen. **(c)** Some tumour cells are critically dependent on autocrine or paracrine growth factors for their sustained proliferation. Interruption of the stimulatory signal transduction pathway by mabs which compete for ligand binding can effectively inhibit tumour cell growth. The effect is cytostatic, but may be followed by apoptotic death or terminal differentiation.

activate C1. A variety of different cell types have been shown to be capable of mediating ADCC under different conditions, including natural killer (NK) cells, monocytes and lymphokine-activated killer (LAK) cells – in fact most cells expressing Fc receptors (CD64, CD32 and CD16) (Stötter and Lotze, 1990). It has been suggested that some of the apparent benefits obtained in colorectal cancer patients by use of the mab 17.1A may be due directly or indirectly to its ability to invoke ADCC with human effector cells (Riethmüller, 1994).

4.5.2   INDIRECT EFFECTS – CARRIERS OF EFFECTOR MOLECULES

(a)   Immunotoxins

Immunotoxins consist of a monoclonal antibody linked to a toxic protein; the antibody selectively targets the toxin to cells by binding to a cell surface antigen expressed uniquely or at elevated levels on the target compared with normal tissues. The toxin must then enter the cell in order to kill it by irreversibly blocking an essential metabolic process such as protein synthesis in ribosomes (Figure 4.3(a)). Common toxins employed are of bacterial or plant origin, and consist of an alpha chain (the toxin moiety) linked to a beta chain which is concerned with binding to cell membranes and internalization. Smaller single chain ribosome-inactivating proteins exist, such as the 30 kDa gelonin and saporin and the 17 kDa α-sarcin (Table 4.2).

Clinical trials of systemic immunotoxin therapy were first conducted in patients with B-cell chronic lymphocytic leukaemia; there followed attempts to treat T-cell lymphoma, melanoma, colon, ovarian, breast and small cell lung cancer, with varying degrees of success (Wawzynczak, 1991). Toxic side-effects and development of humoral immune responses to both components of the immunotoxin were problems common to all studies. Most trials now in progress are concentrating on lymphoid malignancies where access to

target cells is less of a problem than with solid tumours, and where the often reduced immunocompetance of the host may minimize antibody responses to the conjugates.

(b)   Radioimmunotherapy (RAIT) and photoimmunotherapy

Radionuclides have been used as therapy for selected malignancies for many years, and it was a logical progression to link such agents to monoclonal antibodies in attempts to increase their selectivity and the types of cancers that could be treated. A variety of radionuclides, including alpha emitters, low, medium, and high range beta emitters, and those acting through electron capture and/or production of Auger electrons are available, each with its own advantages and drawbacks (Table 4.3).

Much useful scientific information has emerged from such studies, including the biodistribution of differentially labelled mabs, and estimation of the cumulative radiation dose in tumours and normal tissues. One major theoretical advantage compared with some other forms of targeted therapy is that the isotope (if a beta-emitter) does not have to be delivered to every cell; thus tumour cells not expressing antigen or in a portion of the tumour not immediately accessible to mab may yet be susceptible to radiation 'crossfire' (Figure 4.3(b)). To date, most attempts to treat tumours by systemic delivery of radiolabelled mabs have been limited by toxicity in sensitive normal tissues such as bone marrow. In addition, certain tumours may be radio-resistant by virtue of innate properties or the presence of hypoxic areas. Good results have been obtained with ^{131}I-labelled mabs directed against antigens on B-cell lymphomas and leukaemias since such targets are generally radiosensitive and easily accessible.

A further problem with solid tumours is that mab penetration may be limited to the outer, well vascularized regions by increasing interstitial pressure and by an 'antigen

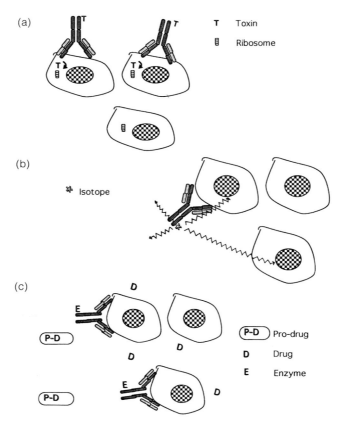

Figure 4.3   Indirect (effector targeting) mechanisms by which mabs may be used to kill tumour cells. **(a)** Immunotoxin therapy. Mabs are used to deliver to tumour cells a toxic protein which must then be internalized by receptor-mediated endocytosis before being routed to ribosomes where it inhibits protein synthesis. **(b)** Radioimmunotherapy. Mabs are used to target alpha or beta emitting isotopes to tumours; if the latter, antigen-negative cells may be damaged by radiation 'crossfire'. **(c)** ADEPT. Mab–enzyme conjugates are delivered to a tumour, then a prodrug is administered which will be converted by the enzyme at the tumour site into an active drug.

barrier' whereby bound mab impedes the progress of other molecules to deeper regions. Both of these factors would tend to concentrate radioactive energy in the outer areas of tumours, increasing the probability of damage to surrounding normal tissue. A novel suggestion to overcome this has been the development of mabs directed against antigens (nuclear histones) accessible only in necrotic and ischaemic regions of tumours. In experimental models such radiolabelled TNT (tumour necrosis targeting), mabs have been shown effectively to penetrate to the centre of xenograft tumours where they remained for extended periods and produced regressions in 88% of mice without evidence of normal tissue toxicity. Pilot clinical studies showed that the same mabs were capable of detecting necrotic regions in human tumours (Epstein *et al.*, 1991), and their future therapeutic applications are awaited with interest.

Table 4.2 Features of immunotoxin therapy

Advantages:	*Disadvantages:*
Conjugation of toxins to mabs relatively simple	A minority of mabs yield effective immunotoxins
Internalization of a single molecule can kill a cell	Conjugates are cleared more rapidly than mabs
Normal cells (if antigen negative) will be spared	Efficient endocytosis and correct intracellular routing required
Potent cytocidal action independent of secondary agent or host accessory mechanism	No effect on antigen-negative tumour cells
	If intact toxin used – danger of release and damage to normal cells
	Variable susceptibility of cells expressing same antigen

Examples of effector molecules for immunotoxin therapy:

Bacterial	*Plant*	*Fungal*
Diphtheria toxin	Ricin toxin	α-Sarcin RIP
Pseudomonas exotoxin	Abrin toxin	Restrictocin RIP
	Gelonin RIP	
	Saporin RIP	(Trichothecenes)
	Pokeweed antiviral protein	(Calicheamycin)

RIP = single chain ribosome-inactivating protein.

Labelled mabs may also be delivered directly into a body cavity (e.g. intra-peritoneally, intrapleurally or intrathe-cally), directly into tumour deposits (e.g. melanoma, glioma) or into afferent blood or lymphatic vessels in attempts to increase availability of mab to tumour before it is diluted in the peripheral circulation. Although such approaches have produced some positive results (Maraveyas and Epenetos, 1991), it is an intellectually unsat-isfying strategy, and one which does not address the major problem of disseminated micrometastases. A further possibility which is being explored, and which loosely falls into the category of radiation based im-munotherapy, is the use of mab targeted photosensitizers such as haematoporphyrin. Although applications are again limited to tumours accessible to laser light (if necessary delivered by fibre-optics), early results are promising.

Future developments may include the use of two-step strategies (as discussed below for ADEPT), perhaps based on the extremely high affinity of molecules such as streptavidin and biotin (Kd = 10^{-15}M). Mab–avidin conju-gates could be pre-injected, allowed to local-ize, and after an appropriate period be followed by inoculation of the small easily diffusible biotin molecule radiolabelled with an isotope of choice.

(c) Chemoimmunotherapy

The aim of chemoimmunotherapy is to achieve site-specific delivery of chemo-therapeutic drugs to minimize normal tissue damage. It was hoped that this approach would increase the stability (and therefore

Table 4.3   Features of radioimmunotherapy (RAIT)

Advantages:	Disadvantages:
Antigen-negative tumour cells may be killed by crossfire	Hypoxic tumour cells are radioresistant
Radioisotope conjugation methods are advancing rapidly	Mab in blood will irradiate sensitive normal tissues
Availability of wide variety of suitable isotopes	Nearby source of short half-life radionuclides required
	Facilities for handling isotopes and 'hot' patients required

Suitable radionuclides for RAIT:

Isotope	Half-life	Emissions/range		Notes
Astatine-211	7 h	α	50–90 μm	Cyclotron-produced; dehalogenation problem
Bismuth-212	1 h	α	50–90 μm	
Gold-199	3.2 d	β	< 200 μm	Produced carrier-free from Pt-198; γ for imaging
Iodine-131	8 d	$\beta + \gamma$	< 100 μm–2 mm	Dehalogenation problem
Copper-67	2.5 d	β		Requires chelation
Rhenium-186	3.5 d	β	100 μm–1 mm	Requires chelation; γ for imaging
Rhenium-188	17 h	β	< 1 mm	
Yttrium-90	2.5 d	β	~ 11 mm	Requires chelation; free Y-90 goes to bone; Y-86 for imaging
Iodine-125	2.5 d	Auger few nm		Dehalogenation; no imaging; requires internalization

half-life) of the drugs, and result in an enhanced therapeutic index (Juliano, 1991). However, the chemical conjugation of mainly hydrophobic drugs to hydrophilic mabs is difficult, and requires that the molecules contain appropriate chemical groups for linking. In most cases (except with alkylating agents such as melphalan and chlorambucil) the procedures were found to decrease the activity of both the drug and the antibody carrier (Pietersz and McKenzie, 1992). Also, the efficacy of single agent chemotherapy is generally far less than can be achieved with modern multi-drug regimens, and hence this approach awaits the development of new drugs which are more active as single agents, or perhaps ultra-cytotoxic drugs which are currently too dangerous to administer in an unconjugated form; e.g. aminopterin, idarubicin derivatives and podophyllotoxin.

(d)   ADEPT

Problems associated with the direct delivery of chemotherapeutic agents linked to antibodies has led to the development of an indirect approach with the acronym of ADEPT; Antibody Directed Enzyme Prodrug Therapy (Bagshawe, 1989). This is a two-step approach: it involves the use of tumour selective mabs to deliver enzymes to antigens present on the surface of tumour cells. Once unbound conjugate has cleared sufficiently from blood and normal tissues, a non-toxic prodrug is administered which should only be converted to an active toxic drug by catalytic activity of the enzyme at the tumour site (Figure 4.3(c)). This strategy has many theoretical advantages (Table 4.4), but careful consideration must be paid to the choice of enzyme and drug. Enzymes of mammalian origin may be less immunogenic than bacterial enzymes, but their prodrug targets may also act as substrates for endogenous enzymes. Clinical trials are underway using anti-CEA F(ab')$_2$ linked to carboxypeptidase G2 followed by a mustard prodrug in colorectal cancer, and further refinements may need to be introduced as the data emerge. For example, it may be found that strategies are required to increase the clearance rate of the mab–enzyme conjugate to reduce the possibility of systemic toxicity and minimize the opportunity for generation of immune responses to the foreign proteins. It is likely that new generations of agents will combine target specificity plus catalytic function in a single molecule, either by the production of 'abzymes' – antibodies with intrinsic enzymic activity – (Green, 1989) or by the generation of recombinant molecules from genes spliced to encode antigen-binding mab regions and catalytic domains of enzymes.

Table 4.4 Features of antibody directed enzyme prodrug therapy (ADEPT)

Advantages:	*Disadvantages:*
Suitable for membrane-bound or secreted antigens	Dependent on high antigen density
Antigen-negative tumour cells may be killed by diffusible drug	Possibility of prodrug activation by endogenous enzymes
Alkylating agents generally used are: non-cycle specific; diffuse well in tissues; equally toxic to oxygenated and hypoxic cells; rarely induce multi-drug resistance	Conjugates may be highly immunogenic
	Tumours must be drug sensitive
	Conjugate loss from blood may be too slow and may require 'clearing' agent

Examples of prodrugs activatable by enzymes:

Prodrug	*Enzyme*
5-Fluorocytosine	Cytosine deaminase
Etoposide phosphate Mitomycin phosphate Phenol mustard phosphate	Alkaline phosphatase
Mono-chloro mono-mesyl benzoic acid mustard	Carboxypeptidase G2
Doxorubicin phenoxyacetamide	Penicillin amidase
Cephalosporin doxorubicin Cephalosporin mustard	β-Lactamase

4.6   CELLULAR EFFECTORS AND MOLECULAR MESSENGERS IN CANCER THERAPY

The specificity and strength of the immune system is amply demonstrated by the phenomenon of tissue transplant rejection, and its potential in cancer treatment by the anecdotal responses of small numbers of patients in pioneering immunotherapeutic trials with LAK or TIL cells and/or cytokines. Preliminary studies have suffered from the lack of defined antigens, toxicity of systematically administered therapy, and the inability to accurately identify determinants of response (Lotze and Finn, 1990). The challenge of the next decade is to harness and direct the undoubted power of these reactions towards more feasible and rational therapies against the common cancers, and in particular the problem of disseminated disease.

Definitive evidence that potential tumour rejection antigens exist on the majority of human cancers is now emerging (Boon, 1993), and the means of stimulating T-cell responses to them is becoming available. Recognition of these antigenic determinants is now known to be regulated by HLA haplotypes; i.e. T-cell receptors will only respond to certain peptides presented in association with particular MHC class I antigens. Thus candidates for immunotheraphy or vaccination must be 'typed' for both tumour antigen expression and HLA subtype in order to ensure their responsiveness. Cytokines are by their nature designed to be short-range, rapidly acting cellular messengers, hence it is not surprising that systemic infusion of high doses is associated with toxic side-effects. The future use of these molecules as amplifiers of an anti-tumour immune response will depend upon finding the means to target either the gene or protein to sites of metastasis, or their incorporation into vaccines (Patel and Collins, 1992). In general terms, the use of vaccines as active specific therapy is likely to be more effective than 'passive' infusion of cells or cytokines; the immunity produced has the potential to be long lasting rather than transient, should be relatively non-toxic and may ultimately be used as prophylactic treatment in groups at high risk of developing primary or secondary cancers (Bystryn, 1990).

4.7   SUMMARY

We are at an early stage in the development of monoclonal antibodies as therapeutic agents, yet they have already proved their worth in diagnostic and prognostic applications, and the new generations of engineered molecules show great promise in a wide variety of novel approaches. New and better defined categories of human tumour antigens have been described, and the mechanisms of induction of cellular and humoral responses (and reasons for their failure) are rapidly being elucidated. The availability of cloned genes and recombinant products is allowing a better analysis of the potential interactions of various cytokines, and hence their more effective deployment *in vivo*. Although many formidable problems remain in the development of safe and effective immunotherapies for cancer, there is now a rational basis on which to build future experimental and clinical work, and every reason for optimism.

REFERENCES

Adair, J.R. (1992) Engineering antibodies for therapy. *Immunological Reviews*, **130**, 5–40.

Allan, S.M., Dean, C.J., Fernando, I. *et al.* (1993) Radiolocalisation in breast cancer using the gene product of the c-erbB-2 as the target antigen. *British Journal of Cancer*, **67**, 706–12.

Bagshawe, K.D. (1989) Towards generating cytotoxic agents at cancer sites. *British Journal of Cancer*, **60**, 275–81.

Bakir, M.A., Eccles, S.A., Babich, J.W. *et al.* (1992) C-erbB-2 protein overexpression in breast cancer as a target for P.E.T. using ^{124}I labelled monoclonal antibodies. *Journal of Nuclear Medicine*, **33**, 2154–2160.

Ball, E.D., Mills, L.E., Cornwell, G.G. *et al.* (1990) Autologous bone marrow transplantation for acute myeloid leukaemia using monoclonal antibody purged bone marrow. *Blood*, **75**, 1199–206.

Bicknell, R. and Harris, A.L. (1991) Novel growth regulatory factors and tumour angiogenesis. *European Journal of Cancer*, **27**, 781–5.

Bolhuis, L.H., Sturm, E. and Braakman, E. (1991) T cell targeting in cancer therapy. *Cancer Immunology and Immunotherapy*, **34**, 1–8.

Boon, T. (1993) Teaching the immune system to fight cancer. *Scientific American*, **266**, 32–9.

Bystryn, J-C. (1990) Tumor vaccines. *Cancer and Metastasis Reviews*, **9**, 81–91.

Clark, M.R., Gilliland, L. and Waldman, H. (1988) Hybrid antibodies for therapy. *Progress in Allergy*, **45**, 31–49.

Dyer, M.J.S. (1992) Antibody therapy of malignancy. *European Journal of Cancer*, **28**, 276–80.

Epstein, A.L., Chen, F.M., Ansari, A. *et al.* (1991) Radioimmunodetection of necrotic lesions in human tumours using I-131 labelled TNT-1 F(ab')$_2$ monoclonal antibody. *Antibody Immunoconjugates Radiopharmaceuticals*, **4**, 151–61.

Fanger, M.W., Segal, D.M. and Romet-Lemonne, J-L. (1991) Bispecific antibodies and targeted cellular cytoxicity. *Immunology Today*, **12**, 51–4.

Green, B.S. (1989) Monoclonal antibodies as catalysts and templates for organic chemical reactions. *Advances in Biotechnological Processes*, **11**, 359–93.

Gusterson, B.A. (1992) Identification and interpretation of epidermal growth factor and c-erbB-2 over-expression. *European Journal of Cancer*, **28**, 263–7.

Harris, A.L., Nicholson, S., Sainsbury, R. *et al.* (1992) Epidermal growth factor receptor and other oncogenes as prognostic markers. *Journal of the National Cancer Institute Monograph*, **11**, 181–7.

Herberman, R.B. and Mercer, D.W. (eds) (1990) *Immunodiagnosis of Cancer*, Marcel Dekker, New York.

Humphrey, P.A., Wong, A.J., Vogelstein, B. *et al.* (1990) Anti-synthetic peptide antibody reacting at the fusion junction of deletion mutant epidermal growth factor receptors in human glioblastoma. *Proceedings of the National Academy of Sciences USA*, **87**, 4207–11.

Juliano, R.L. (ed.) (1991) *Targeted Drug Delivery*, Handbook of Experimental Pharmacology, Springer-Verlag, Berlin.

Leitzel, K., Teramoto, Y., Sampson, E. *et al.* (1992) Elevated soluble c-erbB-2 antigen levels in the serum and effusions of a proportion of breast cancer patients. *Journal of Clinical Oncology*, **10**, 1436–43.

Lemoine, N. and Epenetos, A. (eds) (1993) *Mutant Oncogenes: Targets for Therapy*, Chapman & Hall Medical, London.

Lotze, M. and Finn, O. (eds) (1990) Cellular immunity and the immunotherapy of cancer, *UCLA Symposia on Molecular and Cellular Biology*, New Series, vol. 135 Wiley-Liss, NewYork.

Maraveyas, A. and Epenetos, A.A. (1991) An overview of radioimmunotherapy. *Cancer Immunology and Immunotherapy*, **34**, 71–3.

Martin, E.W., Mojzisik, C.M., Hinkle, G.H. *et al.* (1988) Radioimmunoguided surgery using monoclonal antibody. *American Journal of Surgery*, **156**, 386–92.

McMichael, A.J. Bodmer, W.F. (eds) (1992) A new look at tumour immunology, *Cancer Surveys*, vol. 13, Cold Spring Harbor Laboratory Press.

Modjtahedi, H., Eccles, S.A., Box, G. *et al.* (1993) Immunotherapy of human tumour xenografts overexpressing the EGF receptor with rat antibodies that block growth factor-receptor interaction. *British Journal of Cancer*, **67**, 254–61.

Patel, P. and Collins, M.K.L. (1992) Cytokine modulation of cell growth and role in tumour therapy. *European Journal of Cancer*, **28**, 298–302.

Pietersz, G.A. and McKenzie, I.F.C. (1992) Antibody conjugates for the treatment of cancer. *Immunological Reviews*, **129**, 57–80.

Plowman, G.D., Culouscou, J-M., Whitney, G.S. *et al.* (1993) Ligand-specific activation of HER4/p180 erbB4, a fourth member of the epidermal growth factor receptor family. *Proceedings of the National Academy of Sciences USA*, **90**, 1746–50.

Portoukalian, J., Carrel, S., Dore, J-F. *et al.* (1991) Humoral immune response in disease-free advanced melanoma patients after vaccination with melanoma-associated gangliosides. *International Journal of Cancer*, **49**, 893–9.

Reber, S., Matzku, S., Gunthert, U, *et al.* (1990) Retardation of metastatic growth after immunisation with metastasis-specific monoclonal antibodies. *International Journal of Cancer*, **46**, 919–27.

Riethmüller, G., Schneider-Gädicke, E., Schlimak, G. *et al.* and The German Cancer Aid 17–1A Study Group (1994) Randomised trial of monoclonal antibody for adjuvant therapy of resected Dukes' C colorectal carcinoma. *Lancet*, **343**, 1177–83.

Stötter, H. and Lotze, M.T. (1990) Cytolytic effector cells against human tumors: distinguishing phenotype and function. *Cancer Cells*, **2**, 44– 55.

Tilby, M.J., Newell, D.R., Viner, C. *et al.* (1993) Application of a sensitive immunoassay to the study of DNA adducts formed in peripheral blood mononuclear cells of patients undergoing high-dose melphalan therapy. *European Journal of Cancer*, **29A**, 681–6.

Van der Bruggen, P., Traversari, C., Chomez, P. *et al.* (1991) A gene encoding an antigen recognised by cytolytic T-lymphocytes on a human melanoma. *Science*, **254**, 1643–7.

Wawrzynczak, E.J. (1991) Systemic immunotoxin therapy of cancer: advances and prospects. *British Journal of Cancer*, **64**, 624–30.

Wels, W., Harwerth, I-M., Mueller, M. *et al.* (1992) Selective inhibition of tumour cell growth by a recombinant single chain antibody-toxin specific for the c-erb B-2 receptor. *Cancer Research*, **52**, 6310–17.

Winter, G. and Milstein, C. (1991) Man-made antibodies. *Nature*, **349**, 293–9.

HISTOPATHOLOGY AND THE CLINICAL ONCOLOGIST

Richard L. Carter

This chapter considers two topics: the scope of histopathology in clinical oncology, and its general mode of operation. Specific issues in diagnostic histopathology are not discussed.

5.1 THE SCOPE OF HISTOPATHOLOGY IN CLINICAL ONCOLOGY

Histopathology impinges on many aspects of clinical oncology, ranging from the initial diagnosis of malignancy through to appraisal of end-stage disease. A tissue diagnosis based on morphology – histopathology and/or cytology – is an absolute requirement which can be waived in only exceptional circumstances. A small, deeply seated tumour may, for example, be deemed inaccessible for safe biopsy and the oncologist's diagnosis of neoplasm will rest on other categories of evidence.

5.1.1 STANDARD HISTOPATHOLOGICAL DIAGNOSIS

A standard histopathological diagnosis includes basic morphological features such as the degree of differentiation which form the basis for grading schemes. Large resections provide additional data on the extent of local spread, lymphovascular invasion, and the presence of metastases in regional lymph nodes, while examination of separate biopsies may reveal distant metastases. Much of this information is incorporated into staging schemes. The grading and staging of malig-

nant tumours should be regarded as two generally separate but complementary processes.

(a) Tumour grading

Grading of tumours is based on their histopathological appearances. Most malignant tumours showing any signs of morphological differentiation are characterized in purely descriptive terms by the histopathologist as well, moderately or poorly differentiated, according to a combination of architectural and cytological features. The former might include evidence of glandular or tubular organization, the formation of extracellular keratin masses or the production of osteoid or chondroid matrix. Cytological features include cellular and nuclear pleomorphism, the presence of binucleate or multinucleate elements, and the numbers and characteristics of mitotic figures. The degree of morphological differentiation provides for most (but not all) tumours a rough prognostic guide, particularly for likely future recurrence and/or dissemination. It is, therefore, important that the various descriptive criteria should be standardized as far as possible. Formal grading systems have been devised for several tumour types, such as those in current use for carcinomas of the breast, bladder and prostate and for chondrosarcomas (Figure 5.1). Precise description and delineation of tumour subtypes without grading can, however, provide important prognostic information. Examples include the well differentiated, myxoid, round cell and pleomorphic

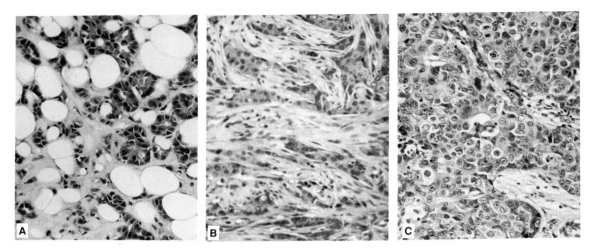

Figure 5.1   Grading of malignant tumours, exemplified by ductal carcinomas of the breast. The scheme devised by Bloom and Richardson uses three distinguishing criteria, based on architectural and cytological features – tubule formation, cellular and nuclear pleomorphism and mitotic figures. The three grades are illustrated: (**a**) Grade 1; (**b**) Grade 2; (**c**) Grade 3.((**a**)–(**c**) haematoxylin and eosin, × 210.)

forms of liposarcoma; sclerosing and non-sclerosing variants of Hodgkin's disease together with the separate categories of lymphocyte predominant, mixed cellularity and lymphocyte depleted; and the numerous forms of non-Hodgkin's lymphoma segregated according to growth pattern (follicular or diffuse) and predominant cell type (small, mixed, large); astrocytomas subdivided into categories of astrocytoma (NOS), anaplastic astrocytoma and glioblastoma multiforme; and the 'favourable' and 'unfavourable' histological forms of Wilms' tumour.

(b)   Tumour staging

Staging of tumours, by contrast, combines all available data – clinical, pathological, radiological – to give an overall categorization of the extent of malignant disease. Various staging schemes are in use such as those promulgated by UICC, AJCC and FIGO. Certain tumour types – Hodgkin's disease, the non-Hodgkin's lymphomas, most paediatric neoplasms – have their own staging systems. There are several tumours where the

histopathologist can provide direct information for staging as well as grading. The best known example is the Dukes' staging scheme (Dukes' A, B and C) for colorectal carcinomas which was devised in 1940, but similar pathological staging is also used for reporting major resections of tumours at sites such as the stomach, bladder and uterus. Cutaneous melanoma exemplifies the interesting situation where staging information is obtained from the initial excision biopsy by measuring tumour thickness (Breslow) and the level of invasion (Clark) down into the papillary dermis, reticular dermis or subcutaneous fat.

5.1.2   HISTOLOGICAL FEATURES

Rare tumour entities identified by the histopathologist may occasionally point to probable aetiological factors – clear cell adenocarcinomas of the vagina or cervix in young women exposed in utero in high doses of stilboestrol, adenocarcinomas of the paranasal sinuses in wood-workers, and mesotheliomas in individuals occupationally exposed to asbestos – but aetiological factors for the common tumours are difficult to infer with certainty in an individual patient. Lung cancer in cigarette smokers, for example, may be of any histological type, although squamous and small cell anaplastic carcinomas predominate in most series. Equally, histopathology provides no specific guidance for the initial choice of therapy although the effects of previous treatment can be assessed morphologically when residual tumour is excised after cytotoxic drugs and/or irradiation. Examples include treated osteosarcomas, Ewing's sarcomas, round cell tumours in children such as neuroblastoma and rhabdomyosarcoma, teratomas and various carcinomas (Molenaar *et al.*, 1984; Picci *et al.*, 1985) (Figure 5.2). Necrosis, haemorrhage and inflammation may be found in responsive tumours with little or no evidence of intact neoplastic cells despite examination of many tissue blocks. Residual tumour in teratomas and other embryonal malignancies sometimes show striking differentiation when compared with their pretreatment biopsies. Whether such maturation is brought about directly by therapy, or whether treatment has eliminated sensitive undifferentiated elements, remains unclear.

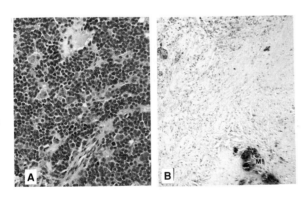

Figure 5.2 The effects of treatment on tumours. (**a**) Diagnostic (pretreatment) biopsy of an adrenal neuroblastoma. (**b**) Residual adrenal mass excised after chemotherapy. No intact tumour was identified in 18 blocks. M = microcalcification. ((**a**), (**b**) haematoxylin and eosin, × 210.)

The histopathologist will also corroborate the development of subsequent recurrent tumour on occasions where morphological confirmation is necessary, usually because results from other investigations such as cytology or radiological imaging are ambiguous. Tumour may return many years after the initial diagnosis – notably carcinomas of the breast and kidney, and melanoma – but late recurrences need to be distinguished from the second primary tumours which arise in various clinical contexts. Multiple or multifocal carcinomas, simultaneous or sequential, are familiar in the urothelium, mucosal surfaces of the head and neck, breast and skin. Second, separate primary tumours are increasingly recognized in patients previously treated with intensive chemotherapy and radiotherapy for their original cancers. Acute (usually non-lymphocytic) leukaemias and non-Hodgkin's lymphomas predominate among these second, treatment-related neoplasms, together with skeletal or soft tissue sarcomas developing in or near previous irradiation fields. Smaller increases in certain squamous and adenocarcinomas are recorded in some series. Two or more additional primary tumours may develop as part of the natural history of the original neoplasm, examples being the malignancies that may develop in children with the genetic form of retinoblastoma and the multiple malignancies encountered in families with the Li–Fraumeni syndrome.

5.1.3 HISTOPATHOLOGY IN AUTOPSIES

Histopathology plays an important part in autopsies performed on patients who have died from cancer, an investigation which clinical oncologists persistently undervalue. Dissection and microscopy will demonstrate the extent of residual tumour which, in certain circumstances, can provide clues for treatment failure (Carter, 1987). Such information can also be used to monitor conclusions based on investigations carried out in life such as

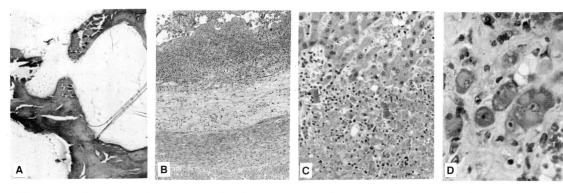

Figure 5.3 Examples of treatment-related tissue toxicity demonstrated at autopsy. (**a**) Complete aplasia of bone marrow. (**b**) Necrotizing enterocolitis. (**c**) Hepatic necrosis. (**d**) Cytomegalovirus pneumonia. ((**a**)–(**d**) haematoxylin and eosin. (**a**), (**b**), × 60; (**c**) × 210; (**d**) × 600.)

radiological imaging, ultrasonography and radionuclide scans. Infections, haemorrhage or organ failure, previously unsuspected or incompletely documented, may become obvious. Morphological abnormalities in the liver, kidneys, bowel, lungs, heart, brain and bone marrow can provide valuable insight into various forms of treatment-related toxicity (Figure 5.3). The recognition of such changes in patients who have received either new forms of treatment, or existing forms in new protocols, is particularly important.

5.1.4   APPLICATIONS OF HISTOPATHOLOGY

A final comment should be made on the applications of histopathology (often combined with cytology) in various prevention and screening programmes for detecting early cancer and its precursors at sites such as the cervix uteri, endometrium, large bowel, breast and skin. Biopsies are sometimes repeated over several years. The morphological changes of impending or actual early malignancy can be subtle, and close correlation of microscopy with endoscopic and/or radiological appearances is essential.

5.2   THE BASIS FOR HISTOPATHOLOGICAL DIAGNOSIS

5.2.1   BIOPSIES/DOCUMENTATION/FIXATION

The histopathologist's starting point is a piece of tissue, removed either as a small biopsy or as part of a larger surgical procedure, accurately documented and promptly submitted, fixed or unfixed according to local requirements.

(a)   Biopsies

Biopsies are conventionally separated into excisional and incisional categories. Material is removed by cold knife, cautery, needle or curettage, usually under direct vision or by endoscopy – which is now extremely versatile. Hitherto inaccessible tumours in the brain can be approached by stereotactic procedures, and the scope of needle biopsies has been widened by the development of biopsies guided by computed tomography or ultrasound. Correct sampling is crucial. Large masses need to be biopsied at several places. Ulcers should be sampled at the edges, but not too peripherally. Thick lesions must be biopsied at an appropriate depth. Degenerate or necrotic zones should be avoided. The most common reasons for a failed biopsy are faulty selection of small, degenerate or non-representative fragments of tissue, and distortion from avoidable artefacts due to the use of cautery, rough handling of tissues and inadequate or inappropriate fixation (see below). Surgical excisions, performed as elective rather than emergency procedures, are undertaken as planned operations in which a tissue diagnosis of cancer has already been established. The questions for the histopathologist are directed more to the extent of local spread, the involvement of draining lymph nodes and any distant organs that are sampled, and the establishment of tumour-free excision margins – a common indication for intraoperative frozen sections. All material, irrespective of size, should be submitted to the pathologist whole and intact: it should never be divided and distributed to different laboratories.

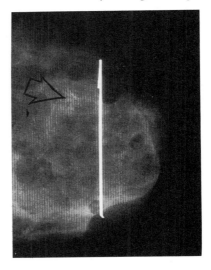

Figure 5.4 X-ray of localization biopsy of breast tissue. The arrow points to a zone of calcification close to the guidewire.

(b) Documentation

Although familiar, the necessary basic information which should accompany excised tissues bears repetition.

1. Specimens must be adequately identified with the patient's name, sex, age/date of birth and hospital number. An error may have catastrophic consequences. Anonymous specimens cannot be accepted for processing.
2. Accompanying request cards must provide adequate clinical details. Major coexisting diseases with health implications for laboratory staff such as infections by human immunodeficiency viruses, hepatitis B virus and *Mycobacterium tuberculosis* must always be specified.
3. References to previous biopsy reports should be quoted, together with relevant information from other laboratory or radiological investigations.

Histopathologists may initially examine their biopsy slides 'blind', but the data listed here must be available before a final report is formulated. It is axiomatic that radiology films are always examined before reporting bone biopsies. Mammograms should accompany all mammogram-directed breast biopsies unless the specimen itself is X-rayed in the laboratory (Figure 5.4).

Large resections must be clearly orientated by the surgical staff, particularly when no normal anatomical structures are included in the dissection. Simple diagrams are helpful. Small normal structures should be identified with sutures (not clips). Recognition of different nodal groups is sometimes difficult in an excised specimen and it is useful if the surgeons identify each group separately.

(c) Fixation

Tissues should be sent to the laboratory unfixed or fixed, according to anticipated diagnostic needs and local practice.

1. Fresh unfixed material has the advantage that samples can also be taken for special requirements such as microbial culture,

frozen sections, electron microscopy, short-term tissue culture, molecular biology and storage in tissue banks. It is, however, perishable, and must be submitted as soon as possible. A dried-out specimen is useless.

2. Large resections are usually fixed directly. Prompt fixation is essential for all material obtained from patients with high-risk infections (see above): no frozen sections or tissue storage can be undertaken. Buffered (10%) formol-saline is the most widely used fixative, the tissues being completely immersed in a large (×10) volume. Special fixatives may be required for the histopathologist's special needs.

5.2.2   LABORATORY PROCEDURES

A detailed account of laboratory methods in histopathology (Bancroft and Stevens, 1990) is not appropriate here, but the basic procedures can be summarized very briefly. The histopathologist examines the material macroscopically, a process which may involve a considerable amount of dissection. Surgical margins are marked with indian ink or similar material. Radiographs are sometimes required on the intact specimen. Tissues are selected for routine microscopy and, where necessary, for other investigations: frozen section immunohistochemistry, electron microscopy and molecular biology. Fresh material is fixed, embedded as tissue blocks, and sections are cut and stained. The standard histopathology processing schedules take 16–24 hours, but longer if tissues have to be decalcified or if the newer techniques of embedding in plastic (instead of paraffin wax) are used.

The final diagnostic material consists of tissue sections cut at 3–5 μm and stained initially with haematoxylin and eosin. Microscopic appearances may be straightforward but, in difficult cases, extensive investigations will be required. The histopathologist's conclusions can thus be forthcoming in a few minutes or may take several days depending on the complexity of the additional procedures and the skill and experience of the observer. Once a diagnosis is reached it is coded according to a standard scheme (usually SNOMED or SNOP) and a report is issued. Computerized systems are increasingly used to disseminate, store and recall histopathological data.

It is appropriate for the clinical oncologist to have at least a general idea of the different histopathological approaches that have been outlined.

(a)   Frozen sections

Frozen sections (Holaday and Assor, 1974; Dankwa and Davies, 1985) may be required in various circumstances. They are cut in a cryostat operating at –20°C to –30°C, and a routinely stained section can be produced within 6–10 minutes. The advantage of speed is offset by difficulties in preparation and interpretation: both architecture and cytology are distorted (Figure 5.5). The main application of frozen sections is to provide a rapid preliminary diagnosis of tumour in the course of a surgical procedure. Such diagnoses are often difficult and sometimes impossible, even for an experienced observer, and final opinions may have to await examination of the routinely processed sections which are always prepared in parallel. It may, however, be sufficient at the time merely to confirm that the material does indeed consist of intact tumour which is adequate for diagnostic purposes. Frozen sections give valuable intraoperative confirmation that resection margins are clear of tumour, provided that the specimen has been appropriately orientated by the surgeons.

In addition to immediate surgical needs, the histopathologist increasingly requires frozen sections for detailed investigation of biopsy material, notably for certain procedures in immunohistochemistry and molecular biology which cannot be carried out on routinely fixed tissues.

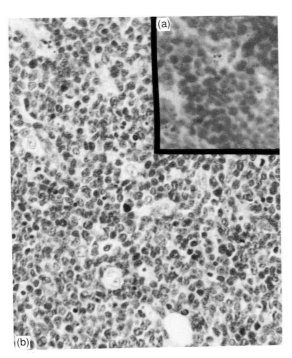

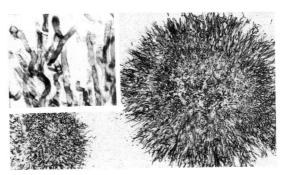

Figure 5.6 Special stains illustrated by fungal colonies demonstrated in lung tissue from a patient with acute monocytic leukaemia. The organism was subsequently identified as Trichosporon beigelii. (Methenamine silver (Grocott), × 220; insert, × 840.)

Figure 5.5 Anterior mediastinal mass: lymphoblastic lymphoma of T lineage. The insert (**a**) shows an intraoperative frozen section of the tumour for comparison with the definitive paraffin section, (**b**) (haematoxylin and eosin, × 380.)

(b) Special stains

The traditional 'special stains' still have a place in the diagnostic histopathology of tumours. They include methods to demonstrate glycogen, mucins, various forms of connective tissues, crystals, pigments (melanin, haemosiderin, bile), amyloid, neurosecretory granules and micro-organisms. Examples are shown in Figure 5.6.

(c) Immunohistochemistry

Diagnostic histopathology has been transformed in the last 10–15 years by the introduction of immunohistochemical techniques (Mason, 1992), many of which can be applied to routinely processed biopsy material. Immunohistochemistry can be thought of es-

sentially as in situ antigenic analysis: the practical details do not need to be discussed here, but the clinical oncologist should be aware of some of the problems, as well as the advantages, that may arise.

It is essential to use standard methods, well-characterized (preferably monoclonal) antibodies and rigorous controls. Limitations of individual antibodies with respect to specificity and sensitivity need to be recognized. Negative results are important. Reliance on staining with a single antibody is sometimes risky, and histopathologists prefer to use a panel of several different antibodies to demonstrate (for example) epithelial, myoid or neural differentiation. Caution is always indicated if an immunophenotype is at variance with other pathological and/or clinical findings: it may be prudent to repeat the tests. Some epitopes are damaged or destroyed by formalin fixation: individual subsets of T lymphocytes, for example, cannot at present be identified in routinely processed tissues and it may be necessary to perform some or all of the immunohistochemistry on cryostat sections. If frozen material is not available, the clinicians will have to consider repeating the biopsy to establish a definitive diagnosis.

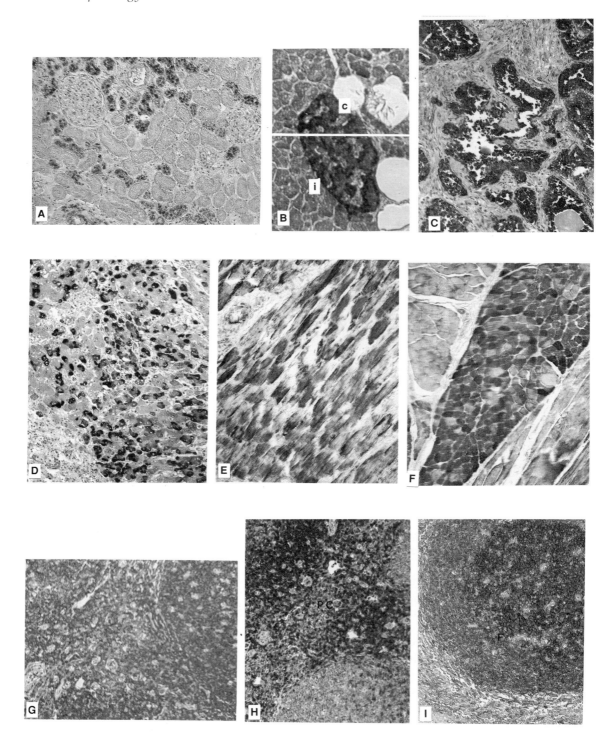

◀ **Figure 5.7** Immunohistochemistry. (**A**) Staining for epithelial membrane antigen (EMA) in the proximal convoluted tubules of the kidney. (**B**) Two pancreatic islets stained for chromogranin, an acidic glycoprotein located in the soluble fraction of neurosecretory granules (**c**), and for insulin (**i**). (**C**) Hyperplastic prostatic epithelium stained for prostate-specific antigen, PSA. (**D**) Liver parenchyma stained for Au antigen of hepatitis B. (**E**) Skeletal muscle stained for the intermediate filament desmin. (**F**) Skeletal muscle stained for fast myosin. Fibres containing slow myosin are not stained, resulting in a mixed 'chequer-board' effect. (**G**)–(**I**) Examples of lymphocyte markers in lymph nodes. (**G**) Uniform staining of all lymphoid populations with leucocyte common antigen, CD45. (**H**) Selective staining of T-lineage lymphocytes with CD3 in the paracortex (PC). The follicles are unstained. (**I**) Selective staining of B-lineage lymphocytes with CD20 in the follicles (F). The paracortex is unstained. ((**A**)–(**I**) × 130)

The practical applications of immunohisto-chemistry in diagnostic histopathology are very extensive. Immunohistochemical staining is illustrated in Figure 5.7, and some examples are listed below:

1. Distinction between undifferentiated carcinoma, amelanotic melanoma and lymphoma.
2. Characterization of spindle cell neoplasms: carcinoma, amelanotic melanoma, sarcoma.
3. Confirmation of gonadal and extragonadal germ cell tumours.
4. Analysis of undifferentiated round cell ('blue cell') tumours in children: identification of neuroblastoma, rhabdomyosarcoma, Ewing's sarcoma, primitive neuroectodermal tumour (PNET), non-Hodgkin lymphoma (especially at extranodal sites).
5. Identification/more precise characterization of endocrine and neuroendocrine neoplasms.
6. Distinction between neoplastic and non-plastic lymphoid proliferations.
7. Characterization of Hodgkin's disease and non-Hodgkin lymphoma.
8. Detection of micrometastases, particularly in lymph nodes and bone marrow.

(d) Electron microscopy

The diagnostic role of electron microscopy in tumour pathology (Ghadially, 1985) has de-clined with the emergence of immunohisto-chemistry. It is most appropriately used to clarify a differential diagnosis which has already been established in the light microscope. Appearances, for example, may point to two or three different entities, and the demonstration of particular ultrastructural features may solve the dilemma (Figure 5.8). Examples include the presence of melanosomes, premelanosomes or neurosecretory granules which, for various reasons, were not demonstrable by immunostaining. All three structures will survive routine processing to some extent and can be demonstrated after formalin fixation and even wax embedding. More exotic examples of diagnostically useful

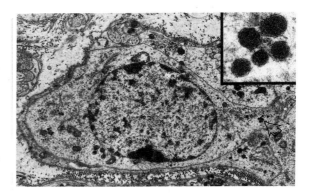

Figure 5.8 Electron micrograph of neuroblastoma cell. The arrow marks a cluster of neurosecretory granules which are shown at a higher magnification in the insert.

features in the electron microscope include Birbeck granules (Langerhans cell histiocytosis), crystals (alveolar soft part sarcoma), ribosomal–lamellar complexes (hairy cell leukaemia) and giant mitochondria (oncocytes).

(e) Molecular biology

The use of molecular biology as an adjunct to diagnostic histopathology is already becoming established, and it is likely that this area will develop rapidly in the next few years. The two outstanding advances are the development of *in situ* nucleic acid analysis and the polymerase chain reaction (Burns and McGee, 1992). In situ nucleic acid analysis involves the demonstration of mRNA or genomic DNA by forming an in situ hybrid between single-stranded, denatured, endogenous DNA or mRNA and an exogenous, complementary, single-stranded nucleic acid sequence or probe. The probe is labelled with a radioactive isotope, a fluorochrome or a chemical such as biotin, and the hybrid can be visualized by autoradiography, immunofluorescence or immunohistochemistry. Various types of test material can be used, and routinely processed surgical tissues are suitable for some applications such as the demonstration of microbial genomes. The prime examples are viruses (HPV, herpes simplex virus, EBV, CMV) but others include *Pneumocystis carinii*, *Legionella spp.* and *Mycobacteria. In situ* hybridization is increasingly used in cytogenetics to localize specific genes and their derangements in metaphase spreads, and chromosomal abnormalities such as translocations, amplifications and deletions can now be demonstrated in interphase nuclei: suitable methods are not yet generally available for interphase cytogenetics in routinely processed tissues.

The polymerase chain reaction (PCR) provides a simple method for amplifying many times a short sequence of DNA, defined by a pair of appropriate synthetic oligonucleotide primers. The technique can be automated and DNA simply extracted from a routinely processed tissue block. The method is already in use to demonstrate sequences from various viral genomes and to identify clonal gene rearrangements in non-Hodgkin lymphomas – affecting the Ig heavy chain gene in B lineage proliferations and the antigen receptor β- and γ-chain genes in T-cell proliferations.

5.2.3 GENERAL ASPECTS OF HISTOPATHOLOGICAL DIAGNOSIS

A final comment may be made on certain general aspects of histopathological diagnosis in clinical oncology (Rambo, 1962). The effective clinical histopathologist cannot operate in isolation, and access to all the relevant clinical information is essential. Problematical tissue diagnoses require close cooperation and discussion with the oncologists, and second opinions (Sissons, 1978) will be desirable in a proportion of cases. The clinicians may then have to accept a delay before a definitive diagnosis is reached, and the pathologist needs to be fully aware of the therapeutic implications. In practice, a provisional working diagnosis can often be made in such circumstances with the clear understanding that it may have to be revised. Equivocal biopsies may need to be repeated if clinical conditions permit. Histopathology is no more infallible than any other diagnostic procedure in clinical medicine. It is (unavoidably) subjective, descriptive, qualitative and dependent on the technical quality of the material examined. Interobserver variation is still wide for some entities, and histopathology in isolation has clear limitations. The recent advances in immunohistochemistry and now molecular biology indicate some of the directions for future development of the subject which will enhance its already central role in clinical oncology.

REFERENCES

Bancroft, J.D. and Stevens, A. (1990) *Theory and Practice of Histological Techniques*, 3rd edn, Churchill Livingstone, Edinburgh.

Burns, J. and McGee, J.O'D. (1992) Tissue nucleic acid analysis, in *Oxford Textbook of Pathology*, vol. 2b, (eds J.O'D. McGee, P.G. Isaacson and N.A. Wright), Oxford University Press, Oxford, pp. 2284–301.

Carter, R.L. (1987) The role of limited, symptom-directed autopsies in terminal malignant disease. *Palliative Medicine*, **1**, 31–6.

Dankwa, E.K. and Davies, J.D. (1985) Frozen section diagnosis: an audit. *Journal of Clinical Pathology*, **38**, 1235–40.

Ghadially, F.N. (1985) *Diagnostic Electron Microscopy of Tumours*, 2nd edn, Butterworths, London.

Holaday, W.J. and Assor, D. (1974) Ten thousand consecutive frozen sections. A retrospective study focusing on accuracy and quality control. *American Journal of Clinical Pathology*, **61**, 769–77.

Mason, D.Y. (1992) Immunocytochemical analysis of human tissues, in *Oxford Textbook of Pathology*, Vol. 2b, (eds J.O'D. McGee, P.G. Isaacson and N.A. Wright), Oxford University Press, Oxford, pp. 2275–84.

Molenaar, W.M., Oosterhuis, J.W. and Kamps, W.A. (1984) Cytologic 'differentiation' in childhood rhabdomyosarcomas following polychemotherapy. *Human Pathology*, **15**, 973–9.

Picci, P., Bacci, G., Campanacci, M., Gasparini, M., Pilotti, S. and 12 others (1985) Histological evaluation of necrosis in osteosarcoma induced by chemotherapy. Regional mapping of viable and nonviable tumor. *Cancer*, **56**, 1515–21.

Rambo, O.N. (1962) The limitations of histologic diagnosis. *Progress in Radiation Therapy*, **2**, 215–24.

Sissons, H.A. (1978) On seeking a second opinion. *Journal of Clinical Pathology*, **31**, 1121–24.

FURTHER READING

GENERAL TEXTS

MacSween, R.N.M. and Whaley K. (eds) (1992) *Muir's Textbook of Pathology*, 13th edn, Edward Arnold, London.

Rosai, J. (ed.) (1989) *Ackerman's Surgical Pathology*, Vols 1 and 2, 7th edn, C.V. Mosby, St Louis.

Sternberg, S.S. (ed.) (1989) *Diagnostic Surgical Pathology*, Vols 1 and 2, Raven Press, New York.

MORE SPECIALIZED TEXTS

Atlas of Tumor Pathology (Second and Third Series), Armed Forces Institute of Pathology, Washington DC.

Biopsy Pathology Series, Chapman & Hall Medical, London.

Dehner, L.P. (1987) *Pediatric Surgical Pathology*, C.V. Mosby, St Louis.

Fox, H. (ed.) (1987) *Haines & Taylor Obstetric and Gynaecological Pathology*, Vols 1 and 2, Churchill Livingstone, Edinburgh.

McKee, P.H. (1989) *Pathology of the Skin*, Gower Medical, London.

Morson, B.C., Dawson, I.M.P., Day, D.W. *et al.* (eds) (1990) *Morson & Dawson's Gastrointestinal Pathology*, 3rd edn, Blackwell Scientific Publications, Oxford.

Russell, D.S. and Rubinstein L.J. (eds) (1989) *Pathology of Tumours of the Nervous System*, Edward Arnold, London.

Stansfeld, A.G. and d'Ardenne, A.J. (eds) (1992) *Lymph Node Biopsy Interpretation*, 2nd edn, Churchill Livingstone, Edinburgh.

NEW IMAGING TECHNIQUES IN RADIOLOGY

6

Rosie Guy

Radiology has become of increasing importance in the management of patients with cancer. Radiological techniques are used not only in the initial diagnosis and staging of patients with cancer, but also in the planning of treatment and in monitoring response and evaluating possible relapse.

Basic techniques such as plain radiography and barium investigations still have an important role to play. However this chapter will focus on the role of more specialized radiological techniques in patient management.

6.1 MAMMOGRAPHY

Continuing improvements in equipment, together with the replacement of xeroradiography by film-screen techniques, have greatly improved the resolution of mammography and it is the technique of choice for imaging the breast. Mammography is used both in the assessment of the symptomatic patient and in screening for carcinoma of the breast.

A carcinoma appears as a mass which is usually spiculate with an ill-defined margin and may contain irregular microcalcification. There may be associated distortion of the breast architecture, skin tethering and nipple retraction. Ultrasound can be helpful in differentiating benign from malignant masses.

Impalpable mammographic abnormalities can be localized with a wire under mammographic or ultrasound guidance prior to excision by the surgeon (Evans and Cade, 1989). Following surgery and radiotherapy, serial mammography is a useful method of evaluating suspected local tumour recurrence (Stomper *et al.*, 1987).

One in 12 women will develop breast carcinoma. The national breast screening programme in the UK recommended by the Forrest report (1986) now offers 3-yearly mammography to all women aged between 50 and 64 years. The hope is that earlier detection of carcinomas will lead to a reduction in patient mortality, although this remains a controversial issue.

6.2 ULTRASOUND

The use of ultrasound in diagnostic imaging has progressed rapidly over the past 20 years since the development of the grey scale display which gave an image of the tissues for the first time. The next development was 'real-time' ultrasound which enabled dynamic rather than just static images to be obtained.

Ultrasound uses high frequency sound waves transmitted through a probe or transducer. These sound waves are reflected back from tissues in their path and this information is used to generate an image. Hence fluid in a simple cyst does not reflect any ultrasound waves and appears black, whereas soft tissues reflect the ultrasound beam and appear grey.

Many ultrasound scanners now incorporate colour Doppler ultrasound which further increases the potential to provide tissue characterization. Blood flow is superimposed as a colour-coded display on the real-time ultrasound image. The ability to identify abnormal tortuous blood vessels feeding a mass may help to confirm that it is malignant.

Ultrasound has particular advantages over other imaging techniques. In addition to being an excellent modality for investigating soft tissues, no ionizing radiation is involved, no sedation is needed to examine children and the equipment is portable and relatively inexpensive.

Ultrasound does however have certain limitations. The quality of the examination is dependent on the skill of the sonographer and images are less reproducible than with computed tomography (CT) or magnetic resonance imaging (MRI). In addition, the ultrasound beam is reflected back at interfaces with air and bone so it cannot be used to image gas-containing structures such as the lung or structures enclosed within bone such as the brain, except during the first year of life when the anterior fontanelle is patent or when a burr hole has been created surgically.

Ultrasound is widely used as a screening test for liver metastases. Most adenocarcinomas such as breast, bronchus and pancreas produce metastases which are hypoechoic and appear dark. A similar appearance is also seen in sarcoma metastases and in lymphoma. Metastases from carcinoid tumours and from vascular or mucinous carcinomas such as colorectal, stomach or bladder carcinoma are more likely to appear hyperechoic and bright. In addition, adrenal metastases and lymphadenopathy may be seen at the time of scanning.

Several studies have reported that contrast-enhanced CT has a slightly higher sensitivity for detection of liver metastases than trans-abdominal ultrasound (Alderson *et al.*, 1983). However intraoperative ultrasound of the liver is superior to any other available method of preoperative evaluation for the detection of liver metastases (Clouse, 1989). Intraoperative ultrasound may also be used to accurately define the segmental anatomy of the liver at the time of resection of liver metastases.

Ultrasound is being increasingly used as the primary investigation in patients with haematuria. It also has an important role as a problem-solving technique, for example in assessing whether a mass lesion identified on an intravenous urogram (IVU) is cystic or solid. Renal cell carcinoma may be effectively staged with ultrasound to evaluate the extent of local tumour, the presence of tumour in the renal vein and inferior vena cava (Schwerk *et al.*, 1985) and local retroperitoneal lymphadenopathy. Ultrasound is the first-line investigation for suspected hydronephrosis, for example in patients with carcinoma of the ovary or prostate.

The jaundiced patient should initially be evaluated with ultrasound to assess whether the jaundice is hepatic in origin or whether it is due to obstruction of the biliary tree. Carcinoma of the pancreas may be seen on ultrasound although overlying bowel gas may preclude optimal examination of the retroperitoneum.

The facility to scan in any plane gives ultrasound a definite advantage over CT for evaluating pelvic pathology. The patient can be scanned transabdominally with a full bladder or transvaginally. The close proximity of the ultrasound probe to the area being investigated enables detailed high resolution images to be obtained although there is a reduced field of view. Transvaginal scanning can be used to detect carcinoma of the endometrium and carcinoma of the cervix (Bourne *et al.*, 1990) and for screening for ovarian carcinoma.

Transrectal ultrasound is a valuable technique for staging peripheral carcinomas of the prostate, and in particular for detecting breach of the prostatic capsule (Hamper *et al.*, 1991). It is also helpful in detecting tumour recurrence following radiotherapy. Ultrasound has a low specificity if used as a screening test for carcinoma of the prostate, but evaluation of the vascularity of a lesion with colour Doppler ultrasound may help to assess whether it is malignant.

High frequency probes are used for scanning superficial structures such as the breast, thyroid and testes. Mammography and ultrasound are complimentary in the diagnosis of breast pathology. Breast carcinomas are frequently scirrhous and this fibrous tissue strongly reflects the ultrasound beam to give characteristic shadowing distal to the tumour (Ueno *et al.*, 1986). It may also be possible to identify abnormal tortuous feeding vessels to a breast carcinoma with colour Doppler ultrasound.

Ultrasound is the modality of choice for evaluating testicular masses. It is particularly helpful when a hydrocele is present and the underlying testis is impalpable or to diagnose a small impalpable tumour.

Endoscopic ultrasound has a high degree of accuracy in the assessment of the depth of invasion from oesophageal carcinoma and local lymphadenopathy (Shorvon, 1990). Local recurrence at the anastomotic site following surgery may also be detected. Endoscopic ultrasound may also be used to assess tumours of the stomach and rectum.

A number of interventional techniques can be carried out using ultrasound guidance, including tissue biopsies, drainage of fluid or abscesses and nephrostomy insertion. Ultrasound may also be used to position therapeutic agents such as ethanol or radioactive seeds within a tumour or to guide placement of a laser probe within the centre of liver metastases for photocoagulation treatment.

6.3 COMPUTED TOMOGRAPHY

The technique of computed tomography (CT) has advanced rapidly in the 20 years since the first scanner was developed. A narrow X-ray beam is used with an array of detectors mounted in a gantry surrounding the patient to produce an axial cross-sectional image. The scanning gantry may be angled by up to 25 degrees to make the scanning plane a little more versatile.

Gas-containing structures have a low attenuation or density and appear black, whereas bony structures have a high attenuation and appear white. Soft tissues have an intermediate attenuation and appear as varying shades of grey according to how the image is displayed. Iodine based contrast media are used routinely to opacify the bowel for scanning the abdomen and pelvis. Intravenous contrast media are used for brain scanning to show breaches in the blood barrier due to tumour and for body scanning to differentiate vessels from adjacent lymph nodes and to increase the detection rate for liver metastases.

Major technical developments have had relatively less impact on CT than on other imaging modalities in recent years. The most important innovation has been the production of less expensive scanners so that CT is now available in most district general hospitals. Ultrafast scanners have scan times of less than 100 milliseconds and are excellent for examining pulmonary and cardiac pathology. However they are expensive and such highly developed technology is not needed in a general oncology practice.

The major role of CT in oncology is in the staging of tumours and in assessing the response to treatment and possible disease relapse. CT is able to provide a far more comprehensive assessment of the chest, abdomen and pelvis than either ultrasound or MRI and gives good soft tissue definition. The main disadvantage of CT is the radiation dose – CT examinations are only 5% of all X-ray examinations requested but they contribute 20% of the total dose from all radiological examinations.

The advent of CT had a major impact on the diagnosis of tumours of the central nervous system (CNS) and it remains the most important investigation, although this is largely due to lack of availability of MR scanners. CT does have certain advantages over MRI in the CNS. It is more sensitive to the presence of calcification within a lesion and it is superior for showing bone destruction and reactive bone formation.

CT has a high sensitivity for the detection of intracranial masses (Baker *et al.*, 1980). The appearance of gliomas varies according to the tumour grade. Lower grade gliomas are more likely to exhibit calcification whereas higher grade gliomas are more likely to be associated with mass effect and show enhancement with intravenous contrast. Hydrocephalus and haemorrhage, seen as an area of high attenuation on an unenhanced scan, are readily identified. Artefact from bone causes image degradation in the posterior fossa and MRI should be used if possible for evaluating suspected posterior fossa lesions.

Contrast enhanced CT is an important screening investigation for cerebral metastases. CT myelography is used in conjunction with conventional myelography to evaluate cord compression, although MRI is the optimal technique for this.

The use of CT has significantly increased the accuracy of staging for tumours of the head and neck (Gatenby *et al.*, 1985). Local soft tissue spread, bony destruction at the skull base and associated lymphadenopathy are all well seen, particularly if contrast enhancement is used.

Plain chest radiography is still the most important method of diagnosing carcinoma of the bronchus and may be the only investigation necessary. However if surgery is being considered and more accurate staging is needed, CT is the imaging method of choice (Graves *et al.*, 1985). Collapsed lung enhances strongly, enabling the primary tumour to be distinguished from distal collapse. Extension into the mediastinum, chest wall involvement and regional lymphadenopathy are all readily evaluated (Figure 6.1).

Pulmonary metastases may be apparent on a chest radiograph but CT is a more sensitive technique for detecting lung metastases and assessing their response to treatment. It is particularly important to know the extent of pulmonary metastatic disease if surgical resection of the metastases is being considered.

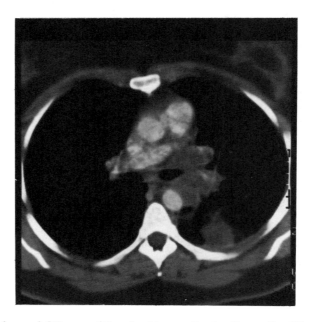

Figure 6.1   Contrast enhanced CT scan of the chest in a patient with small cell lung cancer. The tumour extends into the mediastinum and there is segmental collapse of the left lower lobe.

Abdominal CT scanning, performed during a dynamic injection of intravenous contrast, is the most comprehensive method of staging primary tumours of the liver and biliary tree, gastrointestinal tract, pancreas and kidney, although ultrasound is the most commonly used first-line investigation. The extent of local tumour, regional lymph node involvement and metastases to liver (Figure 6.2), spleen and adrenal glands are readily seen. Abdominal CT is also the best means of screening for abdominal spread of disease from other tumour sites such as breast and lung.

Although CT is widely used for staging primary tumours of the pelvis and for detecting pelvic spread of disease from other primary sites, MRI and ultrasound may be more helpful. CT is broadly equivalent to MRI for staging carcinoma of the bladder (Husband *et al.*, 1989), but carcinoma of the cervix and prostate are more accurately staged with MRI and endoluminal ultrasound.

CT has a particular role in the management of certain tumours. Careful CT surveillance of patients with testicular teratomas who have stage 1 disease at presentation enables early detection of small volume relapse so that these patients can then receive curative chemotherapy (Peckham *et al.*, 1982). CT is also important in the staging of lymphomas, where the precise stage of disease is pivotal in deciding the most appropriate form of treatment.

Although CT is widely used in the evaluation of bony and soft tissue tumours, more information is available from MR scanning. However CT still has an important role if surgery is being contemplated both to exclude lung metastases and to assist in calculating the appropriate size and shape of prosthetic implants.

CT can also be used for radiotherapy planning to accurately define the extent of tumour so that the treatment volume can be precisely defined (Hunter, 1990). Biopsy of both

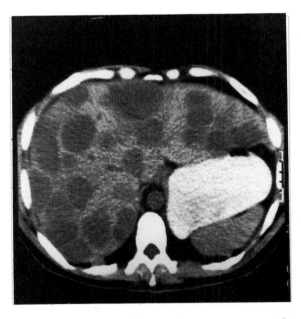

Figure 6.2 Unenhanced CT scan of the upper abdomen in a young man with testicular teratoma. There are multiple low attenuation metastases in the liver and a pulmonary metastasis at the base of the right lung.

primary tumours and recurrent masses where the histology is in doubt may be carried out under CT guidance. A CT-guided biopsy has the advantage of enabling the precise needle path to be visualized, although it is a rather slower technique than ultrasound-guided biopsy.

6.4 MAGNETIC RESONANCE IMAGING

Magnetic resonance imaging (MRI) has evolved as an important technique over the past 10 years. Its value in the management of patients with cancer is becoming widely recognized and it promises to play an increasingly important role as MR scanners become more widely available.

The MR signal, from which the image is created, is derived from radiofrequency energy released from hydrogen nuclei when they are submitted to a radiofrequency pulse within a magnetic field. The energy released can be measured as relaxation time. There are two types of relaxation, T1 and T2, which are based on the sensitivity of the hydrogen ions to their local environment. The relaxation times of different tissues depend on their water content – long for fluids and short for solids.

Tumours have a relatively high water content and therefore tend to have longer relaxation times than adjacent normal tissues. T1-weighted or T2-weighted images can be generated, which emphasize differences in T1 or T2 relaxation between tissues. On T1-weighted images tumours have a low signal and look darker than surrounding tissues. On T2-weighted images tumours have a higher signal and look brighter.

Newer sequences enable the signal from specific tissue components, for example fat, to be selectively suppressed. Intravenous contrast media, such as gadolinium DTPA, may also be used with T1-weighted images. Breaches of the blood–brain barrier and vascular tissues enhance, giving a high signal.

MRI has particular advantages over other imaging techniques. No ionizing radiation is used and images may be obtained in any plane, unlike the limited cross-sectional plane of CT. Soft tissue contrast is superior, although initial hopes that MRI would be tissue specific have not been fulfilled. MRI is not a sensitive technique for assessing bony destruction and calcification.

The main limitations of MRI have been the cost and limited availability. There are also a few contraindications to MR scanning, including pacemakers that might malfunction in the magnetic field, ferromagnetic clips on intracranial aneurysms, cochlear implants and the presence of metallic particles in the eye. Special equipment is needed if anaesthetics are used in MRI and some patients find the enclosed tunnel in the bore of the magnet in which they have to lie rather claustrophobic.

Although CT was a major advance in the evaluation of primary and secondary malignant disease of the central nervous system, MRI has definite advantages over CT. The posterior fossa is not degraded by artefact from bone on MR images and the facility to obtain images in the sagittal plane enables the relationship of tumours to the fourth ventricle to be readily demonstrated on MRI (Figure 6.3).

Infiltrating low grade gliomas are often difficult to identify on CT and the extent of tumour involvement is much easier to see with MRI. Enhanced T1-weighted scans are helpful in assessing tumour recurrence, although enhancement of granulation tissue following surgery may be misleading (Hesselink and Press, 1988). In addition it must be remembered that active tumour cells extend out into the oedema beyond the area of enhancement.

Enhanced MR images are the most sensitive technique for demonstrating intracranial metastases (Sze *et al.*, 1990). Demonstration of multiple metastases may be of particular importance if surgical resection or targeted

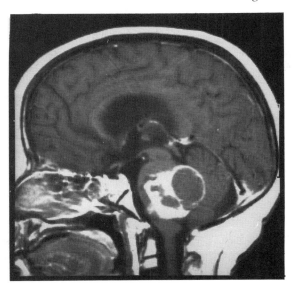

Figure 6.3 Midline sagittal enhanced T1-weighted MR scan of the brain in a child. There is an enhancing brain stem glioma compressing the fourth ventricle.

radiotherapy are being considered for an apparently solitary metastasis. Enhanced MRI is also a sensitive technique for detecting meningeal tumour involvement.

MRI has made it possible for the first time to directly image long segments of the spinal cord in the sagittal plane. The axial plane is helpful for assessing specific abnormalities and the coronal plane is used to evaluate paraspinal masses and suspected intraspinal extension, for example with neuroblastomas.

Infiltrating intramedullary gliomas of the cord are particularly difficult to evaluate with other modalities but are clearly seen with MRI, and an associated syrinx which may be amenable to surgical drainage can be demonstrated (Sze, 1992).

Where MRI is available it has replaced CT myelography as the technique of choice for patients with suspected cord compression (Williams *et al.*, 1989). The patient does not have to be moved, as in a myelogram, and there is no risk of the neurological deterio-ration which may occur following a lumbar puncture. Unsuspected multiple levels of cord compression may be demonstrated and these are of particular importance if surgical decompression is being considered.

Although radionuclide bone scanning is the best screening test for suspected bone marrow metastases, MRI is even more sensitive and is very helpful in equivocal cases (Jones *et al.*, 1990). MRI can also be valuable in monitoring treatment response and suspected relapse in patients with bone marrow malignancy such as leukaemias, although its precise role in this area has not yet been defined.

The multiplanar capability of MRI is particularly helpful for assessing the extent of head and neck malignancies and the presence of intracranial extension, although CT is superior for detecting bony destruction.

The plain radiograph still holds the key to the diagnosis of bone tumours, but MRI is the technique of choice for local tumour staging (Zimmer *et al.*, 1985). It is the best method

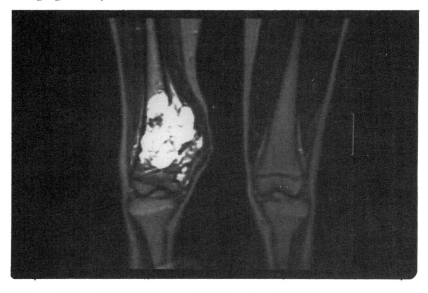

Figure 6.4   Coronal T2-weighted MR scan of the legs in a child. There is an osteosarcoma involving the lower right femur with an extensive high signal soft tissue mass.

for assessing the extent of bone marrow involvement, the associated soft tissue mass and the relationship of the tumour to the epiphyseal plate and adjacent joints (Figure 6.4). This knowledge is of particular importance with the advent of new chemotherapy regimens and limb salvage surgical techniques.

Conventional MR scans take several minutes and movement artefacts from respiration and peristalsis have been a major obstacle to the development of MRI of the abdomen. In addition a gastrointestinal contrast medium has only recently been available. New pulse sequences enable good quality scans to be obtained in a single breath hold and this will no doubt increase the use of MRI in the abdomen. Some studies suggest that enhanced MRI is more sensitive than either CT or ultrasound for assessing liver lesions (Nelson *et al.*, 1989). In addition the coronal plane helps to define the relationship of tumour to surrounding blood vessels, which is helpful in surgical planning.

Movement artefacts do not cause the same problems in the pelvis and MRI is already a well-established technique for the staging of pelvic malignancy. The internal anatomy of organs such as the prostate, cervix and uterus is well demonstrated on T2-weighted images and this has been further enhanced by the development of new surface coils and endorectal coils (Rifkin *et al.*, 1990). Pelvic lymphadenopathy is also well seen on MRI.

Accuracy rates of 80–90% can be obtained with MRI for the staging of carcinoma of the cervix and prostate. The benefits of MRI over CT for staging carcinoma of the bladder are less clear but some studies suggest that MRI more clearly demonstrates extravesical spread and possibly the depth of tumour invasion within the bladder wall.

MRI is an excellent technique for evaluating chest wall masses and intraspinal extension of thoracic tumours but intrapulmonary lesions such as metastases are poorly visualized and CT remains the best technique for identifying pulmonary metastases.

An important area of current research is MR spectroscopy. Some tissue characterization is possible and the technique is promising as a method of investigating drug pharmacokinetics and distribution *in vivo* and monitoring response of tissues to chemotherapy. However MR spectroscopy does not yet have a clinical role.

Recent developments in MRI include new fast pulse sequences that enable scans to be performed in seconds rather than minutes, greatly reducing movement artefacts. New endorectal coils and 'phased array' surface coils aligned in series greatly improve the resolution of MR images. The role of MRI in radiotherapy treatment planning is currently being evaluated.

6.5 NUCLEAR MEDICINE

Nuclear medicine techniques are used both in the imaging and treatment of oncology patients. Unlike CT and MRI, which give excellent displays of anatomical detail, radionuclide scans have a much lower resolution but are able to give valuable information about metabolic function.

A radionuclide image is obtained by measuring the emission of gamma rays from radiopharmaceuticals, which have usually been injected intravenously into the patient, using a gamma camera. Single photon emission computed tomography (SPECT) scanning involves a modified gamma camera which rotates around the patient. Sections can be reconstructed through the body in any plane, usually axial, increasing anatomical definition. Positron emission tomography (PET) is discussed in a subsequent chapter.

The most common radionuclide imaging test requested in oncology is the technetium-99m methylene diphosphonate bone scan as a screen for the presence of bony metastatic disease. It is cheap and sensitive and involves a significantly lower radiation dose than a plain radiographic skeletal survey. An area of increased uptake simply reflects increased osteoblastic activity and is not specific for malignancy – it may also be seen in inflammation or infection, fractures or degenerative disease (Roberts *et al.*, 1976). Metastases which are still visible on plain radiographs may be rendered bone scan negative following treatment.

In some conditions, such as myeloma, the plasma cells do not excite an osteoblastic response and a bone scan is usually negative even in the presence of widespread bone marrow disease. A radiographic skeletal survey is then a more appropriate method of detecting bone marrow deposits.

A number of other radionuclide scans are also used in oncology. CT and ultrasound are the most widely used techniques for detecting liver metastases but technetium-99m colloid scans of the liver may be helpful in some equivocal cases. The colloid is taken up by the normal Kupffer cells in the liver so metastases appear as focal areas of decreased uptake. The resolution of colloid scans cannot approach that of other imaging modalities and the specificity is low, for example cysts will also cause a focal defect. The use of SPECT increases the detection rate for deep liver metastases (Brendal *et al.*, 1984).

Renal scanning is mainly used in oncology to study renal function, for example when a nephrectomy is being considered. Lymphoscintigraphy with technetium-99m antimony sulphide can be used to evaluate possible nodal masses, but has largely been replaced by CT scanning supplemented by formal lymphography in equivocal cases.

Uptake of gallium-67 citrate is increased in a range of tumours, in particular lymphoma. By using increased amounts of radioactivity and SPECT it is possible to improve the accuracy of gallium scanning (Anderson *et al.*, 1983). Although it can be used in the staging of lymphoma, it is of more value in assessing whether there is still active disease present in a residual mass following treatment.

Both technetium-99m diethylene triamine pentacetate (DTPA) (planar and SPECT) and technetium-99m hexamethyl propylene amine oxime (HMPAO) scans show increased uptake in primary brain tumours and metastases. However CT and MRI are the first-line methods of evaluating such patients and radionuclide imaging would only be used if these techniques were not available.

The development of monoclonal antibody techniques has made imaging with radionuclide-labelled antibodies a real possibility although at present this remains a research tool. A range of primary malignancies and their metastases can currently be imaged using radioimmunoscintigraphy and these include melanoma, neuroblastoma and ovarian, colonic and thyroid carcinomas.

The noradrenaline analogue meta-iodobenzyl guanidine (MIBG) is taken up in tissues with an increase in neurosecretory granules (Chapter 2). Uptake is high in neuroblastoma and phaeochromocytoma and may also be seen in carcinoid tumours and medullary cell carcinoma of the thyroid. I-123 MIBG (a gamma emitter) is now routinely used in the staging of children with neuroblastoma. MIBG readily demonstrates metastases to liver, lung and bone marrow (Bomanji *et al.*, 1988) and it can be used to evaluate response to treatment and possible recurrence following treatment. In addition to its use in diagnostic imaging, the beta emitting isotope I-131 MIBG is used for targeted therapy of neuroblastoma metastases.

6.6   INTERVENTIONAL TECHNIQUES IN RADIOLOGY

Plain radiography, CT, ultrasound and more recently MRI can all be used to guide biopsy and drainage. Interventional radiological techniques can also be used in the treatment of patients with cancer. Selective hepatic artery cannulation has been used to selectively deliver chemotherapy in patients with hepatoma. Selective arterial embolization of hepatic lesions can also result in significant amelioration of patients' symptoms.

REFERENCES

Alderson, P.O., Adams, D.F., McNeil, B.J. *et al.* (1983) Computed tomography, ultrasound and scinitigraphy of the liver in patients with colon or breast carcinoma: a prospective study. *Radiology*, **149**, 225–30.

Anderson, K.C., Leonard, R.C.F., Cannelos, G.P. *et al.* (1983) High dose gallium scanning in lymphoma. *American Journal of Medicine*, **75**, 327–31.

Baker, H.L., Houser, O.W. and Campbell, J.K. (1980) National Cancer Instutite Study: evaluation of computed tomography in the diagnosis of intracranial neoplasms. *Radiology*, **136**, 91–6.

Bomanji, J., Conry, B.G., Britton, K.E. *et al.* (1988) Imaging neural crest tumours with I-123 meta-iodobenzyl guanidine and X-ray computed tomography: a comparative study. *Clinical Radiology*, **39**, 502–6.

Bourne, T.H., Campbell, S., Whitehead, M.I. *et al.* (1990) Detection of endometrial carcinoma in postmenopausal women by transvaginal sonography and colour flow imaging. *British Medical Journal*, **301**, 369.

Brendal, A.J., Leccia, F., Drouillard, J. *et al.* (1984) Single photon emission computed tomography (SPECT), planar scintigraphy, and transmission computed tomography: a comparison of accuracy in diagnosing focal hepatic disease. *Radiology*, **153**, 527–32.

Clouse, M.E. (1989) Current diagnostic imaging modalities of the liver. *Surgical Clinics of North America*, **69**, 193–234.

Evans, W.P. and Cade, S.H. (1989) Needle localisation and fine-needle aspiration biopsy of nonpalpable breast lesions with use of standard and stereotactic equipment. *Radiology*, **173**, 53–6.

Forrest, P. (1986) Breast cancer screening, Report to the Health Ministers of England, Wales, Scotland and Northern Ireland, HMSO, London.

Gatenby, R.A., Mulhern, C.B., Strawitz, J. *et al.* (1985) Comparison of clinical and computed tomographic staging of the head and neck tumours. *American Journal of Neuroradiology*, **6**, 399–401.

Graves, W.G., Martinez, M.J., Carter, P.L. *et al.* (1985) The value of computed tomography in staging bronchogenic carcinoma: a changing role for mediastinoscopy. *Annals of Thoracic Surgery*, **40**, 57–60.

Hamper, U.M., Sheth, S., Walsh, P.C. *et al.* (1991) Capsular transgression of prostatic carcinoma: evaluation with transrectal ultrasound with pathological correlation. *Radiology*, **178**, 791–5.

Hesselink, J.R. and Press, G.A. (1988) MR contrast enhancement of intracranial lesions with Gd-DTPA. *Radiologic Clinics of North America*, **26**, 873–87.

Hunter, R.D. (1990) Radiotherapy treatment planning, in *Radiology in the Management of Cancer*, (eds R.J. Johnson, B. Eddleston and R.D. Hunter), Churchill Livingstone, London, pp. 443–55.

Husband, J.E.S., Olliff, J.F.C., Williams, M.P. *et al.* (1989) Comparison of computed tomography and magnetic resonance imaging at 1.5 Tesla for staging bladder cancer. *Radiology*, **173**, 435–40.

Jones, A.L., Williams, M.P., Powles, T.J. *et al.* (1990) Magnetic resonance imaging in the detection of skeletal metastases in patients with breast cancer. *British Journal of Cancer*, **62**, 296–8.

Nelson, R.C., Chezmar, J.L., Sugarbaker, P.H. *et al.* (1989) Hepatic tumours: comparison of CT during arterial portography, delayed CT and MR imaging for pre-operative evaluation. *Radiology*, **172**, 27–34.

Peckham, M.J., Barrett, A., Husband, J.E. *et al.* (1982) Orchidectomy alone in testicular stage 1, non-seminomatous germ cell tumours, *Lancet*, *ii*, 678–80.

Rifkin, M.D., Dahnert, W., and Kurtz, A.B. (1990) State of the art: endorectal prostate ultrasound. *American Journal of Roentgenology*, **154**, 691–700.

Roberts, J.G., Bligh, A.S., Gravelle, I.H. *et al.* (1976) Evaluation of radiography and isotopic scintigraphy for detecting skeletal metastases in breast cancer. *Lancet*, **i**, 237–9.

Schwerk, W.B., Schwerk, W.N. and Rodeck, G. (1985) Venous renal tumour extension: a prospective US evaluation. *Radiology*, **156**, 491–5.

Shorvon, P.J. (1990) Endoscopic ultrasound in oesophageal cancer: the way forward? *Clinical Radiology*, **42**, 149–51.

Stomper, P.C., Recht, A., Berenberg, A.L. *et al.* (1987) Mammographic detection of recurrent cancer in the irradiated breast. *American Journal of Roentgenology*, **148**, 39–43.

Sze, G., Milano, E., Johnson, C. *et al.* (1990) Detection of brain metastases: comparison of contrast-enhanced MR and enhanced CT. *American Journal of Neuroradiology*, **11**, 789–91.

Sze, G. (1992) MR imaging of the spinal cord: current status and future trends. *American Journal of Roentgenology*, **159**, 149–59.

Ueno, E., Tohno, E., Hirano, Y. *et al.* (1986) Ultrasound diagnosis of breast cancer. *Journal of Medical Imaging*, **6**, 178–88.

Williams, M.P., Cherryman, G.R. and Husband, J.E. (1989) Magnetic resonance imaging in suspected metastatic cord compression. *Clinical Radiology*, **40**, 286–90.

Zimmer, W.D., Berquist, T.H., McLeod, R.A. *et al.* (1985) Bone tumours: magnetic resonance imaging versus computed tomography. *Radiology*, **155**, 709–18.

POSITRON EMISSION TOMOGRAPHY APPLICATIONS TO ONCOLOGY

Robert J. Ott

7.1 INTRODUCTION

One of the primary objectives of any medical imaging procedure is to provide accurate and, if possible, quantitative information to aid the diagnosis and treatment of disease. In oncology, X-ray CT, ultrasound and most recently MRI all provide high quality morphological information. Conventional radioisotope imaging (scintigraphy) whilst providing unique functional information is often limited by poor spatial resolution and sensitivity. The development of tissue malignancy can be detected in its early stages through biochemical processes and similarly the effects of treatment can be seen by changes in these processes. For the measurement of these changes to be used for diagnosis and treatment non-invasively, a high spatial resolution, quantitative, functional imaging technique is required. The only technique presently satisfying these criteria is positron emission tomography (PET).

7.2 POSITRON EMISSION TOMOGRAPHY

7.2.1 THE TECHNIQUE

PET is a technique for imaging the *in vivo* distribution of radioactively labelled pharmaceuticals. A large number of readily made radionuclides decay via the emission of a positron (a positive electron). The positron from a radioactive decay will travel a millimetre or so in tissue before coming to rest. At this point the positron will combine with a nearby atomic electron and annihilate. The mass destroyed in the annihilation is turned into two collinear gamma rays each with an energy of 511 keV (equal to the mass of the electron-positron pair). These annihilation gamma rays can be detected by surrounding the patient with the appropriate detectors (a positron camera). If both gamma rays are detected simultaneously (in time coincidence) the line joining the two detection points can be assumed to pass through the position of the radioactive decay. A large number of detected gamma ray pairs can, thus, be used to reconstruct, via CT techniques, the distribution of the radioactive tracer and hence the attached drug (Phelps *et al.*, 1986).

Certain physical effects combine to affect the quality of the images formed by PET. The use of short lived isotopes means that the tracer is decaying during imaging. At high count rates accidental coincidences can occur between gamma rays emitted from different radioactive decays. Also at high count rates the gamma ray detectors may suffer 'dead-time' losses if a second event arrives before the previous one has been processed. Finally gamma rays may be scattered or absorbed in tissue or the detectors themselves. The effects of radioactive decay, camera dead-time, accidental coincidences (sometimes known as random) must be corrected for to ensure that the images formed are quantitative. The corrected images can then be used to extract physiological parameters relating to the utilization of the tracer.

7.2.2 THE POSITRON CAMERA

There are two major types of positron camera. The most commonly used is based on surrounding the patient with large numbers (500–4000) of scintillating crystal/ photomultiplier combinations (Figure 7.1) (Phelps *et al.*, 1986). Figure 7.1 shows a typical configuration of a single section of a multiring positron camera with (a) a plan of a hexagonal array of detectors, (b) details of the scintillator/photomultiplier com-

binations and (c) a side view. These multicrystal cameras have high spatial resolution and detection sensitivity to 511 keV gamma rays but at a cost in excess of that of a gamma camera, ultrasound scanner, MRI unit or X-ray CT scanner. However, they provide images with more than 50 times the sensitivity of a gamma camera (used for scintigraphy) with better spatial resolution.

An alternative technology using large area multiwire cameras is under development (Marsden *et al.*, 1989). The advantages of such systems are their large axial field-of-view and lower cost. Present multiwire cameras suffer from low sensitivity, but new developments of these techniques (Wells *et al.*, 1992) should provide a competitive positron camera for the price of a top of the market gamma camera. PET will only be widely available for clinical use when the costs of the cameras are brought down to this level.

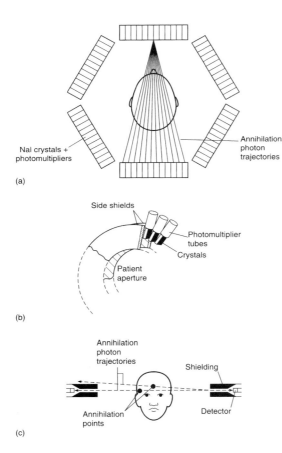

Figure 7.1. Schematic diagram of a multicrystal PET camera showing: (**a**) a single hexagonal ring of detectors; (**b**) details of the scintillator/photo-multiplier combinations; (**c**) a plan view of a single ring.

7.2.3   THE RADIOACTIVE TRACERS

PET has been established on the use of short lived radionuclides such as ^{11}C, ^{13}N, ^{15}O and ^{18}F as these can be readily labelled to a wide range of 'biologically interesting' pharmaceuticals. These tracers are easily made using a compact cyclotron, offer the possibility of studying the basic physiology of human cancer and allow laboratory and *in vitro* methods to be extended to patients non-invasively. The short half-life of these radionuclides limits their use to sites with an on-site cyclotron except for ^{18}F (Table 7.1).

Longer-lived nuclides (^{124}I, ^{66}Ga, ^{55}Co) can be produced by cyclotrons remote from the site of use. Others can be produced from bench-top radioisotope generators in which a long lived radionuclide is used to provide a supply of short lived decay products daily. Examples of useful positron emitting radio-

Table 7.1 Examples of radionuclides used in the applications of positron emission tomography to oncology and the percentage of radioactive decay via positron emission

Tracer	Half-life	Source	% Positron emission
Carbon-11	20 min	On-site cyclotron	99.8
Nitrogen-13	10 min	On-site cyclotron	100
Oxygen-15	2 min	On-site cyclotron	99.9
Fluorine-18	110 min	Remote cyclotron	96.9
Gallium-68	68 min	Ge/Ga generator	90
Copper-62	9.9 min	Zn/Cu generator	97.8
Rubidium-82	75 s	Sr/Rb generator	96
Iron-52	8 h	Remote cyclotron	56.5
Cobalt-55	18 h	Remote cyclotron	77
Gallium-66	9.5 h	Remote cyclotron	56.5
Bromine-75	1.6 h	Remote cyclotron	76
Strontium-83	33 h	Remote cyclotron	76
Yttrium-86	15 h	Remote cyclotron	66
Iodine-124	4.2 d	Remote cyclotron	25

nuclide generators are ^{68}Ge/^{68}Ga, ^{82}Sr/^{82}Rb and ^{62}Zn/^{62}Cu. This large number of radionuclides provide (Table 7.1) a useful range of labels for physiological probes for use at centres than cannot afford the on-site cyclotron. For many cancer studies, the longer lived tracers are proving to be as useful as the more conventionally used short lived variety because of the extended nature of the physiology of interest.

7.2.4 THE RADIOPHARMACEUTICALS

The obvious advantage of using the isotopes of carbon, nitrogen and oxygen is the ability to label agents specifically utilized by the bodies tissues. Examples of these are given in Table 7.2. Oxygen can be used either in its molecular gaseous form or as a label for carbon dioxide, carbon monoxide and water. These tracers allow the measurement of tissue perfusion, vascularity and oxygen utilization. Nitrogen can be incorporated into ammonia, amino acids and fatty acids and carbon into amino acids, glucose, pyrimidines, etc. Similarly fluorine can be used analogously to hydrogen as a label for deoxyglucose, amino acids, pyrimidines and receptor ligands. The

halogens, particularly iodine and bromine, can label proteins and pyrimidines whilst the radio-metals can be used as protein labels and with a range of ligands (Table 7.3). The broad range of available isotopes allows the possibility of labelling tracer quantities of anti-cancer drugs which could then be used in clinical studies to examine the drug pharmacokinetics in humans prior to treatment.

7.2.5 THE PHYSIOLOGICAL MEASUREMENTS

PET images can provide information relating to the use of a radiopharmaceutical by the body tissues. These range from agents which localize in particular organs or tissues to those which enable cellular processes to be measured, by labelling DNA/RNA for instance. Extraction of physiological parameters from PET images requires 'calibration' of images so that the data represent quantitative measurements for tracer uptake. It is then possible to apply mathematical models (Phelps *et al.*, 1986) based on laboratory studies with the tracer to clinical images to extract values for regional measurements of, for example, perfusion, glucose metabolism, etc. Absolute quantification of images may

Table 7.2   Examples of radiopharmaceuticals labelled with short lived positron emitting tracers

Tracer	Radiopharmaceutical	Application in tumour studies
Carbon-11	Carbon monoxide	Blood volume
	Methionione	Amino acid transport and metabolism
	Thymidine	Proliferation and metabolism
	Methylspiperone	Receptor localization
	Raclopride	Receptor localization
Nitrogen-13	Ammonia	Perfusion
	Glutamate	Metabolism
Oxygen-15	Water	Perfusion
	Carbon dioxide	Perfusion
	Carbon monoxide	Blood volume
Fluorine-18	Deoxyglucose	Glucose metabolism
	Tyrosine	Amino acid transport and metabolism
	Uracil	Drug uptake and metabolism
	Deoxyuridine	Proliferation and metabolism
	Oestradiol	Receptor localization
	Fluoride	Skeletal imaging

Table 7.3   Examples of radiopharmaceuticals labelled with medium half-life and generator produced positron emitting tracers

Tracer	Radiopharmaceutical	Application in tumour studies
Gallium-68	Red blood cells	Blood volume
	EDTA	Tissue permeability
	Colloid	Hepatic tumour localization
Copper-62	PTSM	Perfusion
Rubidium-82	Chloride	Perfusion
Iron-52	Citrate	Bone marrow imaging
Cobalt-55	Bleomycin	Drug uptake and tumour localization
	Monoclonal antibody	Tumour localization
Gallium-66	Citrate	Tumour localization
	Monoclonal antibody	Tumour localization
Bromine-75	Deoxyuridine	Proliferation and metabolism
Strontium-83	Chloride	Skeletal tumour function
Yttrium-86	Monoclonal antibody	Tumour localization and dosimetry
Iodine-124	Sodium iodide	Thyroid cancer localization and dosimetry
	Deoxyuridine	Proliferation and metabolism
	Iodotamoxifen	Drug uptake and metabolism
	Methyltyrosine	Amino acid transport and metabolism
	Monoclonal antibody	Tumour localization and dosimetry
	Metaiodobenzylguanadine	Neural crest tumour uptake/dosimetry

PTSM, is pyruvaldehide bis (*N*-methylthiosemicarbazone); EDTA, is ethylene diamine tetra-acetic acid.

require arterial blood sampling so that values of perfusion and metabolism can be obtained in absolute units (e.g. ml/min, ml/mg/min).

Semiquantitative measurements of tissue function can be obtained by determining standard uptake values (SUVs), for instance, which is the ratio of the uptake per unit mass of target tissue to the injected tracer dose per unit patient mass.

Measurement of glucose metabolism has been the most extensively used PET study in cancer because the majority of tumours show hypermetabolism of glucose in comparison to normal or benign tissues. Amino acid metabolism (Mazoyer *et al.*, 1993), especially using methionine or tyrosine, has been shown in the laboratory to be related to protein synthesis and thus presents a potential method for measuring synthesis rates in human tumours. Similarly DNA/RNA precursors such as thymidine or the deoxyuridines may provide tools for determining the cellular proliferation rate of tissues, possibly the most sensitive measure of tumour viability and function. Studies using amino acids and proliferation markers are increasing in number in attempts to extract useful biological parameters from the PET images obtained.

Other measurements of specific interest in oncology are related to hypoxia and receptor/antigen density. Isotopes of fluorine or bromine can be attached to radiosensitizers like misonidazole or its derivatives and may allow the measurement of hypoxic cell fraction in human tumours. Studies using halogen isotopes are underway to determine receptor density in tissues (breast for example) and there have been several recent applications of PET to monoclonal antibody imaging.

Future applications include the labelling of anticancer drugs. The important factors here are the incorporation of the radiolabel into the drug without modifying the drug action and identification of the metabolic processes involved in drug action. Good examples of this are ^{18}F in fluorouracil and ^{124}I in the tamoxifen derivatives. Studies with trace quantities of these agents will allow 'drug dosimetry' to be performed in tumour and non-target tissues and provide invaluable information on the efficacy of the drugs.

The sensitivity of PET allows nmol and pmol levels of tracers to be used, minimizing the chance of affecting the system being examined. PET is therefore almost unique in determining quantitatively from images the non-perturbed function of body processes not available from morphological techniques.

7.3 CLINICAL APPLICATIONS

Until recently PET studies have been carried out predominantly in patients with neurological and cardiological disorders (Phelps *et al.*, 1986). However the high spatial resolution (~5 mm) and sensitivity to a range of unique physiological agents is ideally suited to applications in oncology where quantitative measurements of biochemical processes are of clinical value in the management of patients.

PET has been used to measure physiological processes in a wide range of cancers, some with obvious clinical application others to increase the understanding of basic human tumour physiology. Some examples of PET applications to different tumour types are given below.

7.3.1 CEREBRAL TUMOURS

PET studies of cerebral tumours have been by far the greatest in number because of the limited axial field-of-view of most PET cameras (typically 10 cm). The majority of studies have been performed using fluorodeoxyglucose (FDG) to evaluate its application as a measure of tumour status and response to treatment. A smaller number of studies have measured tumour perfusion, oxygen metabolism, amino acid metabolism, blood– brain barrier permeability and the role of receptor ligands in pituitary adenomas. A recent review of the clinical applications of PET in brain tumours is given by Coleman *et al.* (1991).

FDG metabolism has been used to assess the degree of malignancy because of the difference in glucose metabolism between different tumour grades. Results indicate a high degree of correlation between FDG uptake in primary cerebral tumours and tumour grade. Further studies show that measurement of FDG uptake can be used as a prognostic marker, particularly survival time, as well as or better than histological grading. It has also been shown that malignant degeneration in low grade tumours can be detected via a switch from hypo- to hypermetabolism of FDG.

FDG has also been used to monitor the effects of brain tumour treatment. In the early postoperative period where MRI and CT are inaccurate FDG does not accumulate in surgical sites and raised FDG uptake is indicative of persistent tumour. Patients treated with radiotherapy and/or chemotherapy have been evaluated for response using FDG, and it was concluded that glucose metabolism was a good indicator of therapeutic effectiveness. Also, following radiotherapy or chemotherapy, FDG scanning has been shown to differentiate between recurrent glioma and necrosis. Figure 7.2 shows an example of a patient with radiation induced necrosis with reduced FDG uptake (a) and a recurrent glioma with enhanced FDG uptake in comparison to normal cortex (b). Validation of this will provide a valuable tool to determine whether post-treatment symptoms are related to tumour regrowth or normal tissue damage.

Measurements in cerebral tumours of blood flow (perfusion) with ^{15}O labelled CO_2 or H_2O and oxygen metabolism with O_2 have shown that both are highly variable with no apparent correlation to tumour status, grade, prognosis, etc. However the role of blood flow in tracer accumulation in tissue is important and perfusion often needs to be determined when physiological parameters are to be extracted from images.

Amino acid metabolism, particularly with [^{11}C]L-methionine, can produce high contrast images of primary brain tumours. The tumour (glioma)/normal brain uptake ratio is in the range 1.2–3.5 with a high degree of correlation with malignancy and grade (Mazoyer et al., 1993). Whilst initial results have been encouraging, the complex metabolism of these agents has made it difficult to obtain values for protein synthesis rates which might be accurate markers of tumour status. In pituitary adenomas [^{11}C]methionine has been shown to be an accurate marker of response to bromocriptine within hours of the start of treatment (Bergstrom et al., 1991).

Simple tracers such as RbCl and Ga-EDTA have been used to study the role of blood–brain barrier permeability in the treatment of cerebral tumours (Ott et al., 1991). Significant changes in permeability during chemotherapy for primary cerebral lymphoma have been measured at a level which would affect the access of the drugs to the tumour. No effect was seen in normal brain following conventional cerebral irradiation. These results have affected the management of patients undergoing drug therapy.

Valk et al. (1992) have shown that the uptake of the hypoxic cell tracer [^{18}F]fluoromisonidazole in glioma significantly exceeds that of normal cortex. Tumour uptake falls into two groups with different retention times. The authors speculate that tumour uptake of this agent may be proportional to hypoxic cell fraction but provide no evidence for this assumption.

An area of growing interest is the possibility of measuring cellular proliferation rates using DNA/RNA binding ligands. Gill et al. (1990) have shown a strong correlation between [^{18}F]fluorodeoxyuridine uptake (FUdR) in glioma and the histopathology of the tumour. In particular the growing edge of tumours is well defined by this agent. However the complex metabolism of FUdR again makes it difficult to establish the fraction of RNA labelling. Interest has now moved to the possible use of [^{11}C]thymidine. Specifically efforts are being made to label the

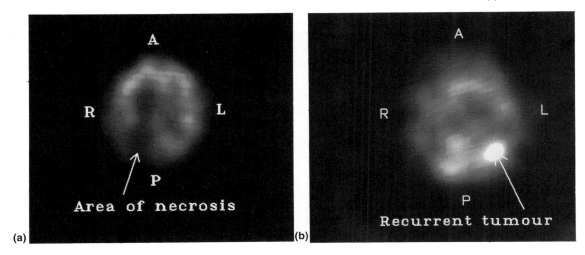

Figure 7.2 Transaxial PET brain sections following radiotherapy for glioma showing: (a) hypo-metabolism of FDG in necrotic tissue; (b) hypermetabolism of FDG in recurrent tumour.

tracer in such a way that there is minimal signal from metabolites.

Studies with the dopamine receptor ligands [^{11}C]raclopride and [^{11}C]methylspiperone (Muhr *et al.*, 1986) have been carried out in patients with pituitary adenomas. Tracer uptake seems to be proportional to receptor binding. These tracers may be useful for determining the sensitivity of prolactinomas to dopamine agonists and also to determine response to such treatment.

7.3.2 HEAD AND NECK CANCER

Planar scintigraphy has been used to measure FDG metabolism in patients with malignant head and neck tumours before and during radiotherapy. Tumours were shown to be FDG positive prior to treatment and reduction in FDG uptake after radiotherapy correlated with response. Non-responders showed a constant level of uptake. FDG uptake also seemed to correlate with radiotherapy dose given and the half-life of FDG in tumour returned to normal tissue values following treatment. It has been proposed that FDG imaging be used as a method of

follow-up of head and neck tumours after radiotherapy.

A comparison of FDG uptake with DNA flow cytometry via nuclear DNA content and percentage of proliferative cells shows no relationship with histological grade but positive correlation with cells in S+G2/M and with S-phase percentage. Haberkorn *et al.* (1991) compared FDG uptake in head and neck tumours (both primary and metastases) with flow cytometric DNA content and proliferation rate. Two patient groups with different levels of FDG uptake were both seen to correlate with proliferation. No correlation was found between perfusion and proliferation. The authors propose that the two patient groups may represent different oncogenic transformations.

Leskinen-Kallio *et al.* (1992) have imaged head and neck patients with the amino acid [^{11}C] methionine and measured tumour influx constants (Ki) and SUV values. All tumours showed positive uptake and a strong correlation was found between Ki, SUV measurements and histological grade. The authors hypothesize that this agent may be useful for delineating tumour boundaries prior to radiotherapy.

Head and neck tumours have been imaged with [¹¹C] thymidine (van Eijkeren *et al.*, 1992) as a possible method of determining cellular proliferation rates. All tumours showed positive uptake with a rapid initial decrease followed by plateau. Their data show a possible influence by both blood flow and cellular metabolism. However there is much competing uptake in normal tissues, particularly salivary glands, making tumour delineation difficult.

An interesting result comes from Koh *et al.* (1990) who have used the tracer [¹⁸F] fluoromisonidazole in an attempt to determine the hypoxic cell fraction in patients with head and neck tumours. Positive uptake of the tracer in excess of blood activity levels has been seen but the relationship to hypoxic cell fraction has yet to be ascertained.

7.3.3   THYROID CANCER

Flower *et al.* (1989) have shown how imaging with [¹²⁴I] sodium iodide in patients with thyroid cancer can give both improved tumour localization and allow accurate dosimetry for treatment with [¹³¹I] sodium iodide to be carried out. Figure 7.3(a) is a transverse section through the thorax of a patient with thyroid cancer showing high uptake of tracer quantities of [¹²⁴I] sodium iodide in rib metastases. These images can be used to determine the tissue concentration of iodine in tumour and hence the radiation dose that could be achieved with high activities of [¹³¹I] sodium iodide. Preliminary results (Figure 7.3(b)) show the radiation dose–response relationship for normal thyroid tissue and tumour, indicating a real difference in the dose achieved for successful treatment and continuing tumour growth. These data may help to explain the variation in response between metastases in the lungs and skeleton.

7.3.4   LYMPHOMA

FDG metabolism measurements again play the major role in the application of PET to

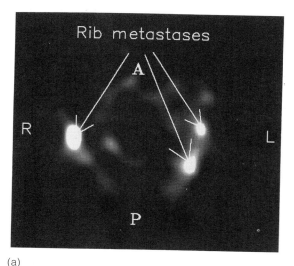

(a)

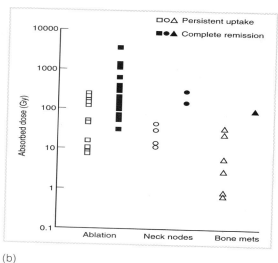

(b)

Figure 7.3   (**a**) Transaxial section through the thorax of a patient with rib metastases from thyroid cancer showing uptake of [¹²⁴I] sodium iodide in the tumours. (**b**) Preliminary radiation dose–responses data for [¹³¹I] sodium iodide therapy of thyroid cancer. □ ○ △, Persistent uptake; ■ ● ▲, complete remission.

lymphoma. Early studies indicated that FDG uptake was a more sensitive tumour detection method in non-Hodgkin's lymphoma (NHL) than the historical 'gold standard' [67Ga]citrate scintigraphy. A more recent study by Okada *et al.* (1991) confirmed this finding and showed that high tumour accumulation of FDG indicated poor prognosis with greater sensitivity than gallium scanning. A further study by the same group (Okada *et al.*, 1992) has investigated the relationship between FDG metabolism and pathology in NHL. The authors claim a correlation between FDG uptake and proliferation as measured by mitotic cell counts and Ki-67 monoclonal antibody.

Two further studies have investigated the role of [11C]methionine and [11C]thymidine (TdR) in NHL. The first (Leskinen-Kallio *et al.*, 1991a) compares the amino acid with FDG imaging and concludes that whilst the former is better at detecting all grades of tumour, FDG is superior in distinguishing between high grade NHL and other grades. The second (Martiat *et al.*, 1988) suggests that [11C]TdR may be suitable for directly measuring cell proliferation in NHL but the high level of uptake in abdominal tissues limits the application.

7.3.5 BREAST CANCER

FDG planar imaging has been shown to localize successfully in primary, lymph node and soft tissue metastases. Increased FDG uptake following treatment correlated with clinical progression. Wahl *et al.* (1991) confirmed these findings in soft tissue using PET but also showed good localization of skeletal metastases. Their data include several examples of FDG positive metastases and primary tumours previously undetected by X-ray techniques, and claim substantial potential for FDG PET scanning as an accurate detector of widespread disease. This application has been confirmed by Tse *et al.* (1992) who claim

a high level of sensitivity to primary tumours in radiodense breasts and for preoperative identification of axillary lymph node metastases.

A study of the efficacy of amino acid uptake in both primary and metastatic breast tumours has been reported by Leskinen-Kallio *et al.* (1991b). These data show a correlation between lesion size, [11C]methionine uptake and S-phase fraction as measured by flow cytometry. The authors claim that [11C] methionine uptake may correlate with proliferative rate in breast carcinoma.

Mintun *et al.* (1988) have developed several steroid receptor ligands to quantify oestrogen and progestin receptors in breast cancer. Using [18F]fluoroestradiol they show that the uptake in primary breast masses correlates well with tumour oestrogen receptor concentration determined *in vitro*. They have also shown that this tracer successfully localizes involved nodes and metastases and suggest that this tracer may be of value in assessing the likely sensitivity of these sites to hormone therapy. Effort is now directed to the labelling of tamoxifen and its derivatives allowing the possibility of pretherapy tracer studies for dosimetry.

Positron emitter labelled monoclonal antibodies should add improved sensitivity and spatial resolution to the purported tumour specificity of these agents. Bakir *et al.* (1992) report successful *in vitro* and laboratory based studies using [124I]ICR12, a c-*erb*B2 proto-oncogene product antibody. This may prove to be a useful prognostic tool in breast cancer.

7.3.6 LUNG CANCER

In common with other malignant tumours lung cancers show high levels of metabolic activity and several studies have examined the role of FDG imaging in the lung. Strauss and Conti (1991) report on the evaluation of 100 patients prior to therapy. SUVs for all lung malignancies were significantly higher than for benign lesions but there was no difference in FDG uptake with different histology. The data show a clear role for FDG in staging lung primaries, especially in cases where CT failed to differentiate between benign and malignant tissue. No correlation was found between tumour perfusion and metabolism. A group of patients with small cell carcinoma were followed up after a range of the therapies. Again FDG PET was found to be the most accurate method of determining tumour response. Continued intense metabolism after treatment correlated with residual tumour growth. Similar results were obtained in patients with mesotheliomas.

Fujiwara *et al.* (1989) have used [^{11}C]methionine in patients with lung tumours with four different histologies. This study indicates a possible correlation between amino acid uptake and tumour histology in squamous cell carcinoma and large cell carcinoma.

7.3.7   COLORECTAL CANCER

FDG has been used to localize metastatic disease in the liver from colon cancer. Strauss and Conti (1991) report the results of an extensive study which shows how FDG SUV clearly differentiates between tumour and scar tissue although there is significant FDG uptake in inflammatory disease. FDG scanning has also been used to monitor palliative radiotherapy of non-resectable colorectal carcinoma. Data show a significant reduction of tumour uptake in some patients and long term retention in others. These results are thought to correlate with the palliation status of the disease. In about half of the cases studied normal CEA plasma levels were seen with elevated FDG SUV levels in residual or recurrent tumour, showing that CEA was a poor marker of disease status in comparison to FDG imaging.

The radiolabelling of anticancer drugs enables measurements of *in vivo* drug kinetics to be made using PET imaging. Strauss and Conti (1991) have reported the use of tracer doses of [^{18}F]5-fluorouracil (5-FU) in patients with liver metastasis from colon carcinoma. These data show a strong correlation between the initial uptake of the tracer in metastases and the response to 5-FU therapy. The study also shows that increased tumour uptake of 5-FU can be achieved via regional (intra-arterial) application of the drug and that there is a strong correlation between 5-FU uptake and metabolism. The use of 5-FU as a pretherapy tracer also identified groups of patients for which 5-FU treatment was not viable.

7.3.8   SOFT TISSUE AND BONE TUMOURS

Skeletal imaging prior to the introduction of technetium-99m was carried out using ^{18}F-labelled fluoride ion. A revival of this method has been reported by Hawkins *et al.* (1992). They demonstrate that whole body skeletal imaging with PET is viable and have produced parametric images of the ion rate constant which can be used as a 'bone metabolic index' to improve the objective evaluation of focal bone disease.

As with most other cancers, FDG metabolism has been measured in several studies of musculoskeletal tumours. Adler *et al.* (1991) report that the uptake of FDG in these tumours correlates strongly with grade. A PET evaluation of soft tissue masses with FDG has been carried out by Griffeth *et al.* (1992). Their data show that a semiquantitative assessment of FDG uptake can differentiate accurately between benign and malignant tumour.

7.3.9   NEURAL CREST TUMOURS

The synthetic physiological guanethidine analogue meta-iodobenzylguanidine (mIBG) has been used to diagnose and treat neural crest tumours in both adults and children. Ott *et al.* (1992) have shown that it is possible to use tracer doses of [^{124}I]mIBG in patients with neural crest tumours to plan the treatments with [^{131}I]mIBG.

Pheochromocytoma has also been imaged using [^{11}C]hydroxyphedrine and PET (Shulkin *et al.*, 1992). This tracer is shown to localize all lesions previously identified by mIBG scintigraphy. It is proposed that this technique may be promising as a sensitive detector of 'more elusive' tumours.

7.3.10 OTHER TUMOURS

There have been a few isolated studies, mostly with FDG, in other cancers which indicate the potential use of PET in the management of patients. These include cancer of the prostate, pancreas, melanoma, testicular carcinoma and paediatric tumours.

One study (Hoffman *et al.*, 1992) involving a large number of patients has evaluated FDG in paediatric posterior fossa brain tumours. They conclude that increased FDG uptake is correlated with the more malignant and aggressive tumours and see a role for FDG

scanning in the patient management similar to that with adults.

An amino acid study using [^{11}C]methionine (Syrota *et al.*, 1982) has shown that PET scanning has a higher sensitivity, specificity and accuracy than CT scanning in pancreatic disease, although it was not possible to differentiate between cancer and chronic pancreatitis.

Finally a study of the uptake of FDG in testicular carcinoma (Ott *et al.*, 1994) shows a strong correlation between changes in FDG uptake and tumour response to chemotherapy. Figure 7.4, below, illustrates how (1) the hypermetabolism of FDG in an abdominal mass from malignant teratoma is turned to hypometabolism (2) in the necrotic mass (still visible on X-ray CT) following treatment and the return of normal kidney function. Preliminary results show high uptake in active germ cell tumours but none in differentiated tissue. The sensitivity of FDG is 78% with a specificity of 100%. The limit on

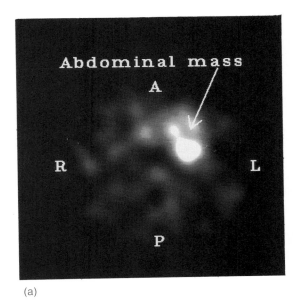

(a)

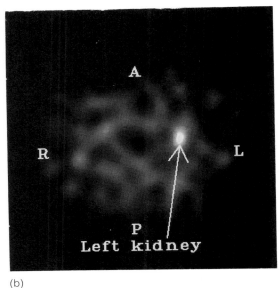

(b)

Figure 7.4 Transaxial PET sections though the abdomen of a patient with a mass from testicular carcinoma showing: (**a**) high FDG metabolism prior to chemotherapy; (**b**) zero FDG metabolism in remnant non-viable mass (as seen on X-ray CT). Note the return of normal kidney function.

sensitivity was caused by the non-detection of small tumours of 1 cm or less in diameter.

7.4   CONCLUSIONS

There are already some areas in which PET has direct clinical input into oncology. The differentiation between benign conditions such as radiation induced necrosis and tumour regrowth is of obvious importance in a wide range of tumour sites. Studies have shown that both [^{18}F]FDG and amino acids are appropriate tracers here. It has also been shown that tumour grading and response to therapy can be determined from PET scanning. Measurements of protein synthesis or cellular proliferation *in vivo* could in the near future provide important methods for determining those patients most likely to benefit from accelerated radiotherapy or high dose chemotherapy. However parameters related to these tissue properties have yet to be successfully extracted from PET images. Anticancer drug dosimetry could well target expensive treatment to responding patients and save non-responders from the worst of the side-effects. Studies here are just beginning.

Overall it seems likely that PET will play an important role in the management of individual cancer patients as the technique becomes more readily available. Whilst PET is still an expensive technique there should be further possibilities to expand on a broader front (Ott, 1989) by sharing radiopharmaceutical facilities on a regional basis. The unique, quantitative, functional information provided by PET makes it an exciting addition to the imaging tools available to the oncologist to help improve overall patient management.

REFERENCES

Adler, L.P., Blair, H.F., Makley, J.T. *et al.* (1991) Noninvasive grading of musculoskeletal tumours using PET. *Journal of Nuclear Medicine,* **32**, 1508–12.

Bakir, M.A., Eccles, S.A., Babich, J.W. *et al.* (1992) c-erbB2 protein overexpression in breast cancer as a target for PET using iodine-123-Labelled monoclonal antibodies. *Journal of Nuclear Medicine,* **33**, 2154–60.

Bergstrom, M., Muhr, C., Lundberg, P.O. *et al.* (1991) PET as a tool in the clinical evaluation of pituitary adenomas. *Journal of Nuclear Medicine,* **32**, 610–15.

Coleman, R.E., Hoffman, J.M., Hanson, M.W. *et al.* (1991) Clinical applications of PET for the evaluation of brain tumours. *Journal of Nuclear Medicine,* **32**, 616–22.

Flower, M.A., Schlesinger, T., Hinton, P.J. *et al.* (1989) Radiation dose assessment in radioiodine therapy. 2. Practical implementation using quantitative scanning and PET with initial results on thyroid carcinoma. *Radiotherapy and Oncology,* **15**, 345–57.

Fujiwara, T., Matsuzawa, T., Kubota, K. *et al.* (1989) Relationship between the histologic type of primary lung cancer and carbon-11-methionine uptake with Positron Emission Tomography. *Journal of Nuclear Medicine,* **30**, 33–7.

Gill, S., Wilson, C., Heather, J. *et al.* (1990) Brain-tumour imaging with positron emission tomography (PET) using F-18-5-fluoro-2-deoxyuridine (FUdR). *British Journal of Cancer,* **61**, 166.

Griffeth, L.K., Dehdashti, F., McGuire, A.H. *et al.* (1992) PET evaluation of soft-tissue masses with fluorine-18 fluorodeoxyglucose. *Radiology,* **182**, 185–94.

Haberkorn, U., Strauss, L.G., Reisser, C. *et al.* (1991) Glucose uptake, perfusion, and cell proliferation in head and neck tumours: relation of positron emission tomography to flow cytometry. *Journal of Nuclear Medicine,* **32**, 1548–55.

Hawkins, R.A., Choi, Y., Huang, S. *et al.* (1992) Evaluation of skeletal kinetics of fluorine-18 fluoride ion with PET. *Journal of Nuclear Medicine,* **33**, 633–42.

Hoffman, J.M., Hanson, M.W., Friedman, H.S. *et al.* (1992) FDG-PET in paediatric posterior fossa brain tumours. *Journal of Computer Assisted Tomography,* **16**, 62–8.

Koh, W.J., Rasey, J.S., Evans, M.L. *et al.* (1990) Imaging of hypoxia in human tumours with (F-18)fluoromisonidazole. *Journal of Nuclear Medicine,* **31**, 756.

Leskinen-Kallio, S., Ruotsalainen, U., Nagren, K. *et al.* (1991a) Uptake of carbon-11-methionine and fluorodeoxyglucose in non-Hodgkin's lymphoma: a PET study. *Journal of Nuclear Medicine*, **32**, 1121–18.

Leskinen-Kallio, S., Nagren, K., Lehikoinen, P., *et al.* (1991b) Uptake of C-11-methionine in breast cancer studies by PET. An association with the size of S-phase fraction. *British Journal of Cancer*, **64**, 1121–4.

Leskinen-Kallio, S., Nagren, K., Lehikoinen, P. *et al.* (1992) Carbon-11-methionine and PET is an effective method to image head and neck cancer. *Journal of Nuclear Medicine*, **33**, 691–5.

Marsden, P.K., Ott, R.J., Bateman, J.E. *et al.* (1989) The performance of a multiwire proportional chamber positron camera for clinical use. *Physics in Medicine and Biology*, **34**, 1043–62.

Martiat, Ph., Ferrant, A., Labar, D. *et al.* (1988) *In vivo* measurement of carbon-11 thymidine uptake in non-Hodgkin's lymphoma using Positron Emission Tomography. *Journal of Nuclear Medicine*, **29**, 1633–7.

Mazoyer, B.M., Heiss, W.D. and Comar, D. (1993) *PET Studies on Amino Acid Metabolism and Protein Synthesis*, Kluwer Academic Publishers, Dordrecht.

Mintun, M.A., Welch, M.J., Siegel, B.A. *et al.* (1988) Breast cancer: PET imaging of oestrogen receptors. *Radiology*, **169**, 45–8.

Muhr, C., Bergstrom, M., Lundberg, P.O. *et al.* (1986) Dopamine receptors in pituitary adenomas: PET visualisation with C-11-N-methyl-spiperone. *Journal of Computer Assisted Tomography*, **10**, 175–80.

Okada, J., Yoshikawa, K., Imaseki, K. *et al.* (1991) The use of FDG-PET in the detection and management of malignant lymphoma: correlation of uptake with prognosis. *Journal of Nuclear medicine*, **32**, 686–91.

Okada, J., Yoshikawa, K., Itami, M. *et al.* (1992) Positron emission tomography using fluorine-18-fluorodeoxyglucose in malignant lymphoma: a comparison with proliferative activity. *Journal of Nuclear Medicine*, **33**, 325–9.

Ott, R.J. (1989) Nuclear medicine in the 1990's. A quantitative physiological approach. *British Journal of Radiology*, **62**, 421–32.

Ott, R.J., Brada, M., Flower, M.A. *et al.* (1991) Measurements of blood–brain-barrier permeability in patients undergoing radiotherapy and chemotherapy for primary cerebral lymphoma. *European Journal of Cancer*, **27**, 1356–61.

Ott, R.J., Tait, D., Flower, M.A. *et al.* (1992) Treatment planning for I-131-mIBG radiotherapy of neural crest tumours using I-124-mIBG positron emission tomography. *British Journal of Radiology*, **65**, 787–91.

Ott, R.J., Wilson, C., Young, H. *et al.* (1994) Role of PET imaging with F^{18}-deoxyglucose in the management of testicular germ cell tumours. *Nuclear Medicine Communications*, **15**, 228.

Phelps, M.E., Mazziotta, J.C. and Schelbert, H.R. (eds) (1986) *Positron Emission Tomography and Autoradiography; Principles and Applications to the Brain and Heart*, Raven Press, New York.

Shulkin, B.L., Wieland, D.M., Schwaiger, M. *et al.* (1992) PET scanning with hydroxyphedrine: an approach to the localisation of pheochromocytoma. *Journal of Nuclear Medicine*, **33**, 1125–31.

Strauss, L.G. and Conti, P.S. (1991) The applications of PET in clinical oncology. *Journal of Nuclear Medicine*, **32**, 623–48.

Syrota, A.S., Duquesnoy, N., Paraf, A. *et al.* (1982) The role of positron emission tomography in the detection of pancreatic disease. *Radiology*, **143**, 249–53.

Tse, N.Y., Hoh, C.K., Hawkins, R.A. *et al.* (1992) The application of Positron Emission Tomographic imaging with fluorodeoxyglucose to the evaluation of breast disease. *Annals of Surgery*, **216**, 27–34.

Valk, P.E., Mathis, C., Prados, M.D. *et al.* (1992) Hypoxia in human gliomas: demonstration by PET with fluorine-18-fluoromisonidazole. *Journal of Nuclear Medicine*, **33**, 2133–7.

van Eijkeren, M.E., De Schryver, A., Goethals, P. *et al.* (1992) Measurements of short-term C-11-thymidine activity in human head and neck tumours using positron emission tomography (PET). *Acta Oncologica*, **31**, 539–43.

Wahl, R.L., Cody, R.L., Hutchins, G.D. *et al.* (1991) Primary and metastatic breast carcinoma: initial clinical evaluation with PET with the radiolabelled glucose analogue 2-[F-18]-fluoro-2-deoxy-D-glucose. *Radiology*, **179**, 765–70.

Wells, K., Ott, R.J., Suckling, J. *et al.* (1992) The status of the ICR/RAL BaF_2-TMAE Positron camera. *IEEE Transactions on Nuclear Science*, **39**, 1475–9.

PRINCIPLES OF SURGICAL ONCOLOGY 8

Tim Davidson and Nigel P.M. Sacks

8.1 INTRODUCTION

The surgical oncologist plays an important role in the multidisciplinary approach to the management of cancer at every stage of the disease. Surgeons have a clear idea of the natural history of the disease as they are often involved in the initial evaluation of patients with common malignancies and until recently surgery was the only curative treatment for patients with cancer. Cancer screening, the initial diagnosis and staging of the disease, locoregional control, treatment of complications of disease progression such as bowel or urinary tract obstruction, the control of pain, reconstruction, rehabilitation, and, in occasional circumstances, treatment of distant metastatic disease, may all involve the surgeon. In addition to the curative treatment that can be offered for many patients, the surgical oncologist plays a central role in the palliation of the disease.

Some 30% of the work of any general surgeon (even those without a specialist interest in cancer) involves patients with cancer. Whether surgical oncology should be recognized as a strictly separate speciality within surgery remains a contentious issue (Beahrs, 1991). What is certain, however, is that surgeons dealing with cancer today must possess a much broader set of clinical and technical skills to participate as an effective member of a multidisciplinary cancer care team to ensure that each patient benefits from the full range of diagnostic and treatment options available (Balch, 1990).

8.2 SCREENING AND PREVENTION

The surgeon is increasingly called upon to give educational advice both to patients in the clinic and people in the community about reducing risk factors, such as smoking for lung cancer or sun exposure for melanoma. Early detection of cancer not only has the potential to improve cure rates but may enable the surgeon to limit the extent of surgery. For example, most melanomas are now detected at an early stage and can usually be treated by relatively narrow excision margins.

Successful cancer screening programmes must have the following characteristics:

1. The tumour should be an important health problem.
2. There should be a detectable preclinical phase of the tumour.
3. The natural history of precursor lesions should be known.
4. There should be effective treatment for the disease.
5. The screening test should be acceptable, 102safe, reliable and cost-effective.

Cervical cytology screening is now widely accepted as instrumental in reducing mortality from cervical cancer although it has never been tested by controlled randomized trials (Skrabanek, 1988). With regard to breast cancer, there are no reliable data to suggest that screening mammography reduces mortality in the youngest or oldest age groups (Dixon, 1993) but population screening for breast cancer for women aged 50–64 years fulfils these criteria (Frisell *et al.*, 1991) and has been shown to lead to a relative reduction in the cause-specific mortality of up to 30% in the screened population.

Population based screening for other malignancies (e.g. gastric cancer using photofluorographic barium meal, ovarian cancer using pelvic ultrasound and the tumour marker CA125, or colonic cancer using occult blood testing) remain of unproven benefit. Screening should also be offered to individuals who have an inherited susceptibility to cancer, such as familial polyposis of the colon, dysplastic naevus syndrome or families with multiple endocrine neoplasia predisposing to medullary thyroid carcinoma. If identified, these individuals can be cured by preventive surgery (Table 8.1).

8.3   EVALUATION OF PRIMARY DISEASE

8.3.1   CLINICAL EXAMINATION

The initial diagnosis and staging of a patient with cancer is usually in the hands of a surgeon. Careful history-taking and physical examination remain paramount, together with a high index of suspicion that a symptom or sign may indicate malignant disease. Surface lesions such as melanoma or basal cell carcinoma may be immediately recognized. Examination of deeper tissues (such as the prostate, rectal tumours or breast masses) may be aided by ultrasound probe at the time of clinical examination.

Initial evaluation may require upper or lower gastrointestinal endoscopy, cystoscopy, bronchoscopy or nasendoscopy, all of which may involve tissue sampling for diagnosis. The advent of flexible fibreoptic endoscopes has made many of these investigations rapid and minimally traumatic for the patient and they seldom necessitate inpatient admission or general anaesthesia.

8.3.2   IMAGING

The oncologist relies increasingly on radiological imaging to provide staging information about the presenting cancer. In deep-seated or extensive lesions such as soft-tissue sarcoma, MRI or CT scanning of the tumour site are mandatory prior to any surgical planning (Figure 8.1). Such imaging can accurately predict the relationship of the tumour to bone, viscera, neurovascular structures and tumour extension beyond compartmental boundaries (Davidson *et al.*, 1987a) and so allow evaluation for feasible radical surgery. Mammography in suspicious breast lesions may be diagnostic and may provide evidence of multifocal or bilateral disease or of extensive microcalcification beyond the palpable lesion which may preclude breast conserving surgery.

8.3.3   TISSUE BIOPSY

Adequate biopsy of any malignancy is essential before a diagnosis can be confirmed and definitive treatment commenced. The surgeon

Table 8.1 Operations that can prevent cancer

Underlying condition	Associated cancer	Prophylactic operation
Cryptorchidism	Testis	Orchidectomy
Familial adenomatous polyposis Ulcerative colitis	Colon and rectum	Proctocolectomy ± anal pouch
Multiple endocrine neoplasia	Medullary thyroid	Thyroidectomy
Familial breast cancer	Breast	Bilateral mastectomy ± reconstruction

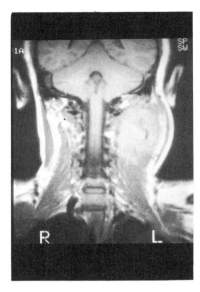

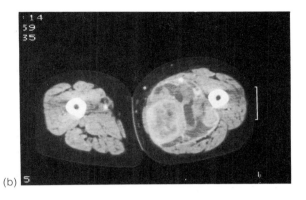

(a)

(b)

Figure 8.1 Tumour imaging: (a) MRI scan of malignant fibrous histiocytoma of occipital region arising in left trapezius muscle; (b) CT scan of rhabdomyosarcoma arising in left adductor compartment of thigh.

must be capable of securing tissue suitable for histological or cytological interpretation and the pathologist must be capable of a confident opinion on the small sample he or she receives. Fine needle aspiration (FNA) cytology and needle core biopsy are now widely used for diagnosis in accessible solid tumours, often under local anaesthetic and as an outpatient procedure.

(a) FNA cytology

FNA cytology performed with a 21 G needle and 20 ml syringe is quick, safe, relatively inexpensive and can easily be repeated if the first aspirate proves inadequate for cytological diagnosis. FNA cytology has been used in the diagnosis of breast tumours for over 10 years (Wanebo *et al.*, 1984) and in the hands of a trained cytopathologist provides specificity and sensitivity greater than 90%. With experienced cytological interpretation the false-positive rates are in the range 0–3%, allowing treatment decisions to be made with

confidence on the 'triple assessment' of clinical, mammographic and cytology findings. FNA cytology is of value in assessing enlarged lymph nodes where it may confirm metastatic melanoma or carcinoma but is unsuitable for accurate diagnosis in lymphoma. The accuracy of FNA cytology in thyroid, pancreatic and soft tissue malignancies is less consistent but many centres routinely perform it (Kissin and Williamson, 1990).

(b) Needle core biopsy

Histological assessment from needle core biopsy obtained with a cutting needle (such as Trucut, Corecut, Bioptycut or similar type) or high-speed drill biopsy is adequate for most accessible cancers. Crushing or charring of removed tissue must be avoided. Tissue cores should be representative of the whole tumour and zones of haemorrhage and necrosis avoided. The routine use of Trucut biopsy does not appear adversely to affect local or distant recurrence in breast cancer (Fentiman *et al.*, 1986). In soft tissue sarcoma, Trucut biopsy achieves a diagnostic accuracy of up to 90% (Kissin *et al.*, 1986).

For deep-seated tumours (retroperitoneal, intra-abdominal or intrapleural sites) ultrasound or CT guided needle biopsy or FNA cytology makes open biopsy avoidable in the majority of such patients. Tumour seeding down the needle tract, although reported in a handful of cases, does not pose a problem of any significance (Burn, 1989).

(c)   Incision vs excision biopsy

Where open surgical biopsy is required, excision of the whole lesion is usually preferable to incision and sampling of only a part of the tumour. In melanoma, excision of the whole lesion allows accurate microstaging of the primary lesion by Breslow thickness or Clarke's level which may not be the case if an incision biopsy is performed; in many thinner lesions excision biopsy will also be sufficient treatment. Excision biopsy of lymph nodes may establish a diagnosis of lymphoma or be of value in the staging of common solid tumours, including bronchogenic carcinoma and intra-abdominal adenocarcinoma. To allow greatest accuracy of histological subtyping in lymphoma, removal of a whole node and with minimal crushing artefact is necessary.

In some cancers however, incision biopsy may be necessary when tumour fixity from local extension or irradiation fibrosis makes attempted excision too hazardous or extensive a procedure. In large soft tissue tumours (e.g. where Trucut biopsy has failed to provide diagnostic material) incision biopsy may cause less violation of tissue planes than an inexperienced attempt at excision which might compromise subsequent chances of radical surgery. The placement of the biopsy incision in such cases is critical so that it may be included in subsequent definitive surgery and is best left to the surgeon ultimately responsible for surgical resection.

8.4   STAGING

The planning of primary therapy requires full information about the extent of the disease. A clinical diagnosis together with the result of tissue biopsy and non-invasive staging investigations may determine whether the case is inoperable or potentially curable. The recognition of clearly incurable states will avoid the use of inappropriate local therapies including surgery and radiotherapy. Computerized imaging of potential metastatic sites has now become the foremost modality for identifying distant disease spread. CT scanning or MRI have largely replaced modalities such as lymphangiography, lung tomography and isotope brain and liver scanning.

Surgical staging techniques such as mediastinoscopy or staging laparotomy are seldom indicated today. The morbidity of invasive staging procedures needs to be balanced against the potential advantage that such staging information may confer, particularly where a decision needs to be made regarding available adjuvant therapy. In melanoma prophylactic or elective regional node dissection provides staging information but is less widely advocated because of the surgical morbidity, particularly following groin dissection, and the lack of demonstrable advantage over a 'wait and see' policy of therapeutic node dissection (Scott and McKay, 1993). In contrast, axillary dissection in breast cancer at the time of primary surgery serves both as a staging procedure, allowing a more rational decision whether to advise adjuvant chemotherapy, and as treatment for the axilla, reducing both the potential problem of uncontrolled axillary disease and the need to include the axilla in the breast irradiation field (Sacks *et al.*, 1992).

8.5   SURGICAL CURE VS LOCAL CONTROL

The intent of potentially curable surgery is to eliminate all gross tumour with safe normal tissue margins. Surgery is the main locoregional therapeutic modality to have a major impact on cancer management (Elias, 1989). The pathological staging of the disease is the most important factor in establishing whether cure is possible. Examples of curative surgery range from local excision of a basal cell carcinoma or early melanoma, to anterior resection for Dukes' A rectal carcinoma, gastrectomy for early gastric cancer, and radical nephrectomy for a localized renal carcinoma.

Whilst preoperative staging prior to planning major surgery is routine, complete operative exploration is essential and suspicious lesions in liver, peritoneum, pleura or nodes must be biopsied at the time of surgery. Exhaustive investigations to exclude asymptomatic metastases are not indicated when surgery is indicated in any event, e.g. for colonic carcinoma, and the detection of disease spread, e.g. liver metastases at laparotomy, does not alter the decision to operate but might influence the radicality of the colonic resection performed. Metastatic

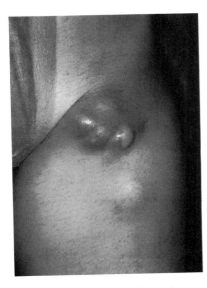

Figure 8.2 Extensive regional involvement of left inguinofemoral nodes by melanoma. Wide excision with repair of the defect using a fasciocutaneous rotation flap was necessary to prevent imminent tumour fungation.

disease should be confirmed histologically and where there is doubt frozen section may be required to determine the extent of resection that is appropriate.

Even when not curative, surgery is essential to gain symptomatic control of local disease causing obstruction to hollow viscera such as gut, biliary tract and urinary system. Removing a locoregional tumour, even in the presence of distant metastases, may control discharges, fungation and haemorrhage (Figure 8.2). Debulking a primary tumour may also enhance the effectiveness of radiotherapy and chemotherapy. Once a tumour has infiltrated nerve roots it is difficult for surgery in itself to relieve pain but this complication should always be anticipated and attempts to control the disease before it infiltrates nerve roots, especially around the brachial and sacral plexus, may prevent the development of intractable pain.

8.6 RELATIONSHIP BETWEEN LOCAL RECURRENCE AND SURVIVAL

For some tumours, such as those arising around the head and neck or in the pelvis, local recurrence has an obvious impact on survival through direct extension to involve vital structures. Meticulous surgical technique in performing mesorectal excision for rectal cancer is claimed to improve not only local control rates but also overall survival (MacFarlane *et al.*, 1993). For other tumours such as breast cancer, melanoma or sarcoma arising in the limbs, local recurrence seldom has direct lethal consequences but might affect survival if it resulted in an increased chance of distant metastasis (Barr *et al.*, 1991).

The demonstration of an apparent relationship between local recurrence and decreased survival in many types of tumour could be due to a common prognostic factor and not necessarily infer a causal relationship. Local recurrence for example after breast conservation surgery is usually considered a predictor but not a cause of metastatic progression

(Fisher *et al.*, 1991). Others have argued that locoregional recurrence correlates with an additional hazard for survival (Stotter *et al.*, 1990) and for it to be simply a marker for a risk already present at initial treatment is not consistent with the data on the natural history of breast cancer (Tubiana, 1992).

In the absence of trials of sufficient statistical power, opinion remains divided on this major point, with many authors now considering that in most tumours the appearance of systemic disease is independent of local recurrence and that local disease can be satisfactorily salvaged without impairment of survival. Clearly, such different philosophies are reflected in different locoregional management of the primary tumour. The philosophy in a particular unit will for instance influence the mastectomy rate in breast cancer patients, the extent of primary surgery in cutaneous and mucosal melanoma (Davidson *et al.*, 1987b) or the amputation rate in the primary management of limb sarcomas.

8.7 SURGICAL RADICALITY AND MORBIDITY

In recent decades surgical oncology has witnessed the progressive abandonment of mutilating surgery and the constant search for safe conservative techniques where appropriate. In areas of treatment, collaboration between the radiotherapist, medical oncologist and reconstructive surgeon has led to fewer ablative procedures such as limb amputation, radical vulvectomy or radical mastectomy in an attempt to contribute as much to the quality of survival as to its duration (Veronesi, 1989). In areas of diagnosis, too, this evolution has led to closer collaboration with the pathologist, radiologist and endoscopist to reduce the need for staging laparotomy in lymphoma, mediastinal biopsy in chest tumours, and 'second look' surgery in patients with pelvic tumours.

This move away from mutilating surgery has been in response to two general perceptions. First, there has been the recognition that multimodality treatment, such as radiotherapy and chemotherapy with limb-sparing surgery in osteosarcoma, or hormonal therapy with breast conservation in elderly patients with breast cancer, may be just as effective as ablative surgery in terms of patient survival. Further progress is being made to tailor treatment to individual patients by identifying those patients with a poor prognosis where adjuvant therapies are most appropriate and so reduce further the morbidity from overtreatment (Blamey, 1989). Secondly, the observation that local recurrence, when it occurs, does not necessarily correlate with poorer patient survival, has led surgeons to a reappraisal of the Halstedian centrifugal theory of tumour spread and to look more critically at the grounds on which major surgical morbidity might be justified. Philosophical and cultural differences exist between the USA and UK in these areas, an example being the different attitudes to radical prostatectomy on either side of the Atlantic.

8.8 RECONSTRUCTION

Reconstruction should be considered at the initial stages of treatment as well as later in the course of the disease. A patient facing a limited expectation of life should not carry the added burden of physical or functional morbidity and surgeons have moved away from the concept that patients have to 'earn' their reconstruction by proving to be free from recurrence for a set period. Where surgical facilities permit, immediate reconstruction is often in the patient's best interest, and for major soft tissue resection involving chest wall, abdominal wall, limbs or limb girdles, collaboration between oncological and reconstructive surgeons is routine.

Reconstructive surgery involving the head and neck region and the breast may be of vital importance in allowing a patient to face an uncertain future with equanimity.

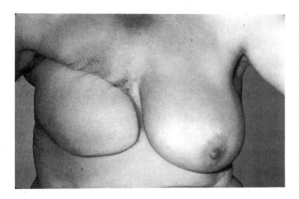

Figure 8.3   Reconstruction using a pedicled latissimus dorsi myocutaneous flap following full-thickness chest wall resection for locally advanced recurrent right breast cancer.

Although reconstruction adds to the extent and time of the surgical procedure, it may expedite the patient's discharge from hospital by achieving rapid healing following resection within irradiated tissues. Pedicled or free myocutaneous flaps, muscle flaps and omentum introduce well-vascularized and compliant tissue into rigid postirradiation defects and are now widely used to reconstruct wounds in the perineum, groin and chest wall (Figure 8.3).

8.9   SURGERY FOR METASTASES

Surgical treatment of metastatic disease is by definition rarely considered to be curative, but in selected patients may return the patient to a disease-free state for long enough to justify the morbidity of surgical intervention. The widest experience of surgical treatment of metastatic tumour spread has been gained with colorectal secondaries in the liver as discussed in Chapter 45. Patient survival in selected series is 40% at 5 years and 27% at 10 years, and operative mortality in the region of 5% (Nagorney, 1991). Criteria for patients likely to benefit from surgery with respect to size and distribution of metastases have been established, but individual judgement on the wisdom of resection in each patient is essential (Scheele, 1993). The biological behaviour of the metastatic disease must be borne in mind, and tempering surgical enthusiasm with a 3–6 month 'test of time' is advisable, particularly for synchronous metastases, small or multiple lesions (Cady and Stone, 1991).

For tumours where the natural history is more aggressive (gastric, adrenal, breast cancer) the likelihood of long-term survivors following hepatic resection is too low to justify this approach, although anecdotal successes have been reported. In patients with endocrine malignancies (carcinoid, islet cell carcinoma, gastrinoma) the opposite approach is often justified; hepatic secondaries from these tumours may be compatible with a natural history of 10 years or more and are often symptomatic and any effort at resection, where feasible, is worthwhile.

Metastatic disease may require thoracic, orthopaedic or neurosurgical expertise. In patients with solitary lung metastases, e.g. from soft tissue sarcoma, colorectal or renal carcinoma, with no evidence of disease spread elsewhere and where the biological behaviour of the tumour indicates slow disease progression, thoracotomy may prolong survival. Pathological fractures of the long bones need emergency reduction and internal fixation but ideally this complication should be anticipated with prophylactic pinning for radiolucent secondaries in weight-bearing bones. Symptoms suggesting cord compression from secondary disease should be urgently investigated and emergency decompression performed if appropriate. Similarly the neurosurgeon may be called upon for symptom relief by decompressing nerves, removing solitary cerebral metastases where appropriate and performing tractotomies for pain.

The surgical team managing cancer patients may be required to provide venous access, both for safe and reliable delivery of cytotoxic agents and for nutritional support. Long-term venous access is best provided by tunnelled silicone rubber central venous catheters (e.g. Hickman) which have the advantages of low thrombogenicity and minimal tissue reaction, and in the absence of line infection can remain *in situ* for months or years. Totally implantable venous access devices (Soo *et al.*, 1984) have a subcutaneous port which is placed surgically to allow the cancer patient to bathe and swim whilst providing regular central venous access for chemotherapy. Surgical placement is required too for vascular catheters to deliver regional cytotoxics, e.g. hepatic arterial infusion chemotherapy using either a subcutaneous port or an implantable Infusaid pump.

Detailed management, including surgical procedures, for individual types of cancer will be covered in following chapters, but some of the principles of surgical oncology discussed here, and the ways in which they may need to be modified, can be illustrated in the remainder of this chapter with reference to some of the common solid tumours.

8.10   BREAST CANCER

In advising patients (or relatives) about screening and prevention of breast cancer, the surgical oncologist must also be aware of the limitations of techniques which are not of proven benefit, for instance breast self-examination or ultrasound screening have not been shown to reduce mortality from breast cancer. Mammographic screening is in fact secondary prevention aimed at detecting the cancer at a subclinical stage with hopefully a higher chance of cure; hopes for true primary prevention of breast cancer currently lie in identifying (and treating) the underlying genetic disorder and possibly the use of tamoxifen in high risk women.

In the clinic the surgeon has responsibility for the diagnosis and staging of the disease before determining rational therapy. Outpatient diagnosis is usually easy to achieve using triple assessment (clinical, mammography and FNA cytology) or needle core histopathology. If the patient has clini-cally operable breast cancer then extensive further evaluation to exclude asymptomatic distant metastases is unnecessary before undertaking definitive surgery. However with more locally advanced disease (e.g. chest wall fixity, supraclavicular node involvement) then staging investigations may be indicated.

When distant disease is suspected because of the patient's symptoms, staging investigations are appropriate prior to planning surgery. Patients presenting with distant metastases where the primary focus in itself is not a problem should initially be treated with systemic therapy as they are likely to succumb to metastatic disease before the primary needs local treatment. Therefore locoregional therapy with surgery, radiotherapy, or in combination, should be kept in reserve.

Radical mastectomy in the days before the availability of radiotherapy or chemotherapy achieved the objective of local control in approximately 70% of all cases (Halsted, 1907). Today most patients with operable breast cancer can be offered breast conservation with no increased risk of dying. The choice in locoregional surgery for operable breast cancer usually lies between modified radical mastectomy or quadrantectomy, axillary node dissection and radiotherapy to the breast (Cady, 1991). The decision over which approach is to be preferred is determined by the position and size of the primary in relation to the size of the breast, and, when either option is appropriate, by the preference of the individual patient. There are no good data to support the commonsense notion that breast conservation in itself improves psychological morbidity of the treatment of the disease (Fallowfield *et al.*, 1986).

Techniques for breast reconstruction have improved enormously over recent years and this has largely depended upon the availability of implantable prostheses. For relatively small busted women, having had a simple or modified radical mastectomy in the past, a subpectoral tissue expander can produce pleasing results that will satisfy most patients. However women who have undergone radical mastectomy or mastectomy plus radiotherapy in the past usually require a myocutaneous flap to improve wound healing or produce sufficient volume to match up with the contralateral breast. These flaps can be based on the latissimus dorsi pedicle or the rectus abdominis muscle (TRAM flap). Often an adjustment mammoplasty of the contralateral breast is necessary to achieve perfect symmetry. Most surgical oncologists now agree that there is no logic in delaying reconstruction for a finite period, e.g. 2 years, following mastectomy to avoid local recurrence complicating or being masked by reconstructive surgery, nor excluding those patients with the poorer prognosis as indicated by local recurrence who might thereby be denied reconstruction for their limited remaining years.

Initial failure to control the disease in the axillary nodes can result in the very worst complications of breast cancer, where the uncontrolled disease grows to obstruct the lymphatics, the axillary vein and the brachial plexus (Danforth, 1992). This can lead to a painful, useless and swollen arm. Most locally advanced breast cancer (Figure 8.4) can be conventionally managed by chemotherapy, endocrine therapy or radiotherapy. However radical surgery still has a role where local control of the disease has not been possible with combinations of systemic therapy and radiotherapy yet the patient is not obviously dying of distant metastases. Under these circumstances a wide resection of the breast, underlying muscles and chest wall may provide effective palliation. Reconstruction of the defect is possible using myocutaneous flaps or an omental graft covered by split skin. This approach may be necessary for the late effects of radionecrosis as well as controlling the ulcerating malignancy.

8.11 GASTROINTESTINAL TRACT

A high proportion of patients with upper-gastrointestinal malignancy – oesophageal and gastric cancers in particular – have advanced disease at presentation and the disappointing survival figures of those regarded as potentially curable suggest that many of them already have occult metastases. Whilst surgery can undoubtedly cure patients with early stage invasive tumours, its chief contribution lies in control of local disease and the relief of symptoms of obstruction, tumour bulk, acute or chronic blood loss and occasionally perforation.

The most effective way to relieve symptoms is to excise the primary tumour completely, even when metastases are present. If this is technically feasible there may be little practical difference in surgical terms between curative and palliative procedures. When complete excision is impossible, symptoms due to obstruction can still be relieved by surgical bypass, or by establishing a channel through the tumour by various means. Unless the primary tumour is removed, however, symptoms of obstruction may recur and others such as bleeding may become more prominent. However, surgery may not always succeed in achieving

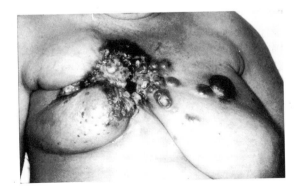

Figure 8.4 Failed local control with extensive skin and chest wall involvement by breast cancer following surgery and radiotherapy.

palliation: certain symptoms, such as the pain of malignant infiltration, may not be alleviated by surgery at all; others may be due to metastatic disseminated disease rather than the primary tumour itself. Under these circumstances, surgical intervention of any kind may be entirely inappropriate. Preserving an intact gastrointestinal and urogenital tract may spare the dying patient the additional burden of a colostomy, ileostomy or urostomy bag.

8.11.1   OESOPHAGEAL CANCER

Surgical excision is possible in over 50% of cases of oesophageal cancer but despite a substantial fall in operative mortality, largely due to improved anaesthesia and postoperative care, the complication rate particularly following anastomotic dehiscence remains high and the 5 year survival despite adequate excision is only 15%. Undisputedly the best results of surgery are achieved by experienced teams in carefully selected cases.

Oesophageal intubation is the standard way of relieving dysphagia in patients with unresectable tumours or malignant tracheo-oesophageal fistulas, although laser ablation is a safe alternative where facilities exist. Intubation is achieved either by traction at open operation using the Mousseau-Barbin tube or by pulsion through an endoscope (Nottingham or Atkinson tube). Endoscopic intubation under fluoroscopic control is safer and recovery is swifter if a laparotomy can be avoided (Earlham and Cuhna-Melo, 1982).

8.11.2   GASTRIC CANCER

The main aim of surgery for gastric cancer is to effect a cure but this succeeds in only a minority of patients (Table 8.2). The palliative role of surgery should not be underestimated and patients with symptomatic gastric cancer have better palliation, particularly of symptoms caused by mechanical obstruction, and a longer life expectancy after resection than after bypass procedures or no treatment at all. Adenocarcinomas of the cardia show virtually no response to irradiation, and the quality of swallowing is poor after intubation and only temporarily improved by laser therapy. Likewise, simple bypass of antral tumours offers little useful palliation as vomiting returns when the stoma becomes occluded.

The mortality rate of gastric resection is related to the type of operation performed. Partial gastrectomy for antral tumours has a lower mortality rate while total gastrectomy for tumours of the body and cardia has a higher mortality rate. Extending the resection to include *en bloc* regional node clearance increases the morbidity of the surgery (Dent *et al*, 1988) but does not produce a survival benefit in most Western series where the majority of patients have serosal involvement with likely intraperitoneal micrometastases at the time of presentation (Cunningham, 1990).

8.11.3   MALIGNANT OBSTRUCTIVE JAUNDICE

Most patients with carcinoma of the head of pancreas have unresectable tumours and present with obstructive jaundice. Relief of

Table 8.2   Results of surgery in gastric cancer, taken from seven studies 1952–87

Patients (no.)	Operation rate (%)	Resection rate (%)	5-year survival (%)
7044	79	62	12

Reproduced from Cunningham, 1990.

biliary obstruction results in a prolonged and more comfortable survival, free of distressing pruritus. Biliary decompression can be achieved by inserting a stent endoscopically or radiologically (Speer *et al.*, 1987), with a mortality rate and subsequent mean survival time similar to those for surgical bypass. As duodenal obstruction eventually occurs in up to 30% of patients most surgeons perform a gastroenterostomy at the time of surgical biliary bypass. Though recovery is quicker after endoscopic decompression, early occlusion and infection of the stent is not uncommon and may require further admission to hospital for antibiotics or stent change; even so, the total period spent in hospital may still be less than after surgery, especially if the survival time is short (Shepherd *et al.*, 1988).

8.11.4 COLORECTAL CARCINOMA

The majority of colonic tumours are resectable and even in the presence of metastases their excision is worthwhile to prevent obstruction developing. Carcinoma of the lower third of rectum, however, may be difficult to remove without sacrificing intestinal continuity. Although a colostomy is undesirable in a patient with metastatic disease, excision of the rectum should still be undertaken if this is the best way to ensure local control.

Endoscopic transanal resection (ETAR) for rectal cancer is suitable for local curative resection in selected patients with small well-differentiated Dukes' A carcinoma. Palliation is the main indication for ETAR in frail patients where the burden and risks of major surgery involving a colostomy outweigh the risks of failure to control or cure the disease (Kettlewell, 1991). Patients with rectal carcinoma who are unsuitable for anaesthesia or surgery can be helped by palliative radiotherapy which is effective in reducing bleeding and mucous discharge. Diathermy fulguration, cryosurgery or laser photocoagulation are alternative ways of controlling local symptoms.

8.12 HEAD AND NECK CANCER

The cure rate for patients suffering from cancer in the head and neck region (excluding the skin and central nervous system) is around 30% of those treated for cure. These disappointing figures emphasize the reality of the slow progress made in the past 30 years. More than in all cancer surgery, local control of the disease must be the primary object of treatment. Rehabilitation is of paramount importance and it is in this field that there has been the greatest advance in the management of these patients.

The head and neck region is more complex than many others as there is a multiplicity of essential and social functions that challenge the surgeon – breathing, mastication, swallowing, speech, and last but not least appearance is a prime consideration. Each function may require separate and multiple surgical procedures: an end tracheostome may alleviate breathing difficulties but will limit communication unless a technique for the restoration of speech is available and offered. The services of a specialist speech therapist are essential for all laryngectomy patients. Likewise a gastrostomy or jejunostomy will relieve the need for the patient to masticate and swallow.

Advanced local disease in the head and neck is debilitating and will without doubt affect one or more of the essential functions of the region (Pettarel *et al.*, 1989). If the removal of advanced disease is considered, yet it is felt that adequate clearance is impossible, the balance between surgical excision, reconstruction and the prospect of early local recurrence in relation to morbidity and life quality must be appreciated by both patient and surgeon alike. Loss of the ability to converse and eat are a high price for a patient to pay if the duration of life is limited. Reconstruction is usually performed at the time of excisional surgery to achieve tissue cover, promote healing, cosmesis and function. The replacement of the whole tongue with a platform of tissue (e.g. a latissimus dorsi myocutaneous flap) can restore the ability to swallow and maintain intelligible speech and yet relieve the severe pain of a tongue tumour.

Reconstructive techniques must achieve an adequate replacement of those tissues excised, dead space must be eliminated and normal anatomical relationships must be maintained. When the mucosa of tongue, floor of mouth or pharynx has to be replaced, the tissue to be chosen for repair will be influenced by the space available for the repair. Many of the pedicled flaps, e.g. pectoralis major and latissimus dorsi myocutaneous flaps, are bulky. Free tissue transfer, e.g. radial or lateral forearm flaps, allows a higher degree of accuracy in the ability to effect a repair of limited tissue loss but may lack the bulk required to eliminate a tissue dead space.

8.13   GYNAECOLOGICAL CANCER

In ovarian cancer, tumour debulking is carried out: to improve the response to chemotherapy and on occasion radiotherapy; to prevent complications that will inevitably arise involving the gastrointestinal and urogenital tracts; to help to prevent the development of ascites and excessive uncomfortable abdominal distension; and, finally, the psychological advantages of removing a huge abdominopelvic mass are enormous when viewed in the overall context of treatment of an individual patient's cancer.

Intestinal obstruction is common and may be recurrent or subacute in nature. At presentation it is important to consider the various possible causes: recurrent abdominal or pelvic cancer with a single or multiple areas of metastatic obstruction, adhesions which may be benign, postoperative or on occasions related to radiotherapy or a radiation-induced bowel stricture. Initial conservative treatment is with intravenous fluids, nasogastric aspiration to defunction the gastrointestinal tract, analgesia, antiemetics and antispasmodic agents; total parenteral nutrition may need to be considered whilst assessing the response.

Where obstruction persists, more active treatment should be considered. Internal bypass, bowel resection, the creation of a colostomy or other stoma for palliative reasons may well be indicated, but to perform this for prophylactic purposes should not be necessary (Walsh and Schofield, 1984). Repeated surgical exploration for obstruction may ultimately necessitate gastrostomy for palliation of vomiting but prolonged parenteral nutrition once there is no prospect of tumour remission should be avoided.

The development of a fistula occasionally complicates cervical carcinoma and presents as either a vesicovaginal or rectovaginal fistula; on occasions a 'three-way' fistula may develop. This may be due to a primary tumour but more usually is a result of tumour progression following radiotherapy and radionecrosis. Although the ideal management of excision of the fistula with primary repair should be considered, it is rarely practical. A small fistula may be dealt with in this way, utilizing healthy non-irradiated tissue such as omentum. More usually, urinary diversion will be necessary; rarely an indwelling catheter will relieve incontinence from a vesicovaginal fistula. A fistula involving the large bowel may similarly be managed with diversion by colostomy usually proving the most practical solution.

Ascites is much less of a problem now with more effective chemotherapy, especially when treating ovarian cancer. However it may still lead to troublesome abdominal distension and paracentesis may be required for symptomatic relief. The use of diuretics, especially spironolactone, is of value. With rapidly recurring symptomatic ascites, peritoneovenous shunts (e.g. LeVeen) offer good short-term improvement if the ascites is not loculated. Shunts have recognized major complications (sepsis, coagulopathy) and may lead to further rapid dissemination of tumour particularly with ovarian cancer (Moskovitz, 1990).

8.14 RELIEF OF URETERIC OBSTRUCTION

Many malignant tumours are capable of ureteric obstruction either from retroperitoneal metastases, lymphadenopathy or direct invasion. Relief of obstruction seldom confers a significant survival advantage and quality of life may indeed be impaired both by the effects of the tumour and the morbidity of the urinary diversion required. Death from renal failure appears (at least to the observer) to be less distressing than death with uncontrolled pelvic malignancy. Ureteric obstruction in the presence of untreatable malignancy should in general not be relieved unless relief of obstruction will permit effective palliative chemotherapy or radiotherapy.

Once a decision to undertake relief of obstruction is made, the method employed should be as minimally invasive as possible. The optimal technique is the endoscopic insertion of a ureteric stent under radiological control. This has the advantage of requiring no external appliance or stoma, but may be technically impossible if the ureteric orifices are obscured or the course of the ureter distorted by tumour masses.

Less satisfactory is the insertion of a percutaneous nephrostomy tube under radiological or ultrasound control. Nephrostomy drainage can rarely be maintained for longer than 6 weeks; there are frequent problems with infection and blockage or displacement of the nephrostomy tube. However, it may be indicated in patients with relatively acute obstruction in whom other treatment offers a reasonable prospect of tumour regression or in those in the early stage of radiotherapy where oedema may have made a partial obstruction complete. 'Permanent' methods of diversion (e.g. ileal conduit or catheterizable stoma) are rarely indicated.

8.15 CONCLUSIONS

The role of local treatment remains paramount in the cure of cancer. Most patients who are cured of cancer are cured by surgery. In patients without metastases at the time of diagnosis the cure depends upon the effectiveness of local treatment, and many patients both with and without distant metastases die as a consequence of failure to control their locoregional disease. As a partner in a multidisciplinary team the surgeon must be able to coordinate surgery, radiation therapy and systemic therapy to achieve the best results in the surgical patient.

The primary aims of cancer surgery must therefore remain as improving lifespan and maximizing local disease control. In addition the surgical oncologist is constantly striving to reduce surgical mortality and morbidity and to contribute to the rehabilitation and quality of life of the cancer patient. To accomplish this the cancer surgeon must continue to participate in clinical trials, to pursue research into the understanding of tumour biology, and to work in close collaboration with colleagues in other disciplines within the field of cancer treatment.

REFERENCES

Balch, C.M. (1990) The surgeon's expanded role in cancer care. *Cancer*, **65**, 604–9.

Barr, L.C., Stotter, A.T. and A'Hern, R.P. (1991) Influence of local recurrence on survival: a controversy reviewed from the perspective of soft tissue sarcoma. *British Journal of Surgery*, **78**, 648–50.

Beahrs, O.H. (1991) Surgical oncology – a speciality or just special? *Archives of Surgery*, **126**, 1408–10.

Blamey, R. (1989) Does biological understanding influence surgical practice? *British Journal of Cancer*, **60**, 271–4.

Burn, I. (1989) Principles of surgery in the primary treatment of cancer, in *Surgical Oncology: A European Handbook*, (ed. U Veronesi), Springer-Verlag, Berlin, pp. 123–30.

Cady, B. (1991) Choice of operations for breast cancer: conservative therapy versus radical operations, in *The Breast: Comprehensive Management of Benign and Malignant Conditions*, (eds K.I. Bland and E.M. Copeland), Saunders, Philadelphia, pp. 753–69.

Cady, B. and Stone, M.D. (1991) The role of surgical resection of liver metastases in colorectal carcinoma. *Seminars in Clinical Oncology*, **18**, 399–406.

Cunningham, D. (1990) The management of gastric cancer, in *Surgical Oncology: Current Concepts and Practice*, (ed. C.S. McArdle), Butterworth, London, pp. 28–52.

Danforth, D.N. (1992) The role of axillary lymph node dissection in the management of breast-cancer. *Principles and Practice of Oncology*, **6**, 1–16.

Davidson, T., Cooke, J., Parsons, C. *et al.* (1987a) Pre-operative assessment of soft-tissue sarcomas by computed tomography. *British Journal of Surgery*, **74**, 474–8.

Davidson, T.I., Kissin, M. and Westbury, G. (1987b) Vulvo-vaginal melanoma – should radical surgery be abandoned? *British Journal of Obstetrics and Gynaecology*, **94**, 473–6.

Dent, D.M., Madden, M.V. and Price, S.K. (1988) Randomised comparison of R1 and R2 gastrectomy for gastric cancer. *British Journal of Surgery*, **75**, 110–12.

Dixon, J.M. (1993) Screening for breast cancer. *British Journal of Surgery*, **80**, 141–2.

Earlam, R. and Cuhna-Melo, R.C. (1982) Malignant oesophageal strictures: a review of techniques for palliative intubation. *British Journal of Surgery*, **69**, 61–8.

Elias, E.G. (1989) *CRC Handbook of Surgical Oncology*, CRC Press, Boca Raton, pp. 5–7.

Fallowfield, L.J., Baum, M. and Maguire, G.P. (1986) Effects of breast conservation on psychological morbidity associated with the diagnosis and treatment of early breast cancer. *British Medical Journal*, **293**, 1331–4.

Fentiman, I.S., Millis, R.R., Chaudary, M.A. *et al.* (1986) Effect of the method of biopsy on the prognosis of and reliability of receptor assays in patients with operable breast cancer. *British Journal of Surgery*, **73**, 610–12.

Fisher, B., Anderson, S., Fisher, E.R. *et al.* (1991) Significance of ipsilateral breast tumour recurrence after lumpectomy. *Lancet*, **338**, 327–31.

Frisell, J., Eklund, G., Hellstrom, L. *et al.* (1991) Randomised study of mammography screening: preliminary report on mortality in the Stockholm trial. *Breast Cancer Research and Treatment*, **18**, 49–56.

Halsted, W.J. (1907) The results of radical operations for the cure of cancer of the breast. *Annals of Surgery*, **46**, 1–27.

Kettlewell, M.G.W. (1991) Endoscopic transanal resection for rectal cancer. *International Journal of Colorectal Disease*, **6**, 82–3.

Kissin, M.W., Fisher, C., Carter, R.L. *et al.* (1986) The value of trucut needle biopsy in the diagnosis of soft tissue tumours. *British Journal of Surgery*, **73**, 742–4.

Kissin, M.W. and Williamson, R.C.N. (1990) The role of surgery, in *Treatment of Cancer*, 2nd edn, (eds K. Sikora and K.E. Halnan), Chapman & Hall, London, pp. 29–52.

MacFarlane, J.K., Ryall, R.D.H. and Heald, R.J. (1993) Mesorectal excision for rectal cancer. *Lancet*, **341**, 457–60.

Moskovitz, M. (1990) The peritoneovenous shunt: expectations and reality. *American Journal of Gastroenterology*, **85**, 917–29.

Nagorney, D.M. (1991) Opinion: resection of hepatic metastasis for colorectal cancer. *Journal of Surgical Oncology Supplement*, **2**, 74–5.

Pettavel, J., Costa, J., Douglas, P. *et al.* (1989) Surgery in the treatment of recurrent and metastatic cancer, in: *Surgical Oncology: A European Handbook*, (ed. U. Veronesi), Springer-Verlag, Berlin, pp. 131–41.

Sacks, N.P.M., Barr, L.C., Allen, S.M. *et al.* (1992) The role of axillary dissection in operable breast cancer. *The Breast*, **1**, 41–9.

Scheele, J. (1993) Hepatectomy for liver metastases. *British Journal of Surgery*, **80**, 274–6.

Scott, R.N. and McKay, A.J. (1993) Elective lymph node dissection in the management of malignant melanoma. *British Journal of Surgery*, **80**, 284–8.

Shepherd, H.A., Royle, G., Ross, A.P.R. *et al.* (1988) Endoscopic biliary endoprosthesis in the palliation of malignant obstruction of the distal common bile duct: a randomised trial. *British Journal of Surgery*, **75**, 1166–8.

Skrabanek, P. (1988) Cervical cancer screening: the time for reappraisal. *Canadian Journal of Public Health*, **79**, 86–9.

Soo, K.C., Davidson, T.I., Selby, P. *et al.* (1985) Long-term venous access using a subcutaneous implantable drug delivery system. *Annals of the Royal College of Surgeons of England*, **67**, 263–5.

Speer, A.G., Cotton, P.B., Russell, C.G. *et al.* (1987) Randomized trial of endoscopic versus percutaneous stent insertion in malignant obstructive jaundice. *Lancet*, **i**, 57–62.

Stotter, A., Atkinson, E.N., Fairston, B.A. *et al.* (1990) Survival following locoregional recurrence after breast conservation therapy for cancer. *Annals of Surgery*, **212**, 166–72.

Tubiana, M. (1992) The role of local treatment in the cure of cancer. *European Journal of Cancer*, **28A**, 2061–9.

Veronesi, U. (1989) The role of surgery in cancer treatment, in: *Surgical Oncology: A European Handbook*, (ed. U. Veronesi), Springer–Verlag, Berlin, pp. 1–6.

Walsh, H.P.J. and Schofield, P.F. (1984) Is laparotomy for small bowel obstruction justified in patients with previously treated malignancy? *British Journal of Surgery*, **71**, 933–5.

Wanebo, H.J., Feldman, P.S., Morton, C. *et al.* (1984) Fine needle aspiration cytology in lieu of open biopsy in management of primary breast cancer. *Annals of Surgery*, **199**, 569–79.

David P. Dearnaley

9.1 INTRODUCTION

Irradiation has been used in the management of cancer since the turn of the century. Currently radiotherapy is given to about half of the 200 000 patients who develop cancer in the UK each year (Welsh Office, 1989). It has a curative role in two-thirds of these patients, either used alone or in conjunction with surgery or chemotherapy. In addition radiotherapy has an important palliative role in those patients who go on to develop recurrent or metastatic disease, particularly for the relief of pain, bleeding or symptoms from compression of vital structures such as the spinal cord.

The role of radiotherapy for a particular tumour type is determined partly by the average radiosensitivity of the tumour relative to adjacent normal tissues and partly by the probability that the tumour is localized, as listed below:

Radiotherapy has a curative role for squamous cell carcinomas of the head and neck, cervix, anal canal and skin. Localized carcinomas of the bladder and prostate may also be eradicated using radiotherapy alone, as may more radiosensitive tumour types such as early stage Hodgkin's and non-Hodgkin's lymphoma, seminoma and some brain tumours such as medulloblastoma and ependymoma.

1. Curative as sole treatment for:
   (a) Head and neck cancers
   (b) Cancer of the cervix
   (c) Anal and skin cancer
   (d) Bladder cancer
   (e) Prostate cancer
   (f) Early lung cancer
   (g) Seminoma
   (h) Hodgkin's disease and non-Hodgkin's lymphoma
   (i) Meduloblastoma and some other brain tumours
   (j) Thyroid cancer.
2. Component of multimodality curative treatment:
   (a) Breast cancer
   (b) Rectal cancer
   (c) Soft tissue sarcoma
   (d) Advanced head and neck cancer
   (e) Whole body radiotherapy before bone marrow transplants.
3. Palliative radiotherapy:
   (a) Pain, especially bone metastases
   (b) Bleeding, e.g. haemoptysis, haematuria
   (c) Spinal cord compression
   (d) Brain metastases
   (e) Venous or lymphatic obstruction
   (f) Primary brain tumour, e.g. high and low grade astrocytomas.

Radiotherapy may be used as an adjunct to conservative surgery to secure local disease control in the treatment of breast cancer, rectal cancer and soft tissue sarcomas, and needs to be integrated into multimodality curative treatments when adjuvant chemotherapy is to be used in addition.

Judgements as to the most appropriate treatment for an individual require a detailed clinical and radiological assessment of each patient and their tumour so as to be able to accurately define the extent and stage of disease as well as the suitability of an individual patient for a particular treatment approach.

For many cancers the balance between different treatment modalities is still being evaluated and a clear understanding of the results of clinical trials is important in view of the speed and frequency with which treatment advances are brought into clinical practice. Treatment decisions for an individual patient are compounded by the requirement for medical and psychological support for co-incidental or treatment related problems and attention must also be given to the anxiety and stress experienced by patients and their relatives at the prospect of a life threatening illness. All of these facets of patient management are the remit of the radiotherapist. In the UK radiotherapists are often also responsible for chemotherapy and the breadth of management responsibility has lead to the renaming of the speciality as clinical oncology.

9.2   THE BASIS OF IRRADIATION PRACTICE

9.2.1   X-RAY PRODUCTION AND RADIOACTIVITY

X-rays are emitted when high speed electrons hit high atomic weight targets such as a tantalum. The early kilovoltage machines produced electrons from heated metal filaments but modern megavoltage (MV) linear accelerators use a radiowave guide to further accelerate electrons produced in this way to bombard the target at high energy producing X-rays in the range of 4–24 MeV (million electron volts). Alternatively suitable radionuclides may be utilized for therapeutic purposes. These radioactive atoms have unstable nuclei which release energy in the process of spontaneous disintegration. This may be in the form of gamma rays which are identical to X-rays or in the form of high speed electrons or other particles. A variety of isotopes are available for medical usage (Tables 9.1, 9.2). Cobalt-60 produces gamma rays of approximate energy of 1,2 MeV and is suitable for both external beam irradiation or intracavitary treatment and other isotopes such as iridium-192, caesium-137 and gold-198 are used for interstitial and intracavitary purposes. The final possibility is to administer isotopes systemically or onto body cavities. Localization of the isotopes in or around the tumour may be on a metabolic basis, for example, iodine-131 to treat thyroid cancer or localization may be attempted by tagging the radionuculide to monoclonal anti-

Table 9.1   Radionuclides used in brachytherapy

Isotope	Caesium-137	Cobalt-60	Gold-98	Iodine-125	Iridium-192	Radium-226
Half-life	30 yr	5.3 yr	2.7 d	60 d	74 d	1600 yr
Emission used in therapy	Photon	Photon	Photon	Photon	Photon	Photon
Energy (MeV)	0.66	1.17,1.33	0.41	0.027–0.032	0.3–0.6	0.18-2.2

Table 9.2   Radionuclides used in unsealed sources

Isotope	Iodine-131	Phosphorus-32	Strontium-89	Rhenium-186	Yttrium-90
Half-life	8.0 d	14.3 d	50.5 d	3.8 d	2.7 d
Emission used in therapy	Electron/photon	Electron	Electron	Electron	Electron
Energy (MeV)	0.19*/0.36*	0.70*	0.58	0.36	0.93

* Most abundant radiation.

bodies, although the dream of this 'magic bullet' approach has not been fulfilled due to a range of practical and technical difficulties.

Radiation dose is defined as the amount of energy absorbed per unit mass of tissue. This is measured in Gray (Gy) which represents the absorption of 1 joule per kilogram the previous used unit of absorbed dose was the rad, 100 rad = 1 Gray.

9.2.2 BIOLOGICAL EFFECTS OF IONIZING RADIATION

Irradiation with photons (X-rays or gamma rays), electrons or high energy particles such as neutrons or pions interact indirectly or directly with tissue to produce short lived ion radicals. These damage nuclear DNA leading eventually to cell death, which may occur rapidly, or after several cell divisions when disturbance of DNA synthesis has led to abnormal mitosis. Cells whose mitotic cycle time is short will show signs of radiation damage more quickly than those whose cycle time is long. Considerable variation exist in the radiosensitivity of different tumours. For example, with conventionally fractionated radiotherapy a dose of about 25 Gy is required to control a 2 cm seminoma, a dose of 35–40 Gy to control a 2 cm lymphoma and 60–65 Gy to control a squamous cell carcinoma. Doses of 70 Gy would not control an astrocytoma of similar size. Radiosensitivity can be similarly ranked in the laboratory with cell lines derived from human tumours and can be conveniently expressed as the proportion of cells surviving after a 2 Gy fraction of irradiation (Table 9.3) (Deacon, *et al.*, 1984). The biological basis for this intriguing variation is complex and imperfectly understood. In the laboratory, cell survival curves show an initial 'shoulder' region followed by a more rapidly falling exponential component (Figure 9.1). This shoulder region represents an ability to accumulate and repair an amount of 'sublethal' radiation damage. Differences in this repair capacity between tumours may be part of the explanation for the different radioresponsiveness of different tumours, particularly during fractionated treatment using relatively low radiation doses when the shoulder on the cell survival curve is reconstituted after each radiation dose (Figure 9.1) (McMillan, 1989). However, it has been suggested by some authors that the level of DNA damage induction by radiation may be the primary determinant of radiosensitivity (Radford, 1986). It is also clear that the rate

Table 9.3 Radio responsiveness of human tumours

Clinical radio responsiveness			In vitro *radio responsiveness of human tumour cell lines* (*Surviving fractions after 2 Gy*)
Radiosensitive	A.	Lymphoma, myeloma, neuroblastoma	0.19
	B.	Small cell lung cancer, medulloblastoma	0.22
	C.	Cervix, bladder, breast carcinoma	0.46
	D.	Colorectal, pancreas, squamous lung carcinoma	0.43
Radioresistant	E.	Renal carcinoma, melanoma, osteosarcoma, glioblastoma	0.52

Modified from Deacon *et al.*, 1984.

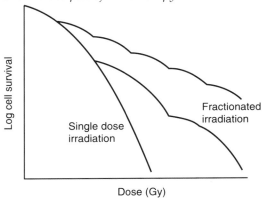

Figure 9.1 Multidose compared with single dose irradiation survival curves. The proportion of cells surviving for a given dose increases with decreasing fraction size dose due to repair of sublethal damage between irradiation exposures. Increasing fractionation 'dissociates' early and late normal tissue reactions and may improve the therapeutic ratio.

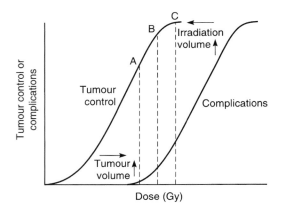

Figure 9.2 Dose–response curves for tumour control and complications. Small changes in dose have major effects on steep part of sigmoid curves. Optimal dose (B) gives high tumour control with low complication rate – further increases in dose (C) produce little improvement in control at expense of high complication rate. Suboptimal dose (A) significantly reduces tumour control.

at which a tumour can regrow or repopulate, the degree of oxygenation and cell cycle effects (cells are most radiosensitive in mitosis and G2 phase and most resistant in late S and G1) have significant influences on the radio-responsiveness of tumours. Similarly, normal tissues show varying sensitivity both to the degree and timing of radiation damage. Generally 'acute' reactions occur within 3 months of treatment, 'late reactions' occur at more protracted intervals. Tissues having a high proliferative rate, such as skin and mucosal surfaces, express damage more rapidly (acute reacting), whereas slowly dividing tissue are late reacting. In particular it is possible that damage to endothelial cells is responsible for many of the late radiation effects apparent clinically (Hopewell *et al.*, 1989).

The dose–response curves for both normal tissues and malignant tumours are sigmoid in shape (Figure 9.2) and relatively small changes in dose can have major implications for both tumour control or normal tissue complications. In clinical practice we wish to judge the optimum dose to obtain complica-

tion-free control, but of course in reality the exact position of these dose–response curves is not known for any individual patient or their tumour. The relative position of these curves depends critically on the tumour and target volume irradiated. The probability of local control decreases with increasing tumour volume and the incidence of complications rises as large volumes of normal tissue are included in the radiation fields. The situation can readily be envisaged when dose–effect curves cross with increasing tumour volume and therefore radiotherapy target volume. Dose limitation due to the radiosensitivity of normal tissues such as small bowel, lung or spinal cord, limits the total dose that can be safely given, so limiting the radiocurability of tumours.

9.2.3 DOSE AND FRACTIONATION

It was realized by pioneering French radiotherapists in the 1920s that the effects of a given total dose of irradiation on tumours as well as normal tissues could be dramatically modified by dividing it into smaller parts or fractions. Empirically fractionated treatment regimes were developed which allowed for higher total doses to be delivered obtaining better local tumour control but without a high incidence of normal tissue damage. Why should using shall fraction sizes 'spare' normal tissue rather than tumour? A simple explanation is based on the four **r**'s of radiobiology:

1. Repair of sublethal damage
2. Re-assortment of cells within the cell cycle
3. Repopulation
4. Re-oxygenation.

Fractionated treatment spares normal tissue because sublethal damage is repaired between daily fractions of treatment and normal tissues are allowed to repopulate if the overall treatment time is sufficiently long. Many tumours have a relatively poor blood supply and contain hypoxic regions which are relatively resistant to radiotherapy. Increasing the treatment time using a fractionated regimen allows surviving hypoxic tumour cells to re-oxygenate and additionally cells are allowed to re-assort into the more radiosensitive phases of the cell cycle.

In general the dose of radiotherapy given in clinical practice is determined by the tolerance of normal tissues rather than the tumour control probability. The tolerance dose for late and acutely reacting normal tissues are 'dissociated' in that a severe acute tissue reaction is not necessarily followed by severe late tissue damage. Late tissue damage is more sensitive to increases in fraction size than acutely reacting tissues (Hall, 1988) and this has led to the adoption of 'conventional' 2 Gy treatment fractions in many centres. However, it must be admitted that there is by no means consensus on optimal radiotherapy regimens for any particular tumour type or site. '**Conventional**' radical radiotherapy to an epithelial tumour would be with a total dose of 60–70 Gy given in 2 Gy daily treatments, five times per week.

Accelerated treatment aims to overcome tumour repopulation as a potential cause of radioresistance. The same total and number of radiation fractions are used but treating twice per day so as to reduce the overall treatment time. **Hyperfractionated** treatment aims to improve the therapeutic ratio by reducing the dose given in each treatment, thereby relatively reducing late side-effects and permitting an increase in total dose to increase tumour control. So that the overall treatment time is not prolonged two or more treatments need to be given each day. **Hypofractionated** treatment gives a smaller number of radiation fractions but the dose per fraction is increased. However, the total dose delivered must be lower than with 'conventional' fractionation because of enhanced late normal tissue reactions. This potentially deleterious effect on tumour control may be balanced in some circumstances by the overall shortened duration of treatment as radical hypofractionated treatments, if given on a daily basis, will also be accelerated (Sutton and Hendry, 1985). Hypofractionated treatments are convenient for radiotherapy departments and patients alike and are recommended for almost all palliative treatments. Examples of standard and investigational treatment schedules are given in Table 9.4.

9.3 RADIATION TECHNIQUES

Radiotherapy treatments aim to deliver an homogeneous dose of irradiation to an accurately localized tumour volume and to minimize the effect on the surrounding normal tissue. This requires the target volume to be defined as accurately as possible from clinical examination, radiological investigations which frequently includes CT scans, and from a knowledge of the natural history and patterns of spread of any particular type of malignancy. The choice of the most appropriate management strategy for an individual patient

Table 9.4 Examples of standard and investigational[†] radiotherapy schedules for radical and palliative treatments

Radical treatments	Dose (Gy)	Fraction (no.)	Time	
Conventional fractionation	64	32	6.5 wk	Head and neck tumours, bladder cancer, prostate cancer
Hypofractionation (Manchester School)	50–55*	16	21 d	
Accelerated treatment[†] (RMH Trial)	60.8	32	26 d	Bladder cancer
Hyperfractionated treatment[†] (Horiot, *et al.*, 1992)	80.5	70	7 wk	Oropharygeal cancer
CHART[†] (Continuous Hyperfractionated Accelerated Radiotherapy)	54	36	12 d	Head and neck tumours Lung tumours
(Saunders and Dische, 1990; Saunders, *et al.*, 1989)				
Palliative treatments‡				
Conventional	30	10	2 wk	Control of pain from bone metastases
hypofractionated (Price *et al.*, 1986)	8	1	1 d	
Conventional	30	10	2 wk	Brain metastases
hypofractionated (RCR § Trial)	12	2	2d	
Conventional	30	10	2 wk	Lung cancer
hypofractionated (Medical Research	17	2	7 d	
Council, 1991; Bleehen, *et al.*, 1992)	10	1	1 d	

* Dependent on volume treated (Sutton and Hendry, 1985).
† Investigational.
‡ Randomized studies have shown clinical equivalence between these radiotherapy schedules.
§ Royal College of Radiologists.

requires close cooperation between the clinical oncologist and colleagues in histopathology and diagnostic radiology. The successful implementation of a radiation treatment depends critically on the cooperation and team work between clinician, medical physicists, therapy radiographers and the support of the mould room technicians.

9.3.1 EXTERNAL BEAM IRRADIATION

(a) Photons

Radiation beams are produced by small targets or sources usually 1 m from the patient. The dose at any point within the tissue is determined both by the distance from the target or source (following an inverse square relationship) and the attenuation of the irradiation within the tissue. Figure 9.3 shows a typical isodose distribution produced from a linear accelerator. Photons are described as indirectly ionizing. They do not produce chemical and biological damage themselves but give up their energy when absorbed to produce fast moving electrons. The process of absorption varies with the photon energy. At low energies the photoelectric process dominates which varies with the cube of the atomic number (Z^3) of the tissue and results in the clear distinction between bone, soft tissue and air interfaces

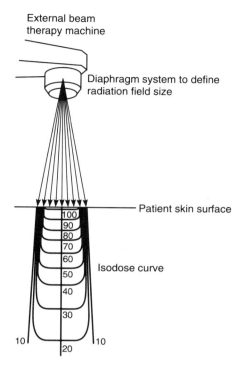

External beam
therapy machine

Diaphragm system to define
radiation field size

Patient skin surface

Isodose curve

100
90
80
70
60
50
40
30
10   10
20

Figure 9.3 Typical dose distribution from a linear accelerator. The radiation field size is defined by collimators and diaphragms close to the target. Note the `skin sparing effect', the 100% isodose is below the skin surface.

treatment. Higher photon energies penetrate tissue more deeply and so megavoltage beams are essential for the optimal treatment of deeply seated tumours. Additionally there is no increase in bone absorption at megavoltage energies, as is the case with lower energies, and megavoltage treatments are associated with 'skin sparing' meaning that the maximum dose is delivered just below the surface. This is because electrons created by the interaction of photons with tissue travel some distance before they deposit their energy; these distances are very small with superficial and orthovoltage energies and skin frequently becomes the dose limiting normal tissue.

(b)   Radiotherapy planning

Superficial X-rays are used to treat, for example, skin cancers. Megavoltage irradiation is used to treat more deeply sited tumours, for example tumours within the abdomen, pelvis and thorax. It is important that the tumour dose is relatively homogeneous as the minimum dose in the target volume determines the probability of treatment failure and the maximum dose, the probability of radiation induced complications. This is achieved by using two or more radiation beams which treat the patient from predetermined fixed positions; alternatively rotational or arcing techniques may be employed. A composite isodose plan is drawn up from the isodose distributions from the individual beams (Figure 9.6). Beam characteristics may be modified by using wedges or compensators (Figures 9.5 and 9.6). This is necessary when angled fields are used or when there are significant changes in the patient's outline or contour. The dimensions of the rectangular radiation treatment beam are determined by the thick secondary collimators on the therapy machine head. These beams may be further shaped by placing lead or alloy blocks in the beam path of the irradiation portals to follow

visible on diagnostic X-rays. At megavoltage energies photons are absorbed by the Compton process which is dependent on electron density rather than atomic number and explains why at these energies there is little difference in absorption between bone and soft tissues. In clinical practice the term superficial irradiation is used to describe photon energies up to approximately 150 KeV, orthovoltage treatment uses photon energies of approximately 300 KeV and megavoltage treatment uses cobalt sources (1.2 MeV) or now more commonly 4–18 MeV photons produced from linear accelerators. Typical dose distributions are shown in Figures 9.4 and 9.5. There are important difference between these classes of radiation

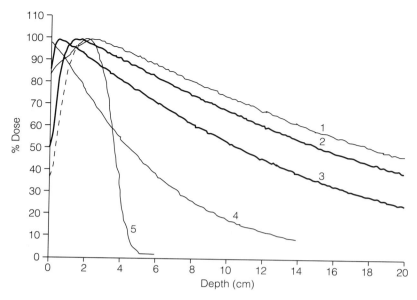

Figure 9.4 Dose distributions for photon and electron beams: 1, 10 MV photon beam; 2, 6 MV photon beam; 3, ^{60} Co; 4, 160 KV photon beam; 5, 10 MeV electron beam.

the intended treatment volume. This is a routine procedure when treating with anterior and posterior opposing beams, e.g. in the treatment of lymph nodes in seminoma or Hodgkin's disease (Chapters 18 and 34), but more sophisticated techniques are required for the shaping of complex field arrangements to cover irregularly shaped tumour and target

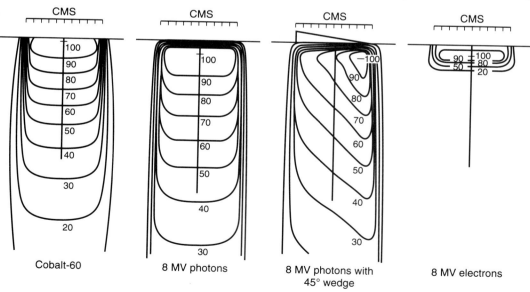

Isodose distributions for megavoltage photon and electron beam treatment

Figure 9.5 Isodose distributions for megavoltage photon and electron beam treatment.

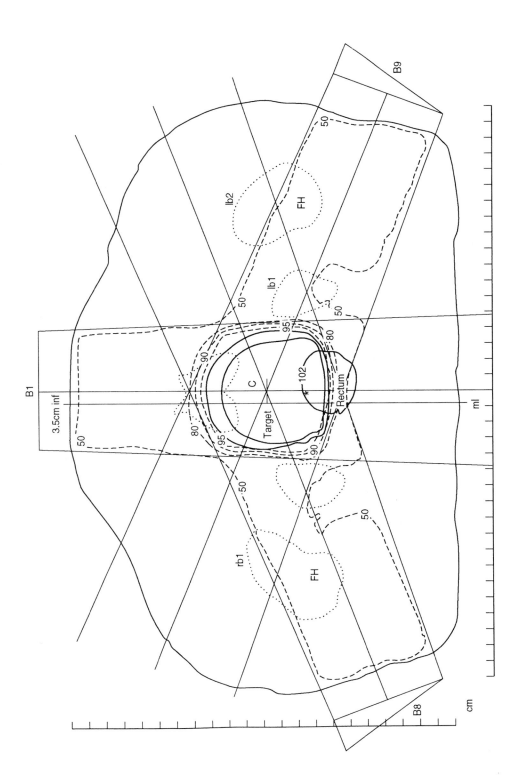

Figure 9.6 Three field plan for treatment of prostate cancer using anterior and posterior oblique treatment fields. Dose at isocentre (C) is 100%. Dose to the posterior rectal wall and femoral heads (FH) is limited to 50%.

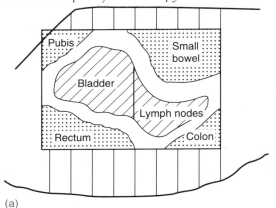

(a)

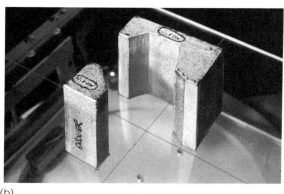

(b)

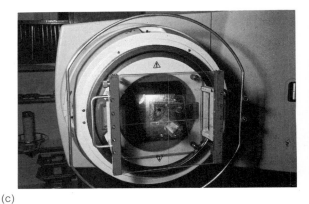

(c)

Figure 9.7 (**a**) Schematic representation of 3-D planning for bladder cancer and pelvic lymph nodes from several CT slices. Lateral view is shown. Customized blocks are made from low melting point alloy (cerrobend) (**b**) and (**c**) mounted on templates to shape radiation fields (**c**).

volumes which require the three-dimensional reconstruction of tumour and target volumes from CT images (Figure 9.7).

The steps involved in the implementation of external beam irradiation treatment are:

1. Tumour localization
2. Determination of target volume
3. Localization of target volume with reference to patient contour and skin markers
4. Production of radiation isodose plan
5. Dose prescription
6. Simulation of planned fields
7. Verification of radiotherapy fields on linear accelerator (LINAC)
8. Treatment delivery.

Clinical examination and radiological methods, most particularly including CT and more recently MRI, are used to gain full informa-

tion on the local site and extent of tumour spread. The volume of tissue to be irradiated is determined from these findings and from a knowledge of the patterns of spread and sites of recurrence for each tumour type. The target volume includes the tumour and margin of surrounding tissue which might be expected to contain microscopic spread. Additionally the margin must allow for a variety of technical factors. These include:

1. The limitation in accuracy of radiological techniques in defining tumour.
2. The accuracy of definition of the target volume within an outline of the body contour.
3. The accuracy and reproducibility of simulator and linear accelerator positioning.
4. An allowance for patient movement during planning and treatment, as well as

5. Movement of the tumour within the patient.

The reproducibility of patient positioning is a crucial factor in delivering accurate treatments and when sensitive normal tissue structures, such as spinal cord or brain, are adjacent to the treatment areas, such as in head and neck and brain tumours, fixation devices are used to hold the patient as still as possible (Figure 9.8).

Following the definition of an appropriate target volume this must be localized within an outline of the patient's contour with reference to readily identifiable skin markers or tattoos (Figure 9.9). This is essential as the positioning of radiation beams must always be made with reference to fixed and identifiable marks on the patient's surface. A radiation isodose plan is then produced (Figure 9.6) where the beam positions can be related to surface marks on the patient. The radiotherapy dose prescription is then defined detailing the radiation dose to be delivered

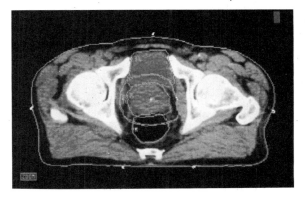

Figure 9.9 CT localization of prostate cancer. The prostate (P) has been outlined and the target volume (TV) drawn with a 1 cm margin. Sensitive normal tissue structures bladder (BL) and rectum (R) are additionally outlined. Anterior and lateral tattoos are marked with barium paste to aid localization.

from each beam during the radiotherapy treatment. It is now standard practice to take the reference point for dose prescription to be at the isocentre (i.e. at the point of intersection) of the radiation beams rather than prescribing to an arbitrary 'maximum' or 'minimum' dose. The size, shape and orientation of the planned radiation fields are then checked on the simulator and the patient proceeds to treatment on the linear accelerator. To ensure that the correct dose and field arrangements are used on each treatment, computerized verification sustems have been developed; additionally 'check' films may be taken on the linear accelerator using either films or more recently electronic portal imaging devices (EPID). The quality of these images is poor because of the lack of discrimination of megavoltage beams between bone and soft tissue interfaces; nevertheless, they give a final check on the accuracy of treatment delivery.

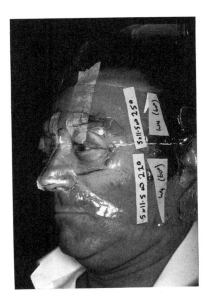

Figure 9.8 Immobilization cast or shell used to ensure accurate patient positioning for radiotherapy of head and neck or brain tumours. The position of radiation fields is marked on the cast.

(c) Electrons

Linear accelerators may be also used to produce therapeutic electron beams. The narrow primary electron beam in linear accelerator is scattered by foil rather than hitting the usual target and is then collimated to produce a beam of the required shape. Electrons are directly ionizing and have a finite rage in tissue (Figures 9.4 and 9.5). Unlike photons the dose distribution of electrons shows a well-defined plateau, and the distance of the 90% isodose from the skin surface in centimetres is approximately one-third of the electron beam energy in MeV. There is a 'tail' on the dose distribution due to the secondary production of low energy X-rays (bremmstrahlung effect) which increases at higher energies. The well-defined peak of energy distribution is useful if a rapid fall off in dose distribution is required (e.g. in boost treatments in breast cancer and in the treatment of tumours adjacent to the spinal cord), but it must be noted that electron beams give a small degree of 'skin sparing' which unlike X-rays is more pronounced with low energies. This must be remembered when treating superficial tumours where wax 'build-up' may be required to shift the 100% isodose to the skin surface.

9.3.2 BRACHYTHERAPY

In this type of treatment radioactive sources are placed immediately adjacent to or within a tumour. High dosage is given to the immediate area, with a rapid fall off in intensity with increasing distance from the sources (Figure 9.10) which follows an inverse square law. Accurate placement of sources is therefore essential if the tumour volume is to be adequately encompassed whilst sparing surrounding critical normal tissue structures. Radium was initially used and dose expressed in mg radium hours (i.e. amount of radium × time of treatment). Subsequently systems have been developed which describe the appropriate positioning and activity of sources to achieve a particular dose at defined reference points. For endocavitary treatment of cervix cancer the Manchester system (Cole and Hunter, 1985) defines point A in the paracervical triangle as being 2 cm lateral to the central canal of the uterus and 2 cm proximal to the lateral fornix with the second reference dosage point, point B, as being 3 cm lateral to point A and in the same plane.

Increasing awareness of the radiation protection difficulties caused by radium, and in particular its daughter product radon gas, led to the search for safer artificial isotopes. Additionally, in order to reduce the radiation dosage to operator, theatre and nursing staff, 'after-loading' systems have been developed which allow more careful placement of the interstitial or intracavitary devices whose position can be checked radiographically before the radioactive sources are inserted into the applicators (Figures 9.10 and 9.11). This may be done manually, which has advantages for those working in theatre, but does nothing to reduce the radiation exposure of nursing staff. Alternatively, and preferably, radioactive sources are remotely introduced from a protective safe. Many such systems are now commercially available and suitable isotopes include caesium-137, cobalt-60 and iridium-192 (Table 9.1). The Paris system of dosimetry (Pierquin *et al.*, 1978) was developed for use with iridium sources of uniform linear activity, and now modern systems can provide computer generated isodose distributions. The previous radium based treatments used a low dose rate of approximately 0.5 Gy per hour to point A, and in the Manchester system two insertions of approximately 70 hours were given over a total time of 10 days to give a total point A dose of 75 Gy (Cole and Hunter, 1985). A variety of high dose rate (1–2 Gy/min) remote after-loading devices are now available which allow the total treatment to be given in a matter of minutes rather than several days. This has the advantage of allowing treatments to be given on a out-patient basis and minimizes the movement of sources and applicators during therapy. Dis-

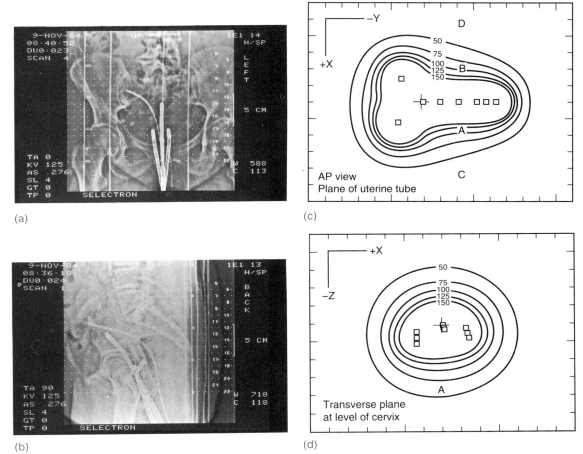

Figure 9.10 Intracavitary irradiation of cervix cancer with uterine tube and vaginal ovoids. Anteroposterior (**a**) and lateral (**b**) radiographs. Rectal catheter containing lithium fluoride has been placed to measure dose. Note proximity of anterior rectal wall and sigmoid colon to sources. Rapid fall off in dose is seen in isodose distributions (**c**) and (**d**).

advantages include the need for special shielding around the high dose rate sources, which is similar to that required for tele-therapy cobalt-60 sources, and additionally it is essential that treatments are fractionated and that adjustments in total dose are made to account for the increased radiobiological effect of high dose rate therapy (Perez and Glasgow, 1987; Hall and Brenner, 1992). With these adjustments results appear equivalent both in terms of disease control and com-plication rate to conventional low dose rate systems (Utley *et al.*, 1984).

9.3.3 IRRADIATION FROM UNSEALED SOURCES

There is a limited place in clinical practice for the use of systematically administered radionuclides. The best example is of the use of iodine-131 in the treatment of thyroid cancer and thyrotoxicosis. Well-differentiated primary and metastatic thyroid cancer takes up radio-iodine avidly and very high local activities may be obtained provided any normal thyroid remnant has been ablated. Such treatment is the best clinical example of

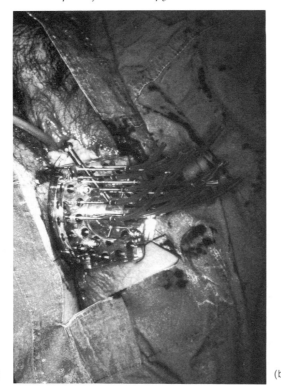

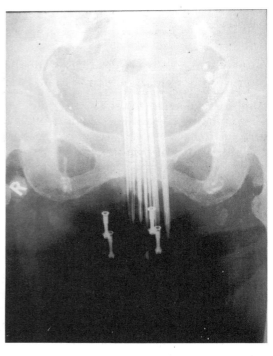

(a) (b)

Figure 9.11 Interstitial implant for vaginal carcinoma. Lucite template is sewn to perineum and guide wires introduced (**a**). Check films show satisfactory positioning (**b**) prior to loading with iridium-192. Similar techniques are suitable for treatment of carcinomas of anal canal, prostate and parametrial infiltration from cervix cancer.

a 'targeted' isotope therapy which localizes in and around tumours following a natural metabolic pathway. Other examples of 'metabolic targeting' include phosphorus-32 for the treatment of polycythemia rubra vera, strontium-89 which localizes to areas of osteoblastic bone metastases and MIBG which is metabolized and taken up by neuroendocrine tumours such as neuroblastoma. Radioactive colloids such as phosphorus-32 or gold-198 may be of value in the palliation of patients with ascites and have been used to treat patients with early stage ovarian cancer instilling the isotope into the abdominal cavity. The distribution of activity achieved by these techniques is, however, very variable. Much hope was centered on the expectation that monoclonal antibodies conjugated to isotopes

would prove of significant value in targeting therapy but these hopes have not yet been realized due to the relatively low affinity and poor uptake of antibody isotope conjugates in and around tumours.

9.3.4 DRUG AND RADIATION INTERACTIONS

Pharmacological agents may interact with radiation in a variety of ways, and much current interest centres on how drugs and irradiation can be combined in an optimal fashion (Steel and Peckham, 1979). The aim of such combinations may be either to produce an improvement in the therapeutic ratio of local treatment or to produce 'spatial cooperation' where the intention is for systemic chemotherapy to eradicate generalized micrometastases, using local irradiation to control the tumour at the primary (or sanctuary) site.

(a)   Drug and radiotherapy interactions for improvement of local tumour control

Although the combination of drugs and irradiation may well have an enhanced effect on tumour control, the therapeutic ratio will only be improved if less enhancement is seen in normal tissues than the tumour. In studies of combined modality treatments it is therefore essential to document both tumour control and normal tissue toxicity.

Cytotoxic chemotherapy and radiotherapy

Many studies have been undertaken to assess the possible benefits of combined modality treatments in advanced localized tumours, but few have as yet shown any convincing evidence of improvement in therapeutic ratio. There is an extensive literature on the combination of radiation and chemotherapy using methotrexate, 5FU and cisplatinum, but despite undoubted clinical responses to chemotherapy results have generally been negative (Carter *et al.*, 1987; Stell and Rawson, 1990). These studies have most commonly used sequential drug and radiation protocols, but using concomitant treatment with methotrexate the Christie Hospital Group have suggested an advantage for this approach in advanced head and neck cancers (Gupta *et al.*, 1987). Concomitant chemo-irradiation may also be advantageous at other sites and a randomized study in squamous cell carcinoma of the oesophagus (Herskovic *et al.*, 1992) using concomitant cisplatin and 5FU showed a significant improvement in local control and survival despite an increase in treatment toxicity. Further studies are being undertaken, e.g. with 5FU in cancer of the anal canal and with concomitant cisplatin and irradiation for bladder cancer.

(b)   'Spatial cooperation'

If the desired interaction is one of spatial co-operation it seems probable that drug and irradiation should be separated as far as possible in time so as to avoid adverse toxicity and that the correct strategy is to give optimal chemotherapy and radiotherapy independently to the relevant areas of disease. It appears that it is safer to give chemotherapy first, so as to reduce adverse reactions that can be seen, e.g., following concomitant administration of methotrexate and brain irradiation (Bleyer, 1981) or the sequence of initial abdominal pelvic irradiation followed by cisplatinum combination chemotherapy (Yarnold *et al.*, 1983). A good example of the value of this type of combined modality treatment approach is in the use of prophylactic brain irradiation in acute leukaemia, the central nervous system being a 'sanctuary' site from most chemotherapy agents. For the common 'solid' tumours meta-analysis has shown reduction in the development of distant metastases and improved survival following adjuvant treatment with both hormone and chemotherapy for breast cancer (Early Breast Cancer Trialists' Collaborative Group, 1992a,b) and currently multicentre studies are assessing the impact of adjuvant chemotherapy in, for example, bladder and cervical cancer.

9.4   FUTURE DEVELOPMENTS IN RADIOTHERAPY

Current radiotherapy practice gives excellent results for many patients; nevertheless failure to obtain local tumour control remains a significant problem, particularly for tumours which present at an advanced stage of disease. In the USA, it has been estimated that approximately 200 000 patients per year do not have their primary tumour successfully controlled, the equivalent number for the UK being approximately one-fifth of this or 40 000 patients per year (Suit and Urie, 1992).

There is considerable scope for improving survival rates from cancer by increasing the effectiveness of local treatment using radiotherapy alone or in combination with other treatment modalities (Suit, 1982). Improvements in results can be expected to develop from two complementary approaches, first the 'biological' optimization of radiotherapy dose and fractionation and secondly from improvements in technology of treatment delivery and in particular 'conformal' radiotherapy.

9.4.1 BIOLOGICAL OPTIMIZATION

An important goal of current research is to determine the molecular basis for underlying differences in radiosensitivity for both tumours and normal tissues. It seems there may be differences in both induction of damage to DNA, and capacity to accurately repair and rejoin DNA strand breaks (Powell and McMillan, 1990). Study of radiosensitivity syndromes such as ataxia telengiectasia (Cox *et al.*, 1986) may be informative and cloning of the responsible gene should help to identify at least one mechanism of radiosensitivity. In the future it may be possible to predict both the sensitivity of tumour and normal tissues on an individual basis using clonogenic or DNA damage assays (Parkins and Horwich, 1989) (Burnet *et al.*, 1992). It is clear that one mechanism of radiation resistance is the rapid proliferation of tumour stem cells during radiotherapy treatment (Trott and Kummermehr, 1985; Withers, 1985). The potential doubling time of tumours may be as short as 2–4 days (Wilson *et al.*, 1988) and during a 7 week course of radiotherapy this allows the number of tumours stem cells to increase by a factor of more than 10^4. Tumour cell repopulation may be particularly efficient at the start of radiotherapy and this has lead to the strategy of exploring 'accelerated' treatment schedules using multiple doses of radiotherapy per day in order to shorten the overall treatment time. Clinical studies using CHART (Continuous Hyperfractionated Accelerated Radiotherapy; Table 9.4) (Saunders *et al.*, 1989; Saunders and Dische, 1990) show potential improvements in local control and this treatment approach is now being tested in multicentre randomized studies. The alternative approach of hyperfractioned treatment (Table 9.4) has also been tested in clinical trials and favourable results reported for both head and neck cancers (Horiot *et al.*, 1992) and bladder cancer (Edsmyr *et al.*, 1985).

9.4.2 PHYSICAL OPTIMIZATION

Conventional radiation planning produces regular geometrically shaped treatment volumes which are defined by the shape of the collimators on the head of the linear accelerator. Cancers have irregular shapes with the result that radiation treatment volumes frequently contain relatively large amounts of normal tissues. Technological developments in imaging using either CT or MRI have made it possible to reconstruct tumours in three dimensions. These advances have been complimented by developments in computer planning software which can produce accurate dose maps in three dimensions. Shaping of the radiotherapy beams produced by linear accelerators can be achieved either by using customized shaped blocks made of low melting point alloy or preferably by multileaved collimators to treat more complex target volumes. These technical advances will allow intricately shaped target volumes to be achieved (Tait, 1990; Webb, 1993). Such precision methods of treatment lead to at least a 50% reduction in the volume of normal tissues treated to high dose. In consequence there is scope for significant improvement in the therapeutic ratio producing either a decrease of acute and late complications for a given dose of radiotherapy or permitting dose escalation with improved local tumour control for the same incidence of side effects. The gain in tumour control probability depends upon the slope of the dose–response curve (Figure 9.2).

Typically a 10% increase in dose results in a 20% increase in local control probability. The expected increase in normal tissue tolerance as a result of conformal dose distributions should permit dose escalations of 10–20% compared with current conventional treatment (Suit and Urie, 1992) and this should therefore translate into a 20–40% improvement in local control rates.

Further clinical studies are needed to confirm the benefit of these exciting developments in radiotherapy technology and biology. It is realistic to expect that such refinements in radiotherapy methods should lead to further improvements in the control of primary tumours and translate into an overall increase in the survival of patients with cancer.

REFERENCES

Bleehen, N.M., Girling, D.J., Machin, D. *et al.* (1992) A Medical Research Council (MRC) randomised trial of palliative radiotherapy with 2 fractions or a single fraction in patients with inoperable non-small-cell lung cancer (NSCLC) and poor performance status. *British Journal of Cancer*, **65**, 934–41.

Bleyer, W.A. (1981) Neurologic sequelea of methotrexate and ionising radiation: a new classification. *Cancer Treatment Reports*, **65** (Suppl 1), 89–98.

Burnet, N.G., Nyman, J., Turesson, I. *et al.* (1992) Prediction of normal-tissue tolerance to radiotherapy from *in-vitro* cellular radiation sensitivity. *Lancet*, **399**, 1570–1.

Carter, S.K., Bakowski, M.T. and Hellmann, K. (1987) Head and neck cancer, in *Chemotherapy of Cancer*, 3rd edn, (eds S.K. Carter, M.T. Bakowski and K. Hellmann), Churchill Livingstone, Edinburgh.

Cole, M.P. and Hunter. R.D. (1985) Female genital tract, in *The Radiotherapy of Malignant Disease*, (eds: E.C. Easson, and R.C.S. Pointon), Springer-Verlag, Berlin.

Cox, R., Debenham, P.G., Masson, W.F. *et al.* (1986) Ataxia-telangiectasia: a mutation giving high frequency of misrepair of DNA double-strand scissions. *Molecular Biology of Medicine*, **3**, 229–44.

Deacon, J., Peckham, M.J. and Steel, G.G. (1984) The radioresponsiveness of human tumours and the initial slope of the cell survival curve. *Radiotherapy and Oncology*, **2**, 317–24.

Early Breast Cancer Trialists' Collaborative Group. (1992a) Systemic treatment of early breast cancer by hormonal, cytotoxic, or immune therapy (Part I). *Lancet*, **339**, (8784), 1–15.

Early Breast Cancer Trialists' Collaborative Group. (1992b) Systemic treatment of early breast cancer by hormonal, cytotoxic, or immune therapy (Part II). *Lancet*, **339**, (8785), 71–85.

Edsmyr, R.F., Anderson, I., Esposti, P.L., *et al.* (1985) Irradiation therapy with multiple small fractions per day in urinary bladder cancer. *Radiotherapy and Oncology*, **4**(3), 197–203.

Gupta, N.K., Pointon, R.C.S. and Wilkinson, P.M. (1987) A randomised clinical trial to contrast radiotherapy with radiotherapy and methotrexate given synchronously in head and neck cancer. *Clinical Radiology*, **38**, 575–81.

Hall, E.J. (1988) Time, dose and fractionation in radiotherapy in, *Radiobiology for the Radiologist*, 3rd edn (eds E.J. Hall, J.B. Lippincott), Philadelphia, pp. 239–59.

Hall, E.J. and Brenner, D.J. (1992) The 1991 George Edelstyn Memorial Lecture: needles, wires and chips – advances in *Brachytherapy*. *Clinical Oncology*, **4** (4), 249–56.

Herskovic, A., Martz, K., al-Sarraf, *et al.* (1992) Combined chemotherapy and radiotherapy compared with radiotherapy alone in patients with cancer of the esophagus. *New England Journal of Medicine*, **326**, 1593–8.

Hopewell, J.W., Calvo, W. and Reinhold, H.S. (1989) Radiation effects on blood vessels: role in late normal tissue damage, in *The Biological Basis of Radiotherapy*, 2nd edn. (eds G.G., Steel, G.E., Adams and A. Horwich), Elsevier, Amsterdam, pp. 101–12.

Horiot, J.C., Le Fur, R., N'Guyen, T. *et al.* (1992) Hyperfractionation versus conventional fractionation in oropharyngeal carcinoma: final analysis of a randomised trial of the EORTC cooperative group of radiotherapy. *Radiotherapy and Oncology*, **25**, 231–41.

McMillan, T.J. (1989) The molecular basis of radiosensitivity, in *The Biological Basis of Radiotherapy*, 2nd edn, (eds G.G., Steel, G.E. Adams and A. Horwich), Elsevier, Amsterdam, pp. 29–44.

Medical Research Council, L.C.W.P. (1991) Inoperable non-small-cell lung cancer (NSCLC): a Medical Research Council randomized trial palliative radiotherapy with two fractions. *British Journal of Cancer*, **63**, 165–70.

Parkins, C. and Horwich, A. (1989) Prediction of tumour response to treatment, in *The Biological Basis of Radiotherapy* (eds G.G. Steel, G.E. Adams and A. Horwich), Elsevier Science, Amsterdam, pp. 305–17.

Perez, C.A. and Glasgow, G.P. (1987) Clinical applications of brachytherapy, in *Principles and Practice of Radiation Oncology*, (eds C.A. Perez, and L.W., Brady), J.B. Lippincott, Philadelphia, pp. 252–90.

Pierquin, B., Dutreix, A., Paine, C.H. *et al.* (1978) The Paris system in interstitial radiation therapy. *Acta Radiologica Oncology*, **17**, 33–48.

Powell, S. and McMillan, T.J. (1990) DNA damage and repair following treatment with ionizing radiation. *Radiotherapy and Oncology*, **19**, 95–108.

Price, P., Hoskin, P.J., Easton, D. *et al.* (1986) Prospective randomized trial of single and multi-fraction schedules in the treatment of painful bone metastases. *Radiotherapy and Oncology*, **6**, 247–55.

Radford, I.R. (1986) Evidence for a general relationship between the induced level of DNA double-strand breakage and cell killing after X-irradiation of mammalian cells. International *Journal of Radiation Biology*, **49**, 611–20.

Saunders, M.I. and Dische, S. (1990) continuous hyperfractionated accelerated radiotherapy (CHART) in non-small cell carcinoma of the bronchus. *International Journal of Radiation Oncology, Biology, Physics*, **19**, 1211–15.

Saunders, M.I., Dische, S., Hong, A. *et al.* (1989) Continuous hyperfractionated accelerated radiotherapy in locally advanced carcinoma of the head and neck region. *International Journal of Radiation Oncology, Biology, Physics*, **17**, 1287–93.

Steel, G.G. and Peckham, M.J. (1979) Exploitable mechanisms in combined radiotherapy–chemotherapy: the concept of additivity. *International Journal of Radiation Oncology, Biology, Physics*, **5**, 85–91.

Stell, P.M. and Rawson, N.Z. (1990) Adjuvant chemotherapy in head and neck cancer. British *Journal of Cancer*, **61**, 779–87.

Suit, H. and Urie, M. (1992) Proton beam in radiation therapy. *Journal of the National Cancer Institute*, **84**, 155–64.

Suit, H.D. (1982) Potential for improving survival rates for the cancer patient by increasing the efficacy of treatment of the primary lesion. The American Society of Therapeutic Radiologists Presidential Address: October 1981. *Cancer*, **50**, 1227–34.

Sutton, M.L. and Hendry, J.H. (1985) Applied radiobiology, in *The Radiotherapy of Malignant Disease*, (eds E.C. Easson and R.C.S. Pointon), Springer-Verlag, Berlin, pp. 33–55.

Tait, D. (1990) Conformal therapy. *British Journal of Cancer*, **62**, 702–04.

Trott, K.R. and Kummermehr, J. (1985) What is known about tumour proliferation rates to choose between accelerated fractionation or hyperfractionation? *Radiotherapy and Oncology*, **3**, 1–9.

Utley, J.F., von Essen, C.F., Horn, R.A. *et al.* (1984) High-dose-rate afterloading brachytherapy in carcinoma of the uterine cervix. *International Journal of Radiation Oncology, Biology, Physics*, **10**, 2259–63.

Webb, S. (1993) *The Physics of Three-Dimensional Radiation Therapy*, IOP Publishing, Bristol.

Welsh Office (1989) *Review of the Provision of Cancer Services to the People of North Wales.*

Wilson, G.D., McNally, N.J., Dische, *et al.* (1989) Measurement of cell kinetics in human tumours *in vivo* using bromodeoxyuridine incorporation and flow cytometry. *British Journal of Cancer*, **58**, 423–31.

Withers, H.R. (1985) Biological basis for altered fractionated ion schemes. *Cancer*, **55**, 2986–95.

Yarnold, J.R., Horwich, A., Duchesne, G. *et al.* (1983) Chemotherapy and radiotherapy for advanced testicular non-seminoma. 1. The influence of sequence and timing of drugs and radiation on the appearance of normal tissue damage. *Radiotherapy and Oncology*, **1**, 91–9.

PRINCIPLES OF MEDICAL ONCOLOGY 10

Tamas Hickish

10.1 INTRODUCTION

Cancer is frequently a disseminated disease and requires systemic treatment. The history of modern chemotherapy is short and stems from the Second World War and what can now be seen as a serendipitous accident, when seamen, exposed to mustard gas as the result of an explosion in Bari harbour, were observed to develop marrow and lymphoid hypoplasia. The challenge of chemotherapy is to produce effective tumour kill with the minimum impact on normal tissues. With time a variety of parameters have emerged to guide the application of chemotherapeutic agents. These relate their mechanisms of action and pharmacology to tumour cell and normal cell biology and to the clinical context with the identification of realistic and meaningful clinical endpoints.

10.2 TREATMENT OBJECTIVES AND CLINICAL ENDPOINTS

The assessment of the extent of disease determines the treatment strategy, the likely outcome and hence the objectives of treatment. The traditional methods used to stage disease – examination; radiology, X-ray, CT and MRI scanning; bone marrow histology and peripheral blood film – are now been complemented by new ultrasensitive molecular techniques. Integral to the assessment is the identification and quantification of prognostic indicators (e.g. Shipp *et al.*, 1992), com-

prising histological, immunocytochemical and molecular features along with aspects such as age and the bulk of disease. They are becoming increasingly important in defining patient subgroups who are being failed by current therapeutic approaches. Additionally, positron emission tomography and magnetic resonance imaging may enable the early identification of patients who will fail to respond to an implemented treatment (Chapter 7).

Clinical practice has identified the tumour types which when metastatic are either curable or incurable with current therapies. In the latter group chemotherapy is palliative and its use should be judicious and ideally in the context of a clinical trial assessing the utility of a regimen in terms of activity and impact on quality of life. The issues of quality of life and survival benefit are paramount. Randomized trials performed to address these matters have demonstrated how palliative chemotherapy can indeed enhance quality of life and prolong survival (e.g. Nordic Gastro-Intestinal Tumour Adjuvant Therapy Group, 1992).

10.2.1 DEFINING THE RESULTS OF CANCER TREATMENT

A World Health Organization initiative generated a format for reporting the results of cancer treatment (Miller *et al.*, 1981). It outlined the minimum data required about the patient population, tumour, treatment, toxicity, response, duration of response and results of therapy in terms of intention to treat and patients actually treated. The standardization and definition (i.e. of response and toxicity) of data has enabled the comparison and evaluation of clinical trials (Tables 10.1, 10.2).

10.2.2   TREATMENT SCENARIOS

(a)   Induction chemotherapy

When disease is advanced chemotherapy often represents the only appropriate therapeutic option and when it is initiated as the first treatment it is termed induction

Table 10.1   WHO grading of some key toxicities

	Grade 0	Grade 1	Grade 2	Grade 3	Grade 4
Granulocytes 1000/mm^3	> 2.0	1.5–1.9	1.0–1.4	0.5–0.9	< 0.5
Platelets 1000/mm^3	> 100	75–99	50–74	25–49	< 25
Oral	None	Soreness/ erythema	Erythema, ulcers, can eat solids	Ulcers, requires liquid diet only	Alimentation not possible
Nausea/ vomiting	None	Nausea	Transient vomiting	Vomiting requiring therapy	Intractable vomiting

Table 10.2   Some key WHO definitions of response

Complete response (CR) – The disappearance of all known disease determined by two observations not less than 4 weeks apart.
Partial response (PR) – A 50% or more decrease in total tumour by two observations not less than 4 weeks apart (lesions are measured by multiplication of the longest diameter by the greatest perpendicular diameter). In addition there can be no appearance of new lesions or progression of any lesion
No change (NC) – A 50% decrease in tumour size cannot be established nor has a 25% increase in the size of one or more measurable lesions been demonstrated
Progressive disease (PD) – A 25% or more increase in the size of one or more measurable lesions or the appearance of new lesions

Duration of response
The duration of CR lasts from the date the complete response was first noted to the date progressive disease was first noted. PR is the period of overall response and lasts from the first day of treatment to the date of the first observation of progressive disease.

Cure
Three definitions are proposed:
1. When a group of patients has a survival experience identical to that of the general population with the same distribution of demographic factors
2. When there is a low probability of subsequent death from initial neoplasm
3. When a patient has survived in a disease-free state long enough to enter a group with known low probability of developing a recurrence

chemotherapy. The major marker for the potential utility of treatment is the complete remission (CR) rate – cures begin with CRs. Following this the disease-free survival (DFS) represents the quality of the CR and the likelihood it will translate into cure.

(b) Adjuvant chemotherapy

Chemotherapy which is initiated when disease is localized and has been controlled by another therapeutic modality is termed adjuvant chemotherapy. The key marker of response, the CR, is lost and therefore DFS is an initial endpoint representing the efficacy of therapy.

(c) Primary chemotherapy

Chemotherapy is also used when disease is localized to enhance the efficiency of subsequent radiotherapy and/or surgery and is termed primary or neo-adjuvant chemotherapy. This approach can only be adopted when there is a significant probability of response to the treatment regimen. In animal models preoperative chemotherapy has been shown to prevent the increase in tumour cell proliferation consequent upon incomplete resection and thereby to prolong survival (Fisher *et al.*, 1983). This approach may enable the identification of subgroups at high risk of relapse since the quality of the histological response may reflect the impact of treatment on micrometastatic disease.

The evaluation of primary chemotherapy is at its most advanced in breast and head and neck cancer (e.g. Bonadonna *et al.*, 1993). Whilst there is a lack of survival data from randomized trials, in breast cancer the reduction in tumour size in responding patients is associated with an increase in the probability that the definitive surgical procedure will be breast conserving (Smith *et al.*, 1993).

(d) Salvage chemotherapy

Chemotherapy implemented after failure of prior treatment is termed salvage therapy. This group of patients is self selected and for most tumour types has a poor prognosis. Treatment options are generally limited.

10.3 THE KINETICS OF TUMOUR GROWTH: A CRUCIAL PARAMETER IN RATIONAL SYSTEMIC THERAPY

Skipper and Schabel demonstrated how the magnitude of tumour cell kill achieved with a pulse of chemotherapy coupled with the population doubling time determined the duration of survival of mice carrying a leukaemia xenograft. In this system the tumour cell population kill produced by a given dose of chemotherapy followed log-kill kinetics independent of the initial tumour burden. Furthermore, cures were obtainable if the dosage and scheduling of chemotherapy was tailored to the tumour growth and characteristics.

Human tumour growth appears to be better described in terms of Gompertzian kinetics. The growth fraction (the proportion of the tumour cell population in the cell cycle) is considered to exponentially fall as tumour volume increases. Hence when there is significant tumour burden the growth fraction is small and the magnitude of cell death induced by chemotherapy is small. This analysis has been applied to the adjuvant setting (Norton, 1988) and accurately predicts that if occult disease remains, whatever its volume, the DFS will be the same since the growth fraction is inversely geared to tumour volume. The biological basis for this descriptive model is unknown; however the implication is that unless adjuvant therapy produces complete tumour eradication or sterilization it will not produce a survival benefit. This concept in tandem with the proven activity of chemotherapy regimens in a range of solid tumours forms the basis of the current interest of dose-intensive chemotherapy strategies in the adjuvant setting.

10.4   MECHANISM OF ACTION AND RESISTANCE

10.4.1   MECHANISM

The currently available anticancer drugs can be categorized into three broad groups: those that interact with DNA, those that associate with membrane receptors and those that bind to antigen expressed at the cell surface.

The drugs that act at the level of DNA are loosely termed the cytotoxics although properly any drug that produced this effect would merit the name. Table 10.3 lists the mechanistic classes to which the most commonly used of these drugs (along with three new drugs which are showing promising activity in clinical trials: taxol, taxotere and camptothecin) belong. The principal mechanism of action for each drug is uncertain although all produce DNA damage. The alkylating agents appear to predominantly produce methylation of the N^7 position of guanine, thereby possibly inducing arrest of DNA transcription/replication. Cisplatin and carboplatin produce intrastrand DNA crosslinks between neighbouring N^7-O^6 guanines and N^3 cytosines and are currently thought to act as alkylating agents. A number of mechanisms have been implicated in antimetabolite-induced DNA injury including thymidylate synthetase inhibition, purine synthesis inhibition and inhibition of DNA repair. The anthracyclines are thought to produce DNA damage by intercalating with DNA, the production of semiquinone free radicals, or by interacting with the DNA modifying enzyme topoisomerase II to produce a stable enzyme–DNA complex leading to DNA cleavage. The latter may initiate endonucleocytic DNA cleavage–apoptosis (Wyllie, 1993). The epipodophyllotoxins also interact with topoisomerase II to cleave DNA although at a different site. Camptothecin interacts in an apparently similar manner with topoisomerase I. The tubulin binding agents produce DNA damage by perturbing DNA replication. Since some of these drugs are active at certain points in the cell cycle they are denoted phase specific. The DNA in cells in G0 is relatively inaccessible to those drugs which interact with DNA and since obviously DNA synthesis and division processes are inactive, cells in G0 are invulnerable to the cytotoxics.

The mechanism of action for some drugs in certain situations remains elusive. For example, BCNU is cytotoxic to cells in G0 – it is a stem cell poison. This may be the result of DNA–protein cross-links. Similarly alkylating agents frequently produce rapid responses in myeloma, follicular low grade non-Hodgkin's lymphoma and chronic lymphocytic leukaemia (CLL) where the measurable population of cells is in G0. Additionally the toxicity profile of these drugs is not completely predictable with current knowledge. For example, the reason for the difference in myelotoxicity between cisplatin and carboplatin is unexplained.

Membrane active drugs include hormonal agents used in breast and prostate cancer and retinoic acid. The exact mechanism of action of the most extensively used of them all, tamoxifen, is still undecided. Its proven efficacy in premenopausal breast cancer is consistent with an anti-oestrogenic effect yet it is active against oestrogen-receptor negative tumours (Chapter 35).

The production of antibodies which selectively bind tumour specific antigen has led to the hope that these may form the basis of a tumour targeted therapy. Various strategies for achieving tumour kill have been developed. For example, the antibody can be used unadulterated to stimulate a cytopathic immune response when bound to antigen. Another approach is to use the antibody to deliver a cytopathic agent by linking it to either a toxin (e.g. ricin) or a radionucleotide. A sophistication of this approach is to link the antibody to an enzyme which catalyses the activation of a prodrug thereby producing a high concentration of a cytotoxic drug at the site of the tumour. These strategies are

Table 10.3 Acute toxicity

Class and drug	WBC	Platelets	Nausea/vomiting	Some other toxicities
Antimetabolites				
2-chlorodeoxyadenosine	++	++	+	None
Methotrexate	++/+++	++/+++	+	Hepatic dysfunction, mucosity
5-Fluorouracil	+	+	+	Mucositis, diarrhoea
5-Fluorodeoxyuridine	+	+	++	Intra hepatic arterial complications
6-Mercaptopurine	++	++	+	Cholestasis
6-Thioguanine	++/+++	++/+++	+	Cholestasis
Cytarabine	+++	+++	++	Cholestasis, mucositis
Deoxycoformycin	+	+	+	None
Fludarabine	++	++	+	Neurotoxicity at high dose
Alkylating agents				
BCNU	+++	+++	+++	Leukaemia, pulmonary fibrosis, renal failure
Busulphan	+++	+++	+	Pulmonary fibrosis
CCNU	+++	+++	++	Leukaemia, pulmonary fibrosis, Nephro-hepato toxicity
Cyclophosphamide	+++	++	+	Cystitis, alopecia
Ifosfamide	++/+++	++	+	Neurotoxicity, urothelial alopecia, rarely leukaemia
MeCCNU	+++	+++	++	Leukaemia, pulmonary fibrosis, renal failure
Melphalan (low dose)	++/+++	++	++	None
Streptozotocin	+	+	++/+++	Renal failure, hypoglycaemia (but less than cisplatin)
Carboplatin	+++	+++	+	
Chlorambucil	++	++	+	Leukaemia, pulmonary fibrosis
Cisplatin	+	+	+++	Neuro-, nephro-, oto- toxicity
Antibiotics				
Actinomycin D	+++	+++	++/+++	Alopecia, mucositis
Bleomycin	+	+	+	Skin, pulmonary fibrosis fever, allergic reactions
Daunorubicin	+++	+++	++	Alopecia, cardiomyopathy
Doxorubicin	+++	+++	++	Alopecia, cardiomyopathy
Mitomycin C	+++	+++	++	Haemolytic uraemic syndrome, rarely leukaemia

Table 10.3 *contd*

Class and drug	WBC	Platelets	Nausea/vomiting	Some other toxicities
Plant alkaloids				
Vincristine	+	+	+	Distal neuropathy, rarely SIADH
Vinblastine	+++	+++	+	Mucositis, neuropathy
Vindesine	++	+	+	Mucositis, Alopecia, neuropathy
Taxenes				
Taxol	++	++	+	Neuropathy, allergic reactions
Taxotere	++	++	+	Neuropathy, allergic reactions
Epipodophyllotoxins				
Etoposide	++/+++	++	+	Alopecia, mucositis, leukaemia
Tenoposide	++/+++	++	+	Alopecia, leukaemia
Topoisomerate I inhibitors				
CPTII	+	+	+	Diarrhoea
Miscellaneous				
DTIC	+	+	+++	Flu-like syndrome
Procarbazine	++	++	+	Flu-like syndrome, sensitivity to tyramines
Mitoxantrone	++	++	+	Cardiotoxicity, Cholestasis

Key: +, mild; ++, moderate; +++, marked.

currently being evaluated in the phase I and II clinical trials and the use of antibodies as a systemic therapy remains experimental.

In summary, the rational use of oncolytic drugs is limited by significant information gaps. Their use has to be tempered with a degree of empiricism.

10.4.2   RESISTANCE

The major cause for failure of chemotherapy to produce a cure is the presence of resistant tumour cells. These may exist at presentation or may develop during or following chemotherapy. A biological explanation for the emergence of drug resistance is provided by the Goldie–Coldman hypothesis which proposes that mutations result in the genesis and subsequent overgrowth of resistant tumour cell clones. The mathematical description of this process assumes that the rate of mutation to a resistant phenotype is a function of the genetic plasticity of the tumour. Hence, if resistance-mutation occurs in only one in 10^6 cells, the model predicts a significant probability of the presence of resistance tumour cells even in the setting of minimal tumour volume.

DNA repair is thought to underly resistance to many cytotoxics (reviewed in Epstein, 1990). For example, the level of the DNA repair enzyme O_6 alkylguanine DNA alkyltransferase has been found to be elevated in some alkylating resistant tumours and cell lines. Similarly increased DNA repair has been demonstrated in some cisplatin resistant tumours. More drug specific mechanisms include resistance to alkylating agents by conjugation with glutathione and resistance to topoisomerase interactive agents by the production of a mutated enzyme or suppression of enzyme production.

10.4.3   MULTIPLE DRUG RESISTANCE PHENOTYPE

The characterization of one mechanism of resistance began with the generation of cell lines which after exposure to one anticancer drug display resistance to a variety of other agents – the multiple drug resistance (MDR) phenotype. The MDR phenotype results from expression of 170 kDa membrane glycoprotein (P-gp) which is integral to the energy dependent efflux of 'MDR drugs' (Ueda *et al.*, 1987). The gene encoding P-gp, mdr 1, belongs to a multi gene family which includes a number of membrane transport proteins. There is evidence that P-gp is a channel for the influx of ATP under normal physiological conditions. Additionally, since P-gp is expressed in the secretory epithelium of a variety of normal tissues (gut, biliary tract, kidney, pancreas), its role may extend to the secretion of metabolites and toxic substances into the bile, renal and upper gastrointestinal tracts (Arceci, 1993).

Expression of P-gp has been demonstrated across the range of solid and haemopoietic malignancies and a number of retrospective and prospective studies have indicated that expression is an adverse prognostic feature. *In vitro* P-gp can be suppressed by a number of membrane active drugs (verapamil, cyclosporin A, FK506, tamoxifen) and the possibility that this may also be achieved *in vivo* to reverse drug resistance has formed the basis of a number of clinical trials.

Therapeutic benefits from this approach have been demonstrated in lymphoma and refractory myeloma (Miller *et al.*, 1991; Sonnveld *et al.*, 1992); however, overall the likely gains of this strategy are uncertain. Indeed other constructions can be placed upon the P-gp expression data (Kaye, 1993). For example there is evidence indicating P-gp expression is associated with an enhanced metastatic potential. Additionally elevated P-gp expression may be a manifestation of heightened expression of other genes themselves responsible for the MDR phenotype.

10.4.4   COMBINATION CHEMOTHERAPY

The objective of combination chemotherapy is to devise a cytotoxic regimen in which each drug has proven activity as a single agent against the tumour type to be challenged. The selected line-up should comprise the best of the drugs available with each drawn from a different mechanistic class so as to circumvent tumour resistance. Ideally the drugs would interact synergistically (Lotan and Nicolson, 1988). Examples of synergy between cytotoxics include that between cytarabine and etoposide and 5FU and cisplatin (e.g. Chresta *et al.*, 1992). Modulation of 5FU by leucovorin and interferon-α is discussed in Chapter 42.

Ideally the toxicity profile for each drug should not be superimposed, thereby limiting the severity of a given toxicity. Furthermore, when the aim is cure the potential impact of any drug used on longevity should be considered. This issue is particularly stark in the cohort of patients cured of Hodgkin's disease 10–20 years ago and who are now developing secondary malignancies as a consequence of alkylating agent based chemotherapy along with radiotherapy (Chapter 18, and see Chapter 16 for the effect of chemotherapy on fertility).

10.5 DOSE AND TIME

10.5.1 THE DOSE–RESPONSE CURVE AND CONCENTRATION X TIME

The dose–response curve, which describes the relationship between the received dose of a drug and the degree of cell kill, and the effect of duration of exposure on efficiency of the drug are key parameters in cancer chemotherapy. The dose–response curve defines the potential antitumour effect achievable with a given dose of a cytotoxic agent. The dose–response curve also holds for the impact of the drug on normal tissues – the toxicity of the drug. The challenge is to utilize a drug at a dose that is optimally tumorcidal yet acceptably toxic. The shape of the curve is generally sigmoidal with threshold, lag, linear and plateau phases. The gradient of the linear phase is generally specific to the class of drugs. The alkylating agents have a linear-log dose–response relationship over many logs of drug dose whereas for antimetabolites the dose–response curve is linear-log over a limited dose range.

Preclinical experiments show that the shape of the curve for a given drug alters as a function of tumour type and proliferation rate (reviewed in Henderson *et al.*, 1988). The magnitude of response is also a function of the time (T) of exposure to the cytotoxic drug. Hence, equivalent tumour kill can be achieved with different concentrations (C) of drug when C $\times$ T is constant. Duration of exposure is also a key parameter in relation to the mechanism of action of the cytotoxic and the cell cycle characteristics of the tumour. Hence, antimetabolites and topoisomerase I and II interactive drugs are phase specific (e.g. Waits *et al.*, 1992). As such the antitumour response may be schedule dependent. For example, in a randomized comparison of 36 hour intermediate dose versus 4 hour high dose methotrexate infusions for remission induction in children with relapsed acute lymphoblastic leukaemia, the two doses were equivalent in inducing bone marrow remission. This was despite the intermediate dose having a 24-fold AUC (area under the concentration–time curve) (Wolfrom *et al.*, 1993). Synergy between drugs will also have an impact on the dose–response curve shifting it to the left.

Therefore for any cytotoxic there is potentially a schedule and a dose which is optimal in terms of tumour response and toxicity profile.

10.5.2 DOSE INTENSITY

Data from both experimental tumour systems and clinical studies indicate that the delivered dose is vital in determining the probability of tumour eradication when schedule, drug combination and interval of treatment are optimal. Skipper *et al.* (1964)

evaluated the impact of reducing the average dose of a two drug combination on response and cure rate in a mouse xenograft model and demonstrated that there was a major decrease in the percent cure rate despite maintenance of a 100% complete remission rate. This principle appears to hold in the clinical setting. Hrynuik *et al.* have examined the impact of variations in delivered dosage over time – dose intensity – on treatment outcome in breast cancer and other tumours (Hryniuk and Bush, 1984; Hryniuk and Levine, 1986; Levin and Hryniuk, 1987). Specifically, dose intensity was defined as the dose in milligrams per meter square per week. They demonstrated a consistent correlation between the planned (and delivered) dose intensity on median survival and response rate seen in the randomized clinical trials analysed. The dose intensity model may not be all encompassing; it does not include the effects of synergy between drugs or scheduling (Evans *et al.*, 1991; Weitman *et al.*, 1993) and its general applicability has been questioned (Henderson *et al.*, 1988; Hryniuk, 1989). However the positive relationship between dose intensity and response rate has been demonstrated in randomized trials in advanced ovarian, breast and colon cancers and in the lymphomas (e.g. Kaye *et al.*, 1992). The principle has also been shown to hold in the adjuvant setting where relapse is due to the progression of the occult, usually metastatic disease. For example in a study of adjuvant chemotherapy as primary treatment for primary breast cancer, doubling the dose intensity of the CAF (cyclophosphamide, adriamycin and 5-FU) regimen significantly improved disease free survival and overall survival for all pretreatment subgroups (Budman *et al.*, 1992).

Hence the evidence is consistent with the dose intensity proposition; more is better. Conversely the evidence indicates that dose reductions should be restricted as they may adversely affect outcome.

10.5.3 MYELOTOXICITY: A KEY DETERMINANT IN THE DESIGN OF CYTOTOXIC REGIMENS

Following the intravenous delivery of myelosuppressive chemotherapy there is a rapid killing of cell-cycling stem cells in the bone marrow. Otherwise healthy bone marrow has a storage compartment sufficient to maintain peripheral blood levels of mature and functional neutrophils and platelets for 10 days. Hence, blood counts generally reach a nadir between the 10th and 18th days following chemotherapy. The stem cell pool thereafter regenerates and replenishes the neutrophil and platelet compartments from the 10th day onward so that recovery is usually complete by day 21. The stem cell pool appears to be relatively resistant to cytotoxics on day 8, thereby enabling the delivery of further myelosuppressive drugs with little effect on bone marrow recovery.

The scheduling of myelosuppressive chemotherapy is therefore restricted by bone marrow recovery. However, scheduling also has to be appropriate to the growth characteristics of the tumour type. The frequency of cytotoxic delivery needs to be sufficient to prevent tumour regrowth. Hence, for rapidly growing tumours such as intermediate and high grade non-Hodgkin's lymphomas cytotoxic regimens have been devised which sequence myelosuppressive with non-myelosuppressive agents. The ability to maintain the planned regimen has been enhanced by the introduction of cytokines (e.g. G–CSF, GM–CSF, IL3 – Chapter 12). Cytotoxic regimens potentially made feasible by cytokine support are currently under evaluation in randomized clinical trials.

10.5.4 HIGH DOSE INTENSIFICATION

Escalation of dose along the linear phase of the dose–response curve is limited by the attendant toxicities. The prospect of severe treatment related morbidity and mortality has hitherto restricted high dose chemotherapy with autologous bone marrow or peripheral stem cell (PSCR) rescue (HD + ABMT) to use as a salvage therapy. The most extensive experience is with the lymphomas, germ cell tumours and breast cancer. Linch *et al.* have demonstrated a survival benefit for HD (BEAM regimen) + ABMT compared to the same drugs at lower dose without ABMT in relapsed Hodgkin's disease (Linch *et al.*, 1993). Unfortunately the majority of the trials have not been randomized and therefore the precise role of HD + ABMT remains uncertain. They have established CR rates and DFS curves and criteria for the further evaluation of HD + ABMT on a clinical trial basis. The continually improving technology enabling successful support of patients through the period of toxicity to recovery has led to the initiation of randomized trials of HD + PSCR (ABMT) has largely been superceded as part of front-line treatment in poor prognosis intermediate grade non-Hodgkin's lymphoma and primary breast cancer.

10.5.5   CHRONOTHERAPY

Cell cycling of normal tissues including bone marrow appears to be organized on a 24 hour time scale with cell rest at night. Malignant cells appear to be oblivious as to the time of day. Additionally the pharmacokinetics of many drugs including cytotoxics varies as a function of the circadian rhythm (Hassan *et al.*, 1991; Reinberg, 1991). A number of animal and clinical studies have shown that the toxicity and efficacy of a variety of anticancer drugs is circadian dependent. Scheduling of anticancer therapy to exploit circadian resistance of normal tissues relative to tumour (chronotherapy) is currently being evaluated in clinical trials. Studies with 5FU and interferon-α indicate it may be possible to achieve increments in dose intensity without consequent toxicity (Depres-Brunner *et al.*, 1991).

10.5.6   MAINTENANCE THERAPIES

Total tumour eradication may not be feasible with current therapies; however, it may be possible to extend remission using maintenance therapies. Since such treatment would be used long term their toxicities should be minimal. This approach is being explored in a number of tumour types. The use of interferon-α to extend remission following ABMT for multiple myeloma is discussed in Chapter 22.

10.6   FUTURE DIRECTIONS

The disease orientated chapters in this book describe in detail the success of systemic therapy in the various tumour types. Clearly further developments are required.

A fuller understanding of the mechanisms of drug action and cell resistance are required to enable the rational design of treatment regimens. This in part will depend on the development of techniques to directly measure both the activity of drugs at their targets and the degree of DNA damage produced. For example, the extent to which alkylating agents produce DNA adducts in responding and resistant tumours. Furthermore detailed knowledge of mechanisms of action may lead to innovations in agents to protect normal tissues (e.g. WR 2721, a bone marrow protective agent (Glover *et al.*, 1986)).

There is increasing evidence that the final common pathway of cytotoxic induced cell death is via apoptosis (Wyllie, 1993). A complete biochemical description of this process may reveal points at which it can be selectively activated in tumours, perhaps as a single agent approach or in combination with established drugs (Evans and Dive, 1993). The large information gaps in the relationship between peak dose, dose rate, schedule, relation to circadian rhythm and cumulative dose need to be resolved to ensure that maximum activity has been achieved with the available drugs (e.g. Henderson *et al.*, 1988).

The development of a comprehensive prognostic indicator profile will result in the accurate identification of patients at high risk and is likely to lead to the further evaluation of high dose strategies in the adjuvant/neo-adjuvant setting.

The increasing detail of the molecular biology of cancer has yet to have an impact in therapeutics. A full description of the biochemistry associated with a defective gene in terms of abnormal protein(s) and perturbed pathway(s) may reveal points at which altered function can be abrogated (e.g. Gibbs, 1991). The targeting of genes themselves by antisense and triple helix agents may result in a new generation of specific systemic therapies (e.g. Carter and Lemoine, 1993), while a variety of gene therapy strategies have already entered clinical trials.

REFERENCES

Arceci, R.J. (1993) Clinical significance of P-glycoprotein in multidrug resistance malignancies. *Blood*, **81**, 2215–22.

Bonadonna, G., Valagussa, P., Brambilla C. *et al.* (1993) Preoperative chemotherapy in operable breast cancer. *Lancet*, **341**, 1485.

Budman, D.R., Wood, W., Henderson, I.C. *et al.* (1992). Initial findings at CALGB 8541: a dose and dose intensity trial of cyclophosphamide, doxorubicin and 5 fluorouracil as adjuvant treatment in stage II, node positive, female breast cancer. *Proceedings of the American Society of Clinical Oncology*, **11**, (abstr. 29).

Carter, G. and Lemoine, N.R. (1993) Antisense technology for cancer therapy: does it make sense? *British Journal of Cancer*, **67**, 869–76.

Chresta, C.M., Hicks, R., Hartley, J.A. *et al.* (1992) Potentiation of etoposide-induced cytotoxicity and DNA damage in CCRF-CEM cells by pretreatment with non-cytotoxic concentrations of arabinosyl cytosine. *Cancer Chemotherapy and Pharmacology*, **31**, 139–45.

Depres-Brunner, P., Levi, F., Di-Palma, M. *et al.* (1991) A Phase I trial of 21 day continuous venous infusion of alpha interferon at circadian rhythm modulated rate in cancer patients. *Journal of Immunotherapy*, **10**, 440–7.

De Vita, V.T. (1978) The evolution of therapeutic research in cancer. *New England Journal of Medicine*, **298**, 907–10.

Epstein, R.J. (1990) Drug-induced DNA damage and tumor chemosensitivity. *Journal of Clinical Oncology*, **8**, 2062–84.

Evans, D.L. and Dive, C. (1993) Effects of cisplatin on the induction of apoptosis proliferating hepatoma cells and nonproliferating immature thymocytes. *Cancer Research*, **53**, 2133–9.

Evans, W.E., Rodman, J.H., Relling, M.U. *et al.* (1991) Concept of maximum tolerated systemic exposure and its application to phase 1–11 studies of anticancer drugs. *Medical and Pediatric Oncology*, **19**, 153–9.

Fisher, B., Gunduz, N. and Saffer, E.A. (1983) Influence of the interval between primary tumor removal and chemotherapy on kinetics and growth of metastases. *Cancer Research*, **43**, 1488–92.

Gibbs, J.B. (1991) Ras c-terminal processing enzymes – new drug targets? *Cell*, **65**, 1–4.

Glover, D., Glick, J.H., Weiler, C. *et al.* (1986) WR-2721 protects against the hematologic toxicity of cyclophosphamide: a controlled phase II trial. *Journal of Clinical Oncology*, **4**, 584–8.

Goldie, J.H. and Coldman, A.J. (1979) A mathematic model for relating the drug sensitivity of tumour to the spontaneous mutation rate. *Cancer Treatment Reviews*, **63**, 1727–33.

Hassan, M., Oberg, G., Bekassy, A.N. *et al.* (1991) Pharmaco-kinetics of high dose busulphan in relation to age and chronopharmacology. *Cancer Chemotherapy and Pharmacology*, **28**, 130–4.

Henderson, I.C., Hayes, D.F. and Gelman, R. (1988) Dose–response in the treatment of breast cancer: a critical review. *Journal of Clinical Oncology*, **6**, 1501–15.

Hryniuk, W.M. (1989) Dose intensity: a critique of critical review. *Journal of Clinical Oncology*, **7**, 681–2. 682 (1989) [Reply by Henderson, I.C. *et al.* (1989) *Journal of Clinical Oncology*, **7**, 682–3.]

Hryniuk, W. and Bush, H. (1984) The importance of dose intensity in chemotherapy of metastatic breast cancer. *Journal of Clinical Oncology*, **2**, 1281–8.

Hryniuk, W.M. and Levine, M.N. (1986) Analysis of dose intensity for adjuvant chemotherapy trials in stage II breast cancer. *Journal of Clinical Oncology*, **4**, 1162–70.

Kaye, S.B. (1993) P-glycoprotein (P-gp) and drug resistance – time for reappraisal? *British Journal of Cancer*, **67**, 641–3.

Kaye, S.B., Lewis, C.R., Paul, J. *et al.* (1992) Randomised study of two doses of cisplatin with cyclophosphamide in epithelial ovarium cancer. *Lancet*, **340**, 329–33.

Levin, L. and Hryniuk, W. (1987) Dose intensity analysis of chemotherapy regimens in ovarian cancer. *Journal of Clinical Oncology*, **5**, 756–67.

Linch, D.C., Winfield, D., Goldstone, A.H. *et al.* (1993) Dose intensification with autologous bone-marrow transplantation is relapsed and resistant Hodgkin's disease: results of a BNLI randomised trial. *Lancet*, **341**, 1051–4.

Lotan, R. and Nicolson, G. (1988) Can anticancer therapy be improved by sequential use of cytotoxic and cytostatic (differentiating or immuno-modulating) agents to suppress tumor cell phenotypic diversification? *Biochemical Pharmacology*, **37**, 149–54.

Miller, A.B., Hoogstraten, B., Staquet, M. *et al.* (1981) Reporting results of cancer treatment. *Cancer*, **47**, 207–14.

Miller, T.P., Grogan, T.M., Dalton, W.S. *et al.* (1991) P-glycoprotein expression is malignant lymphoma and reversal of clinical drug resistance with chemotherapy plus high dose verapamil. *Journal of Clinical Oncology*, **9**, 17–24.

Nordic Gastrointestinal Tumor Adjuvant Group (1992) Expectancy or primary chemotherapy in patients with advanced asymptomatic colorectal cancer: a randomized trial. *Journal of Clinical Oncology*, **10**, 904–11.

Norton, L.A. (1988) A Gompertzian model of human breast cancer growth. *Cancer Research*, **48**, 7067–71.

Reinberg, A.G. (1991) Concepts of circadian chronopharmacology. *Annuals of the New York Academy of Sciences*, **618**, 102–15.

Shipp, M., Harrington, D., Anderson, J. *et al.* (1992) Development of a predictive model for aggressive lymphoma: the international NHL prognostic factors project. *Proceedings of the American Society of Clinical Oncology*, **11**, (abstr 1084).

Skipper, H.E., Schabel, F.M. and Wilcox, W.S. (1964) Experimental evaluation of potential anti cancer drugs XII. On the criteria and kinetics allocated with curability of experimental leukaemia. *Cancer Chemotherapy Reports*, **35**, 1–111.

Smith, I.E., Jones, A.L., O'Brien, M.E.R. *et al.* (1993) Primary medical (neo-adjuvant) chemotherapy for operable breast cancer. *European Journal of Cancer*, **29**, 1796–1799.

Sonneveld, P., Durie, B.W., Lokhurst, H.M. *et al.* (1992) Modulation of multi-drug resistant multiple myeloma by cyclosporin. *Lancet*, **340**, 255–9.

Ueda, K., Cardareli, C., Gottesman, M.M. *et al.* (1987) Expression of a full length CDNA for the human mdrl gene confers resistance to colchicine doxorubicin and vinblastine. *Proceedings of the National Academy of Sciences USA*, **84**, 3004–8.

Waits, T.M., Johnson, D.H., Hainsworth, J.D. *et al.* (1992) Prolonged administration of oral etoposide in non-small cell lung cancer: a Phase II trial. *Journal of Clinical Oncology*, **10**, 292–6.

Weitman, S.D., Glastein, E. and Karmen, B.A. (1993) Back to basics: the importance of concentration × time in oncology (editorial). *Journal of Clinical Oncology*, **11**, 820–1.

Wolfrom, C., Hartman, R., Feigler, R. *et al.* (1993) Randomised comparison of 36 hour intermediate dose versus high-dose methotrexate infusions for remission induction in relapsed childhood acute lymphoblastic leukaemia. *Journal of Clinical Oncology*, **11**, 827–33. (1993)

Wyllie, A.H. (1993) Apoptosis (The Frank Rose memorial lecture). *British Journal of Cancer*, **67**, 205–8.

EVALUATION OF NEW ANTICANCER DRUGS

11

Ian R. Judson

11.1 INTRODUCTION

Why should early clinical studies involving new anticancer drugs be regarded as different from other drug trials? What methodological, pharmacological and ethical factors are peculiar to anticancer drugs compared with, for example, a new treatment for hypertension? In the first place, the targets for anticancer drugs are often not accurately defined and the mechanisms by which such drugs induce cancer cell death are still obscure. Secondly, most anticancer drugs have a relatively poor therapeutic index. For this reason the majority of antiproliferative agents in current use are given at very close to the maximum tolerated dose (MTD). This precludes the use of healthy volunteers and makes such studies potentially hazardous.

It has been the standard practice to establish the MTD in rodents and extrapolate to man using some form of stepwise escalation to reach a maximum tolerable dose (phase I) which can then be applied in tumour-specific studies of antitumour activity (phase II). This approach does, in the majority of cases, allow for the safe determination of a suitable dose for phase II investigations. However, agents are now being developed aimed at new targets for which the MTD may not be the appropriate dose. Hence, this traditional approach may not always be suitable.

11.2 FIXING A SAFE STARTING DOSE

Before any new drug can be given to humans, its toxicity must first be thoroughly investigated in animals. This has two purposes in the case of anticancer drugs, the identification of specific toxic side-effects and the determination of a MTD. For the majority of anticancer drugs currently in use, the dose limiting toxicity in rodents results from inhibition of cell division in the bone marrow or gut. This leads to a good correlation between the MTD for acute administration in mice and the MTD in man. However, rodents are less good at predicting specific organ toxicities, e.g. to the heart, lungs or nervous system. In addition, rodents do not predict for emesis, a major problem with anticancer drugs.

A number of investigators have shown that for a variety of anticancer agents the MTD expressed in mg/m^2 is approximately equivalent between species (Freireich *et al.*, 1966). The mouse is second only to the rhesus monkey in successfully predicting human toxicity. Nevertheless, it is quite unsafe to commence the testing of drugs in man at doses which are toxic to rodents. A margin of error is required which will allow the choice of a safe starting dose yet limit the numbers of patients who need to be treated in order to find the maximum tolerated dose.

A number of different schemes have been used for determination of a safe starting dose based on animal toxicology. The National Cancer Institute of the USA reviewed the data from mice, dogs and monkeys, and concluded that one-tenth the LD_{10} in mice is a safe starting dose provided this is tolerated in the dog. While dog toxicology is still required in the USA it is not mandatory in Europe for anticancer drugs. A joint committee of the European Organization for Research and Treatment of Cancer (EORTC) and the Cancer Research Campaign (CRC) of the UK follow published guidelines for preclinical toxicology testing of new anticancer agents, which is usually confined to mice and rats (Joint Steering Committee of the EORTC and CRC, 1989). Under these guidelines the safe starting dose in man will be defined as one-tenth the LD_{10} in the mouse, expressed in mg/m², provided there are no unexpected toxicities in the rat. The protocols are currently under review, with a number of areas receiving critical attention, including the avoidance wherever possible of the intraperitoneal route of administration, which often gives misleading results and the need to collect samples routinely for pharmacokinetics. There may be special requirements for antiendocrine agents (Judson, 1989) or those which will be administered orally. Ideally, the drug should be tested using the formulation to be used in the clinical studies.

Occasionally there may be a specific case for including larger animals. For example, in the case of inhibitors of the enzyme thymidylate synthase (TS), dog toxicology is necessary since rodents are likely to underpredict for toxicity. Rodents have a higher circulating plasma thymidine concentration than higher mammals (Jackman *et al.*, 1984) and since thymidine can be salvaged from the blood via the enzyme thymidine kinase, this may circumvent the toxic and antitumour effects of TS inhibition.

11.3   PHARMACOKINETICS AND DETERMINATION OF OPTIMUM SCHEDULE

The study of pharmacokinetics is a vital part of preclinical development in helping to define optimum dose schedules, and allow for correlations to be made subsequently between plasma levels in man and the likelihood of toxicity or antitumour activity. Certain drugs exhibit marked differences in activity depending on the schedule of administration. For examples, the degree of schedule dependency of etoposide was not fully recognized at the time of its introduction to clinical practice, in spite of preclinical evidence that fractionated dose schedules were superior. The benefit of prolonged exposure was unequivocally demonstrated by a randomized study in small cell lung cancer in which at 24 hour infusion was compared with 5 × daily administration (Slevin *et al.*, 1989). Even more prolonged exposures using 2 × daily oral administration have since been introduced, with improvements in convenience and efficacy. For a number of drugs, continuous infusion protocols have been employed as a means of reducing drug toxicity where this is associated with peak plasma concentration, e.g. cardiotoxicity with doxorubicin (Legha *et al.*, 1982). In the case of 5-fluorouracil, it has been shown that continuous infusion is superior to bolus administration (Lokich *et al.*, 1989).

11.4   AIMS OF PHASE I TRIALS

Phase I studies are carried out in order to identify a dose and schedule which can be recommended for phase II testing against specific tumour types. It is important to discover the side-effects and identify the maximum tolerated dose but it is inappropriate to approach this as a toxicology exercise. Although the chance of therapeutic benefit may be small (Bodey and Legha, 1987), it remains feasible to perform such studies in such a way as to maximize this possibility. Preclinical investigations will have established an appropriate starting dose, usually based on the LD_{10} in mice, and ideally the optimum schedule will have been determined in at least one tumour model. There may be some indications of organ specific toxicity, and pharmacokinetic studies in rodents may suggest that impaired renal or hepatic function could lead to increased toxicity due to poor clearance.

11.5 THE ROLE OF PHARMACOKINETICS IN PHASE I STUDIES

In the same way that preclinical pharmaco-kinetic studies are vital to ensure that a drug will be given at a sensible dose and using the optimum schedule, it is equally important to make use of this information in early clinical trials. Collins *et al.* (1986) emphasized the importance of preclinical pharmacokinetic data in anticancer drug phase I trials by showing that for many drugs the area under the concentration × time curve (AUC) at the mouse LD_{10} correlated more closely with the AUC at the human MTD than did the cor-responding doses themselves. In the case of doxorubicin, a particularly good example, this can be explained by the higher clearance in man, compared with the mouse. With the aid of this information the AUC correspond-ing to a toxic dose in the mouse can be more rapidly approached in man than with conven-tional escalation steps, limiting the number of patients treated at suboptimal doses.

In order to pursue a pharmacokinetically guided dose escalation (PGDE), one must first establish a linear relationship between dose and exposure, usually as defined by the AUC, in the mouse. In other words, elimination is not dependent on a saturable mechanism which could lead to a very rapid increase in plasma concentration above a certain dose threshold. This must then be confirmed in man, requiring great care during the initial dose escalations. There must be an assay of sufficient sensitivity to measure plasma levels accurately at the starting dose in man. Finally, there must be a direct relationship between toxicity and AUC. This sounds obvious but may not hold true for an antimetabolite, in which case maintenance of the plasma con-centration above a minimum inhibitory threshold for a given period of time may be more important than AUC.

In a review carried out by the Phar-macology and Metabolism (PAM) Group of the EORTC, it was advised that a number of

additional precautions be taken. These include the exclusion of species differences in plasma protein binding and the identification of metabolites in the mouse and their con-tribution to toxicity/activity. Retrospective analyses suggest that problems may still be encountered in applying PGDE to drugs which require metabolic activation and those for which toxicity is related to peak con-centration rather than AUC (EORTC PAM Group, 1987).

Where the principles of PGDE have been applied prospectively, there have been many problems including failure to measure the drug in man at the starting dose, as in the case of amphethinile (Smith *et al.*, 1988) and oxantrazole (Hantel *et al.*, 1990). Excessive interpatient variation in AUC at the first dose levels with the anthrapyrazole CI 941 prevented accurate dose escalation based on AUC (Graham *et al.*, 1992). In a phase I trial of the anthracycline iodo-doxorubicin, Gianni *et al.* (1990) successfully used pharmacokinetic data for both the parent drug and an active metabolite to guide dose escalation. Even where there have been no savings in the number of dose escalations, there are many examples where pharmacokinetic data have contributed to a phase I study either by identifying important species differences in metabolism, as in the case of iodo-doxorubicin, or non-linear pharmacokinetics, thus ensuring safer dose escalation.

Important though plasma concentrations may be, pharmacokinetics may be misleading in the case of drugs which require intracellu-lar activation, e.g. nucleoside analogues such as cytosine arabinoside (ara-C), since plasma levels may not directly reflect intracellular levels of the phosphorylated metabolite ara-CTP (Riva *et al.*, 1985). Differences in target cell levels of both activating and inactivating enzymes, and also extracellular levels of nucleic acid precursors, may affect efficacy. For example, genetic variations in levels of thiopurine methyltransferase, an enzyme which inactivates 6-mercaptopurine, may be responsible for large variations in the activity of this drug (Lennard *et al.*, 1990).

11.6 PHARMACODYNAMIC MEASUREMENTS IN EARLY CLINICAL TRIALS

Pharmacokinetics has been defined as the study of what the body does to the drug, whereas pharmacodynamics is the study of what the drug does to the body, i.e. the relationship between dose and toxicity. Both need to be taken into account during the investigation of a new drug. Ideally, we should be studying the link between plasma or tissue concentration and antitumour effect (Ratain *et al.*, 1990).

The preclinical study of toxicity, antitumour activity, optimum schedule of administration, drug disposition and elimination, will help in planning clinical trials but it is important to confirm that the drug is behaving in a similar fashion in man. In addition to its potential use in dose escalation, an adequate pharmacokinetic assay must be available in order to correlate toxicity with plasma and tissue drug levels and examine inter-patient variability. For drugs which undergo extensive metabolic alteration, particularly to active species, it is necessary to investigate metabolism during the phase I study. The phenyltriazene CB10-277 is a good example of such a compound. This analogue of dacarbazine appeared to be activated more efficiently in rodents but proved to be much less potent in man, although a correlation between the levels of the active metabolite and myelosuppression was observed when a 24 hour infusion schedule was employed (Foster *et al.*, 1993).

Pharmacokinetic studies may lead to alternative ways of determining an appropriate dose. Carboplatin is largely excreted unchanged in the urine, hence there is a good correlation between glomerular filtration rate (GFR) and carboplatin clearance. This has led to the development of dosage formulae based on GFR (Egorin *et al.*, 1985; Calvert *et al.*, 1989) which give a much more accurate prediction of subsequent drug exposure (AUC) than dosage based on surface area. The use of such formulae should have the effect of both reducing excessive toxicity in patients with impaired renal function and preventing suboptimal dosage in patients with above average clearance. Horwich *et al.* (1991) showed that patients receiving carboplatin for the treatment of testicular tumours were more likely to relapse if the calculated carboplatin AUC, based on the formula: Dose (mg) = AUC(GFR (ml/min) + 25), was < 4 mg/ ml.min. A retrospective analysis of over 1000 patients with ovarian cancer treated with carboplatin (Jodrell *et al.*, 1992) appeared to show an increase in response rate up to AUC = 5, above which toxicity but not antitumour activity increased. Nevertheless, Jones *et al.* (1992) and Lind *et al.* (1992) have shown apparent benefit from further dose escalation with this drug and the extent of this dose–response relationship remains under investigation.

In addition to determining the appropriate dose of a drug in relation to an individual patient's ability to excrete or metabolize it, we should ask the question: what measurement is likely to be most important for predicting antitumour activity? This may be peak plasma concentration, AUC or steady state concentration during continuous infusion. For example, Evans and colleagues (1986) at the St Jude Children's Hospital, Memphis, investigating the use of high dose methotrexate (MTX) in the treatment of acute lymphoblastic leukaemia (ALL), showed that children with a steady state MTX concentration <16 μM were three times more likely to relapse than those above this level. Individualized doses based on clearance measurements after a test dose are now being tested prospectively in comparison with a standard dose. Evans has suggested (1988) that if the appropriate pharmacokinetic parameter determining toxicity is known, this might lead to a definition of 'maximum tolerated systemic exposure' as an end point for a phase I trial rather than MTD.

Since plasma concentrations may not always predict intracellular drug levels, these should be measured if possible. For example, Plunkett *et al.* (1985) have shown a strong positive correlation between a trough concentration of the phosphorylated metabolite ara-CTP of ≥ 75 μM in leukaemic cells and the likelihood of subsequent remission. This information has been used to develop a pharmacologically guided dosage schedule. The study of platinum-DNA adduct formation in peripheral blood cells in patients with ovarian cancer receiving cisplatin demonstrated a surprisingly good correlation between adduct levels and subsequent response to treatment (Reed *et al.*, 1987). In our laboratories we are developing sensitive radioimmunoassay techniques for the measurement of changes in tissue nucleotide levels in order to monitor inhibition of thymidylate synthase (G.W. Aherne, personal communication).

11.7 ETHICAL PROBLEMS AND PATIENT SELECTION

Two contradictory ethical problems face the phase I study investigator. Patients treated at the starting dose have very little chance of therapeutic benefit, while those treated at the MTD could suffer serious toxicity. Hence the need to expedite dose escalation while limiting the risk of toxicity. The solutions to these problems lie in the use of all the information available for speeding up dose escalation and similar attention to preclinical data, together with appropriate patient selection to limit the risk of side-effects.

The selection of patients for phase I studies must take into account their performance status (PS) and immediate prognosis, since patients whose disease is too far advanced will not only fail to respond but are also more likely to suffer serious side-effects. From the ethical point of view this is clearly unacceptable. Such patients will also bias the determ-

ination of dose limiting toxicity, often leading to an underestimation of the MTD (Bodey and Legha, 1987). This may lead to the conduct of phase II studies at too low a dose, resulting in a false negative result.

Both extensive prior treatment with bone marrow stem cell poisons, such as mitomycin C and chloroethylnitrosoureas, and radiotherapy to the spine and pelvis, are likely to increase the severity and duration of myelosuppression by diminishing bone marrow reserve. These factors need to be taken into account when assessing the MTD.

Although antitumour responses are rarely seen in phase I trials the chances can be maximized by choosing patients with appropriate tumour types who have not been too heavily pretreated. For example, in the phase I trial of carboplatin reported by Calvert *et al.* (1985), a large number of patients had refractory or recurrent ovarian cancer and many responses were observed. It is worth noting that in addition to the possibility of direct benefit, patients with refractory cancer may derive considerable comfort from the knowledge that their participation may benefit others in the future.

11.8 DEFINITION OF THE MTD AND DOSE ESCALATION STRATEGIES

Since a phase I study must try to define the MTD while avoiding serious and irreversible toxicity, serious difficulties may arise if the dose limiting toxicity is other than myelosuppression. The severity of emesis, neuropathy and mucositis are all more difficult to define and may vary more widely between patients. Where toxicities are cumulative or delayed this problem becomes especially difficult. The working definition of MTD used by the Cancer Research Campaign Phase I Committee suggests the 'highest safely tolerable dose', i.e. WHO grade III of any of the following: myelosuppression, diarrhoea, mucositis, skin toxicity, or WHO grades II–III hepatic, renal, pulmonary, cardiac or neurological toxicity. An approximate description of

Table 11.1 Definition of the maximum tolerated dose (MTD): the highest dose causing none of these toxicities

Origin	MTD
Bone marrow	Granulocytes $< 0.5 \times 10^9$, platelets $< 50 \times 10^9/l$, severe haemolytic anaemia
Gut	Diarrhoea requiring i.v. fluid replacement severe mucositis preventing oral intake
Liver	Bilirubin $> 45 \ \mu mol/l$, ALT > 100 iu (international units)/l
Kidney	Creatinine $> 300 \ \mu mol/l$, or irreversible progressive dose-related decrease in glomerular filtration rate
Heart	Left ventricular failure, life-threatening arrhythmias
Central nervous system	Paralysis, mental deterioration, fits, coma
Skin	Severe exfoliative dermatitis

WHO grades I–IV would be mild, moderate, severe and potentially life-threatening respectively, although of course the latter only applies to the bone marrow or essential organs not hair loss. A summary of some of the more common criteria for defining the MTD is given in Table 11.1.

A variety of methods have been used for dose escalation, most commonly a modification of the Fibonacci series using large initial escalations, reducing to 33% (in the true series, $U_{n+1} = U_n + U_{n-1}$, the recurring increment is 61%). Less conservative methods have been employed, e.g. 100% increments until the first signs of biological effect, and the use of pharmacokinetics in expediting dose escalation has been discussed above.

If sporadic toxicities are observed, it is important to treat a larger number of patients at that dose level. If the toxicity does not recur then dose escalation should proceed as planned. Escalation in the same patient may sometimes be allowed. This has the advantage for any individual patient of increasing the likelihood of therapeutic benefit but makes it more difficult to identify cumulative toxicity.

Since the prime purpose of the phase I study is to select a dose for phase II trial, a reasonably large cohort of patients should be treated at just below the MTD in order to study the degree of interpatient variability and to ensure that the dose is suitable. Too high a dose will lead to excessive toxicity, but too low a dose may result in a drug failing to show activity in phase II, especially if the dose–response curve is steep and the therapeutic index low. In our phase I trial of ICI D1694, the quinazoline antifolate TS inhibitor (Judson et al., 1992), a total of 20 patients were treated at 3.0 mg/m² owing to the variable and cumulative nature of the gut and bone marrow toxicities observed, in order to be sure that this was the appropriate dose for phase II investigation. Responses were observed in a number of tumour types including breast and ovarian cancers.

11.9 CLINICAL EVALUATION OF DRUGS WITH NOVEL TARGETS

There is a growing list of new approaches to cancer therapy which do not rely on the ability to block cell replication, summarized below:

1. Immunomodulation, including gene therapy.

2. Promotion of differentiation.
3. Inhibition of angiogenesis and metastasis.
4. Inhibition of cell signalling pathways.
5. Chemoprevention, antiendocrine agents, free radical scavengers.
6. Modulation of anticancer drug resistance.
7. Bioreductive agents to target hypoxic cells.
8. Monoclonal antibody targeting, including antibody directed enzyme prodrug therapy (ADEPT).

These approaches are changing the way we think about testing new drugs and many difficult challenges lie ahead.

11.9.1 IMMUNOMODULATION

Advances in recombinant DNA technology have made available a number of naturally occurring molecules with the ability to modulate the immune system. Biological response modifiers, or cytokines, may act directly on the cancer cell or indirectly via an impact on the immune system. So far only the interferons and IL-2 have found a clearly defined role in cancer therapy. The early experience with the interferons was extremely disappointing, since few patients had tumour regression and those that responded did so only slowly. However, it has gradually become clear that a more appropriate use of interferons may be in patients with minimal residual disease who may experience prolonged remission. The use of interferon-α has been licensed for use in responding patients with multiple myeloma in whom it prolongs remission (Mandelli *et al.*, 1990) and studies are underway in a number of other tumour types including small cell lung and ovarian cancer. Cytokines may display a so-called 'bell-shaped' dose–response curve, hence the most effective dose may be much lower than the MTD. This property is shared by some other new agents such as bryostatin 1, which is thought to act via protein kinase C. This makes it particularly difficult to determine the appropriate dose for phase II study, especially if the precise mechanism of action is unclear. An alternative approach in the future may be to transfer specific cytokine genes into tumour cells. Tumour cells which are made to overexpress cytokines such as tumour necrosis factor alpha (TNFα), or IL-2, by this technique, become more immunogenic and can be used as a vaccine to promote an effective antitumour immune response (Rosenberg, 1992).

11.9.2 PROMOTION OF DIFFERENTIATION

A number of drugs have been identified with potent ability to promote differentiation of experimental cell lines *in vitro*. In the majority of cases such drugs have failed to show any useful activity against established solid tumours. However, all-*trans* retinoic acid has proved very successful in human promyelocytic leukaemia, in which a number of trials have reported successful results including complete remissions (Smith *et al.*, 1988). The mechanism of action appears to involve a specific chromosomal translocation t(15;17) which fuses the retinoic acid receptor-alpha gene with the PML gene. The novel fusion protein is thought to interfere with normal myeloid differentiation (Goddard *et al.*, 1992). Further therapy is required to maintain remission, but the initial complications of disseminated intravascular coagulation, which complicate intensive chemotherapy for remission induction, may be avoided. Another retinoid, isotretinoin, has demonstrated the ability to inhibit squamous metaplasia and appears to reduce the incidence of second tumours in patients with squamous head and neck cancer. This observation is currently being tested in combination with *N*-acetylcysteine in the large multicentre randomized EUROSCAN trial.

11.9.3 INHIBITION OF ANGIOGENESIS AND METASTASIS

The cytokine usually associated with an effect on tumour vasculature is TNFα but tumour angiogenesis itself has become a potential target for anticancer therapy (Denekamp and Hill, 1991). Associated research is also focused on the metastatic process and the role of cellular adhesion molecules. A number of specific markers have been identified which are associated with increased metastatic potential, such as the CD44 antigen which is increased in metastatic malignant melanoma (Hart *et al.*, 1991) and the *nm23* gene which is downregulated in tumours with increased metastatic potential, or patients with poorer prognosis (Hennessy *et al.*, 1991). Conversely, animal experiments using gene transfection demonstrate that restoring normal expression can reduce the incidence of lung metastases in human tumour xenografts. This work suggests that the development of genuine antimetastatic agents may be possible. Testing such drugs will be time consuming and require large randomized trials.

11.9.4 INHIBITION OF CELL SIGNALLING PATHWAYS

The complex sequence of events which occurs following binding of peptide growth factors' specific receptors on the cell surface is becoming better understood. This knowledge has suggested a large number of potential new targets for growth inhibition, such as tyrosine kinases, protein kinase C, phospholipases, growth factor–receptor interactions, calcium flux and many more. A number of drugs which have been discovered through the usual mixture of serendipity and screening turn out to have activities in this area. As yet it is too early to say whether such new targets will offer improved selectivity (Workman, 1990). Bryostatin 1 is a macrocyclic lactone protein kinase C (PKC) activator which leads to subsequent downregulation. Laboratory studies have demonstrated *in vitro* cytotoxic activity against leukaemic cells, including acute myeloid leukaemia (Grant *et al.*, 1990). Some experiments suggest that at least some of the activity may be mediated through

secondary release of cytokines (Lilly *et al.*, 1991). In phase I studies using a single bolus injection every 3 weeks, severe myalgia proved dose limiting (Carmichael and Harris, 1993). Further investigations are continuing using a fractionated schedule at non-myalgic doses. Repeat administration is possible and antitumour responses have been observed.

11.9.5 CHEMOPREVENTION

Most approaches to the prevention of cancer have concentrated on screening and the success of programmes for cervical and breast cancer is well known. The use of drugs to try and prevent cancer is more difficult, since one must be absolutely sure that the intervention is not itself toxic. The trials of tamoxifen in women with a strong family history of breast cancer and increased risk of developing the disease, have aroused great controversy, although the pilot study at the Royal Marsden Hospital (Powles and Jones, 1991) has suggested a reduction in the risk of osteoporotic bone and cardiovascular diseases.

Many promising substances are free radical scavengers, some of which are common vitamins, e.g. C and E. Treatment will need to be prolonged, requiring an effective dose as determined by pharmacokinetics and low toxicity to ensure compliance. Large numbers of patients will need to be treated in randomized trials, such as the one combining *N*-acetylcysteine with isotretinoin in patients with previous head and neck cancer discussed above.

11.9.6 MODULATION OF ANTICANCER DRUG RESISTANCE

Cytotoxic drug resistance may be intrinsic or acquired and represents a major problem in cancer therapy. Many different mechanisms are known, including the P-glycoprotein drug efflux pump conferring the multidrug resistance phenotype (Ling *et al.*, 1988). Inhibitors of P-glycoprotein, such as verapamil and cyclosporin A, have been extensively investigated. Toxicity is a major problem which has so far limited the efficacy of this approach. Another potential issue is the impact of resistance modifiers on the pharmacokinetics of the cytotoxic agent concerned. In the case of platinum anticancer drugs, resistance can occur due to reduced drug uptake, detoxification by thiols such as glutathione and enhanced DNA repair. Glutathione synthesis can be inhibited by the drug buthionine sulfoximine and may enhance the antitumour activity of alkylating agents like melphalan (Bailey *et al.*, 1992), although this would be likely to increase nephrotoxicity with cisplatin. There are also data to suggest that both transport (Basu and Lazo, 1992) and DNA repair (Swinnen *et al.*, 1991) can be modulated. The development of resistance modifiers requires a clear understanding of the mechanisms of resistance, detailed toxicity and pharmacokinetic phase I studies and ultimately large randomized trials.

11.10 PHASE II STUDIES

Having determined a suitable dose and schedule for further study, a new agent will then be tested for activity against specific tumour types. Patient populations vary according to the median age of peak incidence and the aetiology of particular tumour types. This may affect drug tolerance and it may also be necessary to consider the option of choosing separate doses for non-previously treated and heavily pretreated patients. Another approach is to recommend dose escalation if a predetermined level of toxicity is not observed after the first course. Conversely, dose reductions will, of course, be allowed if toxicity is excessive.

11.10.1 PRIOR THERAPY: YES OR NO?

If failure to choose the right dose and schedule can result in a falsely negative phase II study, what about the choice of patients? It is known that previous exposure to cytotoxic

drugs and radiotherapy may lead to the induction of drug resistance, in some cases due to increased expression of P-glycoprotein (Schneider *et al.*, 1989) or via an increase in reduced glutathione levels (de Vries *et al.*, 1989). Because of the impact of acquired resistance on response rates it would be ideal if one could test new drugs in previously untreated patients. However, there are practical and ethical problems with this approach, particularly in disease types where conventional treatment is reasonably effective, at least in the short term.

For example, metastatic breast cancer is generally regarded as incurable, hence the administration of a new drug prior to conventional combination chemotherapy does not involve withholding potentially curative treatment. Therefore, it should be regarded as ethical to investigate new agents first line in advanced breast cancer, with the exception of patients with life-threatening liver or lung disease. Such patients require prompt administration of chemotherapy of known efficacy.

In small cell lung cancer (SCLC) the problem of acquired resistance is clearly illustrated by two of the most active drugs in this disease, etoposide and carboplatin. Etoposide has been reported to give a response rate of 50% in previously untreated patients (Eagan *et al.*, 1976) compared with 3–9% in patients with previously refractory disease (Harper *et al.*, 1982; Issell *et al.*, 1985). Similarly, carboplatin achieved a response rate of 60% in untreated compared with 19% in previously treated patients (Smith *et al.*, 1985).

The practice of testing new drugs in previously untreated patients with SCLC has recently become more widely accepted (Ettinger, 1990), particularly in patients with extensive disease, on the grounds that their survival is so poor. However, the use of ineffective drugs first line may prejudice subsequent treatment. In a phase II study of idarubicin in previously untreated extensive disease patients, the response rate was only 14% (Cullen *et al.*, 1987). This was not unexpected, but these patients subsequently fared badly in spite of switching rapidly to conventional chemotherapy and their median survival was only 6 months. Similar results with mitoxantrone were reported.

If extensive disease SCLC is not a good testing ground for new agents, what about limited disease? These patients have a much worse prognosis than those with metastatic breast cancer (Smith, 1989). However, the majority of such patients show some evidence of response after only one course of treatment. Thus it seems likely that even one course of experimental therapy could give sufficient indication of efficacy to justify further investigation. Alternatively, patients who relapse off treatment, particularly after a long treatment-free interval, have a good chance of a second response with the same treatment, e.g. 67% in a study at the Royal Marsden Hospital (Vincent *et al.*, 1988), a finding which has been confirmed by other groups. These patients should be considered for new drug trials.

In ovarian cancer a similar problem has been identified. In a retrospective study of five phase II trials, it was found that treatment-free interval was the most important prognostic factor for response in a multivariate analysis (Blackledge *et al.*, 1989). The impact of differences in this variable may explain the wide variations in response to certain agents, e.g. 0–26% for mitoxantrone as second line therapy for stage III/IV ovarian cancer. In ovarian cancer as in SCLC, retreatment with the same chemotherapy may be effective after a reasonable time off treatment. In this case, platinum complex based chemotherapy may produce a response rate of about 50% after a treatment-free interval of > 12 months (Gore *et al.*, 1990). For this reason, phase II studies in ovarian cancer should first be performed in patients who have previously had a good response to therapy and relapsed after a long, e.g. 12 months, treatment-free interval. Again, there is concern about the possibility that exposure to an ineffective drug may induce resistance to more effective conventional agents and response assessment is a major problem in this disease (Wiltshaw *et al.*, 1990). Drugs with some indication of activity may be tested first line in stage IV patients who are currently incurable.

11.10.2   SURROGATE MARKERS OF ACTIVITY

In order to limit exposure to the experimental agent tumour markers could be used to give an early indication of activity. Examples are CA-125 in ovarian cancer (Rustin *et al.*, 1989), and prostate specific antigen (PSA) in prostate cancer, a disease where conventional response criteria are extremely difficult to obtain (Dundas *et al.*, 1990). Careful studies are now required to validate the use of such markers as a substitute for objective tumour measurements.

If tumour markers are a useful way of monitoring response, pharmacokinetics should also be considered as an integral part of phase II studies to investigate interpatient variations in toxicity which might be explained by differences in clearance or extent of metabolic activation. Unfortunately, the majority of phase II studies have tended to ignore such issues, which may remain incompletely understood for several years after the introduction of a new drug. As discussed above, techniques to measure drug effect should also be developed, as in the case of thymidylate synthase inhibitors.

11.10.3   RANDOMIZED PHASE II STUDIES

Finally, there are concerns about the uncontrolled nature of phase II studies. This is particularly important in the case of diseases for which even standard therapy is relatively ineffective. For example, the range of reported response rates to single agent 5-fluorouracil in large bowel cancer was 8–85% in one survey (Moertel and Thynne, 1982). Such differences may be due to chance or patient selection and there is clearly a good case to be made for performing randomized phase II studies in order to monitor the quality of patient selection and minimize reporting bias.

11.11 CONCLUSIONS

The successful evaluation of new anticancer drugs increasingly depends on a detailed understanding of mechanism of action and pharmacology. The current generation of antiproliferative agents remains vitally important for the treatment of many cancers and improvements will no doubt continue to be made through the development of analogues with reduced toxicity or enhanced efficacy. Well-proven preclinical toxicology, phase I and phase II protocols exist which work well for these agents. However, drugs are now being developed for a variety of new targets which will require a different approach. Most importantly, it will be necessary to measure biological effect, rather than toxicity, as an end point for phase I trials, and proof of activity is likely to require large randomized trials. This will be a major organizational challenge but these are exciting prospects which could radically alter the way in which cancer is treated in the future.

REFERENCES

Bailey, H., Mulcahy, R.T., Tutsch, K.D. *et al.* (1992) Glutathione levels and γ-glutamylcysteine synthase activity in patients undergoing phase I treatment with L-buthionine sulfoximine and melphalan. *Proceedings of the American Association of Cancer Research*, **33**, 479.

Basu, A. and Lazo, J.S. (1992) Sensitization of human cervical carcinoma cells to *cis*-diaminedichloroplatinum (II) by bryostatin 1. *Cancer Research*, **52**, 3119–24.

Blackledge, G., Lawton, F., Redman, C. *et al.* (1989) Response of patients in phase II studies of chemotherapy in epithelial ovarian cancer: implications for patient treatment and design of phase II studies. *British Journal of Cancer*, **59**, 650–3.

Bodey, G. and Legha, S. (1987) The phase I study: general objectives, methods, and evaluation *Developmental Oncology*, **46**, 153–74.

Calvert, A., H., Harland, S.J., Newell, D.R., *et al.* (1985) Phase I studies with carboplatin at the Royal Marsden Hospital. *Cancer Treatment Reviews*, **12**, 51–7.

Calvert, A., Newell, D., Gumbrell, L., *et al.* (1989) Carboplatin dosage: prospective evaluation of a simple formula based on renal function. *Journal of Clinical Oncology*, **11**, 1748–56.

Carmichael, J. and Harris, A. L. (1993) Problems in evaluation of compounds involved in signal transduction in phase I studies. *European Journal of Cancer*, **29A** (suppl 6), S35.

Collins, J., Zaharko, D., Dedrick, R. *et al.* (1986) Potential roles for preclinical pharmacology in phase I clinical trials. *Cancer Treatment Reports*, **70**, 73–80.

Cullen, M.H., Smith, S.R., Benfield, G.R. *et al.* (1987) Testing new drugs in untreated small cell lung cancer may prejudice the results of standard treatment: phase II study of oral idarubicin in extensive disease. *Cancer Treatment Reports*, **71**, 1227–30.

Denekamp, J., and Hill, A. (1991) Angiogenic attack as a therapeutic strategy for cancer. *Radiotherapy and Oncology*, **20** (suppl. 1), 103–12.

de Vries, E.G., Jeijer, C., Timmer-Bosscha, H. *et al.* (1989) Resistance mechanisms in three human small cell lung cancer cell lines established from one patient during clinical follow-up. *Cancer Research*, **49**, 4175–8.

Dundas, G.S., Porter, A.T. and Venner, P.M. (1990) Prostate-specific antigen: monitoring the response of carcinoma of the prostate to radiotherapy with a new tumor marker. *Cancer*, **66**, 45–8.

Eagen, R.T., Carr, D.T., Frytak, S. *et al.* (1976) VP16 versus polychemotherapy in patients with advanced small cell lung cancer. *Cancer Treatment Report*, **60**, 949–51.

Egorin, M.E.9 Van Echo, D.J., Olman, E.A. *et al.* (1985) Prospective validation of a pharmacologically-based dosing scheme for the cisplatin analogue, carboplatin. *Cancer Research*, **44**, 5432–8.

EORTC PAM Group (1987) Pharmacokinetically guided dose escalation in phase I clinical trials. Commentary and proposed guidelines. *European Journal of Cancer and Clinical Oncology*, **7**, 1083–7.

Ettinger, D.S. (1990) Evaluation of new drugs in untreated patients with small-cell lung cancer:

its time has come. *Journal of Clinical Oncology*, **8**, 374–7.

Evans, W. (1988) Clinical pharmacodynamics of anticancer drugs: a basis for extending the concept of dose-intensity. *Blut*, **56**, 241–8.

Evans, W.E., Crom, W.R., Abromowitch, M. *et al.* (1986) Clinical pharmacodynamics of high-dose methotrexate in acute lymphocytic leukaemia. *New England Journal of Medicine*, **314**, 471–7.

Foster, B.J., Newell, D.R., Gumbrell, L.A. *et al.* (1993) Phase I trial with pharmacokinetics of CB10-277 given by 24 hours continuous infusion. *British Journal of Cancer*, **67**, 369–73.

Freireich, E., Gehan, E., Rall, D. *et al.* (1966) Quantitative comparison of toxicity of anticancer agents in mouse, rat, hamster, dog, monkey and man. *Cancer Chemotherapy Report*, **50**, 219–45.

Gianni L., Vigani, L., Surbone, A. *et al.* (1990) Pharmacology and clinical toxicity of 4′-iodo-4′-deoxydoxorubicin: an example of successful application of pharmacokinetics to dose escalation in phase I trials. *Journal of the National Cancer Institute*, **82**, 469–77.

Goddard, A.D., Borrow, J. and Soloman, E. (1992) A previously uncharacterised gene, PML, is fused to the retinoic acid receptor alpha gene in acute promyelocytic leukaemia. *Leukemia*, **6**(suppl. 3), 1175–95.

Gore, M.E., Fryatt, I., Wiltshaw, E. *et al.* (1990) Treatment of relapsed carcinoma of the ovary with cisplatin or carboplatin following initial treatment with these compounds. *Gynecologic Oncology*, **36**, 208–11.

Graham, M.A., Newell, D.R., Foster, B.J. *et al.* (1992) Clinical pharmacokinetics of the anthrapyrazole CI-941: factors compromising the implementation of a pharmacokinetically guided dose escalation scheme. *Cancer Research*, **52**, 603–9.

Grant, S., Boise, L., Westin, E. *et al.* (1990) *In vitro* effects of bryostatin 1 on the metabolism and cytotoxicity of 1-beta-D-arabinofuranosyl-cytosine in human leukemia cells. *Biochemical Pharmacology*, **42**, 853–67.

Hantel, A., Donehower, R., Rowinsky, E. *et al.* (1990) Phase I study and pharmacodynamics of piroxantrone (NSC 349174), a new anthrapyrazole. *Cancer Research*, **50**, 3284–8.

Harper, P.G., Dully, M.B., Geddes, D.M. *et al.* (1982) VP16-213 in small cell carcinoma of the bronchus resistant to initial combination chemotherapy. *Cancer Chemotherapy and Pharmacology*, **7**, 179–80.

Hart, I.R., Birch, M. and Marshall, J.F. (1991) Cell adhesion receptor expression during melanoma progression and metastasis. *Cancer Metastasis Reviews*, **10**, 115–28.

Hennessy, C., Henry, J.A., May, F.E. *et al.* (1991) Expression of the antimetastatic gene nm23 in human breast cancer: an association with good prognosis. *Journal of the National Cancer Institute*, **83**, 281–5.

Horwich, A., Dearnaley, D.P., Nicholls, J. *et al.* (1991) Effectiveness of carboplatin, etoposide, and bleomycin combination chemotherapy in good-prognosis metastatic testicular non-seminomatous germ cell tumours. *Journal of Clinical Oncology*, **9**, 62–9.

Issell, B.F., Einhorn, L.H., Comis, R.L. *et al.* (1985) Multicenter phase II trial etoposide in refractory small cell lung cancer. *Cancer Treatment Reports*, **69**, 127–8.

Jackman, A., Taylor, G., Calvert, A. *et al.* (1984) Modulation of anti-metabolite effects: effects of thymidine on the efficacy of the quinazoline-based thymidylate synthetase inhibitor, CB3717. *Biochemical Pharmacology*, **33**, 3269–75.

Jodrell, D.I., Egorin, M.E., Canetta, R.M, *et al.* (1992) Relationship between carboplatin exposure and tumour response and toxicity in patients with ovarian cancer. *Journal of Clinical Oncology*, **10**, 520–8.

Joint Steering Committee of the EORTC and the CRC (1989) General guidelines for the pre-clinical toxicology of new cytotoxic anticancer agents in Europe. *European Journal of Cancer*, **26**, 411–4.

Jones, A., Wiltshaw, E., Harper, P. *et al.* (1992) A randomised study of high versus conventional dose carboplatin for previously untreated ovarian cancer. *British Journal of Cancer*, **65**(suppl. XVI), 15.

Judson, I. (1989) New endocrine agents, guidelines for future development. *British Journal of Cancer*, **60**, 153–4.

Judson, I., Clarke, S., Ward, J. *et al.* (1992) A phase I trial of the thymidylate synthase inhibitor ICI D1694. *Annals Oncology*, **3**(suppl. 5), 51.

Legha, S., Benjamin, R., Mackay, R. *et al.* (1982) Adriamycin therapy by continuous intravenous infusion in patients with metastatic breast cancer. *Cancer*, **49**, 1762–6.

Lennard, L., Lillyman, J., Van Loon, J. *et al.* (1990) Genetic variation in response to 6-mercaptopurine for childhood acute lymphoblastic leukaemia. *Lancet*, **336**, 225–9.

Lilly, M., Brown, C., Pettit, G. *et al.* (1991) Bryostatin 1: a potential anti-leukemic agent for chronic myelomonocytic leukemia. *Leukemia*, **5**, 283–7.

Lind, M.J., Millward, M.M, Chapman, F. *et al.* (1992) The use of RH-GCSF to increase the delivered dose of carboplatin in women with advanced epithelial ovarian cancer. *Proceedings of the American Society of Clinical Oncology*, **11**, 230.

Ling, V., Juranka, P.F. and Endicott, J.A. (1988) Multidrug resistance and P-glycoprotein expression, in *Mechanisms of Drug Resistance in Neoplastic Cells*, (eds P.V. Woolley and K.D. Tew), Academic Press, San Diego, pp. 197–209.

Lokich, J.J., Ahlgren, J.D., Gullo, J.J. *et al.* (1989) A prospective randomized comparison of continuous infusion fluroruracil with a conventional bolus schedule in metastatic colorectal carcinoma: a Mid-Atlantic Oncology Program Study. *Journal of Clinical Oncology*, **7**, 425–32.

Malik, S.T., Rayner, H., Fletcher, J. *et al.* (1987) Phase II of mitoxantrone as first-line chemotherapy for extensive small cell lung cancer. *Cancer Treatment Reports*, **71**, 1291–2.

Mandelli, F., Avvisati, G., Amadori, S. *et al.* (1990) Maintenance treatment with recombinant interferon alfa-2b in patients with multiple myeloma responding to conventional induction chemotherapy. *New England Journal of Medicine*, **332**, 1430–4.

Moertel, C.G. and Thynne, G.S. (1982) Large bowel, in *Cancer Medicine*, 2nd edn, (eds J.F. Holland and E. Frei III), Lea and Febiger, Philadelphia, pp. 1830–59.

Plunkett, W., Iacoboni, S., Estey, E. *et al.* (1985) Pharmacologically directed ara-C therapy for refractory leukemia. *Seminars in Oncology*, **12**, 20–30.

Powles, T.J. and Jones, A.L. (1991) Chemoprevention of breast cancer, in *Medical Management of Breast Cancer*, (eds T.J. Pourles and I.E. Smith), Martin Dunitz, New York, pp. 289–95.

Ratain, M.J., Schilsky, R.L., Conley, B.A. *et al.* (1990) Pharmacodynamics in cancer therapy. *Journal of Clinical Oncology*, **8**, 1739–53.

Reed, E., Ozols, R., Tarone, R. *et al.* (1987) Platinum-DNA adducts in leukocyte DNA correlate with disease response in ovarian cancer patients receiving platinum-based chemother-apy. *Proceedings of the National Academy of Sciences USA.*, **84**, 5024–8.

Riva, C., Rustum, Y. and Preisler, H. (1985) Pharmacokinetics and cellular determinates of response to 1-B-d-ara-binofuranosylcytosine. *Seminars in Oncology*, **12**, 1–8.

Rosenberg, S.A. (1992) The immunotherapy and gene therapy of cancer. *Cancer Research*, **10**, 180–99.

Rustin, G.J., Gennings, J.N., Nelstrop, A.E. *et al.* (1989) Use of CA-125 to predict survival of patients with ovarian carcinoma. *Journal of Clinical Oncology*, **7**, 1667–71.

Schneider, J., Bak, M., Efferth, Th. *et al.* (1989) P-glycoprotein expression in treated and untreated human breast cancer. *British Journal of Cancer*, **60**, 815–8.

Slevin, M., Clark, P., Joel, S. *et al.* (1989) A randomized trial to evaluate the effect of schedule on the activity of etoposide in small-cell lung cancer. *Journal of Clinical Oncology*, **9**, 1333–40.

Smith, D., Ewen, C., Mackintosh, J. *et al.* (1988) A phase I and pharmacokinetic study of amphethinile. *British Journal of Cancer*, **57**, 623.

Smith, I.E. (1989) New treatments for small cell lung cancer: when to test. *Chest*, **96**(suppl.), 59S–61S.

Smith, I.E., Harland, S.J., Robinson, B.A. *et al.* (1985) Carboplatin: a very active new cisplatin analog in the treatment of small cell lung cancer. *Cancer Treatment Reports*, **69**, 43–6.

Smith, M.A., Parkinson, D.R., Cheson, B.D. and Freidman, M.A. (1992) Retinoids in cancer therapy. *Journal of Clinical Oncology*, **10**, 839–64.

Swinnen, L.J., Ellis, N.K. and Erickson, L.C. (1991) Inhibition of cis-diammine-1, 1-cyclobutanedicarboxylatoplatinum(II) cytotoxicity by hydroxyurea and 1-β-D-arabinofuranosylcytosine. *Cancer Research*, **51**, 1984–5.

Vincent, M., Evans, B. and Smith, I.E. (1988) First-line chemotherapy re-challenge after relapse in small cell lung cancer. *Cancer Chemotherapy and Pharmacology*, **21**, 45–8.

Wiltshaw, E., Perren, T.J., Fryatt, I.D. *et al.* (1990) Carboplatin and ifosfamide in ovarian cancer phase II and III trials. *Cancer Chemotherapy and Pharmacology*, **26**(suppl) S48–50.

Workman, P. (1990) The cell membrane and cell signals: new targets for novel anticancer drugs. *Annals of Oncology*, **1**, 100–11.

PRINCIPLES OF CYTOKINE THERAPY   12

Anne Taylor and Martin Gore

The last 10–15 years has seen an explosion of information on cytokines and their role or potential role in cancer therapy. Much of the new information has led to more questions than answers and there is still much to be learned.

This chapter will define cytokines, describe their function in clinical practice and their mechanisms of action. The use of individual cytokines for human cancer therapy, response rates and toxicities will also be described. Separate sections will deal with adoptive immunotherapy, biochemotherapy, cytokine gene therapy and the problems associated with the delivery, dosing and scheduling of this treatment modality.

12.1   WHAT ARE CYTOKINES?

The existence of cytokines has been recognized for over 30 years but the ability to study them in detail was only made possible by the advent of improvements in cell culture, development of monoclonal antibodies and the exploitation of recombinant DNA technology allowing the production of large quantities of pure material.

Cytokines are soluble small proteins which are part of the group of biofunctional agents known as the peptide regulatory factors. These are multifunctional mediators of cellular growth and differentiation (Green, 1989). They have been variously called biological response modifiers, biologicals and interleukins, but these terminologies will not be used further in this chapter. Unlike true hormones, cytokines tend to act locally in a paracrine or autocrine fashion. Cytokines form part of a very complex network in which one cytokine influences the production of other cytokines. They are produced by mononuclear cells and have the following characteristics: they are of low molecular weight, usually less than 80,000 kDa, they have specific high-affinity cell surface receptors, they have the ability to affect cellular differentiation and/or proliferation, most are glycosylated and most have multifunctional activity. These characteristics can be summarized as follows:

1. Low molecular weight (< 80 kDa).
2. Soluble.
3. Produced by many cell types.
4. Have specific high-affinity cell surface receptors.
5. Mostly glycosylated.
6. Multifunctional activity.
7. Autocrine/paracrine activity.
8. Affect cellular differentiation/proliferation.
9. Induction of other cytokines.
10. Effects modulated by presence/absence of other cytokines.

The effects of a particular cytokine on a single cell type are dependent on the prevailing intercellular environment, i.e. its effects may be altered by the presence or absence of other cytokines. Cytokines can up- or down-regulate unrelated receptors, this is known as transmodulation. In addition the observed biological effects of a cytokine may be modified indirectly by another cytokine which it in turn may induce.

The original method of naming cytokines was according to their biological actions but this resulted in the same cytokine having several names. The nomenclature was therefore rationalized in 1986 by the 6th International Congress of Immunology. New cytokines are called interleukins and designated a number after they have been cloned and sequenced, older terminologies are now not used. However, it was decided to continue with the old names for a small group of the earliest described cytokines, namely interferons, colony-stimulating factors and tumour necrosis factor, because of familiarity. The cytokines were initially studied because of their role in the control of immunity, infection, differentiation, embryogenesis and growth, but more recently their role in the aetiology and/or control of cancer has been recognized. Structurally there is some cross-species homology with cytokines but results of cancer treatment experiments in animals need careful interpretation before being translated to the human situation. This chapter will deal only with the effects of cytokines and the results of trials in humans.

12.2 BIOLOGICAL ACTION OF CYTOKINES AND THEIR SOURCES

The site of production of individual cytokines and their main actions are listed in Table 12.1 and discussed in more detail in the paragraphs that follow.

12.2.1 INTERLEUKIN 1

This cytokine is produced by macrophages and other cell types in response to mitogens. It occurs in two molecular forms, IL1-alpha and IL1-beta, but the two appear to bind the same receptor and the difference between them is minimal. Numerous biological effects have been attributed to interleukin-1. It induces IL-1 receptor expression on T lymphocytes and the production of interleukin - 2 by these same cells. On its own, IL-1 has no proliferative action on haemopoietic cells but it is a potent inducer of other cytokines and regulatory proteins (interferons, interleukin 6) which result in stimulation of early and late stage haemopoietic progenitor cells. It acts in an autocrine fashion resulting in further IL-1 production and is a chemotaxin for polymorphonuclear cells and macrophages. It induces endothelial and osteoblast proliferation and bone resorption by osteoclasts. It augments NK mediated cytotoxicity. In induces changes in the cell cycle status of non-cycling immature haemopoietic progenitors by increasing the proportion of cells in G2, M and S.

The clinical effects of IL-1 are multiple: it produces fever, anorexia, neutrophilia, secretion of acute phase proteins by the liver and aids in repair of injured tissues. It may also act as a procoagulant.

12.2.2 INTERLEUKIN 2

This cytokine is produced only by activated T lymphocytes, of the helper subset. The interaction of IL-2 with the IL-2 receptor promotes progression of T cells through the S phase of the cell cycle. It induces expansion and activation of T and B cells. The secretion of IL-2 and cell surface expression of the IL-2 receptor are both dependent upon recent antigen-induced activation of the T cell, i.e. the T cell requires two distinct and temporarily separable extracellular signals for growth. The IL-2 receptor consists of two chains, the 55 kDa alpha chain and the 75 kDa beta chain. IL-2 binds to the alpha chain with low affinity and to the beta chain with intermediate affinity. If both chains are present they form a dimer which binds IL-2 with high affinity. Ten per cent of receptors on the cell surfaces are of the dimer or high affinity variety and they are involved in receptor-mediated endocytosis

Table 12.1   Classification of cytokines: sites of production and mechanisms of action

Name	Site of production	Mechanism of action
IL-1	Macrophages, many other cell types	Induction of IL-2 from activated cells Augments NK cytotoxicity Induces acute phase reactants Induces tumour cell lysis by macrophages
IL-2	Activated T cells	Expansion and activation of T and B cells Activates antitumour activity of NK cells
IL-4	Subset of activated T cells	B-cell growth factor (with CSFs) Increases MHC class II antigen expression in resting B cells Enhances production of IgG1 and IgE T-cell growth factor
IL-5	Activated T lymphocytes	Induces eosinophilia
IL-6	Macrophages, stromal cells, some activated T lymphocytes	B-cell growth factor IL-1 and IL-6 accelerate blast colony formation May be an autocrine growth factor in multiple myeloma
alpha-INF	Peripheral blood mononuclear cells	Antiviral Antiparasitic Antitumour activity by both increasing cytotoxicity of macrophages, NK cells and T cells and cytostatic Reverses cytogenic abnormalities
gamma-INF	Fibroblasts Epithelial cells	Controls immune response Antitumour activity
TNF	Activated macrophages Activated T cells	Antiviral activity Directly cytotoxic Mediates shock Induces MHC antigens on epithelial cells
G-CSF	Endothelial cells	Stimulates granulocyte precursors
GM-CSF	Fibroblasts, endothelial cells macrophages and T lymphocytes	Stimulates production of granulocytes and macrophages
M-CSF	Connective tissue cells	Stimulates production of monocytes/macrophages
IL-3	Activated T lymphocytes	Stimulus for production of macrophages, neutrophils, eosinophils, megakarocytes and mast cells

and degradation of IL-2. Internalization is accompanied by a decrease in the number of high affinity IL-2 receptors. The other 90% of receptors do not form dimers and do not appear to mediate any biological activity. The binding of IL-2 to its receptor results in intra-cellular changes, probably via a second messenger which has not yet been identified.

IL-2 has the following biological activities: it causes upregulation of IL-2 gene expression and receptor gene expression. It enhances the cytotoxicity of natural killer (NK), lymphocyte activated killer (LAK) cells and macrophages. It causes proliferation and differentiation of activated T and B lymphocytes and stimulates the production of interferon, tumour necrosis factor and lymphotoxin. It also stimulates oligodendrocyte proliferation.

12.2.3   INTERLEUKIN 3

Refer to section 12.2.9 below.

12.2.4   INTERLEUKIN 4

This cytokine is produced by a subset of activated T helper cells. On its own it has no proliferative effect but it enhances colony formation stimulated by granulocyte colony stimulating factor (G-CSF), macrophage colony stimulating factor (M-CSF) and erythropoietin. Conversely, it inhibits colony formation stimulated by IL-3. Its biological activity is exerted through a specific high affinity receptor expressed on a variety of haemopoietic cells, resting T cells, B cells, macrophages and mast cells. It has the following activities: it upregulates MHC class II expression on resting B cells. It enhances production of IgG, and IgE following stimulation by mitogens. It increases viability and growth of normal resting T cells and some T cell lines. It costimulates growth of mucosal and connective tissue-type mast cells. It has a possible role in thymocyte maturation in the thymus. It has a role in cell-mediated immunity probably by enhancing the development of cytotoxic T lymphocytes and inducing LAK activity.

12.2.5   INTERLEUKIN 5

This cytokine is produced by activated T lymphocytes. It selectively stimulates the proliferation of eosinophil precursors and the functional activity of mature eosinophils. Little other activity is attributed to IL-5 at the present time.

12.2.6   INTERLEUKIN 6

This cytokine is produced by macrophages, stromal cells and some activated T lymphocytes. On its own it has no proliferative effects on haemopoietic cells. In combination with IL-3 it accelerates and enhances blast cell colony formation and potentiates the formation of multilineage granulocyte and macrophage colonies. Some of its activities are thought to overlap with those of IL-1. There is evidence that it may act as an autocrine growth factor in multiple myeloma.

12.2.7   INTERLEUKINS 7 TO 10

These have been identified but will not be discussed here.

12.2.8   ERYTHROPOIETIN

This cytokine is produced predominantly by the juxtaglomerular cells of the kidney, by macrophages and possibly other cells. It stimulates committed erythroid precursors to proliferate and form mature progeny. It is reputed to have a stimulatory action on megakarocytes but it has no other known actions. For complete regulatory control of erythropoiesis other cytokines are required. Levels of erythropoietin in plasma and urine increase in response to blood loss and hypoxia but are subnormal for the degree of anaemia in chronic renal failure. Erythropoietin levels may be increased in some tumours, particularly renal cell carcinoma.

12.2.9   COLONY STIMULATING FACTORS

There are four main CSFs identified so far. These are gramlacyte -macrophage, granulocyte and monocyte colony stimulating factor (GM-CSF), G-CSF, M-CSF and IL-3.

IL-3 is produced exclusively by activated T lymphocytes and acts through a specific receptor. It increases the production of macrophages, neutrophils, eosinophils, megakaryocytes and mast cells. GM-CSF is produced by fibroblasts, endothelial cells, macrophages and T lymphocytes. It is distinguished by its ability to transform both granulocyte precursors and monocytes into granulocytes and macrophages respectively. G-CSF is produced by endothelial cells and activates granulocyte precursors and M-CSF is produced by macrophages and stimulates the development of monocytes and macrophages.

12.2.10 TUMOUR NECROSIS FACTOR

Over 100 years ago the surgeon William Coley recognized that patients with tumours who developed infection or inflammation may experience spontaneous tumour regression which was mediated by a toxin (Coley Nauts *et al.*, 1953). Subsequently, TNF (otherwise known as cachectin) was identified as the elusive toxin (Carswell *et al.*, 1975). Two forms of the cytokine are produced: activated macrophages produce alpha-TNF and activated T cells produce beta-TNF. Both have identical actions and compete for the same receptor. TNF has many recognized activities, some of which overlap with IL-1, and these are as follows: TNF initiates grow thof some cell lines and induces expression of MHC class I and II antigensandlg receptors on secretory epithelialcells.It activates polymorphonuclear cells and has antiviral activity. It activates osteoclasts and causes bone resorption. It is identical to cachectin and is a central mediator of shock in Gram-negative sepsis. It probably has a protective role in some parasitic infections and is implicated in the pathogenesis of cerebral malaria. TNF amplifies the release of IL-1 or CSF.

12.2.11 INTERFERONS

Interferons were the first cytokines to be described. They were identified in 1957 (Isaacs and Lindemann) as proteins produced by the body in response to viral infections and it is now known that they are important in regulating the immune response. Three types of interferon (IFN) are recognized: alpha, beta and gamma. They exert their regulatory activities on cells by interacting with specific high affinity cell surface receptors. Alpha and beta interferons share one receptor and there is another for gamma-IFN. Interferons are produced transiently in response to certain stimuli. Common inducing stimuli for alpha-IFN and beta-IFN include viruses, bacteria and double stranded RNA. Alpha-IFN is mainly produced by peripheral blood mononuclear cells and beta-IFN by fibroblasts and epithelial cells. Inducing stimuli for beta-IFN include nitrogen and antigens. IFNs can also be induced by other protein regulators such as the cytokines TNF, IL-1. IL-2, and CSFs. IFNs can be produced in non-lymphoid sites such as the peritoneum. The IFNs have a number of cell regulatory activities: they protect cells from attack by viruses and other intracellular parasites. They enhance the cytotoxicity of macrophages, neutrophils, NK cells and T lymphocytes. They cause a reversible cytostasis and can lead to tumour stabilization and occasionally regression (i.e. cytotoxic). Interferons stimulate B-cell proliferation and differentiation and may be natural negative growth regulators. Interferons both enhance and inhibit cell differentiation and they may promote the differentiation of some tumour cell lines. They are involved in immune regulation in three major ways: they may alter the cell surface, they may enhance or inhibit effector-cell functional activity or they may alter the production and secretion of other protein mediators.

12.3 CYTOKINES AS CANCER THERAPY

Cytokines have been used as anticancer therapy and may act in a variety of different ways: they

1. Augment the host's defences, thereby acting as effectors or mediators of antitumour response.
2. Increase the individual's antitumour responses through augmentation or restoration of effector mechanisms.
3. Increase tumour cells' sensitivity to an existing biological response.
4. Decrease transformation and/or increase differentiation or maturation of tumour cells.
5. Interfere with growth promoting factors produced by tumour cells.
6. Decrease or arrest the tendency of tumour cells to metastasize to other sites.
7. Increase the ability of the patient to tolerate damage by cytotoxic drugs.
8. Target and bind to cancer cells.

These will be discussed under the following headings:

1. Interferons as cancer therapy
2. CSFs in cancer therapy
3. TNF and cancer therapy
4. IL-2 and cancer therapy
5. Other cytokines
6. Biochemotherapy
7. Future directions, e.g. cytokine gene therapy.

12.3.1 INTERFERONS AS CANCER THERAPY

Interferons were the first cytokines to be used in the treatment of cancer and have a proven role in a number of tumours (Table 12.2). Interferons were first shown to inhibit animal tumours induced by oncogenic viruses and the growth of chemically induced tumours (Balkwill, 1985). There are three main ways in which interferons can affect tumours:

1. They can directly modulate tumour cell growth and differentiation and the tumour's response to growth factors.
2. They can act as immunomodulators. They enhance or even initiate host responses to the tumour. They can also induce cell surface antigens and can directly sensitize

Table 12.2 Phase I/II trial response rates for interferon

	%
Hairy cell leukaemia	80
Lymphoma (low grade)	65
CML	60
Kaposi's sarcoma	34
Lymphoma (all)	25
Melanoma	22
Renal	15

tumour cells to attack by cytotoxic cytokines.
3. They may exert regulatory effects on host/tumour interactions not associated with the immune response, for instance, interferon can inhibit the growth of oncogenic viruses and may interfere with the production of essential host nutritional or angiogenic factors that are locally active.

Currently the interferons have been shown to have antitumour activity in a limited number of relatively uncommon

Table 12.3 Side-effects of IL-2

Common (40–60%)	Nausea and vomiting
	Diarrhoea
	Hypotension
	Creatinine ($\times 2$–6 N)
	Bilirubin ($\times 2$–6 N)
	Fevers
	Wt gain (5–10%)
Uncommon (10–20%)	Hypothyroidism
	Drowsiness
	Respiratory distress
	Arrhythmia
	Bilirubin ($> \times 10$ N)
Rare (<1%)	Coma
	Wt gain (> 20%)
	Creatinine ($> 6 \times 10$ N)
	Myocardial infarction
	Deaths

cancers. They are of proven value in hairy cell leukaemia, chronic myeloid leukaemia, multiple myeloma, Kaposi's sarcoma and some cases of non-Hodgkin's lymphoma especially mycoses fungoides. Their role is less clear in the treatment of carcinoid tumour, renal cell carcinoma and melanoma (Table 12.3)

There are several generalizations that can be made about the use of interferon in cancer therapy:

1. Tumours that are sensitive to interferons are slow growing and relatively well differentiated.
2. Responses to therapy are typically slow.
3. Low dose maintenance therapy to sustain a remission may be a more appropriate strategy in some tumour types.
4. Continuous dosing appears more effective than intermittent dosing.
5. Interferons are more active when there is a small tumour burden.
6. Local or locoregional treatment may be more effective than systemic administration.
7. The maximally tolerated dose is between 5 and $100 \times 10_6 U/m_2$ depending on route of administration, duration of therapy and the performance status of patients.
8. It may not be necessary to use high doses to achieve tumour responses.
9. Beta-IFN appears to be no more effective than alpha-IFN.
10. Gamma-IFN has more potent immunoregulatory activities than alpha-IFN or beta-IFN and interacts more closely with other cytokines. Although it has antitumour activity, its superior immunoregulatory activities do not translate to greater efficacy compared with the two other IFNs.

The current main indications for treatment with interferons are: in chronic myeloid leukaemia and hairy cell leukaemia (HCL) interferon is the treatment of first choice (Golomb, 1987), although recent results suggest pentostatin may be at least as efficacious in HCL. New patients should receive interferon, although the optimum duration of treatment has not yet been established. Studies show that alpha-IFNs induce complete haematological remission in a majority of minimally treated benign phase CML patients (Talpaz *et al.*, 1987). There is a suggestion that long term administration of IFNs may inhibit or delay the development of blast crisis. Furthermore, alpha-IFN can prolong remissions induced by busulphan in CML (Bergsagel, 1988). In multiple myeloma, two studies (Mandelli *et al.*, 1988; Cunningham *et al.*, 1993) have shown a statistically significant advantage to the use of alpha-IFN, prolonging the duration of remission in patients who have responded to chemotherapy. In Kaposi's sarcoma median response rates to alpha-IFN are 34% (Goldstein and Lazlo, 1986) which is comparable to other treatments. In carcinoid tumours studies have shown that there is a reduction in secreted peptides and amines produced by tumours. However, this is not associated with objective reductions in tumour size (Oberg *et al.*, 1983; Eriksson *et al.*, 1987). In malignant melanoma there is no proven role for the systemic administration of IFN. Good responses are seen in malignant melanoma when IFNs are given intralesionally (Von Wussow *et al.*, 1988). However, melanoma is known to respond to a multitude of agents when this route is used. In renal cell carcinoma several trials show antitumour activity; overall the response rate is 15% (Horoszewicz and Murphy, 1989). Patients who have had a prior nephrectomy, no other treatment and no bony metastases are more likely to respond to IFN and many show increased survival (Elson *et al.*, 1988). Provera gives response rates of 10% with less toxicity (reviewed by Gore, 1993). It must also be remembered that renal cell carcinoma undergoes spontaneous remissions in a small proportion of cases (< 1%). The toxicity of IFNs are very dose and route dependent. The following are side-effects of IFN administration:

1. Fever
2. Headache
3. Malaise
4. Nausea/vomiting
5. Hypotension
6. Granulocytopenia
7. Thrombocytopenia
8. Disorientation
9. Depression
10. EEG abnormalities
11. Elevated serum triglycerides.

12.3.2   CSFs IN CANCER THERAPY

Myelotoxicity is a major dose limiting factor in many chemotherapy regimens and the advent of recombinantly produced CSF was hailed as an exciting advance because they would allow dose intensification, higher response rates, faster recovery from neutropenia and fewer complications. Currently, the CSFs are expensive and have not been shown to improve survival in any tumour type and therefore they should not be used routinely. However, randomized studies comparing placebo against G-CSF or GM-CSF have shown reduced requirements for i.v. antibiotics and less hospitalization when CSFs are used with standard dose chemotherapy (Nemunaitis *et al.*, 1991). High dose chemotherapy and autologous bone marrow transplant can be performed with greater safety and less inpatient hospital days, but it is uncertain if this translates to improvements in long term survival. Erythropoietin has recently become available for study in patients with cancer and early results suggest improved quality of life with correction of chronic anaemia (Ludwig *et al.*, 1993). Further studies are underway to assess its usefulness in patients receiving cisplatin based chemotherapy and abdominal-pelvic radio-

therapy. Its use is likely to remain limited because of expense and the ease with which patients can be given blood transfusions. A major problem that remains is thrombocytopenia which is not overcome by the currently available growth factors, although recent studies suggest a beneficial role for IL-3/GM-CSF (Tepler et al., 1993). Growth factors have a role in numerous non-oncological conditions but their discussion is outside the scope of this chapter.

12.3.3   TNF AND CANCER THERAPY

TNF is known to be produced in cancer patients and has both positive and negative aspects. On the positive side it is known to be directly cytotoxic to tumour cells, it activates host immunity, disrupts tumour blood supply and may also synergize with other cytokines. However, it also has detrimental effects, for instance it contributes to cancer cachexia, it is mitogenic for tumour cells, it makes tumour cells resistant to its cytotoxic activity and it promotes bone and cartilage breakdown. Clinical data from phase I and II studies show it is very toxic and has minimal activity in advanced cancer (Jones and Selby, 1989). The side-effects of TNF are:

1. Fever
2. Anaemia
3. Increase in fasting serum triglycerides
4. Decrease in serum albumin and cholesterol
5. Acute reversible lung injury
6. Increase in acute phase reactants
7. Hepatic dysfunction
8. Renal dysfunction
9. Thrombocytopenia
10. Mild hypertension/hypotension
11. Transient neutrophilia
12. Transient lymphopenia
13. Rigors
14. Chills
15. Myalgia
16. Tachycardia

17. Neutropenia
18. Headache
19. Fatigue
20. Anorexia
21. Nausea

To date, there is no trial suggesting that TNF has a role in any cancer treatment when used as a single agent. It may have a place in combination therapies and it is one of the cytokines being used in gene therapy protocols.

12.3.4 IL-2 AND CANCER THERAPY

Adoptive immunotherapy refers to the transfer of cells with specific antitumour activity to tumour bearing hosts. Such cells can be produced by taking lymphocytes from cancer patients and stimulating them *in vitro* with IL-2 to become highly cytotoxic. These cells are non-specifically cytotoxic and are known as lymphokine activated killer (LAK) cells. They have a greater range of targets than NK or cytotoxic T cells and are able to lyse NK resistant targets. LAK cells were first described in 1980 (Yron *et al.*, 1980) and can be generated from any sample of lymphoid tissue (peripheral blood mononuclear cells or lymphocyte cells from the thoracic duct, lymphocytes derived from the spleen, bone marrow or cord blood and tumour-infiltrating lymphocytes). In practice, LAK cells are produced by stimulating lymphocytes taken from patients by leukopheresis. Like NK cells, LAK cells have the morphology of large granular lymphocytes but LAK cells require at least 48 hours' exposure to IL-2 to attain maximal cytotoxic activity whereas NK cells are active immediately after isolation from the spleen or peripheral blood. LAK activity is found *in vivo* only at the site of a local immune response. LAK cells contain cytoplasmic granules that are rapidly cytotoxic and are calcium dependent. They bind to target cells by specific but unidentified receptors on the plasma membrane. They can also be generated from the lymphocytes found in human solid tumours (Rosenberg *et al.*, 1986). These lymphocytes appear functionally deficient, but when isolated and stimulated by IL-2 they have a greater magnitude and range of cytotoxic activity than LAK generated from peripheral blood cells. The disadvantage is that it takes longer to generate LAK from tumour-infiltrating lymphocytes than from peripheral blood cells (10–20 days compared with 2 days).

The first clinical trials of IL-2 and LAK using schedules derived from animal experiments were reported in 1985 (Resenberg *et al.*, 1985). Initial phase 1 studies using low dose IL-2 showed limited antitumour activity but defined its toxicities. Later studies employed higher doses of IL-2 and a 20% overall response rate was reported in patients with melanoma and renal cell carcinoma (Rosenberg *et al.*, 1985, 1987). More importantly, most of the responses were durable for longer than 12 months and several patients were reportedly alive and disease free at 4 and 5 years. Subsequent trials have attempted to define the optimum scheduling, route and dose of IL-2 and to determine if LAK cells are contributing to the response rates seen in earlier studies.

The following results have been found in melanoma: 130 patients in three studies have received high dose bolus IL-2/LAK, 88 patients in one study received high dose bolus IL-2 alone and 73 received low dose bolus IL-2 alone and the overall response rates respectively were 17.3%, 22.5% and 16% with the majority of the responses being partial remissions (PRs) rather than complete remissions (CRs). One randomized study comparing bolus IL-2 alone to IL-2/LAK at both high and low doses of IL-2 failed to show any difference between the two arms. High dose continuous infusion IL-2/LAK has been evaluated in three studies: 73 evaluable patients had an overall response rate of 19.3% (range 3%–50%) all of which were PRs. One randomized trial of continuous IL-2 alone versus IL-2/LAK showed no difference between the two arms (9% versus 6%). The median duration of response for complete responders in all these trials was 24 months with the longest being 52 months (reviewed by Sparano and Dutcher, 1993). Subcutaneous IL-2 has been given in a variety of schedules and doses and response rates range from 0 to 11% (Kirchner *et al.*, 1990; Ratain *et al.*, 1990; Atzopodien *et al.*, 1990). In conclusion, in melanoma IL-2 shows modest activity with response rates of 10% to 20%, a small proportion are complete and there may be durable remissions. On the available evidence bolus IL-2 is probably slightly more effective than continuous IL-2 and subcutaneous IL-2 seems least effective. The addition of LAK cells is not justified on current evidence. Most responses have been reported in skin, lymph nodes and lung, although responses have been seen at most visceral sites.

In renal cell carcinoma initial studies reported response rates of 35% (Rosenberg *et al.*, 1985, 1987). A further six studies have evaluated high-dose IL-2/LAK using both bolus and continuous infusion schedules; in 316 evaluable patients the overall response rate was 22% (24 CRs, 46 PRs) and there was no difference between the two schedules. Five trials have evaluated IL-2 alone in 145 evaluable patients with an overall response rate of 20% (seven CRs, 22 PRs). The median duration of response for complete responders in these 11 trials was 18 months, the longest being 31 months (reviewed by Sunderland and Weiss, 1993). One randomized study of 45 patients showed no difference in response between IL-2/LAK and single agent IL-2 (Bajorin et al., 1990). Subcutaneous IL-2 has also been evaluated and overall is 22% (Ratain *et al.*, 1990; Atzopodien et al., 1990; Kirchner *et al.*, 1990). Many of the remissions have been durable and best responses are seen in skin, lymph nodes and lung.

In other malignancies IL-2 with or without LAK cells appears to be of limited usefulness. In patients with relapsed lymphoma or AML overall response rates of 20–30% have been

seen but none are durable. Responses have been seen in patients with lung, breast, ovary and colon cancer but there is no evidence it is of any benefit over existing treatments. Locoregional IL-2 has been used successfully into the intrapleural, peritoneal, vesical and intrathecal cavities (Urba, 1993) but may produce local fibrosis and there is no convincing evidence for its routine use. IL-2 has been infused into the hepatic, splenic and superficial temporal arteries with a reduction in systemic toxicities (Thatcher *et al.*, 1989; Mavligit *et al.*, 1990; Gore *et al.*, 1992). Minor responses were seen when patients were given intra-arterial IL-2 for metastatic melanoma and two PRs were seen when IL-2 was given through the superficial temporal artery for advanced squamous cell carcinoma of the head and neck. Local complications seen included cellulitis, venous thrombosis/embolism and pain at the site of infusion. These local problems will need to be addressed in any future studies of intra-arterial IL-2.

IL-2 side-effects are very dose and schedule dependent and are increased by the addition of LAK cells. A reversible flu-like syndrome is seen and hepatic and renal dysfunction occurs (Rosenberg *et al.*, 1985). A major side-effect is increased vascular permeability and reduced systemic vascular resistance resulting in hypotension and often requiring vasopressor support. An increase in body weight of up to 10% (Lotze *et al.*, 1986) occurs and is due to the accumulation of extravascular fluid. Patients become hypoalbuminaemic and may develop erythema, pruritus and skin scaling (Orr *et al.*, 1987). IL-2 can also cause serious neurological toxicity ranging from slight disorientation to a severe encephalopathic syndrome. It usually manifests late in the course of treatment and may continue to worsen even after discontinuing IL-2. IL-2 is also myelosuppressive with transient leucopenia, anaemia and thrombocytopenia. However, lymphocytosis and eosinophilia are sometimes seen and may be associated with responses. A variety of electrolyte disturbances may occur, commonly hypo-calcaemia and hypokalaemia, and in addition zinc and ascorbate deficiencies have been noted by some authors (Marcus *et al.*, 1987). All these acute side-effects are generally rapidly reversible once the IL-2 has been stopped. IL-2 may also cause prolonged toxic-ities due to autoimmune phenomena, for instance, hypothyroidism and arthritis, (Atkins, 1993).

Patients receiving IL-2 or IL-2/LAK require supportive measures: non-steroidal anti-inflammatory drugs to control fever and pethidine or morphine to control rigors. A range of antiemetics have been used to control nausea but no single drug is superior. Antihistamines and topical skin preparations are used to alleviate pruritus. The haemo-dynamic disturbances require central venous access, fluid replacement, albumin and some-times vasopressors such as dopamine and dobutamine. Diuretics may be used for fluid overload provided the patient is not hypo-tensive. Electrolytes are monitored daily and replaced as necessary. Patients also require prophylactic antibiotics to avoid infection from their central lines.

12.3.5   OTHER CYTOKINES AS CANCER THERAPY

Recently IL-1 and IL-6 have entered phase I clinical trials. IL-1 when given following chemotherapy has been shown to shorten neutrophil recovery (Wilson *et al.*, 1993). IL-3 in combination with GM-CSF appears to hasten recovery from chemotherapy induced myelosuppression, particularly thrombocytopenia, and appears to be safe (Tepler *et al.*, 1993). IL-6 has been used in a small number of patients and appears to be safe and may also have thrombopoietic ac-tivity (Chang *et al.*, 1993; Samuels *et al.*, 1993). No significant antitumour responses have been seen. Other cytokines are being evaluated in the preclinical setting and are likely to reach the clinic in the near future.

12.3.6   BIOCHEMOTHERAPY

Biochemotherapy refers to the modulation of cytotoxic drugs by the concomitant or sequential use of cytokines. It is hoped that the combination may result in increased response rates and/or increased duration of responses. There are multiple potential levels for cytotoxic/cytokine interactions *in vitro*. The synergistic interaction between cytokines and cytotoxic agents appears to be sequence dependent.

The concept of combining cytokines and cytotoxic drugs to enhance antiproliferative activity is complex. There are several possible interactions between cytokines and cytotoxic drugs, including modulation of target enzymes of drug metabolism, modulation of receptors, alteration of cell cycle phases, and modulation of gene expression. Chemotherapy may potentiate immunotherapy, not only by cytoreduction, but also by functioning as a biomodulator, by influencing membrane fluidity or antigen stability.

(a)   Mechanisms of interactions between interferon and cytotoxic drugs

The best example of chemotherapy– biother-apy interactions is 5-fluoruracil (5-FU) and INF. Within 24 hours of exposure to 5-FU, there is induction of intratumoral thymidylate synthetase (TS) (Wadler and Schwartz, 1990). The main active metabolite of 5-FU is fluorodexyuridylate which forms a stable complex with TS and reduced folates, the complex inhibits TS enzyme activity which is required for synthesis of DNA precursors. INF inhibits the acute induction of TS and increases the level of the active metabolite, fluorodeoxyuridylate, 10-fold, resulting in greater inhibition of the target enzyme TS. INF also inhibits thymidine uptake and thymidine kinase activity, thus re-ducing the salvage pathway of DNA synthe-sis. INF can also alter the pharmacokinetics of 5-FU, increasing the area under the 5-FU concentration curve up to 1.5-fold. In clinical trials, four out of five phase I studies show an advantage for the combination, five phase II studies show variable results and a phase III study is ongoing (Wadler, 1992).

(b)   Mechanisms of interactions between TNF and cytotoxic drugs

Topoisomerases have emerged as a critical site of action of cytotoxic drugs. Recent evidence suggests that recombinant human TNF significantly enhances the *in vitro* cytotoxicity of a number of cytotoxic drugs, including adriamycin, actinomycin, etoposide and teniposide, all of which target this enzyme (Alexander *et al.*, 1987). It appears that TNF enhances the cytotoxicity of these drugs by increasing topoisomerase II levels. The scheduling of the chemotherapy and TNF is crucial in this interaction (Krueser *et al.*, 1991) and enhanced cytotoxicity only occurs if the TNF is given coincidentally or subsequently to the cytotoxic drug, augmenting drug mediated killing. However, clinical trials have failed to demonstrate this effect in patients (Jones and Selby, 1989).

(c)   Mechanisms of interaction between haemopoietic growth factors and cytotoxic drugs

In patients with acute myeloid leukaemia it has been shown that cytosine arabinoside cytotoxicity is enhanced by the concomitant use of CSFs (Cannistra *et al.*, 1989). Both GM-CSF and IL-3 are the most effective CSFs at increasing S-phase fraction, and since cytosine arabinosideis is S-phase specific cytotoxicity is enhanced. These factors also enhance the intracellular metabolism of cytosine arabinoside, inducing higher antileukaemia activity (Brach *et al.*, 1992).

(d)   Mechanisms of interactions between interleukins and cytotoxic drugs

Combination therapy with interleukins and antitumour drugs may be beneficial, increasing the therapeutic effect while decreasing toxicity. IL-1, for instance, alters the cell cycle status so more cells are cycling and less drug may be required for the same effect or the same amount of drug may produce an increased effect. By combining chemotherapy with cytokines it is hoped to prolong the duration of response. For instance in melanoma chemotherapy, platinum especially , can provide significant cytoreduction but this is short lived in most cases. The treatment of disseminated malignant melanoma with monotherapy or combined chemotherapy has disappointingly low objective response rates. Clinical trials with combined interferon and cytostatic drug therapy showed promising initial results (McClay and Mastrangelo, 1988). More than 200 patients in several trials have received dacarbazine and interferon and it is effective in over 50% of patients, leading to complete or partial responses in 27% and stabilization of disease in 28% (Garbe *et al.*, 1992). A randomized study comparing IFN and dacarbazine versus dacarbazine alone shows twice the response rate and survival time for the combination (Falkson *et al.*, 1990), but this has not been confirmed by others. Several clinical trials show no advantage to adding interferon to cisplatin or vinblastine.

The addition of IL-2 to chemotherapy and/or interferon would seem to augment the response rates from preliminary trials (Rosenberg *et al.*, 1988). A recent phase II study of sequential chemoimmunotherapy, combining decarbazine, cisplatin and carmustine with INF and IL-2 showed a response rate of 55%, with a suggestion of durable responses for some patients, but longer follow-up is required (Richards *et al.*, 1992). There are no clinical studies on the combination of INF with fotemustine or the nitrosureas which can cross into the cerebrospinal fluid.

12.3.7 CYTOKINE GENE THERAPY

The most exciting new area of cytokine use is gene therapy. The major problem to date in the use of cytokines has been their systemic toxicity. By molecular engineering it is now possible to modify cells to secrete various cytokines. This strategy aims at producing powerful local effects without the systemic toxicity. The altered immunological environment of the tumour cell may enhance tumour antigen presentation to the immune system or enhance activation of tumour specific lymphocytes, resulting in systemic antitumour activity. Gene transfer using defective retroviral vectors may in the near future allow enhanced antitumour immune responses, but two criteria need to be fulfilled: the tumour must present novel antigens or a neo epitope not found on normal cells and the immune system must be appropriately activated to respond to these novel antigens.

Gene therapy is a form of active immunotherapy. Earlier immunological studies performed in solid tumours used irradiated tumour cells or irradiated-virus infected tumour cells. Another method has been the use of mutagenesis to transform non-immunogenic tumours into immunogenic variants and thereby stimulate an immune response. This form of tumour cell vaccination can be given by various routes – subcutaneous, intravenous and intraperitoneal. Recent advances have allowed cytokine gene transfer into tumour cells (transduction) and cytokine gene transfer has been carried out in mice using IL-2, IL-4, gamma-INF, TNF and IL-7 (Pardoll, 1992). The strategy behind this therapy is to bypass defects in the patient's immune response, specifically helper cells, activation which in turn causes stimulation of cytotoxic T cells. The local and systemic side-effects associated with the introduction of large numbers of cytokine gene transduced tumour cells is unknown from animal models. A potential side-effect is the production of an auto-immune response against tissue specific antigens shared by the tumour. For human tumours, defective retroviral vector systems are the gold standard for high efficiency gene transfer (Mulligan, 1991). Human gene therapy was first performed in 1990 for treatment of adenosine deaminase deficiency. It is hoped in the future to introduce cytokine genes directly into human tumour infiltrating lymphocytes (TILs) which could be carried directly to the site of the tumour. Alternatively, the cytokine genes could be transduced into the human tumour cells themselves and enhance the host immune response.

12.3.8 CYTOKINE DELIVERY, DOSAGE AND SCHEDULING

The biologically active forms of most cytokines have been shown to be rapidly degraded *in vivo* and this may account for the discrepancy between antitumour activity *in vitro* and *in vivo*. Pharmacokinetic studies have shown short half-lives for most cytokines, with a rapid initial fall in serum levels followed by a slower steady state of decline. One way of overcoming such short lived activity is to use either continuous intravenous infusions or the subcutaneous route. Research is underway to develop a second generation of cytokines with structural alterations that will give them greater stability *in vivo*. Local administration of cytokines may produce high therapeutic levels intra-arterially, intraperitoneally, intravesically and intrathecally but this is only applicable to a minority of cancers. Direct antitumour administration has also been used but does not have an impact on disseminated cancer. The usual rules of giving the maximum tolerated dose of an antitumour drug may not necessarily apply to therapy with cytokines in the same way as conventional cytotoxic drugs. If the aim is to directly effect antitumour proliferation, then maximal tolerated dose is required. However, if the aim is to maximize the immune response to the tumour lower doses may be sufficient. A 'bell-shaped' dose–response curve (Figure 12.1) may exist where there is an optimal immunomodulation dose (Jones and Selby, 1990). From the studies so far, the doses of cytokines required to produce a response are unclear. It is also uncertain for how long cytokine therapy should be continued, as there is evidence that responses may occur for some months after treatment is stopped. There may be a role for maintenance treatment with cytokines, especially INFs, but this needs to be further defined by ongoing studies.

12.4   CONCLUSIONS

Cytokine therapy has progressed a long way since the first introduction of INFs to treat human cancer. The availability of large quantities of recombinant cytokines for use in clinical trials is making studies in this area feasible. We know from initial experience with INFs and IL-2 that cytokines can be much more toxic in humans than is readily apparent from animal experiments. For this reason, it is essential for research to find new strategies to deliver cytokines in such a way as to target human tumours selectively and also to develop cytokines that are more stable *in vivo*. In addition, the combination of cytokines with conventional cytotoxic drugs warrants further investigation. It may be that when more selectively targeted cytokine therapies become available this strategy will be more powerful.

REFERENCES

Alexander, R.B., Nelson, W.G. and Coffey, D.S. (1987) Synergistic enhancement by tumour necrosis factor of *in vitro* cytotoxicity fozrm chemotherapeutic drugs targeted at DNA topoisomerase II. *Cancer Research*, **47**, 2403–6.

Atkins, M.B. (1993) Autoimmune disorders induced by interleukin-2 therapy, in *Therapeutic Applications of Interleukins-2*, (eds M.B. Atkins and J.W. Mier), Dekker, New York pp. 389–408.

Atzpodien, J., Korfer, A., Franks, C.R. *et al.* (1990) Out-patient experience with the use of subcutaneous interleukin-2 in 65 cancer patients. Proceedings of the American Society of *Clinical Oncology*, **9**, 758.

Balkwill, F.R. (1985) Antitumour effects of interferons in animals. *Interferon: In vivo and Clinical Studies* **4**, 23–45.

Bajovin, D.F., Sell, K.W. and Richards, J.M. (1990) A randomised trial of interleukin-2 plus

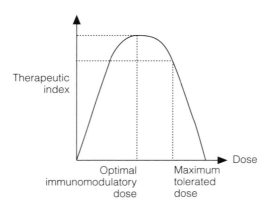

Figure 12.1   Diagrammatic representation of optimum immunomodulatory dose with BRMs for biological therapy. (Adapted from Jones and Selby, 1991.)

lymphokine-activated killer cells versus interleukin-2 alone in renal cell carcinoma. *Proceedings of the American Association of Cancer Research*, 1106.

Bergsagel, D.E. (1988) Interferon - 2B in the management of chronic granulocytic leukaemia. *Cancer Treatment Reviews*, **15**, 15–20.

Brach, M.A., Meulelsmann, R.H. and Hermann, F. (1992) Haematopoeitins in combination with I-beta-D arabinofuranosylcytosine: possible strategy for improved treatment of myeloid disorders. *Seminars in Oncology*, **9**, (suppl.4). 25–30

Cannistra, S.A., Groshek, P. and Griffin, J.D. (1989) Granulocyte – macrophage – colony – stimulating factor enhances the cytotoxic effects of cytosine arabinoside in acute myeloblastic leukaemia and in the myeloid blast crisis phase of chronic myeloid leukaemia. *Leukaemia*, **3**, 328–34.

Carswell, E.A., Old, L.J., Kassel, R.J. *et al.* (1975) An endotoxin induced serum factor that causes necrosis of tumours. *Proceedings of the National Academy of Sciences* USA, **72**, 3666–70.

Chang, A., Boros, L. and Asbury, R. (1993) Effects of interleukin-2 in cancer patients treated with ifosfamide, carboplatin and etoposide. *Proceedings of the American Society of Clinical Oncology*, **12**, 936.

Coley Nauts, H., Fowler, G.A. and Bogatko, R.H. (1953) A review of the influence of bacterial infection and of bacterial products (Coley's toxins) on malignant tumours in man. *Acta Medica Scandinavica*, **274-7** (suppl), 29–97.

Elson, P.J., Witte, R.S. and Trump D.L. (1988) Prognostic factors for survival in patients with recurrent or metastatic renal cell carcinoma. *Cancer Research*, **48**. 7310–13.

Eriksson, B. Oberg, K., Alm, G. *et al.* (1987) Treatment of malignant endocrine pancreatic tumours with human leucocyte interferon. *Cancer Treatment Reports* **71**, 31–7.

Falkson, C.I., Falkson, G., and Galkson H.C. (1990) Improved results with the addition of recombinant interferon alpha-2b to dacarbazine in treatment of patients with metastatic malignant melanoma. *Proceedings of the American Association of Cancer Research* **31A**, 1185 (abstr).

Garbe, C., Kreuser, E.B., Zouboulis, C.C. *et al.* (1992) Combined treatment of metastatic melanoma with interferons and cytotoxic drugs. *Seminars in Oncology*, **19**, (suppl 4), 63–9.

Goldstein, D. and Lazlo, J. (1986) Interferon therapy in cancer: from imaginon to interferon. *Cancer Research*, **46**, 4315–29.

Golomb, H.M. (1987) The treatment of hairy cell leukaemia. *Blood*, **69**, 679–83.

Gore, M. (1993) Advances in the management of renal cell carcinoma, in *Advances in Urology/Andrology*, vol. 6, (eds. W.F. Hendry and R.S. Kirby), Churchill Livingstone, Edinburgh, pp 51–102.

Gore, M., Riches, P. and Maclennan, K. (1992) Phase I study of intra-arterial interleukin-2 in squamous cell carcinoma of the head and neck. *Bnish Journal of Cancer*, **66**, 405–7.

Green, A.R. (1989) Peptide regulatory factors multifunctional mediators of cellular growth and differentiation. *Lancet*, **i**, 705–7.

Horoszewicz, J.S. and Murphy, G.P. (1989) An assessment of the current use of human interferons in therapy of urological cancers. *Journal of Urology*, **142**, 1173–80.

Isaacs, A. and Lindemann J. (1957) Virus interference I. The interferon. *Proceedings of the Society of London (series B)*, **147**, 259–67.

Jones, A.L. and Selby, P. (1989) Tumour necrosis factor: clinical relevance. *Cancer Surveys*, 1989: **8**, 817.

Jones, A., and Selby, P. (1991) Biological therapies. *Radiotherapy and Oncology*, **20**, 211–23.

Kirchner, H., Korfer, A., Palmer, P.A. et al. (1990) Subcutaneous interleukin-2 and interferon alpha 2B in patients with metastatic renal cell. The German out-patient experience. *Molecular Biotherapy* **2**, 145–54.

Krueser, E.D., Keppleu, B.K., Berderl, W.E. et al. (1991) Synergistic antitumour interactions between newly synthesized ruthenium complexes and cytokines in human colon carcinoma cell lines. *Seminars in Oncology*, **18**, 73–81.

Lotze, M.T., Matary, Y.L., Rayner, A.A. et al. (1986) Clinical effects and toxicity of interleukin-2 in patients with cancer. *Cancer*, **58**, 2764–72.

Ludwig, H., Leitgets, C., Pecherstorfer, M. et al. (1993) Quality of life during erythropoietin therapy in chronic anaemia of cancer. *Proceeding of the American Society of Clinical Oncology* **12**, 1375.

Mandelli, F., Tribalto, M., Avvisati, G. *et al.* (1988) Recombinant interferon alpha-2b as post-induction therapy for responding multiple myeloma patients. M84 protocol. *Cancer Treatment*, **15**, 43–48.

Marcus S.L. *et al.* (1987) Micronutrient depletion in patients treated with high-dose (IL-2) and lymphokine–activated (LAK) cells. *Proceedings of ASIO* **6**, 247.

Mavligit, G.M., Zukiwski, A.A. and Gutterman, J.J. (1990) Splenic versus hepatic artery infusion of interleukin-2 in patients with liver metastases. *Journal of Clinical Oncology*, **8**, 319–24.

McClay, E.F. and Mastrangelo, M.J. (1988) Systemic chemotherapy for metastatic melanoma. *Seminars in Oncology*, **15**, 569–77.

Mulligan, R.C. (1991) Gene transfer and gene therapy, in *Etiology of Human Disease at the DNA Level*, (eds J. Lindsten and U. Petterson), Raven, New York, pp 143–89.

Nemunaitis, J., Rabinowe, S., Singer, J. et al. (1991) Rocombinant granulocyte - macrophage colony stimulating factor after autologous bone marrow transplantation for lymphoid cancer. *New England J Journal of Medicine*, **324**, 1773–8.

Oberg, K., Kuna, K. and Alm, G. (1983) Effects of leucocyte IFN on clinical symptoms and hormone levels in patients with mid-gut carcinoid tumours and carcinoid syndrome. *New England Journal of Medicine*, **309**, 129–133.

Orr, D., Yanelli, J., Sharp, E. et al. (1987) Eosinophilia during (IL2) activated killer (AK) cell therapy. *Proceedings of the American Society of Clinical Oncology*, **6**, 247.

Pardoll D. (1992) Immunotherapy with cytokine gene-transduced tumour cells: the next wave in gene therapy for cancer. *Current Opinion in Oncology*, **4**, 1124–9.

Ratain, M.J., Vogelzang, N.J., Janish, L. et al. (1990) Phase I study of subcutaneous interleukin-2 and interferon alpha 2a. Proceeding of the American Society of Clinical Oncology, 9, 774.

Richards, J.M., Mehta, N., Ramming, K. et al. (1992) Sequential chemoimmunotherapy in the treatment of metastatic melanoma. *Journal of Clinical Oncology.* **8**, 1338–43.

Rosenberg, S.A., Mule, J.J., Spiesis, J. et al. (1985) Regression of established pulmonary metastases and subcutaneous tumour medicated by systemic administration of high-dose recombinant interleukin. *Journal of Experimental Medicine*, **161**, 1169–88.

Rosenberg, S.A., Spiesis, P. and La Freniere, R. (1986) A new approach to the adoptive immunotherapy of cancer with tumour infiltrating lymphocytes. *Science*, **233**, 1318–21.

Rosenberg, S.A., Reichhark, C.M. and Schwartz, S.L. (1987) A progress report on the treatment of 157 patients with advanced cancer using lymphokine-activated killer cells and interleukin 2

or high dose interleukin 2 alone. Journal of Mechicism. *New England J Med*. **316**, 889–97.

Rosenberg, S.A., Packard, B.S., Aebersold, P.M. et al. (1988) Use of tumour infiltrating lymphocytes and interleukin-2 in the immunotherapy of patients with metastatic melanoma. New England Journal of Medicime, **319**, 1676–80.

Samuels, B., Bukowski, R. and Gordon, M. (1993) Phase I study of rh IL-6 with chemotherapy in advanced sarcoma. *Proceedings of the American Society of Clinical Oncology*, **12**, 948.

Sparano, J.A. and Dutcher, J.P. (1993) High dose IL-2 treatment of melanoma. in *Therapeutic Applications of Interleukin-2*, (eds M.B. Atkin and J.W. Mier), Dekker, New York, pp. 99–117.

Sunderland, M.C. Weiss, G.R. (1993) High dose IL-2 treatment of renal cell carcinoma, in *Therapeutic Applications of Interleukin-2* (eds M.B. Atkins and J.W. Mier), Dekker, New York, pp. 119–39.

Talpaz, M., Kantarjian, H.M., McCredie, K.B. et al. (1987) Clinical investigation of human alpha interferon in chronic myleogenous leukkaemia. Blood, 65, 1280–8.

Tepler, I., Hamm, J.T., Shulman, L. et al. (1993) Combination cytokine therapy with recombinant human interleukin-3 and granulocyte colony stimulating factor after ICE chemotherapy for lung cancer. *Proceedings of the American Society for Clinical Oncology*, **12**, 1110.

Thatcher, N, Dazzi, H. and Gosh, A. (1989) Recombinant IL-2 given intra-splenically and intravenously in advanced malignant melanoma. *Cancer Treatment Reviews*, **16** (suppl A), 49–52.

Urba, W.J. (1993) Locoregional administration of IL-2 and/or LAK cells, in *Therapeutic Applications of Interleukin-2*, (eds M.B. Atkins and J.W. Mier), Dekker, New York, pp. 189–215.

Von Wussow, P., Block, B., Hartmann, F. et al. (1988) Intralesional interferon therapy in advanced malignant melanoma. *Cancer*, **61**, 1071–4.

Wadler, S., and Schwartz, E.L. (1990) Antineoplastic activity of the combination of interferon and cytotoxic agents against experimental and human malignancies. A review. *Cancer Research*, **50**, 3473–86.

Wadler, S. (1992) Antineoplastic activity of the combination of 5-fluoruracil and interferon: preclinical and clinical results. *Seminars in Oncology*, **19**, (no. 2, suppl 4), 38–40.

Wilson, W.H., Bryant, G. and Fox, M. (1993) Interleukin-1aa administered before high-dose ifosfamide, carboplatin and etoposide with autologous bone marrow rescue shortens neutrophil recovery: a phase I/II study. *Proceeding s of the American Society for Cinical Oncology*, **12**, 937.

Yron, I., Wood, T.A., Spiesis, P.J. *et al.* (1980) *In vitro* growth of murine T cells. V. The isolation and growth of lymphoid cells infiltrating syngeneic solid tumours. *Journal of Immunology*, **125**, 238–45.

FURTHER READING

Atkins, M.B. and Mier, J.W. (1993) Therapeutic Applications of Interleukin-2, Marcel Dekker, New York.

Balkwill, F.R. (1989) *Cytokines in Cancer Therapy.* Oxford University Press, Oxford.

Cytokines as modulators of cytotoxic drugs in experimental and clinical haematology and oncology. *Seminars in Oncology*, (1992) **19** 2 (4).

Interferon: advances in biotherapy. *Seminars in Oncology*, (1991) **18**, 5 (7).

Interleukin-2: advances in clinical research and treatment. *Seminars in Oncology*, (1993) **20**, 6 (9).

Rosenberg, S.A. (1993) Principles and applications of biologic therapy, in, *Cancer: principles and practice of oncology*, 4th eden, (eds V.T. DeVita Jr, S. Hellman and S.A. Rosenberg), Lippincott, Philadelphia, pp. 293–324.

INFECTION IN CANCER PATIENTS

Beryl Jameson

13.1 BACTERIAL

The principal differences between oncology patients and others in their response to bacterial infections occur in those with haematological malignancies and those having intensive cytotoxic chemotherapy, including conditioning for bone marrow transplantation (BMT). Profound neutropenia influences the presentation and diagnosis, as well as the treatment and prevention, of bacterial infections in those patients.

Bacteraemia is likely to be fatal and the basic principle of treatment is to administer a broad-spectrum combination of antibiotics, intravenously, as soon as possible after fever occurs. A blood culture and urine sample, collected before antibiotics are started, may provide useful information from which treatment can be modified later, but it must not be delayed.

Symptoms and signs such as neck stiffness, pyuria or a chest X-ray shadow, which in the non-neutropenic patient are guides to the choice of antibiotic, may be absent in the neutropenic patient. Fever is frequently the only indication. Combinations of antibiotics are chosen to cover a wide range of both Gram-negative and Gram-positive organisms, and to act synergistically if possible.

The combination of a gentamicin plus carbenicillin, which was introduced in the 1960s, is the model from which today's antibiotic regimens have developed. An antipseudomonal broad-spectrum penicillin with an aminoglycoside remains an effective first choice in the majority of circumstances, though the penicillin now is more likely to be piperacillin or azlocillin and the aminoglycoside may be one of a variety of alternatives, such as amikacin, netilmicin or tobramycin.

The carbenicillin–gentamicin combination was directed at Gram-negative (including pseudomonas) septicaemia, which in the 1960s was the cause of death in up to 50% of febrile neutropenic patients (Schimpff *et al.*, 1971). Many other combinations have been investigated in the ensuing 25 years, notably 'third-generation' cephalosporins (e.g. ceftazidime, cefotaxime) and the quinolones (such as ciprofloxacin) in varying combinations with aminoglycosides or broad-spectrum penicillins. Although the non-aminoglycoside combinations have the advantage of less nephrotoxicity, they have disadvantages such as limited spectra of activity or the tendency to induce multiple antibiotic resistance. The same arguments apply to the use of broad-spectrum antibiotics as single agents. Gaya (1988) discusses in depth the principles governing the choice of antibiotic regimens and also the difficulties associated with clinical trials. Studies require very large numbers to achieve statistically reliable results and also, in the past, there have been problems in comparing results because of differing criteria for success and failure of treatment. Several large multicentre collaborative studies have been published since 1981 by the European Organization for Research and Treatment of Cancer (EORTC) International Antimicrobial Therapy Co-operative Group and are the yardsticks upon which many oncology centres base their policies. Stringent guidelines for the performance of clinical trials have been published recently (Hughes *et al.*, 1992).

At present the evidence is in favour of retaining an aminoglycoside as a component of any empirical regimen, to ensure optimal cover for Gram-negative infections (Gaya, 1988). In the past decade, however, Gram-positive organisms have become commoner causes of bacteraemia and in many oncology centres they now slightly outnumber the Gram negatives. *Staphylococcus epidermidis* currently predominates but streptococci including enterococci, *S. pyogenes* and *S. mitis* are all on the increase.

The need for Gram-positive cover is met by the sequential use of antimicrobials, in which each step is based on the likely effect of the previous one (Barnes and Rogers, 1987). Gaya (1988) dubbed this 'planned, progressive therapy'. It is often necessary to re-assess treatment at 48 or 72 hours after the start of empirical antibiotics, because an organism may have been grown from pretreatment specimens, the fever may have failed to respond, or it may have remitted and recurred. If the reason for persistent or recurrent fever is not obvious from cultures, Gram-positive infection must be assumed and treatment be adapted accordingly. The antibiotic of choice is then usually vancomycin or teicoplanin. It is not customary to include either of these in the initial empirical combination as it is widely felt that two nephrotoxic drugs together should be avoided if possible, and the Gram-negative infection is the more likely to be rapidly fatal.

It may not always be so, and there have recently been recorded instances of rapidly fatal streptococcal infections (Burden *et al.*, 1991). This serves to emphasize that no regimen is universally applicable. The type of infecting organism will vary with the patient's disease and general management (see below) and antibiotic resistance profiles within the locality. However, if local data are not available for making local policy, the reader is advised to be guided by the EORTC clinical trials (1991) or the recommendations of the Infectious Diseases Society of America (Hughes *et al.*, 1990).

Prevention plays as great a part as therapy in the management of infection in the neutropenic patient, and methods of prevention have been the subject of investigation and modification ever since the introduction of combination chemotherapy. The earliest methods concentrated on excluding environmental sources of bacteria, and units for nursing patients in strict segregation, supplied with ultra-clean air and food (Bagshaw, 1964), remain the prototypes for many such units which are being built at the present time. Doubts are frequently expressed about whether specially constructed facilities influence the outcome of cancer therapy and whether their cost is justified. Sometimes such doubts result from an assumption that there is a single, very stringent, standard which must be the aim at all times and in all circumstances. The reality is that methods of infection prevention have always been subject to modification in response to changes in the patients' treatment and supportive care.

At the time when exclusion of exogenous sources of infection was the primary consideration, patients were greatly at risk from *Staphylococcus aureus* and *Pseudomonas aeruginosa* infection for which there were few antibiotics. A period of intense interest in the air-borne route of staphylococcus infection drew upon industry's interest in particle-free work areas, and on the use of plastic isolators to breed germ-free animals for veterinary research, and produced the laminar airflow room and the plastic 'Life Island'. Gram-negative bacteria, especially pseudomonads, were commonly found in the moisture left by downward displacement sterilizers and manually washed bedpans, and also in the disinfectants which were used lavishly but in ignorance of their limitations. The environmental improvements which were to reduce the risk from these bacteria were yet to come, but protective isolation facilities decreased patients' acquisition of them.

(Jameson *et al.*, 1971). It is tempting to assume that some effect on infection rates was also obtained, although few studies of the exclusion component of protective isolation *per se* have been published. The reason for this is that it was soon realized that the patient's own microbial flora constitutes a major source of infection, so studies more often compare regimens which include the use of prophylactic antibiotics.

During the past 25 years a number of influences have affected the practice of infection prevention in cancer patients. The use of disposables, more efficient sterilization and more discriminating use of disinfectants have decreased the risk from Gram-negative bacteria in the environment. Both food and medicines have been recognized as sources of cross-colonization of the human intestine (Shooter *et al.*, 1969) and appropriate hygienic measures have been introduced. More therapeutic antibiotics of varying spectra of activity have become available and antibacterial prophylaxis has progressed from oral non-absorbable drugs to co-trimoxazole and the quinolones.

Nevertheless, more patients are being treated more intensively for a wider range of malignant diseases. Severe mucosal ulceration creates a greater opportunity for bacteraemia caused by alimentary organisms, and the increasing use of indwelling venous catheters allows invasion by the staphylococci and corynebacteria which are normal components of the skin flora.

Co-trimoxazole has been shown in over 30 publications to be an effective prophylactic agent (Hughes *et al.*, 1990), but has recently been challenged by ciprofloxacin, whose favourable attributes include better anti-pseudomonad activity and fewer side-effects. Ciprofloxacin in turn is the subject of conflicting evidence for its efficacy, especially with regard to Gram-positive bacteria. Gram-positive prophylaxis is needed to combat the rising frequency of these infections, which result from greater exposure to therapeutic antibiotics.

Thus there is a constant shifting of forces, which will vary according to local circumstances and resources. It is not always poss-ible to find unequivocal support for what may, however, seem a sensible measure to adopt. In the series 'Aseptic methods in the operating theatre' the Medical Research Council classified procedures as 'established', 'ritual' and 'rational'. The last were defined as those which 'seem desirable on the grounds of common sense and some bacteriological evidence, but which cannot be evaluated' (Medical Research Council, 1968). The same useful criteria could be applied to some infection-prevention procedures for the neutropenic patient. Rational precautions which can and should be taken in any oncology unit are scrupulous attention to handwashing, the provision of a clean diet and reduction of contacts to those persons essential for the patient's wellbeing. At the other end of the scale, there is re-emerging evidence in favour of a controlled and filtered air-supply, but to prevent fungal infection rather than bacterial, and in selected circumstances where patients are at high risk (see below). Between these extremes preventive measures will be dictated by the nature of the oncology practice and available resources.

13.2 FUNGI

Cancer patients are prone to opportunistic fungal infection, most often by *Candida* and *Aspergillus* spp. The type of fungus and the clinical findings vary according to the nature of the defence impairment. The interactions are complex (Warnock and Richardson, 1990) but, as a generality, neutropenic patients are predisposed to invasive candida and aspergillus infections, whereas deficient cell-mediated immunity is associated with cryptococcosis and with superficial candidal infections of the skin and mucous membranes. Contributing factors include disturbance of the normal bacterial flora by prolonged antibiotic therapy and invasion via central venous catheters or ulcerated mucosae.

Candida infections are nearly always of endogenous origin, and mucosal ulceration with painful white plaques on the tongue and lips occur frequently in acute leukaemia and the neutropenic phase of bone marrow transplantation (Figure 13.1). Invasive candida and aspergillus infections are often indicated only by fever which fails to respond to antibacterial antibiotics. Blood cultures and bronchoalveolar lavage are only infrequently positive, especially for aspergillosis; as yet there are no serological methods which combine sensitivity and specificity with ready availability to the routine diagnostic laboratory; the patient may be too ill or too thrombocytopenic for tissue diagnoses to be attempted. Consequently empirical or pre-emptive antifungal treatment is commonly employed and will usually be a component of any scheme for planned progressive therapy of infection in neutropenic patients.

The broad antifungal spectrum of amphotericin B makes it the most appropriate choice for empirical use, but it may cause renal toxicity and hypokalaemia or be associated with severe rigors and hypotension. Alternatives under evaluation includes amphotericin B carried in liposomes or lipid complexes and triazole compounds such as fluconazole and itraconazole (Hay, 1991), but clinical trials of new antifungal agents are hindered by a number of factors. Diagnoses and assessments of outcome which rest upon serology or cultures from normally unsterile specimens, such as sputum, are usually unreliable and tissue diagnoses from biopsies or necropsies may not be available. In addition, since most fungi are sensitive to amphotericin B, to justify the use of a possibly less toxic or more convenient drug for a life-threatening infection, the patient must in some way be unable to received the standard treatment.

Thus in some instances the trial antifungal agent is administered only after amphotericin B has been withdrawn, and the possible influence of the earlier treatment has then to be taken into account when the new drug is assessed. Even when this is not the case, small available numbers and low rates of recovery necessitate large multicentre studies.

These drawbacks result in slow accumulation of reliable data, but some general observations are possible. It appears that amphotericin B incorporated into liposomes may be given in higher doses (3–5 mg/kg/day compared with 1 mg/kg/day of the conventional form) and with greatly reduced nephrotoxicity and side-effects; however, evidence of superior efficacy is needed before these very expensive products can be recommended for general use. Fluconazole has good activity against *Candida albicans* infections of the oropharynx, oesophagus and vagina, but it is unproven as effective treatment for deep candida infections and its poor activity against aspergillosis limits its use as empirical therapy. Some candida species, such as *C. krusei*, also are resistant to fluconazole. When it is used for the specific treatment of susceptible candida infections, this drug has the advantage of being available in both oral and intravenous forms and of being easily absorbed and non-toxic. It is water soluble and penetrates well into the cerebrospinal fluid. Intraconazole has a broad spectrum of activity which includes both yeasts and aspergilli. It is as yet only available as an oral preparation which, because it is not water soluble, requires food

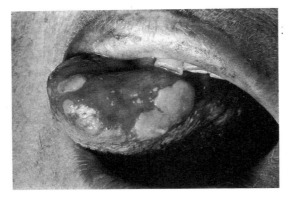

Figure 13.1   Candida infection of the tongue.

for maximal absorption. In cancer patients, itraconazole is chiefly of interest as a non-toxic alternative to amphotericin B for the treatment and prevention of aspergillosis. Studies of small numbers (Denning *et al.*, 1989) have been promising, but an intravenous preparation will be required to demonstrate its value clearly in oncology patients, who may have impaired ability to absorb or swallow for a wide variety of reasons.

There is an increasing need for reliable antifungal therapy. Rates of invasive candidiasis and aspergillosis will vary from one oncology centre to another, but overall fungi are emerging as common and still intractable pathogens. Their occurrence is influenced by the type of immune defect associated with the patient's cancer, with the nature and intensity of the treatment for that disease, and with the resources that are available for supportive care. The price for successful anticancer treatment may be prolonged neutropenia, graft-against-host disease, immunosuppressive treatments or radical surgery. Repeated courses of broad-spectrum antibiotics for the associated bacterial infections mean longer periods when the regulating influence of the normal bacterial flora is disturbed, while the use of intravenous catheters to give drugs and parenteral nutrition offer yet another route for invading pathogens. Thus improved survival creates a greater opportunity for fungal infections to occur.

Recovery rates with currently available treatments are poor (Armstrong, 1993) and attention is being paid to improved chemo-prophylaxis. The non-absorbable polyenes, nystatin and amphotericin B, have been used as oral prophylaxis in leukaemia and bone marrow transplantation for over 20 years, though with little proof of their value. This uncertainty, plus the unpalatability of these drugs, has focused interest on fluconozole. A review of published studies (Warren, 1992) concludes that 50 mg/kg/day effectively prevents *C. albicans* infection, although all

studies record infection with *C. krusei*, which is resistant to fluconazole.

There is no comparable collection of published work related to the prevention of aspergillus infection, although itraconazole is under investigation. On the other hand, since *Aspergillus* spp. are not part of the normal human microflora, some protection may be achieved by mechanical reduction of exposure to its spores. High efficiency particulate air (HEPA) filtration has been shown to prevent infection from environments with a high aspergillus spore count (Barnes and Rogers, 1989) (Scherertz *et al.*, 1987), but if HEPA filtration is installed, the maximum benefit will only be obtained if precautions are also taken to exclude sources other than the air, such as indoor plants and certain food-stuffs.

Invasive fungal infection in cancer patients is not confined to candidiasis and aspergillosis. Increasingly, patients with haematological malignancies are reported with infections due to the Mucorales and to previously unconsidered pathogens such as *Trichosporon* spp. and *Pseudallescheria boydii*. The problems of diagnosis and treatment are similar to those already described (Richardson, 1991).

Cryptococcosis is distinguishable from the infections discussed previously in its presentation, diagnosis and therapy. It is associated with cell-mediated immune deficiencies such as occur in Hodgkin's disease and other lymphomas. *C. neoformans* is the most common infecting species: it is ubiquitous, often being found in large numbers in pigeon-droppings, and is aquired by inhalation. Although lesions may be found in lung, skin and bone, it is usually asymptomatic until it invades the meninges. Even then the presenting symptoms may be non-specific, amounting to no more than severe and persistent headache.

The diagnosis is usually confirmed by the presence of typical budding (and often capsulated) yeasts in the cerebrospinal fluid

(CSF). A latex agglutination test is available for detection of cryptococcal antigen in both CSF and serum. A very valuable application of this test is in monitoring the quantity of antigen in the CSF during and after the treatment. Recurrent relapse is the pattern of this disease and management requires both treatment and prophylaxis. Amphotericin B is regarded by most mycologists as the treatment of choice for the acute phase, possibly supplemented with flucytosine. If this regimen is used, the patient must be observed for signs of bone marrow depression caused by flucytosine. The duration of amphotericin B/flucytosine treatment is usually in the region of 4–6 weeks, and thereafter the patient needs to be given life-long prophylaxis with either low dose amphotericin B or fluconazole. The management of cryptococcosis is discussed in detail by Shaunak and Cohen (1991).

Figure 13.2 shows the hands of a patient whose chronic candida infection of the fingernails responded to amphotericin B which was being given for cryptococcal meningitis. The area of normal growth reflects the long duration of therapy. In fact, this patient had a total of four episodes of cryptococcal infection (without prophylaxis) and in between led an active life until his death due to an unrelated condition.

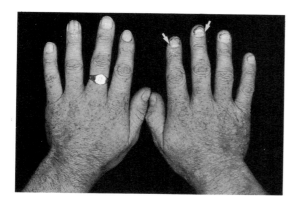

Figure 13.2 Effect of amphotericin B on candida nail infection.

13.3 VIRUSES

13.3.1 HERPES SIMPLEX VIRUS (HSV)

Mucosal ulceration, especially of the mouth and oesophagus, caused by reactivation of latent HSV, is a common complication of cancer chemotherapy and is seen in 70% of seropositive recipients of BMT. Treatment is essential, because of both pain and the fact that the lesions are a portal of entry for bacterial infection.

Acyclovir is the treatment of choice and may be given both orally and intravenously with few side-effects. It is also effective as a prophylactic agent, but the high cost has led to suggestions that the drug should be reserved for symptomatic infections only, as these will respond quickly. A recent finding (Baglin *et al.*, 1989) that HSV is a frequent cause of fever of unidentified origin in neutropenic patients, has influenced opinion in favour of giving acyclovir prophylaxis to seropositive patients at risk, though not to those who are seronegative, in whom the incidence of herpetic ulceration is very much lower.

13.3.2 VARICELLA ZOSTER VIRUS (VZV)

VZV as a primary infection is the cause of chickenpox, and in a reactivated form is the cause of herpes zoster (or 'shingles'). The latter may be limited to a single dermatome or may become generalized and invasive. Both chickenpox and generalized herpes zoster are potentially life-threatening conditions in acute lymphoblastic leukaemia and lymphomas, and during the third to ninth months following BMT. Death results from involvement of vital organs, especially the lungs and central nervous system. Intravenous acyclovir is the treatment of choice.

Cross-infection with VZV is a serious hazard in hospitals where large numbers of immunocompromized patients are treated. A hospital policy for health care workers who have contact with chickenpox, or develop shingles themselves, will ensure that they inform a designated nurse or medical officer and are encouraged to stay away from work if they fall ill during the chickenpox incubation period. Screening of nurses and doctors for VZV seropositivity at the time of employment permits assessment of their risk from contact and also, by the use of seropositive staff to care for patients with zoster and chickenpox, greatly reduces the risk of their contracting the infection and passing it on to other vulnerable patients.

Children with acute lymphoblastic leukaemia, who are receiving maintenance chemotherapy but leading relatively normal lives, are at high risk of contracting chickenpox. Administration of varicella-hyperimmune gamma globulin (Vig/Zig) within 72 hours of contact effectively reduces the severity of the infection. As it does not prevent it completely, it must be remembered that the child may have a mild or atypical attack, during which he or she is infectious. Management must therefore include segregating the child from others at risk (e.g. a clinic, for example) during the incubation period.

The use of acyclovir prophylaxis to prevent zoster following BMT is controversial. Perren *et al.* (1988) showed that while acyclovir was effective prophylaxis when given during the first 6 months following transplantation, the occurence rate in the acyclovir group exceeded that of the control group during the following 6 months. Although it might be argued that there is an advantage in deferring the onset of the infection, the cost-benefit is doubtful, provided that treatment can be given promptly when it is needed.

13.3.3 CYTOMEGALOVIRUS (CMV)

This virus features most prominently in oncology patients as a major cause of fatal pneumonia during the second and third months following BMT. The incidence varies with the type of conditioning regimen used, and is lower after autologous BMT, which does not usually incur graft-against-host disease (Reusser *et al.*, 1990).

Infections occur most often when the BMT recipient is seropositive for CMV, indicating that reactivated latent infection is the likely cause. The infection may also be transmitted by donations of bone marrow or blood products, and seronegative recipients should be given seronegative donations when possible. Leucocyte depleted platelet infusions are also protective (Bowden *et al.*, 1991).

The treatment currently available for CMV pneumonia is ganciclovir, a nucleoside related to acyclovir but with greater *in vitro* activity against CMV. Used alone, it has produced disappointing results, but some improvement has been obtained from combining it with specific hyperimunoglobulin (CMV Ig) (Schmidt *et al.*, 1988).

Ganciclovir has a suppressive effect on the bone marrow which limits its potential application as prophylaxis. Schmidt and colleagues (1991) targeted the prophylactic use of the drug on patients in whom CMV was demonstrated in bronchoalveolar lavage on day 35 following BMT. Five of 20 patients given ganciclovir developed pneumonia, compared with 12/17 lavage-positive patients who were given standard care. Twelve of 59 patients whose lavage did not show the virus also developed CMV pneumonia and since viraemia is also predictive for disease (Goodrich *et al.*, 1991), this may prove to be an easier method for identifying patients for prophylaxis.

The literature on the diagnosis, prevention and therapy of CMV disease is extensive and growing. Readers are recommended to refer to reviews of recent publications, such as are to be found in the journal *Current Opinion on Infectious Disease*.

13.3.4 MEASLES

Immunocompromized children who have been vaccinated in infancy appear not to be at risk from measles. The hazards for those who do aquire the infection while immuno-suppressed are fatal giant cell pneumonia and subacute measles encephalitis, the onset of which may be delayed by up to 6 months. The diagnosis of measles is often obscured by the absence of a typical rash in patients with impaired cell-mediated immunity.

There is no treatment or prophylaxis available, although human immune globulin is sometimes given after exposure to measles in an attempt to modify the attack. The live virus vaccination is contraindicated in immuno-suppressed patients.

13.3.5 OTHER VIRUSES

For many common viruses such as respiratory syncitial virus, adenoviruses, enteroviruses and influenza, prophylaxis and therapy are not available and immunization may be contra-indicated. Avoidance is the chief protective procedure and this includes attention to handwashing and food preparation on the part of carers. These two measures are well recog-nized in the prevention of bacterial infection, but it is less often appreciated that the hands may be vectors even of respiratory viruses.

Live virus vaccines are contraindicated in the immunocompromised, but in the UK, it is possible to obtain an inactivated poliomyelitis vaccine specifically for this group of patients (HMSO, 1992).

13.4 PNEUMOCYSTIS CARINII

This organism, for long regarded as a proto-zoan, has recently been shown by DNA studies to be related to the fungi. Little is in fact known about the life-cycle and pathogenicity of *P. carinii*, because it is difficult to maintain in *in vitro* culture, but it has been recognized for about 50 years as a cause of life-threatening pneumonia in immunodeficient patients, first in malnourished infants after World War II and later as a complication of lymphoblastic leukaemia and BMT.

The successful introduction of co-trimoxa-zole prophylaxis (Hughes *et al.*, 1977) and therapy (Hughes *et al.*, 1975) greatly reduced the danger of this infection in oncology pa-tients, but interest in drug management was re-kindled when it re-appeared in association with HIV infection. Co-trimoxazole side-effects are more severe in AIDS patients and useful in-formation about alternative drugs, such as inhaled pentamidine isethionate, is now being applied to BMT patients in whom co-trimoxa-zole may have an adverse effect on bone marrow recovery.

Absence of sputum is characteristic of *P. carinii* pneumonia (PCP). Athough in expert hands the organisms can be identified in sputum induced by inhaling saline mist, in most circumstances the diagnosis is made by bronchoalveolar lavage (BAL) or, less often, lung biopsy. PCP is usually only one of a number of possible diagnoses in a immuno-compromised patient who presents with a severe respiratory infection, and BAL has the advantage of providing material for bacterial, fungal and viral cultures, and also for rapid identification of pneumocysts, *Legionella* and cytomegalovirus by monoclonal antibody stains. Since more than one pathogen may be present, it is often necessary to treat severe res-piratory infection with a broad-spectrum em-pirical combination of antimicrobials. A typical combination might include erythromycin (for *Legionella* and *Mycoplasma* spp.), amphotericin B and ganciclovir, in addition to the high dose co-trimoxazole regimen appropriate for *P. carinii*.

13.5 FUTURE TRENDS

In the past 10 years or so, the proportion of Gram-positive bacteria isolated from blood cultures has risen to about one-half. At first *S. epidermidis* predominated, but streptococci are also emerging as major pathogens. In the 5th EORTC trial (1991), 64% of all single-organism bacteraemias were due to Gram-positive cocci, with streptococci outnumbering *S. epidermidis.*

Among the Gram-negative infections there is a similar trend towards the appearance of bacteria which were not previously regarded as pathogens. Of 134 Gram-negative isolates at the Royal Marsden Hospital in 1992, 15 were *Pseudomonas* spp. other than *Ps. aeruginosa* (S. Willmott, personal communication). These bacteria are frequently not susceptible to antibiotics in common use and offer a new challenge to policies for empirical therapy.

Haematopoietic growth factors (Lieschke and Burgess, 1992), by reducing the duration of neutropenia and thus the need for frequent courses of antibiotics, may prove to be one means of breaking the pernicious cycle of infection → antibiotic therapy → superinfection and resistance → more infection.

REFERENCES

Armstrong, D. (1993) Treatment of opportunistic fungal infections. *Clinical Infectious Diseases*, **16**, 1–7.

Baglin,T.P., Gray, J.J., Marcus, R.E. and Wreghitt, J.G. (1989) Antibiotic resistant fever associated with herpes simplex virus infection in neutropenic patients with haematological malignancy. *Journal of Clinical Pathology*, **42**, 1255–8.

Bagshaw, K.D. (1964) Ultra-clean ward for cancer chemotherapy. *British Medical Journal*, **2**, 871–3.

Barnes, R.A. and Rogers, T.R. (1987) An evaluation of empirical antibiotic therapy in febrile neutropenic patients. *British Journal of Haematology*, **66**, 137–40.

Barnes, R.A. and Rogers, T.R.F (1989) Control of an outbreak of nosocomial aspergillosis by laminar air-flow isolation. *Journal of Hospital Infection*, **14**, 89–94.

Bowden, R.A., Slichter, S.J., Sayers, M.N., *et al.* (1991) Use of leucocyte-depleted platelets and cytomegalovirus-seronegative red blood cells for prevention of primary cytomegalovirus infection after marrow transplant. *Blood*, **78**, 246–50.

Burden, A.D., Oppenheim, B.A., Crowther, D. *et al.* (1991) Viridans streptococcal bacteraemia in patients with haematological and solid malignancies. *European Journal of Cancer*, **27**, 409–11.

Denning, D.W., Tucker, R.M., Hanson, L.H. and Stevens, D.A. (1989) Treatment of invasive aspergillosis with itraconazole. *American Journal of Medicine*, **86**, 791–800.

EORTC International Antimicrobial Therapy Cooperative Group and National Cancer Institute of Canada Clinical Trials Group (1991) Vancomycin added to empirical combination antibiotic therapy for fever in granulocytopenic patients. *Journal of Infectious Disease*, **163**, 951–8.

Gaya, H. (1988) *Therapeutic Conferences, Planned Progressive Therapy.* Advanced Therapeutic Communications International, Secaucus, New Jersey.

Goodrich, J.M., Mori, M., Greaves, C.A. *et al.* (1991) Early treatment with ganciclovir to prevent cytomegalovirus disease after allogeneic bone marrow transplantation. *New England Journal of Medicine*, **325**, 1601–7.

Hay, R.T. (1991) Antifungal therapy and the new azole compounds. *Journal of Antimicrobial Chemotherapy*, **28** (Suppl A), 35–46.

Hughes, W.T., Armstrong, D., Bodey, G.P. *et al.* (1990) Guidelines for the use of antimicrobial agents in neutropenic patients with unexplained fever. *Journal of Infectious Diseases*, **161**, 381–96.

Hughes, W.T., Feldman, and Sanyal, K. (1975) Treatment of *Pneumocystis carinii* pneumonitis with trimethoprim sulfamethoxazole. *Canadian Medical Association Journal*, **112**, 475–505.

Hughes, W.T., Kohn, S. Chaudhary, *et al.*(1977) Successful chemoprophylaxis for *Pneumocystis carinii* pneumonitis. *New England Journal of Medicine*, **297**, 1419–26.

Hughes, W.T., Pizzo, P.A., Wade, J.C. *et al.* (1992) General guidelines for the evaluation of new anti-infective drugs for the treatment of febrile episodes in neutropenic patients. *Clinical Infectious Diseases*, **15**, (Suppl 1), S206–15.

Jameson, B., Lynch., Gamble, D.R. and Kay, H.E.M. (1971) Five year analysis of protective isolation. *Lancet*, **i**, 1034–40.

Joint Committee on Immunisation and Vaccination (1992) *Immunisation Against Infectious Disease* HMSO, London.

Lieschke, G.J. and Burgess, A.W. (1992) Granulocyte colony-stimulating factor and granulocyte–macrophage colony-stimulating factor. Therapeutic applications. *New England Journal of Medicine*, **327**, 99–106.

Medical Research Council, (1968) Aseptic methods in the operating suite. *Lancet*, **i**, 831–9.

Perren, T.J., Powles, R.L., Easton, D. *et al.* (1988) Prevention of herpes zoster in patients by long term acyclovir after allogeneic bone marrow transplantation. *American Journal of Medicine*, **85**, 99–101.

Reusser, P., Fisher, L.D., Buckner, C.D. *et al.* (1990) Cytomegalovirus after autologous bone marrow transplantation: occurrence of cytomegalovirus disease and effect on engraftment. *Blood*, **75**, 1888–94.

Richardson, M.D. (1991) Opportunist and pathogenic fungi. *Journal of Antimicrobial Chemotherapy*, **28**, (Suppl A), 1–11.

Scherertz, R.J., Belani, A., Kramer, B.S. *et al.* (1987) Impact of air filtration on nosocomial *Aspergillus* infection: unique risk of bone marrow transplant recipients. *American Journal of Medicine*, **83**, 709–18.

Schimpff, S.C., Satterlee, W., Young, V.M. and Serpeck, A. (1971) Empiric therapy with carbenicillin and gentamicin for febrile neutropenic patients with cancer and granulocytopenia. *New England Journal of Medicine*, **284**, 1061–65.

Schmidt, G.M., Kovacs, A., Zaua, A., *et al.* (1988) Ganciclovir/immunoglobulin combination therapy for the treatment of human cyto-megalovirus-associated interstitial pneumonia in bone marrow allograft recipients. *Transplantation*, **46**, 905–7.

Schmidt, G.M., Horak, D.A., Niland, J.C. *et al.* (1991) A randomised, controlled trial of prophylactic ganciclovir for cytomegalovirus pulmonary infection in recipients of allogeneic bone marrow transplant. *New England Journal of Medicine*, **324**, 1005–11.

Shaunak, S. and Cohen, J. (1991) Clinical management of fungal infection in patients with AIDS. *Journal of Antimicrobial Chemotherapy*, **28**, (Suppl A), 67–81.

Shooter, R.A., Cooke, E.M., Gaya, H. and Kumar, P. (1969) Food and medicaments as possible sources of hospital strains of *Pseudomonas aeruginosa*. *Lancet*, **i**, 1227–9.

Warnock, D.W. and Richardson, M. (1990) *Fungal Infection in the Compromised Patient*, 2nd edn, John Wiley, Chichester.

Warren, R.E. (1992) Prevention of infection. *Current Opinion in Infectious Diseases*, **5**, 411.

THE PSYCHOLOGICAL TOLL OF CANCER

Steven Greer

14.1 INTRODUCTION

As one must not try to cure the eyes without the head or the head without the body, similarly (one must not try to cure) the body without the psyche.

> (Socrates in Plato's *Charmides*)

Psychooncology is the name given to the psychological study of persons who develop cancer. A distinguished American oncologist has succinctly outlined the need for this new discipline and its current status:

> ... the treatment of cancer has come to be an extremely technical undertaking, based almost entirely within the busiest and most active wards of the hospital, and involving the strenuous efforts of highly specialized professionals, each taking his or her responsibility for a share of the patient's problem, but sometimes working at a rather impersonal distance from the patient as an individual. To many patients, stunned by the diagnosis, suffering numerous losses and discomforts, moved from place to place for one procedure after another, the experience is bewildering and frightening; at worst, it is like being trapped in the workings of a huge piece of complicated machinery.

It is only in quite recent years that oncologists in general have begun to confront squarely the emotional impact of these ordeals and the fact that emotional states play a large role in the tolerability of treatment and, perhaps, in the outcome as well.

> Within less than a decade, the term psychooncology, viewed at first with deep suspicion by most oncologists, has at last emerged as a respectable field for both application and research. In my own view, having passed through both stages as a skeptical clinician and administrator, the appearance on the scene of psychiatrists and experimental psychologists has so vastly improved the lot of cancer patients as to make these new professionals indispensable'. (Thomas, 1989)

The new discipline of psychooncology encompasses two broad areas of research. The first area comprises studies of the contribution of psychosocial factors to the aetiology and course of cancer. Included here are studies of the role of personality traits, stress and depression in the promotion of cancer as well as studies of the effect of patients' psychological responses to cancer and of psychotherapy on duration of survival. This stimulating, provocative area of research which challenges the orthodox cartesian view of a rigid separation between mind and body is beyond the scope of the present chapter. Interested readers are referred to reviews by Hu and Silberfarb (1988), Greer (1991) and Watson and Ramirez (1991). The other principal area of psychooncology comprises clinical studies of psychological and social morbidity associated with cancer and its various treatments as well as the development and evaluation of psychological therapy designed to improve the quality of life of cancer patients. It is these studies which are considered here.

14.2   CANCER-RELATED PSYCHOSOCIAL MORBIDITY

Faced with a diagnosis of cancer, patients commonly react at first with numbed shock and disbelief followed by anxiety, anger ('why me?') and depression. In the majority of cases, this stress reaction subsides as patients learn to adjust to their disease. But a substantial minority, ranging from 22% (Morris *et al.*, 1977) to 44% (Derogatis *et al.*, 1983), go on to develop psychiatric disorders. Variations in reported prevalence figures are due to differences in site and stage of cancer, in cancer treatments and in the methods used to assess psychiatric disorders. Without psychotherapeutic intervention, such disorders may persist for years, even in the absence of any evidence of disease (Fobair *et al.*, 1986; Irvine *et al.*, 1991). A well-designed study of an unselected series of patients with lung, breast and colorectal cancers reported that there was no improvement in psychological adaptation over time; indeed, a significant decline in mental health scores occurred between baseline assessment and 1–2 years post-diagnosis (Ell *et al.*, 1989). It is not only patients themselves who suffer psychological ill health as a result of cancer; their spouses and family members may be similarly affected (Lichtman and Taylor, 1986). The present discussion, however, will be confined to the patients.

By far the commonest psychiatric disorders among cancer patients are anxiety and depressive states. In a prospective study of 1260 patients attending the Royal Marsden Hospital who were screened psychologically 4–12 weeks after an initial diagnosis of cancer, 23% were found to have clinically significant anxiety or depression (Greer *et al.*, 1992). In anxious patients who are receiving chemotherapy, anticipatory nausea and vomiting (i.e. before the infusions are given) have been reported. At the Royal Marsden Hospital, among outpatients on mild to moderate chemotherapy regimens, 23%

experience anticipatory nausea and 4% anticipatory vomiting (Watson *et al.*, 1992). Patients with advanced cancer may develop confusional states (delirium); these are often mistakenly diagnosed as depression (Levine *et al.*, 1978). Hence, it is important for the clinician to assess cognitive functions of patients with severe psychiatric symptoms or disturbed behaviour (Figure 14.1).

Cancer may also impair social functioning in such areas as work, marriage, relationships with friends and sexual adjustment. As one would expect, marriages which were unsatisfactory before the disease appeared are the ones most likely to deteriorate further. Previously close marriages and similar relationships are rarely damaged by the impact of cancer. Indeed, some marriages actually improve, as the threat to life posed by cancer strengthens the love between the partners (Morris *et al.*, 1977). Difficulties in relationships with friends and neighbours are usually caused by mutual embarrassment and resulting lack of communication; this problem can be overcome by teaching patients how to broach the subject of cancer with other people.

Sexual function has been insufficiently studied. It seems that many oncologists as well as their patients are too embarrassed or regard it as inappropriate to raise this topic in the context of cancer. Be that as it may, it is important for clinicians to inquire about the effect of their treatments on the sexual lives of patients, because such evidence as is available points to considerable impairment of sexual function. Sexual disorders are particularly common in patients with breast and gynaecological cancer, prostatic, penile and testicular cancer, and colorectal and bladder cancers. A combination of psychological causes (e.g. feeling repulsive following disfiguring surgery or ostomies, the partner's reaction) and physical causes (e.g. direct effect of the disease, nerve damage following surgery and irradiation, chemical or surgical castration) underlies cancer related sexual dysfunction.

14.2.1   CAUSES

(a)   Emotional impact of cancer diagnosis

Notwithstanding some recent advances in treatment, cancer still evokes a particular horror and fear second only to that produced by AIDS. McIntosh's (1974) observation nearly 20 years ago that the diagnosis of cancer is, for most people, tantamount to a death sentence, holds good today. The diagnosis of cancer or its recurrence is the most frequent cause of psychiatric disorder (predominantly anxiety and depressive states) as well as social dysfunction among cancer patients.

(b)   Side-effects of treatment

Having faced the emotional trauma of receiving a diagnosis of cancer, the patient will now be required to undergo various kinds of treatment which themselves may produce physical and psychological morbidity.

A cardinal ethical principle within medicine is *primum non nocere* – above all do no harm. Applied to oncology, in which current treatments can cause considerable harm, this principle is taken to mean that any given treatment is justified only when its benefits are demonstrably greater than the harm, i.e. 'side-effects', which it produces. In other words, the prospect of prolonging life must be weighed against impairment in the quality of that life. Of course, in some cancers such as Hodgkin's disease, Wilms' tumour or testicular cancer, treatment has produced such clear-cut improvement in survival rates as to outweigh all other considerations. But for many cancers, the therapeutic and harmful effects of chemotherapy are more finely balanced.

It follows that assessment of quality of life is essential and that such assessment should include psychological and social morbidity. Detailed measures of psychosocial adjustment should be included in all clinical trials for two reasons: first, to provide clinicians with empirical data upon which to base their choice of treatment and, second, to identify those patients who require therapy for psychological disorders.

(c)   Surgery

Mutilating surgery undoubtedly causes emotional distress and may lead to psychiatric disorders and social dysfunction. There is, however, a shortage of systematic controlled studies for many surgical procedures. For example, there are no published data on the psychological effects of surgery for lung cancer. By contrast, the effects of mastectomy have been extensively studied with seemingly contradictory results. In an excellent balanced review of the literature up to 1979, Morris (1979) summarized the evidence as follows:

> It seems likely that about three-quarters of married or older women who have a mastectomy (data on younger single women are inadequate) will recover from the experience within a year of operation; that the marriage relationships may improve, and that most women will return to work. However, a substantial minority of women, between one-quarter and one-third, will be left with feelings of personal inadequacy, anxiety and depression or sexual difficulties, which are not likely to be resolved without intervention, and perhaps not even then.

A criticism of the studies reviewed by Morris is that it was not possible to disentangle the adverse psychological effects of mastectomy from those associated with fear of cancer. When lumpectomy became an acceptable operation for breast cancer, Fallowfield *et al.* (1986) studied a series of patients who were randomly allocated to either lumpectomy or mastectomy. They reported a similar incidence of psychological morbidity in both treatment groups. But a subsequent randomized trial of mastectomy versus segmental resection reported clear psychological advantages for patients who had received segmental resection, namely significantly less anxiety and depression, as well as more positive feelings about their sexuality and body image (Kemeny *et al.*, 1988). In practice, mastectomy has become less common in recent years. Clinical experience indicates that although mastectomy produces psychological distress and sexual dysfunction in many women, there are some who prefer it to less extensive surgery because they fear that cancer cells may still be present in the conserved breast. As a result, some surgeons offer women with primary breast cancer a choice between mastectomy and less extensive surgery. According to a preliminary study, giving patients a choice is psychologically beneficial (Morris and Ingham, 1988).

The psychological effects of surgery for bowel cancer have been documented. A careful study compared the quality of life of patients with rectal cancer who were treated either by abdominoperineal resection (APER) or low sphincter-saving resection (SSR) (Williams and Johnston, 1983). Assessments 1 year after surgery revealed that the quality of life of patients who underwent APER was significantly worse than that of patients treated by SSR: only 40% of APER patients compared with 83% of SSR patients had returned to work, sexual function was impaired in 67% of APER patients compared with 30% of SSR patients; also APER patients were significantly more depressed and their social activities were more restricted as a result of colostomy. Another study which requires mention is that by Sugarbaker *et al.* (1982) who compared the quality of life in patients with osteosarcoma who had undergone either limb amputation or limb salvage. The physical and psychological adjustment of patients was found to be similar in both treatment groups. Where systematic data about post-operative quality of life are lacking, descriptions provided by patients themselves or by their relatives are valuable. Highly recom-

mended are two such publications: Christine Piff's (1985) poignant description of the distressing effects of maxillofacial surgery and an eloquent detailed account by a psychiatrist of his father's quality of life following prostatectomy and hormone therapy for prostatic cancer (Green, 1987).

(d)   Radiotherapy

Emotional distress, clinical anxiety and depression may arise from several sources: the erroneous belief that receiving radiotherapy implies incurable cancer, the claustrophobic surroundings in which radiotherapy takes place, fears of radiation burns or other radiation damage, particularly sterility, contribute to psychological morbidity. During the course of radiotherapy, the peculiarly unpleasant fatigue which many patients report leads, in some cases, to depression. With the exception of radiation damage, psychological symptoms subside within a few weeks of stopping radiotherapy; long-term psychological effects are rare (Danoff *et al.*, 1983).

(e)   Chemotherapy

In the avalanche of published clinical trials of many and various chemotherapy regimens, assessment of quality of life – where it is assessed at all – is usually limited to the occurrence of physical symptoms. In the great majority of trials, measurement of psychological morbidity and social adjustment is conspicuous by its absence. One of the few controlled studies of the psychological effects of adjuvant chemotherapy in women with breast cancer illustrates the clinical value of obtaining such data. In a randomized trial of three forms of treatment following mastectomy for Stage II breast cancer, psychological symptoms were measured over 2 years (Hughson *et al.*, 1986). The treatments were: radiotherapy for 3 weeks; adjuvant cyclophosphamide, methotrexate and 5-fluoruracil

(CMF) for 1 year; radiotherapy followed by chemotherapy.

There were no significant differences in depression or anxiety among patients in the three treatment groups at 1, 3 and 6 months after mastectomy. However at 13 months, patients allocated to chemotherapy had significantly more symptoms, especially depression, than patients receiving radiotherapy alone. Anticipatory (i.e. conditioned reflex) nausea and vomiting increased markedly during the second 6 months of chemotherapy and persisted for up to a year thereafter. The authors concluded that psychological morbidity associated with chemotherapy could be substantially reduced if courses of treatment were restricted to about 6 months. In the absence of any clear survival advantage with more prolonged chemotherapy, Hughson's findings helped to change clinical practice.

In trials which evaluate palliative treatments, measurement of psychosocial adjustment is even more crucial. A valuable study was reported by Silberfarb (1986). Patients with small cell lung cancer were randomly allocated to two different treatment regimens involving chest irradiation, prophylactic cranial irradiation and chemotherapy. Duration of survival and symptoms of physical toxicity were similar in both groups, but the chemotherapy regimen which contained vincristine produced significantly greater depression. The obvious conclusion to be drawn is that vincristine should not be used in these circumstances.

Clinicians need to be aware that the side-effects of chemotherapy are not confined to physical toxicity but include psychosocial morbidity. The undoubted adverse physical and psychological consequences of chemotherapy must be taken into account, together with survival rates, in deciding on the most appropriate treatment regimen. The patient's psychological state should also be considered in deciding when to stop treatment. In cases where there has been no clinical or tumour response, the clinician will stop chemotherapy. Most patients accept this decision, but some become angry or depressed when they realize that active treatment has ceased; they will request further chemotherapy, however experimental and whatever the side-effects. Here, the clinician is faced with a difficult and delicate decision. In coming to that decision, an understanding of the individual patient's psychological attributes and social circumstances is required.

14.2.2 ACUTE PSYCHIATRIC DISTURBANCE

Having considered the causes of *chronic* psychosocial morbidity among cancer patients. We now turn to *acute* psychiatric disturbance. Typically, a patient on the ward becomes restless, noisy, suspicious, angry and apparently confused, with an abnormal mood ranging from euphoria to depression; these symptoms are worse at night. Such a patient requires urgent attention. The clinician's first task is to examine the patient's mental state with particular emphasis on memory, orientation and concentration. A useful standardized clinical measure of these cognitive functions is the Mini-Mental State Exam (Folstein *et al.*, 1984); scores range from 0 to 30 with scores below 24 indicating cognitive impairment. Such impairment (i.e. clouding of consciousness) is a cardinal feature of *acute confusional state* (*delirium*). The main causes of acute psychiatric disturbance among cancer patients are shown in Figure 14.1.

Treatment of acute confusional state will depend on the causes, e.g. lowering the dose or stopping steroids, correcting any metabolic imbalance. Irrespective of the cause, however, the occurrence of an acute confusional state in any patient constitutes an emergency which requires immediate action as follows:

1. Reassure the patient that (s)he will come to no harm. Such reassurance should be carried out by medical and nursing staff who are familiar with and trusted by the

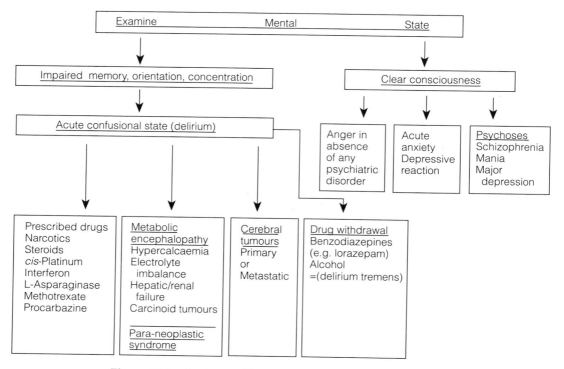

Figure 14.1   Acute psychiatric disturbance in cancer patients.

patient and, where possible, the spouse or a close family member.

2.   Move the patient to a single, well-lit room with a dimmed light at night.

3.   Administer haloperidol orally or i.m. beginning with 1 mg. The psychiatrist or physician should observe the patient closely for extrapyramidal signs. In most cases, 5–10 mg of haloperidol daily is sufficient but up to 20 mg daily can be given. Should extrapyramidal side-effects occur, these can be controlled with anti-cholinergic drugs such as benztropine 0.5–1 mg orally, i.m. or i.v. Usually, haloperidol can be stopped within a few days.

14.3   TREATMENT OF ANXIETY AND DEPRESSIVE DISORDERS

Because anxiety and depression are natural, understandable responses to cancer, some clin-icians – psychiatrists as well as oncologists – assume that psychiatric treatment is neither feasible nor indicated. This assumption is in-correct for two reasons. First, only about 23% of patients suffer from persistent anxiety and depression (i.e. symptoms which persist for more than a month after diagnosis). Second, there is good evidence that psychological dis-tress in cancer patients can be reduced significantly by psychological therapy (Greer *et al.*, 1992). Indeed, psychological therapy can make an important contribution to improving the quality of life of patients.

As mentioned earlier, anxiety and depres-sion are the commonest psychiatric disorders among cancer patients. It must be stressed that approximately 90% of these disorders are a direct reaction to the diagnosis and treat-ment of cancer with no evidence of pre-existing psychiatric illness (Shakin *et al.*, 1991). This has important implications for psychotherapy with cancer patients (see below). Treatment of cancer-related anxiety and depressive disorders can be grouped conveniently under two headings: psychotropic drugs and psychological therapy.

In considering treatment, a basic rule is that psychological therapy of some kind is always required, whereas psychotropic drugs have drawbacks and should be used only occasionally and sparingly.

14.3.1 PSYCHOTROPIC DRUGS

A guide to the use of these drugs is provided in Table 14.1.

(a) Anxiolytics

Although anxiety can be alleviated in most cases by relaxation training and psychological therapy, sometimes the level of anxiety is so great that patients cannot concentrate on psychological procedures. In these circumstances, a brief course of benzodiazepines is indicated. These drugs should not be given for longer than a week in order to avoid drug dependence. Usually, only a few days on benzodizepines are required before patients can learn cognitive and behavioural techniques for reducing their anxiety without recourse to drugs.

(b) Antidepressants

There is a dearth of randomized controlled trials of antidepressant drugs for patients with cancer. The precise indications for antidepressants have not been established empirically. In the opinion of some psychiatrists, these drugs have been underused in oncology and should be given to most, if not all, cancer patients who are depressed (e.g. Massie and Lesko, 1989). There are, however, serious objections to this practice.

Table 14.1 Psychotropic drugs for cancer patients

	Anxiolytics	*Antidepressants*
Indications	Acute severe anxiety and panic attacks	Major depressive illness

Type and dose	Lorazepam 1–2 mg TDS
	Diazepam 2–5 mg TDS
		(a) Tricyclics:
		     Dothiepin
		     Amitryptiline 25–150 mg daily
		     Desipramine
		
		(b) 5HT reuptake inhibitor:
		     Fluoxetine 20 mg daily

Duration	1 week only	If depression improves within 2–3 weeks, continue antidepressant for about 6 months
Drawbacks and side-effects	Drug dependence with withdrawal symptoms Drowsiness, motor incoordination In elderly patients, mental confusion	*Tricyclics*: drowsiness, constipation, dry mouth, postural hypotension, urinary retention, blurred vision, worsening of glaucoma; lowered threshold for epileptic seizures *Fluoxetine*: no anticholinergic effects but nausea, vomiting, diarrhoea, and (rarely) akathisia with agitation, restlessness; convulsions

Antidepressants produce unpleasant side-effects which are particularly distressing for cancer patients. For example, patients receiving chemotherapy and radiotherapy frequently suffer from fatigue and exhaustion; these symptoms are aggravated by the sedative effects of tricyclics. Other troublesome symptoms such as narcotic induced constipation and urinary retention due to prostate carcinoma are made worse by the anticholinergic effects of tricyclics. The newer, much more expensive, 5HT re-uptake inhibitors such as fluoxetine have no anticholinergic properties, but can cause nausea as well as psychomotor restlessness (akathisia) and agitation. Because of the rare risk of fatal systemic vasculitis, fluoxetine should be stopped if a rash develops. Understandably, many cancer patients refuse to take antidepressants or stop these drugs when side-effects occur (Lansky, 1987).

Given these major drawbacks, it is advisable to limit the prescription of antidepressants to patients suffering from a severe type of depression known variously as endogenous depressive illness or major depressive disorder. Diagnosis of this disorder is based on the presence of depressed mood which is usually severe, unrelieved and worse in the mornings, and at least five of the following symptoms: feelings of hopelessness, insomnia (early morning waking), loss of appetite, weight loss, loss of interest and pleasure in usual activities, loss of libido, loss of energy, psychomotor agitation or retardation, impaired concentration, feelings of guilt and worthlessness and suicidal thoughts. Since anorexia, weight loss, loss of energy and libido may be attributable to cancer itself, the diagnosis of depressive illness in cancer patients must be based on the remaining symptoms. Examples of antidepressants are shown in Table 14.1. If a sedative action is required to control psychomotor agitation, dothiepin and amitryptiline are useful; in lethargic patients, on the other hand, fluoxetine and desipramine are preferable. These drugs should be prescribed in lower doses than those recommended for physically healthy patients.

14.3.2 PSYCHOLOGICAL THERAPY

At the Royal Marsden Hospital, we have developed **Adjuvant Psychological Therapy** (APT), a brief structured psychological treatment programme designed specifically for cancer patients.

Aims:

1. To reduce anxiety, depression and other psychiatric symptoms.
2. To improve psychological adjustment to cancer by inducing a positive 'fighting spirit' attitude.
3. To promote in patients a sense of personal control over their lives and active participation in the treatment of their cancer.
4. To teach patients effective coping strategies.
5. To improve communication between the patient and partner by encouraging open expression of feelings.

APT is based upon two premises. First, distressed cancer patients are regarded as psychologically normal – though vulnerable – individuals who have been overwhelmed by the impact of cancer. Second, cancer related psychological morbidity is determined not only by the physical consequences of cancer but also by two crucial factors:

1. The personal meaning of cancer for the individual, i.e. how the patient perceives cancer and its implications.
2. The patient's coping strategies, i.e. what the patient thinks and does to reduce the threat posed by cancer.

It is these topics on which APT is focused. Patients' thoughts and feelings about cancer and their methods of coping are examined closely. Therapy is directed primarily at current problems underlying the emotional distress. Together, the therapist and patient define specific problems which are then tackled by means of various cognitive and behavioural techniques. In order to overcome feelings of helplessness which commonly afflict cancer patients, particular emphasis is placed in therapy upon developing coping skills and fostering patients' personal strengths. Therapy is conducted with individual patients together, where possible, with the spouse or partner. Between 6 and 12 sessions, each lasting 1 hour, are held. A detailed description of APT has been provided by Moorey and Greer (1989). APT has been used successfully in patients with early as well as late stage cancer. A prospective randomized trial has demonstrated that APT results in significant reduction in psychological morbidity among cancer patients (Greer *et al.*, 1992).

14.4 CONCLUSIONS

Cancer exacts a heavy toll not only in terms of death but also in its effect on the quality of life of survivors. At a conservative estimate, nearly one in four cancer patients suffers from distressing psychological disorders and impairment of social functioning. Untreated, such psychosocial morbidity may persist for years, even in the absence of any signs of disease. It follows that closer attention than hitherto must be paid to the psychological adjustment of survivors from cancer. Clinical trials of anticancer treatments should include measures of psychological adjustment. Still more important is a clear recognition by oncologists and psychiatrists alike of the need to provide specific treatment for patients with cancer-related psychological disorders. Psychotropic drugs play only a minor, albeit useful, role. The main treatment is brief psychotherapy on cognitive and behavioural lines. At the Royal Marsden Hospital, we have developed such a therapy programme. It is feasible in a busy hospital, acceptable to patients and its efficacy has been demonstrated in a randomized controlled clinical trial.

REFERENCES

Danoff, B., Kramer, S., Irwin, P. and Gottlieb, A. (1983) Assessment of quality of life in long-term survivors after definitive radiotherapy. *American Journal of Clinical Oncology*, **6**, 339–45.

Derogatis, L.R., Morrow, G.R., Fetting, J. *et al.* (1983) The prevalence of psychiatric disorders among cancer patients. *Journal of the American Medical Association*, **249**, 751–7.

Ell, K., Nishimoto, R., Morvay, T. *et al.* (1989) A longitudinal analysis of psychological adaptation among survivors of cancer. *Cancer*, **63**, 406–13.

Fallowfield, L.J., Baum, M. and Maguire, G.P. (1986) Effects of breast conservation on psychological morbidity associated with diagnosis and treatment of early breast cancer. *British Medical Journal*, **293**, 1331–4.

Fobair, P, Hoppe, R.T., Bloom, J. *et al.* (1986) Psychosocial problems among survivors of Hodgkin's disease. *Journal of Clinical Oncology*, **4**, 805–14.

Folstein, M.F., Fetting, J.H., Lobo, A. *et al.* (1984) Cognitive assessment of cancer patients. *Cancer*, **53**, (Suppl), 2250–5.

Green, R.L. (1987) Psychosocial consequences of prostate cancer – my father's illness – and review of the literature. *Psychiatric Medicine*, **5**, 315–27.

Greer, S. (1991) Psychological response to cancer and survival. *Psychological Medicine*, **21**, 43–9.

Greer, S., Moorey, S., Baruch, J.D.R. *et al.* (1992) Adjuvant psychological therapy for patients with cancer: a prospective randomised trial. *British Medical Journal*, **304**, 675–80.

Hu, D.S. and Silberfarb, P.M. (1988) Psychological factors: do they influence breast cancer? in *Stress and Breast Cancer* (ed. C.L. Cooper), Wiley, Chichester, pp. 27–62.

Hughson, A.V.M., Cooper, A.F., McArdle, C.S. and Smith, D.C. (1986) Psychological impact of adjuvant chemotherapy in the first two years after mastectomy. *British Medical Journal*, **293**, 1268–71.

Irvine, D., Brown, B., Roberts, J. *et al.* (1991) Psychosocial adjustment of women with breast cancer. *Cancer*, **67**, 1097–117.

Kemeny, M., Wellisch, D.K. and Schain, W.S. (1988) Psychosocial outcome in a randomised surgical trial for treatment of primary breast cancer. *Cancer*, **62**, 1231–7.

Lansky, S. (1987) Only a small number of clinically depressed cancer patients can be managed by drugs. *Clinical Psychiatric News*, March 1987, 25.

Levine, P.M., Silberfarb, P.M. and Lipowski, Z.J. (1978) Mental disorders in cancer patients. *Cancer*, **42**, 1385–91.

Lichtman, R.R. and Taylor, S.E. (1986) Close relationships and the female cancer patient, in *Women with Cancer* (ed. B.L. Anderson), Springer, New York, pp. 233–56.

Massie, M.J. and Lesko, L.M. (1989) Psychopharmacological management, in *Handbook of Psychooncology*, (eds J.C. Holland and J.H. Rowland), Oxford University Press, New York, pp. 470–91.

McIntosh, J. (1974) Processes of communication, information seeking and control associated with cancer. *Social Science and Medicine*, **8**, 167–87.

Moorey, S. and Greer, S. (1989) *Psychological Therapy for Patients with Cancer: A New Approach*, Heinemann Medical Books, Oxford.

Morris, J. and Ingham, R. (1988) Choice of surgery for early breast cancer: psychosocial considerations. *Social Science and Medicine*, **27**, 1257–62.

Morris, T. (1979) Psychological adjustment to mastectomy. *Cancer Treatment Reviews*, **6**, 41–6.

Morris, T., Greer, S. and White, P. (1977) Psychological and social adjustment to mastectomy: a two-year follow-up study. *Cancer*, **40**, 2381–7.

Piff, C. (1985) Let's Face It, Gollancz, London.

Shakin, E.J., Heiligenstein, E. and Holland, J.C. (1991) Psychiatric complications of cancer, in *Complications of Cancer Management* (eds P.N. Plowman, T. McElwain and A. Meadows), Butterworth-Heinemann, Oxford, pp. 423–35.

Silberfarb, P.M. (1986) Ensuring an optimum quality of life for lung cancer patients: a psychiatrist's perspective, in *Assessment of Quality of Life and Cancer Treatment: Proceedings of the International Workshop on Quality of Life Assessment and Cancer Treatment* (eds V. Ventafridda, F. van Dam, R. Yancik and M. Tanburimi), Elsevier, New York, pp. 145–50.

Sugarbaker, P.H., Barofsky, I., Rosenberg, S.A. and Gianola, F.J. (1982) Quality of life assessment of patients in extremity sarcoma clinical trials. *Surgery*, **91**, 17–23.

Thomas, L. (1989) Foreword, in *Handbook of Psychooncology*, Oxford University Press, New York.

Watson, M., McCarron, J. and Law, M. (1992) Anticipatory nausea and emesis, and psychological morbidity: assessment of prevalence among out-patients on mild to moderate chemotherapy regimens. *British Journal of Cancer*, **66**, 862–866.

Watson, M. and Ramirez, A. (1991) Psychological factors in cancer prognosis, in *Cancer and Stress: Psychological, Biological and Coping Studies*, (eds C.L. Cooper and M. Watson), Wiley, Chichester, pp. 47–71.

Williams, N.S. and Johnston, D. (1983) The quality of life after rectal excision for low rectal cancer. *British Journal of Surgery*, **70**, 460–2.

Rose Turner

In 1990, the World Health Organization (WHO) adopted the definition of palliative care as 'the total active care of patients whose disease is not responsive to curative treatment. Control of pain, other symptoms and psychological, social and spiritual problems is paramount' (WHO, 1990). This definition effectively unshackled the palliative care physician from the death bed of the cancer patient and allowed them to address the more challenging and rewarding remit of improving and sustaining the quality of life of people with advanced malignancy.

Uncontrolled symptoms in a patient with cancer provide constant witness to the fact of progressive disease. In addition to the physical disabilities imposed on the patient, severe pain, breathlessness or nausea may prove so mentally distracting that the resolution of social or spiritual problems becomes impossible. This in turn may detrimentally affect the way in which the patient dies – the hoped for 'peaceful' end prevented by terminal agitation due to unfinished business. Such a chain of events serves to compound the grief of family and friends who witness it. Paramount then, amongst the aims of a palliative care physician, is to provide comprehensive control of symptoms so that the patient may realize their maximum potential within the temporal and physical constraints imposed by their disease.

15.1 PALLIATIVE CARE – WHEN AND WHERE SHOULD IT START? (FIGURE 15.1)

It is widely accepted that at the time of presentation 55% of patients with malignant disease are technically incurable. After radical therapies – surgery, radiotherapy or chemotherapy – given with curative intent a further 15% of patients will be re-classed as incurable and subsequent treatment will be palliative. With the prospect of cure lost, improved quality of life and symptom control become important end points when assessing the efficacy of any treatment regimen. Constructing therapeutic ratios for such regimens and conveying their potential risks and benefits to the patient, is a vital part of obtaining informed consent for treatment (Ashby and Stoffel, 1991).

Faced with the reality of a malignant disease, many patients will be prepared to accept a treatment of high toxicity for even a small chance of benefit (Slevin *et al.*, 1990). Based on the premise that a reduction in tumour bulk with effective chemotherapy will bring about relief of symptoms, many symptomatic patients will pursue 'active therapies'. In responsive tumours, e.g. small cell lung cancer, breast cancer and lymphomas, low toxicity chemotherapy regimens may provide enduring, comprehensive palliation for the patient. In other, less responsive solid tumours, e.g. mesotheliomas, melanomas and hypernephromas, difficult symptoms frequently develop which are best treated early with palliative medicine.

An integrated approach involving oncologists and palliative care physicians from an early stage in the illness seems to have potential advantages for all involved. The patient receives expert analysis and control of

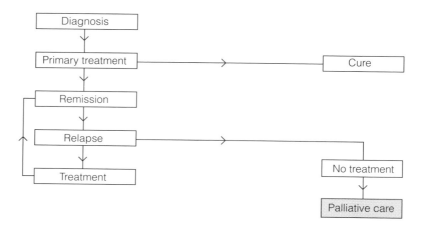

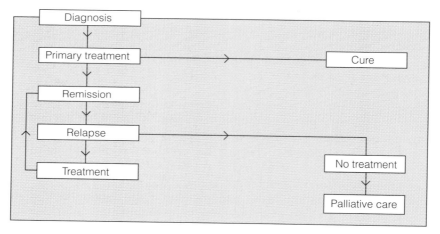

Figure 15.1   The place of palliative care in the management of malignant disease.

symptoms which might shorten inpatient stays and prevent admissions for symptomatic emergencies. The palliative care physician moves away from the traditional place at 'the end of the line' and becomes part of the general supportive services designed to maintain the quality of life and sustain performance status for all cancer patients. The oncologist having no further active therapy to deliver will find it easier to propose continu-ing care by a team already known to the patient rather than referral to an unfamiliar doctor with untested skills. As yet, no large studies exist to confirm or quantify the apparent advantages of this system, but palliative care physicians are present in the breast and urological clinics at the Royal Marsden Hospital and formal research is planned to study the integration of palliative care into the treatment of lung cancer.

15.2 PALLIATIVE CARE – ROUTES OF ACCESS

In the setting of a specialist cancer hospital referrals to palliative care generally fall into two categories. The first group of referrals are elective transfers, seeking continuing care at the stage where all appropriate anticancer treatment has already been given. Developing symptoms from unchecked disease progression may be present. These patients are usually outpatients and assessment and plans for management can be made in an outpatient clinic.

The second group are the palliative care 'emergencies'. Such patients have severe uncontrolled symptoms and need targeted first aid to achieve control of the crisis. These patients have usually been admitted for the purpose of symptom control but the measures employed have proved ineffective or unacceptable, or both.

The group of patients that present in the outpatient clinic are often 'oncology veterans'. Practised in recounting the history of their disease, they describe treatment, symptoms and their medication with considerable accuracy and insight. Patients in this group lend themselves well to the approach outlined by Twycross (Twycross and Lack, 1990). A detailed history is taken to highlight the precise nature of the current symptoms, past medical and psychiatric diseases, family history and current social circumstances. This should be followed by physical examination of the patient. Time taken at this first meeting exploring the case is never wasted. A bond between doctor and patient needs to be established with some urgency and this is helped by listening closely, examining carefully and responding to the patient in an interested, relaxed and unhurried manner. An interpretation of the findings during the initial examination should be offered to the patient and used as a basis for planning further treatment. Involving the patient in his care rather than imposing treatment on him restores some sense of control and choice.

The patient who presents as a 'symptomatic emergency' requires a different approach. Disabled and distracted by uncontrolled pain, vomiting or dyspnoea, the patient is often unable to give a full account of their problem. Clinical information remains the key to understanding and effective control of the symptom. Much information is available from the nursing staff, visiting relatives and the medical records containing results of recent investigations. Often these patients are still receiving active therapy and may have compromised bone marrow or renal function which influences the therapeutic ratio of the many drugs commonly used in symptom control, e.g. steroids, non-steroidal anti-inflammatory drugs and opioids. There is less opportunity for negotiation and choice in such scenarios, although explanation remains important to establish your aims, motives and credentials with patients, relatives and staff. Initially symptomatic emergencies may best be approached in a problem orientated rather than patient orientated way. Simple detailed plans outlining the management for the next 24 hours should be drawn up. (Table 15.1) Control of symptoms allows the re-discovery of the patient beneath. This is graphically illustrated by a failure to recognize the face of a patient treated for intractable vomiting 24 hours previously. The horizon for such a patient lies along the top of his vomit bowl. Only when the sickness is controlled will you see the colour of his eyes!

15.3 PALLIATIVE MEDICINE – A FRAMEWORK FOR SYMPTOM CONTROL

Patients admitted to a palliative care unit for the first time may experience a considerable culture shock. The treatment of cancer with chemotherapy or radiotherapy is an intensive and invasive experience underscored by a myriad of diagnostic and monitoring investigations. With the cessation of active therapies and the shift from tumour orientated medicine to symptom orientated medicine, the need for routine investigation decreases.

Table 15.1 Action plan for a symptomatic emergency

Within 1 hour	Examine patient, notes and drug chart Prioritize control of different symptoms Give first aid: 　analgesics 　antiemetics 　sedation Explain treatment to patient and relatives
Within 3 hours	Institute revised drug regimen Optimize patient's environment, consider: 　urinary catheterization 　specialist bedding/mattressing 　skin traction 　provision of electric fan. If indicated, measure serum electrolytes and calcium. Perform plain 　X-rays to exclude fractures
Within 6–8 hours	Review progress Know results of all investigations and if necessary modify treatment plan 　accordingly
Within 20–24 hours	Review progress If symptom control permits, arrange further investigation of symptom 　when necessary (e.g. plain X-ray, CT or MRI scanning) Plan further maintenance treatment: 　radiotherapy 　bisphosphonates 　nerve blocks
	If symptoms persist, review aims of treatments Review drugs, doses and routes of administration Institute appropriate change

Investigations are performed when the results will influence the patient's future management. This guiding principle is widely used throughout general medicine, but some patients find it difficult to accept.

Any test performed on a patient with advanced cancer has an attendant morbidity. Blood sampling may be difficult in patients who have had chemotherapy or who have lymphodematous limbs, coagulation disorders or skin fragility due to steroid treatment. Patients with pain or dyspnoea may find magnetic resonance scanning traumatic because of the claustrophobic setting and the physical positioning required. Performing such tests, however, may prove to be in the patient's best interest if it leads to correction of symptomatic anaemia, highlights a biochemical abnormality which influences prescribing or defines an incipient cord compression before permanent neurological damage has occurred. Care should be taken to ensure the best possible preparation of the patient for any investigation. Local anaesthetic creams may aid venepuncture (Hanks and White, 1988) and additional analgesia and sedation may be prescribed for patients with symptoms which would make scanning difficult.

After transfer to a palliative care unit the patient may receive unfamiliar treatment for a familiar symptom. In the presence of advanced malignancy the optimal management for a symptom may not be directly extrapolated from practice in general medicine or general oncology. Often patients with advanced cancer are chronically malnourished and disabled through multiple symptoms. The potential for postoperative wound healing and rehabilitation is poor and these factors must be considered before a patient is referred for operation. For these reasons the treatment expected by the patient is often not the treatment prescribed by the physician.

This change in emphasis in treatment is well illustrated by the medical management of bowel obstruction (Baines *et al.*, 1985). In a surgical unit intestinal obstruction would be treated with intravenous fluids and nasogastric suction. If the obstruction does not resolve with conservative measures the patient progresses to surgery after a few days. The approach favoured by palliative care physicians involves subcutaneous infusions of steroids, antiemetics and analgesia. The patient is not kept 'nil by mouth' but is encouraged instead to continue to take small volumes of oral fluid throughout, progressing to a low residue diet when the obstruction resolves. If the obstruction fails to resolve on steroids, the somatostatin analogue, octreotide, which diminishes bowel secretions and motility (Khoo *et al.*, 1992), may be used to minimize the distension and colic. Patients with bowel obstruction managed medically may remain at home if they so wish.

Patients respond to these changes in management policy in different ways. Their premorbid personality, spiritual and cultural beliefs as well as their attitudes and approach to their current illness all influence how easily they are able to make the transition from active to palliative care. Patients who have experienced considerable toxicity from anti-cancer treatment, those with troublesome symptoms or those who are elderly and infirm, may welcome the change of regimen and the provision of intensive supportive medical care. Other patients do not. A nega-tive response from a patient is disappointing but should be respected as the patient's choice. Some of those patients ultimately come to accept palliative care but a few will continue to pursue active treatments until the end.

15.4 PALLIATIVE CARE – WHO PROVIDES IT?

Palliative care has its origins in the work of the hospice movement and has, since its inception, been a multidisciplinary speciality. The involvement of many health care professionals recognizes the wide range of symptoms experienced by patients with advanced cancer and addresses the concept of 'suffering' which 'is experienced by persons, not merely bodies, and has its source in challenges that threaten the intactness of the person as a complex social and psychological entity' (Cassel, 1982). The exact composition of any team will vary according to the resources available locally and the particular skills and motivation of the individual team members. Few teams will contain all the following professionals:

1. Doctor
2. Nurse
3. Pharmacist
4. Physiotherapist
5. Occupational therapist
6. Dietician
7. Macmillan nurse
8. Social worker
9. Chaplain
10. Counsellor/psychologist
11. Speech therapist
12. Stomatherapist,

but the list does emphasize the wide range of skills relevant to the care of patients with advanced malignancy.

Windows of opportunity exist in the care of the patients with advanced malignancy when the introduction of a relevantly skilled member of the multidisciplinary team may make a major impact on the patient's condition and overall quality of life. For example, involvement of the physiotherapist with a patient whose pain control has been optimized before significant muscle wasting has occurred from steroid myopathy, general cachexia and disuse atrophy may result in restored mobility and preserved physical independence. Introduction of the dietician to a patient with dysphagia or nausea, not only provides nutritional expertise for a patient with eating difficulties but may also provide support and information for the relatives who might otherwise be unable to accept a dietary plan for the patient which was appropriate and safe.

Multidisciplinary team work has its critics. However, a strong mandate for a multidisciplinary approach to pain (the commonest symptom in advanced malignancy) can be made through the practical application of the gate control theory of pain transmission first described by Melzack and Wall (1965). This theory proposes that perception of pain resulting from peripheral tissue injury may be controlled at the level of the spinal cord. Transmission of painful stimuli to the higher centres depends on the summation of influences acting on the substantia gelatinosa cell. Inhibitory influences on the cell come from low threshold afferents activated by counter-irritation in the periphery, and from descending fibres arising in the medulla. Activity in the descending fibres is greatest at times of emotional excitement or arousal (Wall, 1978). Counter-irritation may be administered through the application of transcutaneous nerve stimulators, therapeutic massage, hydrotherapy and passive exercises prescribed and controlled by members of the multidisciplinary team. Meanwhile psychological and spiritual support may enhance activity in the descending fibres and inhibit transmission of painful stimuli.

Patients will often define a goal that they are working towards – family weddings, birthdays or anniversaries are common targets. When such a goal has been achieved, review of the symptom control will often show no need for extra analgesia and frequently, distracted by the occasion, the patient may miss regular doses of medication without immediate ill effect. Establishing short term, achievable goals with the patient gives life and treatment a real sense of purpose and focus.

The aims of a hospital based palliative care team are:

1. To provide an expert pain and symptom relief service.
2. To rehabilitate patients within the physical and temporal constraints imposed by their disease.
3. To provide practical and psychological support for the family and friends of the patient, and for the community based health care professionals involved.
4. To provide an educational service.
5. To perform clinical research and medical audit.

If a multidisciplinary team is to work well, good communication is vital if the total package of care is to remain relevant to the patient with his changing needs and expectations. Estimating prognosis is notoriously difficult in patients with advanced malignancies (Murray Parkes, 1972). Often it falls to the palliative care physician to make some estimate of life expectancy, rehabilitative potential or the likelihood of good symptom control to help other members of the team to judge whether major interventions, e.g. re-housing, structural alterations to property, obtaining Power of Attorney, are likely to be in the best interests of the patient and the family.

15.5   PHARMACOLOGY IN PALLIATIVE MEDICINE

Successful management of symptoms with drugs requires:

1. Correct identification of the symptom and its aetiology.
2. Understanding of the drug to be used, including its pharmacokinetics, significant drug interactions and side-effect profile.
3. Correctly evaluating the risk–benefit ratio for each drug, for each symptom in every patient.

For example, a patient complaining of 'diarrhoea' will have his symptoms compounded by treatment with antidiarrhoeal agents if the symptom is spurious and arising in a severely constipated patient. Aperients, as with all drugs, must be prescribed with a knowledge of the patient's past medical history (lactulose may impair diabetic control), and a knowledge of their present physical state (co-danthrusate is contraindicated in immobile patients with urinary catheters and/or faecal incontinence due to the risk of danthron burns).

Polypharmacy is a major problem for patients with advanced cancer and arises in various situations. Many patients may have more than one symptom requiring treatment resulting directly from malignant disease. In the elderly patient, maintenance medication for general medical conditions – e.g. ischaemic heart disease, Parkinson's disease, myxoedema – must be continued. Responsible prescription of certain drugs needs co-prescription of other drugs to prophylax against side-effects, e.g. morphine and aperients, co-prescription of steroids, non-steroidal anti-inflammatory drugs and gastroprotective agents (Piper *et al.*, 1991). Figure 15.2 shows the outpatient medication taken by a patient with multiple myeloma, chronic schizophrenia and ischaemic heart disease.

Awareness of the potential problem of polypharmacy is important. As the disease process progresses, patients often become less capable of managing complicated drug regimens. Memory and concentration may be impaired and swallowing becomes difficult because of dry mouth and neuromuscular weakness affecting the oropharynx and oesophagus. To minimize the number of oral medications required, slow release preparations and drugs with a long half-life may be used. Alternative routes of administration, e.g. rectal, transdermal or subcutaneous injections or infusions, may also improve the lot of the patient who may otherwise be asked to take unacceptable numbers of tablets. Regular review of prescribed medication, specific enquiry as to the efficacy and acceptibility of the drugs, and a conscious effort by the physician helps to construct the simplest regimen possible relevant to the patient's need. Compliance with the prescribed drug regimen may be assisted by the provision of a drug chart or medication presented in a

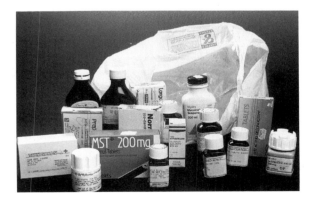

Figure 15.2 Polypharmacy arising through prescribing for multiple pathologies.

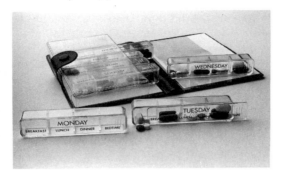

Figure 15.3   Aid to compliance with complicated drug regimens, a dosette box.

dosette box (Figure 15.3). In the days prior to a planned discharge, inpatients can familiarize themselves with the drugs by 'self-medicating' under supervision on the ward, and taking responsibility for the administration of their own drugs. After discharge, many patients prefer to delegate this responsibility to their carer.

This section will not attempt to discuss in detail the treatment strategies available for all symptoms arising as a result of disseminated cancer. This information is available in other texts (Doyle *et al.*, 1993). In the examples below, the principles outlined so far in this section are applied.

15.5.1   PAIN

Research has allowed a good understanding of the pathophysiology of cancer pain (Portenoy, 1992). By careful clinical assessment it is often possible to determine the source of the symptom and thereby predict the most effective type of analgesia for it. The pharmacology of pain management has evolved to address the different underlying mechanisms involved in the generation and appreciation of pain (Hanks and Justins, 1992).

In 1986 the World Health Organization (WHO) published the analgesic ladder

(WHO, 1986) and this provides the backbone of analgesic prescribing, advocating the titration of analgesics against pain, beginning with non-opioid medications (e.g. paracetamol) given regularly and progressing to weak opioids (e.g. co-proxamol, dihydrocodeine) and ultimately to strong opioids (morphine, diamorphine) until pain control is achieved. The majority of patients are able to take their medication orally and morphine is known to be well absorbed from the upper small bowel (Sawe *et al.*, 1985). Only in cases of intractable vomiting, severe dysphagia, upper small bowel obstruction or impaired conscious level will alternative routes of administration need to be considered. Analgesic requirement should be titrated using immediate release preparations. When an effective dose has been established a long acting preparation can be substituted. Approximately two-thirds of patients will have good pain control effected on 30 mg of morphine 4 hourly or less (Twycross and Lack, 1990).

Some pains, particularly those arising from damaged nerve or bone, are unlikely to be completely morphine sensitive and pain control must be established by other means. Radiotherapy (Hoskin, 1988) and nerve blocks may be considered if available. The group of drugs used in these circumstances are collectively known as co-analgesics.

Inflammation plays a key role in the evolution and appreciation of pain. Prostaglandin sensitizes the nerve end plates and begins the propagation of painful nerve impulses. Both steroids and non-steroidal anti-inflammatory drugs (NSAIDs) block prostaglandin synthesis by inhibiting the action of phospholipase A2 and cyclo-oxygenase respectively. Pleuritic pain, pain arising from liver capsule stretch, soft tissue inflammation and bone pain may all respond well to non-steroidal anti-inflammatory drugs. There is a large intersubject variation, however, in the effectiveness of these drugs and many significant side-effects including gastrointestinal haemorrhage, impairment of renal function, diarrhoea and skin rashes which can range from mild erythematous eruptions to toxic epidermal necrolysis. Slow release and suppository preparations of some NSAIDs are available. If after a satisfactory trial no symptomatic benefit has been established the drugs should be withdrawn and consideration given to a trial of steroids which provide a more powerful anti-inflammatory effect.

Steroids are useful when pain arises from a tumour growing in an anatomically confined space, e.g. cerebral, intrapelvic and retroperitoneal tumours. By reducing the halo of inflammatory oedema around the tumour, the volume occupied by the disease is reduced, the pressure lessened and the pain diminished. Pain from hepatic metastases, bone metastases and nerve compression may also improve by the same mechanism (Hanks, 1988). High doses of steroid are prescribed initially (dexamethasone 4 mg t.d.s.) and reduced subsequently in accordance with the patient's symptomatic response, general condition and the evolution of side-effects. The side-effects of steroid adminstration in patients with advanced malignancy appear different from those experienced in patients without a malignancy. Proximal myopathy, oral candida, insomnia, vivid dreams and glucose intolerance predominate. Presumably because of the catabolic state of the metabolism, cushingoid body habitus rarely seems to develop in patients taking steroids in the last weeks of life. Steroids can be given in a once daily dose regimen and dexamethasone and prednisolone are both soluble. Subcutaneous or intramuscular injections of steroid may be painful but subcutaneous infusions appear well tolerated.

Pain described by patients as 'aching', 'burning' or 'shooting' and those pains associated with areas of abnormal sensation or paraesthesiae are usually due to nerve compression or destruction. Of all types of pain these are the least opioid sensitive and the most difficult to control (Hanks and Justins, 1992). The presence of such pain has a profound influence on the patient's quality of life.

Tricyclic antidepressant drugs may improve nerve pain by increasing the levels of serotonin in the spinal cord. Release of serotonin stimulates inhibitory interneurones acting on the transmission cells in the substantia gelatinosa and thereby decreasing the number of painful stimuli rising to consciousness. These drugs can be given as a single night-time dose which often aids sleep. Lower doses are required to effect co-analgesia than to effect antidepression. Co-analgesia occurs after 2–3 days of treatment. Anticholinergic side-effects, including dry mouth, constipation, blurred vision and urinary retention, may prove difficult in some patients.

Anticonvulsant drugs reduce pain by stabilization of the nerve membrane. Damaged nerves are often hyperexcitable and fire in a disorganized, chaotic fashion with the formation of neuropathic eddy currents. By diminishing such activity pain is reduced. Carbamazepine, sodium valproate, phenytoin and clonazepam have all been used in the management or neuropathic pain. Sedation associated with drug doses conferring analgesia is often a problem and the physician must be aware of the numerous potential drug interactions associated with this group of drugs.

Flecainide, the Class Ic antidysrhythmic, is often effective in the management of neuropathic pain. (Dunlop *et al.*, 1988), acting by membrane stabilization. It is a negative inotrope and is known to cause serious or fatal dysrhythmias in the acutely ischaemic myocardium (Cardiac arrhythmia suppression trial (CAST) investigations, 1989). This presents the physician with a difficult therapeutic ratio to construct, weighing the probability of effective symptom control over a short residual life span against the possibility of a severe or fatal adverse drug reaction. In the absence of definite evidence of active ischaemic heart disease and wherever possible a normal ECG, many physicians will try flecainide for refractory neuropathic pain.

15.5.2 VOMITING

Vomiting in advanced cancer is a debilitating and unpleasant symptom. If it continues unchecked it may affect the control of other symptoms when the patient cannot retain and absorb their oral medications. The symptom may be perpetuated by a secondary gastritis and also by psychological phenomena when vomiting becomes 'learned' behaviour and continues long after the physical causes of emesis have been controlled.

Identification of the cause of vomiting is important (Regnard, 1992). It may arise as a direct result of tumour growth, e.g. gastric outflow obstruction, bowel obstruction, cerebral metastases, or metabolic changes that reflect the presence of malignant disease, e.g. hypercalcaemia, liver or renal failure. Morphine, NSAIDs and some antibiotics may cause vomiting in sensitive patients. Other symptoms, e.g. constipation or productive cough, when poorly controlled, may also cause sickness. Vomiting associated with radiotherapy and chemotherapy is well described.

Remediable causes for vomiting should be addressed specifically with the treatment of hypercalcaemia (Ralston *et al.*, 1990), infection, constipation and cough. Vomiting in many patients is multifactorial in aetiology and in such cases treatment should be directed at the most likely cause and the associated mechanism (Peroutka and Snyder, 1982).

Emesis resulting from metabolic disorders or drugs is generally mediated through the chemoreceptor trigger zone in the floor of the fourth ventricle. Antiemetics acting at this site include the phenothiazines and the butyrophenones. Haloperidol is a potent antiemetic with a long half-life which allows a single dose to be taken at night. This class of antiemetic also includes chlorpromazine and

methotrimeprazine which have shorter half-lives and are best reserved for anxious patients where the degree of associated sedation seen may be beneficial. Elderly patients treated with phenothiazine-type medication may develop parkinsonian features.

Gastric stasis, due either to disease or drugs, provides a characteristic clinical picture with a history of infrequent large volume vomits often without significant preceding nausea. On examination, a distended stomach may be visible in a cachectic patient and a succussion splash is sometimes present. In the presence of hepatomegaly a 'squashed stomach syndrome' may arise. Gastropropulsive agents, including metoclopramide, domperidone and cisapride, are often effective in relieving the vomiting associated with both syndromes. In the presence of a complete gastric outflow obstruction, however, they may exacerbate the symptom and should be avoided.

The integrative vomiting centre in the medullary reticular formation contains a high concentration of histamine receptors. Cyclizine is the antihistamine drug most frequently used for its antiemetic action. In many patients it provides effective and acceptable antiemesis but in some dry mouth and constipation are significant side-effects.

Intractable vomiting, refractory to the treatments outlined above, may respond quickly to high dose steroids. Resolution of vomiting in bowel obstruction occurs when the steroids reduce oedema around an obstructing lesion and re-open the lumen of the bowel. When no mechanical obstruction exists the mechanism by which steroids effect antiemesis is uncertain but in many cases a subcutaneous infusion of dexamethasone will bring about a significant improvement within 24–48 hours of starting treatment.

Although their place in preventing sickness post radiotherapy and in some chemotherapy regimens is undisputed, as yet no place has been defined for the new group of $5HT_3$ antagonists in vomiting associated with advanced malignancy. These drugs are very expensive, cause significant constipation and have not been demonstrated to be superior to any of the medications discussed above.

Depending on the severity and frequency of the vomiting, some patients may need to start their treatment using either suppositories or subcutaneous infusions of antiemetics and convert to oral drugs when the vomiting has been controlled. A single antiemetic is sufficient to control vomiting in two-thirds of patients. Trials of additional antiemetics should always be with a drug from a different class based on the supposition that the symptom is multifactorial in aetiology. If the underlying cause for the vomiting can be successfully treated or is likely to recover spontaneously, e.g. radiotherapy gastritis, the antiemetic may ultimately be withdrawn prejudicing the patient's symptom control.

15.5.3 DYSPNOEA

Dyspnoea is a frightening and debilitating symptom which is present in about 50% of all patients with advanced cancer (Heyse-Moore *et al.*, 1991). Breathlessness as with other symptoms may often be multifactorial. In one patient, the contribution from different pathologies, e.g. anaemia, pleural effusion and lymphangitis, may alter with time and the management of the patient must reflect this. After identifying and treating the remediable causes, e.g. diaphragmatic splinting by ascites, heart failure and infection, a large group of patients remain for whom pharmacological palliation of dyspnoea is required.

As the symptom progresses, the patient may have difficulty in drinking, swallowing and speaking and the number of oral medications presented to the patient should be kept to a minimum. The importance of non-pharmacological measures should be recognized and the patient nursed in an environment of calm where there is space, air and light.

Patients physiologically or psychologically dependent on the provision of oxygen may wish to continue with this therapy but many breathless patients feel claustrophobic and suffocated behind a mask. In such circumstances more benefit is often obtained from an electric fan placed close to the patient to create the sensation of free air movement around the face. Drugs given by a nebulizer are better tolerated when given by a mouthpiece for the same reasons.

Breathlessness is frequently associated with anxiety and, in the last stages, with fatigue and exhaustion. When the symptom is severe breathing appears to require constant conscious effort by the patient. The drugs most useful in severe breathlessness are morphine (Bruera *et al.*, 1990) and diazepam.

Given regularly for the relief of pain and titrated to the correct dose, morphine does not appear to cause a degree of respiratory depression that rises to clinical significance (Walsh, 1984). When opioids are given to patients who are breathless, it is observed that it is the patient's perception of breathlessness rather than the respiratory rate which is more significantly affected (Heyse-Moore, 1984). Morphine also reduces the volume of bronchial secretions which may prove troublesome in the terminal phase as a result of hypostatic pneumonia, pulmonary oedema or tumour related exudate or haemorrhage. If further control of this symptom is required, hyoscine given either in the form of a transdermal patch or a subcutaneous infusion is effective. Some patients become agitated on hyoscine which crosses the blood–brain barrier. The alternative is glycopyrronium, which is also compatible with diamorphine in a syringe driver, but which contains an ammonium moiety which polarizes the compound thus preventing any significant central action.

The anxiety and exhaustion of breathlessness is best treated with benzodiazepines. Diazepam has a long half-life and can be given at night with the expectation of continuing anxiolysis the following day. Some patients suffering acute anxiety attacks uncontrolled by relaxation and breathing exercises may be helped by sublingual lorazepam.

15.6 RESEARCH IN PALLIATIVE CARE

Advances in palliative care, as in any speciality, arise through research and the development of new drugs and treatment strategies. However, with the exception of morphine metabolism, practice in palliative care is not yet underscored by scientifically validated studies. Much of the published work is observational and whilst these studies serve to indicate the prevalence of a symptom and its impact on the quality of life, they have not furthered our understanding of the best available treatment.

Why is research in palliative medicine so difficult? Numerous factors contribute:

1. The traditional reluctance of medical and nursing personnel to experiment on 'dying' patients.
2. The short period of time spent by most patients in the palliative care setting does not allow for prospective longitudinal studies.
3. End points are difficult. How do we measure 'quality of life', 'pain control' or 'weakness'?
4. Sometimes a conflict exists between the needs of the patient and the needs of the research protocols. Studies often require hospitalization or increased numbers of outpatient appointments and blood tests at a time when the primary aim of medical management would be to keep the patient at home as much as possible and investigations to a minimum.
5. Pre-existing confounding factors are common in polysymptomatic patients with advanced disease, e.g. prior prescription of steroids for other symptoms, presence of cerebral metastases or bowel obstruction.

6. Obtaining informed consent is often difficult if the patient is confused, distracted or has a short span of concentration due to general weakness.

Often the physician falters at the first hurdle and fails to recognize the opportunity to include a patient in a trial. It is easy to be swept along with the clinical and social undercurrents in an effort rapidly to establish control of symptoms and then miss the chance to enter a patient into a trial.

Obtaining informed consent provides the physician with a mandate to perform the proposed research. When approached, the patients are often willing to participate and their agreement with the trial should relieve the anxieties of the multidisciplinary team about the extra burdens imposed on the patient as a result of the trial.

15.7 CONCLUSIONS

Whilst a cure for cancer is still only available to a minority of patients, the importance of physical and psychological symptom control for all is now being recognized across the range of specialities that provide the continuum of medical cancer care. The further integration of palliative care into mainstream oncology remains a challenge for the future.

Providing total active care for a patient with advanced cancer requires skill and sensitivity to the patient's changing needs. A knowledge of oncology, physiology and pharmacology helps the physician to prescribe the right treatment at the right time for the right patient.

Mercifully few cancer patients are now told 'there is nothing more that can be done for you', yet many patients hear this message implicit in the last discussions with their oncologists. One of the most positive aspects of palliative medicine is that there is always **something** that can be done to help the patient and his family through the difficult phase at the end of a malignant illness.

Through thoughtful, targeted prescribing, the involvement of a dedicated multidisciplinary team and the extension of care to include family and friends, palliative medicine can make a significant difference to the life of a cancer patient.

REFERENCES

Ashby, M. and Stoffell, B. (1991) Therapeutic ratio and defined phases: proposal of ethical framework for palliative care. *British Medical Journal*, **302**, 1322–4.

Baines, M., Oliver, D.J. and Carter, R.L. (1985) Medical management of intestinal obstruction in patients with advanced malignant disease. *Lancet*, **ii**, 990–3.

Bruera, E., Macmillan, K., Pither, J. and MacDonald, R.N. (1990) Effects of morphine on the dyspnoea of terminal cancer patients. *Journal of Pain and Symptom Management*, **5**, 341–4.

Cardiac arryhythmia suppression trial (CAST) investigators (1989) Preliminary report: effect on encainide and flecainide on mortality in a randomised trial of arrhythmia suppression after myocardial infarction. *New England Journal of Medicine*, **321**, 406–12.

Cassel, E.J. (1982) The nature of suffering and the goals of medicine. *New England Journal of Medicine*, **306**, 639–45.

Doyle, D., Hanks, G.W. and MacDonald, N. (eds) (1993) *Oxford Textbook of Palliative Medicine*, Oxford University Press, Oxford.

Dunlop, R., Davies, R.J., Hockley, J. and Turner, P. (1988) Analgesic effects of oral flecainide. *Lancet*, **i**, 420.

Hanks, G.W. (1988) The pharmacological treatment of bone pain, in *Cancer Surveys*, vol. 7, no. 1, (ed. G.W. Hanks), published for the Imperial Cancer Research Fund by Oxford University Press, Oxford, pp. 87–102.

Hanks, G.W. and Justins, D.M. (1992) Cancer pain: management. *Lancet*, **339**, 1031–6.

Hanks, G.W. and White, I. (1988) Local anaesthetic creams. *British Medical Journal*, **297**, 1215–6.

Heyse-Moore, L. (1984) Respiratory symptoms, in *The Management of Terminal Disease*, 2nd edn, (ed. C. Sanders), Edward Arnold, London, pp. 113–19.

Heyse-Moore, L.H., Ross, V. and Mullee Mark, A. (1991) How much of a problem is dyspnoea in advanced cancer? *Palliative Medicine*, **5**, 20–26.

Hoskin, P. (1988) Scientific and clinical aspects of radiotherapy in the relief of bone pain, in *Cancer Surveys*, vol. 7, no. 7, (ed. G.W. Hanks), published for the Imperial Cancer Research Fund by Oxford University Press, Oxford, pp. 69–86.

Khoo, D., Riley, J. and Waxman, J. (1992) Control of emesis in bowel obstruction in terminally ill patients. *Lancet*, **339**, 375–6.

Melzack, R. and Wall, P.D. (1965) Pain mechanisms: a new theory. *Science*, **150**, 971–9.

Murray Parkes, C. (1972) Accuracy of predictions of survival in later stages of cancer. *British Medical Journal*, **2**, 29–31.

Peroutka, S.J. and Snyder, S.H. (1982) Antiemetics: neurotransmitter receptor binding predicts therapeutic actions. *Lancet*, **i**, 658–9.

Piper, J.M., Ray, W.A., Doughterty, J.R. and Griffin, M.R. (1991) Corticosteroid use and peptic ulcer disease: role of non-steroidal anti-inflammatory drugs. *Annals of Internal Medicine*, 735–40.

Portenoy, R.K. (1992) Pathophysiology of cancer pain. *Lancet*, **339**, 1026–31.

Ralston, S.H., Gallacher, S.J., Patel, U. *et al.* (1990) Cancer-associated hypercalcaemia: morbidity and mortality. Clinical experience in 126 treated patients. *Annals of Internal Medicine*, **112**, 499–504.

Regnard, C.F.B. (1992) Nausea and vomiting in advanced cancer – a flow diagram *Palliative Medicine*, **6**, 146–51.

Sawe, J., Kager, L., Svensson, J.O. and Rane, A. (1985) Oral morphine in cancer patients: *in vivo* kinetics and *in vitro* hepatic glucuronidation. *British Journal of Clinical Pharmacology*, **19**, 495–501.

Slevin, M.L., Stubbs, L., Plant, H.J. *et al.* (1990) Attitudes to chemotherapy: comparing views of patients with cancer with those of doctors, nurses and general public. *British Medical Journal*, **300**, 1458–60.

Twycross, R.G. and Lack, S.A. (1990) *Therapeutics in Terminal Cancer*, Churchill Livingstone, Edinburgh.

Wall, P.D. (1978) The gate control theory of pain mechanisms. A re-examination and a restatement. *Brain*, **101**, 1–18.

Walsh, T.D. (1984) Opiates and respiratory function in advanced cancer. *Recent Results in Cancer Research*, **89**, 115–7.

World Health Organization (1986) *Cancer Pain Relief*, World Health Organization, Geneva.

World Health Organization (1990) Cancer Pain Relief and Palliative Care. Report of a WHO Expert Committee. *Tech. Rep. Ser.* **804**, World Health Organization, Geneva.

CANCER THERAPY AND FERTILITY   16

William F. Hendry

After life itself, fertility is probably the most highly prized human possession and cancer threatens both. Yet, while cure of the individual naturally demands priority, relatively little attention is paid to the effects of the tumour, and its treatment, on reproductive function. Perhaps this is partly because it is so complex, so difficult to measure satisfactorily. Life can be quantified by 5 year survival rates, but fertility involves not one but two individuals, and their interaction. Worse, one partner may be, at the time of treatment, only the subject of romantic dreams; but consideration must be given to the day when dreams come true, and the new-found partner has every right to expect that due care was taken of the fertility of his or her loved one. There was a day when the old attitude amongst cancer doctors was a bluff 'well you can't have sex in a coffin, you know'. Increasingly, successful treatment, a more open society and legal precedent (Brahams, 1992) all now demand that reproductive function and future fertility are kept in mind, and fully discussed with both patient and relatives before, during and after treatment.

Fertility is not simply synonymous with gonadal function, although it is obviously dependent on it. Psychological aspects of fertility are affected by fear of the disease, by altered perception of body image, and by age. Normal endocrine function is essential for reproduction, but equally important is an adequate penile blood supply and an intact nervous system (Brindley, 1992) for success-ful erection and ejaculation. Extirpation of the disease with reconstruction, taking care of essential, clearly defined anatomical structures, is the hallmark of contemporary cancer surgery, and the radiotherapist and medical oncologist are equally at pains to achieve maximum therapeutic benefit with minimum toxicity. Cure of the disease and preservation of function must go hand in hand in modern oncology.

16.1 GONADAL FUNCTION AND SPERMATOGENESIS

16.1.1 IMPAIRMENT OF FERTILITY

The relationship between the development and treatment of malignant disease and impaired gonadal function is complex, and varies from individual to individual. Testicular tumours provide a good example of this conundrum, aptly summed up by Schilsky (1989) as 'testis, tumour or treatment?' Is the observed defect in gonadal function inherent in the poor quality of the testis, itself more likely to develop malignancy, is it due to a by-product of the tumour, such as chorionic gonadotrophin, or was it a side-effect of treatment, such as radiotherapy or chemotherapy? Oligozoospermia was found in 37% of men after orchidectomy for testicular tumour by Jewett *et al.* (1983). Testicular biopsies showed pretreatment severe and irreversible impairment of spermatogenesis in the contralateral testes of 24% of such men (Berthelsen and Skakkebaek,

1983). Highly impaired sperm counts have been recorded in 60–70% of testicular cancer patients evaluated soon after orchidectomy (Fossa *et al.*, 1993). Amongst 208 men with testicular tumours after orchidectomy but before any other treatment, we found that only 22% of those with seminomas, and 29% of those with teratomas had sperm counts exceeding 10 million per millilitre (Hendry *et al.*, 1983). Impairment of fertility was not dependent on the stage of the disease at presentation, but it was interesting to note that almost half of the men who had previously fathered children were either azoospermic or severely oligozoospermic, implying that a deterioration had occurred in spermatogenesis, coincident with the development of the tumour. Morrish *et al.* (1990) found that patients with testicular cancer had significantly lower sperm counts than matched normal male volunteers, with higher serum oestradiol levels in those with elevated beta-HCG (human chorionic gonadotrophin) levels. This suggested a paracrine-endocrine mechanism in which tumour-produced HCG stimulated production of oestradiol by normal testicular tissue, thus impairing spermatogenesis. There is, therefore, a potential for recovery of normal sperm output after completion of treatment, even though the sperm concentration was very low at presentation. Indeed, we found that 35% of those starting with poor sperm counts recovered to normal levels when a year or more had elapsed after completion of chemotherapy (Hendry *et al.*, 1983).

16.1.2   TOXICITY OF TREATMENT

It is, therefore, very important to limit toxicity of treatment in these young men, to give every chance for recovery to occur. This is dependent upon the type of chemotherapy used. The alkylating agents cyclophosphamide and chlorambucil have been most commonly associated with infertility. The extent of damage depends on the dose and duration of treatment. Thus, small doses of cyclophosphamide used to treat nephrotic syndrome in childhood have only minor effects on spermatogenesis. On the other hand, the combination chemotherapy regimens used to treat Hodgkins' disease such as MOPP (mustine, vincristine, prednisone and procarbazine) almost always lead to infertility with azoospermia or severe oligozoospermia due to germinal aplasia (Chapman *et al.*, 1979a). Recovery is rare, though not unknown. Similarly, treatment of leukaemia may lead to infertility, although the toxic effects of the alkylating agents can be reduced by using intermittent rather than continuous dosages (Evenson *et al.*, 1984). In the treatment of low-grade non-Hodgkin's lymphoma, azoospermia was observed in all men who received more than 400 mg in total dosage of chlorambucil (Richter *et al.*, 1970). Although some recovery may occur, patients must be warned that damage to the spermatogenic epithelium is likely, and may not recover (for review see Meistrich, 1993). In women, early menopause, dyspareunia, reduced libido and premature osteoporosis may occur (Chapman *et al.*, 1979b).

With the chemotherapy regimens used for metastatic testicular tumours, including cisplatinum, bleomycin and vincristine or etoposide (PVB or BEP), depression of spermatogenesis is temporary (for review see Hansen and Hansen, 1993). Between one-quarter and one-third of our patients recovered normal sperm counts after chemotherapy (Hendry *et al.*, 1983). Drasga *et al.* (1983) noted even better results: 20 of 24 men had recovered spermatogenesis 18 months from completing treatment. The fetal abnormality rate amongst children fathered by these men is no different from matched controls (Senturia *et al.*, 1985). None the less, patients are advised to avoid producing a pregnancy until at least 2 years has elapsed from completion of radiotherapy or chemotherapy.

After paraaortic radiation for stage I seminoma, depression of spermatogenesis is temporary so long as the remaining testicle is shielded with lead (Fossa *et al.*, 1989). However, persistently low sperm counts are likely to follow in the majority of patients if the contralateral testis is not shielded (Hansen *et al.*, 1990). The radiation dose received by the testis is critical in determining the effect on spermatogenesis and time to recovery (for review see Zagars, 1991; Shalet, 1993), and azoospermia is inevitable if scrotal irradiation is given to prevent recurrence after local surgical interference (Thomas *et al.*, 1977). In fact, Kennedy *et al.* (1986) have shown that this is a rare complication and surveillance is now preferred in these circumstances.

16.2   ERECTION AND EJACULATION

16.2.1   NORMAL VS COMPROMISED SEXUAL FUNCTION

Normal sexual function in the male requires intact nervous pathways, adequate blood supply and hormonal stimulation. Erection is primarily under parasympathetic control, via the pelvic nerves which originate principally from the sacral cord segments S2–S3. Ejaculation is controlled by the sympathetic nerve fibres arising from spinal levels T10–L2, travelling down through the sympathetic chain ganglia, the hypogastric plexus, to reach the prostate, seminal vesicles and vasa deferentia. Although there may be some sympathetic control of erection, if the parasympathetic pelvic nerves are cut, for example during radical prostatectomy, the inevitable result is erectile impotence. By contrast, if the sympathetic nerves on both sides of the aorta are cut, or if the hypogastric plexus is divided, e.g. during retroperitoneal lymphadenectomy, then the man is likely to lose his ejaculation while the erections remain normal. Interruption of pelvic blood supply, e.g. during radical cystectomy, will impair the quality of erection. Finally, androgen ablation, e.g. for metastatic carcinoma of prostate, usually results in loss of both erection and

ejaculation. These are obviously of great importance to the man concerned, and his female partner; not only should these matters be fully discussed before selecting treatment, but alternative strategies should also be considered that can avoid these side-effects, or at least ameliorate them.

16.2.2   VULNERABLE NERVOUS PATHWAYS AND 'NERVE SPARING' PROCEDURES

Identification of the nervous pathways which are vulnerable has allowed 'nerve sparing' procedures to be developed. Thus, Lepor *et al.* (1985) showed by serial sections through the entire length of the prostate exactly where the branches of the pelvic plexus run that innervate the corpora cavernosa. Situated posterolateral to the prostate, the autonomic nerves are intimately associated with the vascular structures that form the capsular vessels of the prostate. Based on this knowledge, Walsh and Mostwin (1984) developed a nerve sparing, potency sparing operative technique that is applicable not only to radical prostatectomy, but also to radical cystectomy. This significant advance has made radical prostatectomy more acceptable in the treatment of prostatic carcinoma, leading to a resurgence of interest in this procedure at a time when more and more cases are being discovered early enough to be cured by local methods, detected by screening including routine estimation of serum prostate specific antigen (PSA).

At the same time, nerve sparing techniques have been developed for retroperitoneal lymphadenectomy. Although this operation was never popular for early stage testicular tumours in this country, it was done in some European countries, and became the standard procedure in the USA. Nijman *et al.* (1987) studied the consequences on sexual function, and having reviewed the published literature, concluded that less than one-third of men retained normal antegrade ejaculation after this procedure. Detailed study of 101 patients indicated that of 75 patients who had lost their ejaculation, 55 had retrograde ejaculation and 20 had complete loss of emission into the urethra. Regarding other sexual functions, 17 had loss of libido, 12 had difficulty reaching orgasm and six had erectile dysfunction. A heavy price indeed to pay for an operation that we consider unnecessary, since equally good results can be obtained by surveillance in stage I disease (Freedman *et al.*, 1987). Nevertheless, it was good to observe that the rate of loss of ejaculation could be significantly lowered by modifying the node dissection into a nerve sparing technique, and confining the dissection to one side whenever possible (Jewett *et al.*, 1988; Richie, 1990). Retroperitoneal dissection may be essential for removal of residual nodal masses after chemotherapy when it provides both therapeutic benefit and information of prognostic value in planning future treatment (Hendry *et al.*, 1993). Analysis of ejaculatory function in 186 of these men showed that 22% lost ejaculation, although this was significantly more likely to occur if the dissection was bilateral (45%) or if the mass was very large (greater than 8 cm diameter, 58%). However, careful attention to nerve sparing operative technique led to a reduction in the incidence of loss of ejaculation from 36% before 1984 to 16% since then (Jones *et al.*, 1993).

16.2.3 PRESERVATION OF ERECTION AND EJACULATION

Careful attention to operative techniques, and awareness of the effects of surgery on sexual function, has led to successful preservation of erection and ejaculation by modern nerve sparing techniques. Similarly, avoidance of mass ligature of the internal iliac arteries will preserve enough blood supply to the penis for erection to occur after cystectomy. Endocrine treatment for the younger man with metastatic prostatic cancer can be given in such a way that androgen blockade provides therapeutic benefit whilst sexual func-

tion is preserved. Whereas castration or treatment with superactive analogues of gonadotrophin releasing hormone (GnRH) lead inevitably to loss of sexual function, associated with fall in plasma testosterone levels, a similar response in terms of clinical benefit and fall in serum PSA can be obtained with the pure antiandrogen flutamide, while sexual function is preserved (Sogani and Whitmore, 1979; Lundgren, 1987). Although there is evidence that the duration of response may be shorter when an antiandrogen is used as a single agent as compared to so-called total androgen blockade combining the antiandrogen with castration or GnRH analogue (Crawford and Nabors, 1991), the preservation of sexual function is welcomed by the younger man.

16.3 SEMEN CRYOPRESERVATION

If chemotherapy, radiation treatment or surgery make sterilization of a man inevitable, his semen should be examined to see whether its quality is sufficiently good to allow cryopreservation (Bracken and Smith, 1980; Rhodes *et al.*, 1985). In our experience with over 200 young men with testicular tumours or Hodgkin's disease, one-quarter were suitable (Hendry *et al.*, 1983). Subsequently, 22 men requested artificial insemination of their partners with the banked semen – half of these men had had Hodgkin's disease, and half had had testicular tumours. The women were treated with 1–11 cycles of insemination, leading to a cumulative probability of pregnancy of 45% at 6 months, which can be compared with the normal figure of 71% at this time (Scammell *et al.*, 1985). Nationwide, cryopreservation of semen is available in all except three regions (all in England), and there has been a threefold increase in referrals in recent years (Milligan *et al.*, 1989). Sadly, such laboratories are poorly funded, making adequate provision of such a valuable service difficult.

16.4 ASSESSMENT AND TREATMENT OF INFERTILITY AFTER PREVIOUS CANCER THERAPY

Not uncommonly, the question of fertility arises in patients who have already been treated for malignant disease. All too often, it is disappointing to learn that no pretreatment counselling was given, and loss of fertility comes as a bitter disappointment under these circumstances. The author's experience is confined to men, but women share the same concerns, and these are responsibly addressed by their gynaecological oncologists.

16.4.1 HISTORY TAKING

A careful history, and search of the records, will reveal which drugs have been given, and in what dosage, and this information can be compared with the known reproductive toxicity described above. If radiotherapy was given, the fields are checked and radiation scatter that may have affected the testes is calculated. Details of operative procedures should be obtained, with particular reference to possible damage to the vessels and nerves supplying the genitalia. Pretreatment fertility status is obviously important, and any predisposing conditions such as testicular maldescent or mumps orchitis may be relevant. Continuing medical therapy is reviewed, and it should be remembered that heavy smoking, alcohol abuse and regular cannabis are all potentially damaging to spermatogenesis and sperm function. Any change in erection or ejaculation is defined by sensitive but searching questioning, and the other secondary sexual characteristics should be checked – we once found a large pituitary adenoma in a testicular tumour patient complaining of impotence whilst on follow-up.

16.4.2 CLINICAL EXAMINATION

The man is first examined standing up to see if he has a varicocele (Hendry, 1979). The size and consistency of the testicle or testicles should be measured with Prader's orchiometer and the findings recorded. If more than 15 ml in volume spermatogenesis is likely to be normal, or to have a potential for recovery to normal, whilst if less than 5 ml in volume the prospects are bleak. In between 5 and 15 ml the potential is unknown and biopsy may be required to define spermatogenesis accurately. The prostate and vesicles are palpated with the patient in the left lateral position. If there is clinical suspicion of prostatitis, secretions should be expressed by massage and cultured aerobically and anaerobically. The penis and foreskin are inspected for any defect or tightness. Urine is checked for sugar or protein, examined microscopically and sent for culture and bacterial sensitivities. Plasma testosterone, LH, FSH and prolactin should be measured. Normal Leydig cell function will be reflected by a normal testosterone level. Although both LH and FSH are under the control of GnRH, they do move independently and provide invaluable information on gonadal functions. LH stimulates testosterone production, while FSH controls spermatogenesis with a negative feedback mechanism provided by inhibin. It follows that if the sperm count is low and the FSH is high (normally taken to be at least twice the upper limit of normal), then gonadal failure is likely (Pryor *et al.*, 1976). Low LH and FSH may be found either with normal spermatogenesis releasing plenty of inhibin, or with hypopituitarism. If there is a pituitary tumour, the prolactin is likely to be elevated, and this can usually be detected by appropriate radiological studies.

16.4.3 SEMINAL ANALYSIS

Seminal analysis should be done with a specimen produced after at least 3 days' abstinence, examined within 2 hours of production. Condom collection is not advisable, unless specially designed seminal collection ones are used, which are free of spermicidal substances. Some orthodox Jewish patients will only provide a specimen using such a device. The normal parameters are as follows: a volume of at least 1.5 ml, with more than 20 million spermatozoa per ml, of which at least 40% should be moving actively (Macleod, 1951). The direct mixed antiglobulin reaction (MAR) test is used to see if there are autoantibodies present on the spermatozoa (Hendry, 1992a). If the volume is less than 1.5 ml, the pH and fructose content should be checked: a pH less than 7.2 and absent fructose are indicative of ejaculatory duct obstruction or failure (Pryor and Hendry, 1991). If there is little or no ejaculate, urine should be examined after orgasm to see if there is retrograde ejaculation. Production of a semen sample into a plastic pot is not easy, especially in a draughty hospital toilet, and it is generally sensible to examine at least two samples, one of which may be produced in the comfort and security of the patient's home by whichever means he finds most comfortable.

In cases with erectile dysfunction, colour Doppler ultrasound studies should be done after intracavernosal injection of papaverine. This will distinguish psychological impotence from failure due to lack of arterial inflow, or venous leakage (Rickards, 1993). Neurological damage after radical prostatectomy may take 6–12 months to recover, and the test may need to be repeated in such cases.

In men with severe oligozoospermia or azoospermia, if the testicle is of normal size and serum FSH is normal, scrotal exploration is done under general anaesthetic to take a testicular biopsy to rate spermatogenesis and exclude carcinoma-*in-situ*, and to define any obstruction by vasography.

Hormone deficiency can be corrected by appropriate replacement therapy, but it should be remembered that exogenous testosterone will lead to suppression of both LH and FSH, thus impairing spermatogenesis. If testicular obstruction is present, for example after previous epididymitis or groin surgery, this should be corrected by microsurgical reconstruction (Hendry *et al.*, 1990a). Varicocele causes testicular hyperthermia, and should be treated by high ligation or spermatic vein embolization, especially if only the left testicle is present (Hendry, 1992b). Antisperm antibodies are seldom found in cancer patients in the author's experience, but if present they may be treated by cyclical prednisolone (Hendry *et al.*, 1990b).

16.4.4   LOSS OF EJACULATION

Loss of ejaculation commonly follows paraaortic lymphadenectomy (see above). If retrograde ejaculation is present as shown by the finding of spermatozoa in the urine after orgasm, these can be collected by centrifugation, and after resuspension in suitable tissue culture medium can be used for artificial insemination with successful results (Scammell *et al.*, 1989). Alternatively, drug therapy can be used, employing ephedrine 30–60 mg 1 or 2 hours before intercourse (Lynch and Maxted, 1983) or imipramine 25 mg twice daily (Nijman *et al.*, 1982). If there is complete loss of ejaculation, electroejaculation under general anaesthesia using direct stimulation of the seminal vesicles and ejaculatory ducts with a transrectal probe can be used to obtain semen (Ohl *et al.*, 1991). If the production is less than ideal in quality, spermatozoa can be specially prepared and used for *in vitro* fertilization (IVF) or gamete intrafallopian transfer (GIFT). Modern technology now requires only one healthy sperm for subzonal implantation (SUZI), giving hope to many men previously considered hopeless.

16.4.5   ERECTILE IMPOTENCE

Erectile impotence can be successfully treated by intracavernosal injection of papaverine and/or phenoxybenzamine, or prostaglandin (for review see Gregoire and Pryor, 1992). If this fails, penile implants are now available which allow hydraulic elongation and expansion of the corpora cavernosa when required, but return the organ to its normal dimensions at other times. Although expensive, these products do allow a return to normal sexual function, for example after radical pelvic surgery. Testosterone replacement after removal of bilateral testicular tumours can also allow normal sexual function – we usually recommend Primoteston Depot 250 mg given by intramuscular injection once a month. Penile carcinoma should be managed with due regard to subsequent function. Interstitial radiation of early lesions on the glans penis has been followed by normal erections, and even after partial amputation, sexual intercourse is perfectly possible so long as care is taken in the reconstruction of the abbreviated organ.

16.4.6 TREATMENT IN WOMEN

Women require an adequate vagina for sexual intercourse. Careful reconstruction can provide this after cystectomy for bladder cancer, but after pelvic exenteration, particularly for recurrent gynaecological cancer, vaginoplasty may be preferable: the isolated caecum makes an ideal substitute (Turner-Warwick and Kirby, 1990).

16.5 CONCLUSIONS

Increasing interest in minimizing toxicity whilst obtaining maximum benefit from cancer treatment has led to significant advances in preservation of sexual function and fertility. All patients nowadays have a right to expect these matters to be discussed confidentially with themselves and their partners before treatment proceeds. After treatment has been completed, concern about fertility and prospects for its recovery and treatment should be addressed by logical investigation and appropriate treatment. Much can and should be done to help men and women with these problems in this day and age.

REFERENCES

Berthelsen, J.G. and Skakkebaek, N.E. (1983) Gonadal function in men with testis cancer. *Fertility and Sterility*, **39**, 68–75.

Bracken, R.B. and Smith, K.D. (1980) Is semen cryopreservation helpful in testicular cancer? *Urology*, **15**, 581–3.

Brahams, D. (1992) Chlorambucil, infertility and sperm banking. *Lancet*, **339**, 420.

Brindley, G.S. (1992) Neurophysiology, in *Impotence: diagnosis and management of male erectile dysfunction*, (eds R.S. Kirby, C.C. Carson and G.D. Webster), Butterworth-Heinemann, Oxford, pp. 27–31.

Chapman, R.M., Sutcliffe, S.B., Rees, L.H. *et al.* (1979a) Cyclical combination chemotherapy and gonadal function: retrospective study in males. *Lancet*, **i**, 285–9.

Chapman, R.M., Sutcliffe, S.B. and Malpas, J.S. (1979b) Cytotoxic induced ovarian failure in women with Hodgkin's disease I Hormone function. *Journal of the American Medical Association*, **242**, 1877–81.

Crawford, E.D. and Nabors, W.L. (1991) Total androgen ablation: American Experience. *Urological Clinics of North America*, **18**, 55–63.

Drasga, R.E., Einhorn, L.H., Williams, S.D., Patel, D.N. and Stevens, E.E. (1983) Fertility after chemotherapy for testicular cancer. *Journal of Clinical Oncology*, **1**, 179–83.

Evenson, D.P., Arlin, Z., Welt, S. *et al.* (1984) Male reproductive capacity may recover following drug treatment with the L-10 protocol for acute lymphocytic leukaemia. *Cancer*, **53**, 30–6.

Fossa, S.D., Aass, N. and Molne, K. (1989) Is routine pretreatment cryopreservation of semen worthwhile in the management of patients with testicular cancer. *British Journal of Urology*, **64**, 524–9.

Fossa, S.D., Aabyholm, T. Vespestad, S. *et al.* (1993) Semen quality after treatment for testicular cancer. *European Urology*, **23**, 172 -6.

Freedman, L.S. *et al.* (1987) Histopathology in the prediction of relapse in patients with stage I testicular teratoma treated by orchidectomy alone. *Lancet*, **ii**, 294–8.

Gregoire, A. and Pryor, J.P. (1992) *Impotence: an integrated approach to clinical practice*, Churchill Livingstone, Edinburgh.

Hansen, P.V. and Hansen S.W. (1993) Gonadal function in men with testicular germ cell cancer: the influence of cisplatin-based chemotherapy. *European Urology*, **23**, 153–6.

Hansen, S.W., Berthelsen, J.G. and von der Maase, H. (1990) Long term fertility and Leydig cell function in patients treated for germ cell cancer with cisplatin, vinblastine and bleomycin versus surveillance. *Journal of Clinical Oncology*, **8**, 1695–8.

Hendry, W.F. (1979) Male infertility. British *Journal of Hospital Medicine*, **22**, 47–55.

Hendry, W.F. (1992a) The significance of antisperm antibodies: measurement and management. *Clinical Endocrinology*, **36**, 219 -21.

Hendry, W.F. (1992b) Effects of left varicocele ligation in subfertile males with absent or atrophic right testis. *Fertility and Sterility*, **57**, 1342–3.

Hendry, W.F., Stedronska, J., Jones, C.R. *et al.* (1983) Semen analysis in testicular cancer and Hodgkin's disease: pre and post-treatment findings and implications for cryopreservation. *British Journal of Urology*, **55**, 769–73.

Hendry, W.F., Levison, D., Parkinson, C.M. *et al.* (1990a) Testicular obstruction: clinico-pathological studies. *Annals of the Royal College of Surgeons of England*, **72**, 396–407.

Hendry, W.F., Hughes, L. Scammell, G., Pryor, J.P. and Hargreave T.B. (1990b) Comparison of prednisolone and placebo in subfertile men with antibodies to spermatozoa. *Lancet*, **335**, 85–8.

Hendry, W.F., A'Hern, R.P., Hetherington, J.W. *et al.* (1993) Paraaortic lymphadenectomy after chemotherapy for metastatic non seminomatous germ cell tumours: prognostic value and therapeutic benefit. *British Journal of Urology*, **71**, 208–13.

Jewett, M.A.S., Thachill, J.V. and Harris, J.F. (1983) Exocrine function of testis and germinal testicular tumour. *British Medical Journal*, **286**, 1849–50.

Jewett, M.A.S., Kong, Y.S.P., Goldberg, S.D. *et al.* (1988) Retroperitoneal lymphadenectomy for testis tumor with nerve sparing for ejaculation. *Journal of Urology*, **139**, 1220–4.

Jones, D.R., Norman, A.R., Horwich, A. and Hendry, W.F. (1993) Ejaculatory dysfunction after retroperitoneal lymphadenectomy. *European Urology*, **23**, 169–71.

Kennedy, C.L., Hendry, W.F. and Peckham, M.J. (1986) The significance of scrotal interference in stage I testicular cancer managed by orchiectomy and surveillance. *British Journal of Urology*, **58**, 705–8.

Lepor, H., Gregerman, M., Crosby, R. *et al.* (1985) Precise localization of the autonomic nerves from the pelvic plexus to the corpora cavernosa: a detailed anatomical study of the adult male pelvis. *Journal of Urology*, **133**, 207–12.

Lundgren, R. (1987) Flutamide as primary treatment for metastatic prostatic cancer. *British Journal of Urology*, **59**, 156–8.

Lynch, J.H. and Maxted, W.C. (1983) Use of ephedrine in post-lymphadenectomy ejaculatory failure: a case report. *Journal of Urology*, **129**, 379.

Macleod, J. (1951) Semen quality in 1000 men of known fertility and in 800 cases of infertile marriage. *Fertility and Sterility*, **2**, 115–39.

Meistrich, M.L. (1993) Effects of chemotherapy and radiotherapy on spermatogenesis. *European Urology*, **23**, 136–42.

Milligan, J.W., Hughes, R. and Lindsay, K.S. (1989) Semen cryopreservation in men undergoing cancer chemotherapy – a U.K. survey. *British Journal of Cancer*, **60**, 966–7.

Morrish, D.W., Venner, P.M., Siy, O. *et al.* (1990) Mechanisms of endocrine dysfunction in patients with testicular cancer. *Journal of the National Cancer Institute*, **82**, 412–18.

Nijman, J.M., Jager, S., Boer, P.W. *et al.* (1982) The treatment of ejaculation disorders after retroperitoneal lymph node dissection. *Cancer*, **50**, 2967–71.

Nijman, J.M., Koops, H.S., Oldhoff, J. *et al.* (1987) Sexual function after bilateral retroperitoneal lymph node dissection for non-seminomatous testicular cancer. *Archives of Andrology*, **18**, 255–67.

Ohl, D.A., Denil, J., Bennett, C.J. *et al.* (1991) Electroejaculation following retroperitoneal lymphadenectomy. *Journal of Urology*, **145**, 980–3.

Pryor, J.P. and Hendry, W.F. (1991) Ejaculatory duct obstruction in subfertile males: analysis of 87 patients. *Fertility and Sterility*, **56**, 725–30.

Pryor, J.P., Pugh, R.C.B., Cameron, K.M. *et al.* (1976) Plasma gonadotrophic hormones, testicular biopsy and seminal analysis in men of infertile marriages. *British Journal of Urology*, **48**, 709–17.

Rhodes, E.A., Hoffman, D.J. and Kaempfer, S.H. (1985) Ten years of experience with semen cryopreservation by cancer patients: follow-up and clinical considerations. *Fertility and Sterility*, **44**, 512–16.

Richie, J.P. (1990) Clinical stage I testicular cancer: the role of modified retroperitoneal lymphadenectomy. *Journal of Urology*, **144**, 1160–3.

Richter, P., Calamera, J.C., Morgenfeld, M.C. *et al.* (1970) Effect of chlorambucil on spermatogenesis in the human with malignant lymphoma. *Cancer*, **25**, 1026–30.

Rickards, D. (1993) Recent advances in ultrasound, in *Recent Advances in Urology/Andrology*, 6th edn, (eds W.F. Hendry and R.S. Kirby), Churchill Livingstone, Edinburgh, pp. 17–30.

Scammell, G.E., White, N., Stedronska, J. *et al.* (1985) Cryopreservation of semen in men with testicular tumour or Hodgkin's disease: results of artificial insemination of their partners. *Lancet*, **ii**, 31–2.

Scammell, G.E., Stedronska-Clarke, J., Edmonds, D.K. and Hendry, W.F. (1989) Retrograde ejaculation: successful treatment with artificial insemination. *British Journal of Urology*, **63**, 198–201.

Schilsky, R.L. (1989) Infertility in patients with testicular cancer: testis, tumour or treatment? *Journal of the National Cancer Institute*, **81**, 1204–5.

Senturia, Y.D., Peckham, C.S. and Peckham, M.J. (1985) Children fathered by men treated for testicular cancer. *Lancet*. **ii**, 766–9.

Shalet, S.M. (1993) Effect of irradiation treatment on gonadal function in men treated for germ cell cancer. *European Urology*, **23**, 148–52.

Sogani, P.C. and Whitmore, W.F. (1979) Experience with flutamide in previously untreated patients with advanced prostatic cancer. *Journal of Urology*, **122**, 640–3.

Thomas, P.R.M., Mansfield, M.D., Hendry, W.F. and Peckham, M.J. (177) The implications of scrotal interference for the preservation of spermatogenesis in the management of testicular tumours. *British Journal of Surgery*, **64**, 352–4.

Turner-Warwick, R. and Kirby, R.S. (1990) The construction and reconstruction of the vagina with colocecum. *Surgery, Gynaecology and Obstetrics*, **170,** 132–6.

Walsh, P.C. and Mostwin, J.L. (1984) Radical prostatectomy and cystoprostatectomy with preservation of potency. Results using a new nerve-sparing technique. *British Journal of Urology*, **56**, 694–7.

Zagars, G.K. (1991) Management of stage I seminoma: radiotherapy, in *Testicular Cancer. Investigation and Management*, (ed. A. Horwich, Chapman & Hall, London), pp. 98–101.

Jessica Corner

17.1　INTRODUCTION

Cancer is a complex disease, with the potential to cause major multisystem dysfunction, and is a life threatening illness. Unlike many other diseases, cancer demands that treatment is intense, both in duration and in the number and range of side-effects and sequelae it causes. As already described in earlier chapters, it also requires the sufferer to make profound adjustments to the potential threat to one's life; the mutilating effects of cancer surgery; changes in the ability to perform usual social and occupational roles; to endure prolonged and toxic treatment; and after the treatment phase to live with uncertainty over whether the cancer will return at some later date.

The recognition of the vast range of needs for care and support amongst patients with cancer and their families, the need to have health care professionals skilled in the administration of complex cancer therapies and monitoring and managing the toxic effects of these, led to the development of cancer care as a speciality in nursing. The first extended roles for nurses in cancer care were undertaken by nurses working in clinical trials, administering treatment and collecting patient data. It was soon realized that nurses in clinical research roles contributed greatly to both the research and the quality of patient care, from such roles the identity of the 'cancer nurse' has evolved (Yarbro, 1991). Today cancer nursing has developed way beyond nurses being seen as a junior team members in clinical research.

Nurses themselves provide clinical leadership in cancer care in many instances, and increasingly nursing research is being recognized as making a significant contribution to knowledge in oncology (Corner, 1991).

With the developing recognition of the importance of nursing within cancer care, education for nurses has also developed. In 1974 the Royal Marsden Hospital commenced the first course in the UK which led to a recordable qualification in cancer nursing. Since that time the range and depth of courses in the speciality of cancer nursing have developed enormously in Europe and the USA. Education in cancer care in basic nurse training is recognized to be limited to no more than a few hours or study days; consequently nurses who have received no specialist training in cancer care are known to feel inadequately prepared to deal with the problems of patients (Corner and Wilson-Barnett, 1992). Beyond this level, nurses wishing to specialize in cancer nursing can now study courses in cancer care at undergraduate and masters levels, and can continue their studies by undertaking MPhil and PhD study if they wish.

The development of academic study for nurses in cancer care has meant that the knowledge base for nursing practice has been delineated and different levels of practice identified. On first entering the speciality, nurses need to be provided with education which will equip them with the knowledge and skills necessary to practise as a cancer nurse. As nurses gain experience they frequently wish to extend their knowledge in particular aspects of cancer care such as psychological care, palliative care, breast care or bone marrow transplant nursing. Nurses pursuing careers as clinical nurse specialists or who have important leadership positions in nursing will increasingly be expected to hold a Masters degree in cancer care, and training in research methods is now an inherent part of most nursing courses. In addition nursing in Europe and the USA is developing recognition that different levels of practice exist, and nurses are developing their skills to an advanced level, which involves becoming a clinical expert in a particular aspect of care, utilizing and initiating research, acting as a role model and educator of less experienced nurses and being able to effect change where required (UKCC, 1991; Yasko, 1991). It is clear that these developments have led to the expansion of the roles and responsibilities of cancer nurses, allowing the provision of comprehensive care which goes far beyond optimal medical treatment of the disease. Table 17.1 shows examples of the range of roles that exist for cancer nurses. Among the most important role to develop in cancer nursing is that of the clinical nurse specialist.

The clinical nurse specialist combines the functions of expert practitioner to a narrowly defined client group, acts as an educator to patients, families and nursing staff, is available for other nursing colleagues to consult on the care of patients, and engages in research regarding their area of specialist practice (Siehl, 1982; Storr, 1988). Many examples of such nurses exist in the UK, some of these are identified in Table 17.1.

17.2   THE FOCUS OF NURSING IN CANCER TREATMENT AND CARE

As cancer nursing has evolved as a speciality, and the knowledge required by practitioners has been identified, so too has developed a strong nursing philosophy in cancer care and an understanding of the particular contribu-

Table 17.1   Examples of cancer nursing roles

Areas of care
Health promotion/primary prevention
Acute cancer care
Palliative care
    Community nurse specialist
    Hospital support team
    Hospice

Nursing roles
Breast cancer nurse specialist
Stoma care nurse specialist
Bone marrow transplant nurse
Gynaecological cancer nurse specialist
Head and neck cancer nurse specialist
Community liaison nurse
Patient education nurse
Home chemotherapy nurse
Clinical trials nurse
Paediatric cancer nurse
Rehabilitation nurse
Intravenous therapy nurse
Chemotherapy nurse
Psychological support nurse
Cancer counselling
Complementary therapies nurse
Nurse researcher

tion of cancer nursing within the multidisciplinary team. Medicine in oncology rightly has cure and disease control as its first priority. The focus of medical practice and research therefore is to develop and evaluate new treatment regimens for patients and to work towards developing optimal treatment whilst maintaining maximum life quality. This means that the approaches adopted in medical practice focus on the objective assessment of disease stage and response to treatment using indicators such as duration of survival, treatment toxicity and cost versus quality of life estimates.

Nursing has care as its primary focus in the sense that nursing seeks to assist in the containment of the effects of cancer and its treatment on the person, also to understand the meaning of the disease experience to the

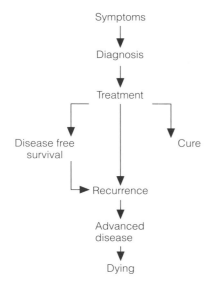

Symptoms

Diagnosis

Treatment

Disease free survival

Cure

Recurrence

Advanced disease

Dying

Figure 17.1   The disease continuum.

individual, and in so doing act as compassionate friend to the patient (Leininger, 1981; Roach, 1984). Nursing is therefore preoccupied with the whole experience of cancer, with not separating mind from body, and with focusing activity around symptoms and problems resulting from the disease or its treatment. This can create tensions for nurses working in acute treatment settings when the goals of active curative treatment and the goals of caring do not always rest easily side by side. It is these very differences that make nursing and medicine ideal partners in finding a pathway through the difficult route cancer patients have to follow.

The experience of cancer for the individual is in general long and complex and cannot be considered as a single illness and treatment episode. Rather the illness career with cancer represents a continuum from first experience of cancer symptoms to either cure or death, and this is illustrated in Figure 17.1. Contact with health carers during this illness career occurs at critical moments such as diagnosis, treatment or recurrence. The nature of this contact can be pivotal in determining the

quality of life for patients, and nurses play an important part in this. The role of cancer nursing throughout the disease experience is varied, but encompasses a number of elements which are listed below:

1. Assisting patients and their families to adjust and adapt to life with cancer.
2. Administering cancer treatment and providing supportive care to patients during intensive cancer treatment programmes.
3. Managing the problems caused by cancer and its treatment.
4. Facilitating rehabilitation to normal life following cancer treatment.
5. Providing support and symptom management to individuals with recurrent and advanced disease.
6. Managing cancer care services to ensure optimal care delivery.
7. Researching and evaluating nursing practice in cancer care.

Each of these areas warrants closer attention, since nurses have been working to articulate the specific contribution they make to each within the multi-disciplinary team, and to extend their work into areas of need identified for patients.

17.2.1   ASSISTING PATIENTS AND THEIR FAMILIES TO ADJUST AND ADAPT TO LIFE WITH CANCER

It is now well established that the meaning of cancer within society is that of a disease which is perceived to be synonymous with death (Sontag, 1979), and a death which involves much pain and suffering. This is in direct contrast to society's beliefs about other conditions such as cardiovascular disease, which is associated with power, success and an 'easy' pain free death (Donovan and Girton, 1984). In a survey of public opinion the fear of cancer was felt to be worse than that of death itself by a significant proportion of the population (Cancer Relief Macmillan Fund, 1988). Such fears are known to extend to health care professionals as well, with non-specialist doctors and nurses being extremely pessimistic about the disease and its treatment (Easson, 1967; Corner and Wilson-Barnett, 1992). The effects of such beliefs are manifested in patients with symptoms of cancer delaying attending for medical attention through fear, and thus worsening their chances of successful treatment (Eddy and Eddy, 1984). The negativity of health carers towards the disease has in the past led to their reluctance to disclose information regarding diagnosis and prognosis, and awkward and inadequate communication with patients (McIntosh, 1977; Bond, 1978). The recognition of these problems has been a catalyst in the development of special training schemes for nurses to help them feel more comfortable about cancer, and to give them communication and counselling skills to equip them to work with patients at all stages of the disease.

A body of research has been undertaken demonstrating the devastating consequences of receiving a diagnosis of cancer to the individual and the occurrence of psychological problems such as anxiety and depression as a result (Holland and Rowland, 1989). Research has demonstrated that specially trained nurse counsellors can identify those at risk of such problems and can be effective in reducing the incidence of adjustment problems amongst patients with breast cancer (Maguire *et al.*, 1980; Watson *et al.*, 1988). This has been influential in encouraging a heavy emphasis of the nursing role in cancer care to be placed upon assisting patients to adapt and adjust to living with cancer. It has also led nurses to re-evaluate the role of nursing in such care and to undertake developmental work to promote understanding of the nursing position with regard to assisting patients in adjusting.

Much of the work in the developing field of psychooncology focuses on the processes by which individuals diagnosed as having cancer cope. In particular coping with the stresses of the knowledge of having a life threatening illness and those imposed by cancer treatment; and in identifying the mechanisms which promote more, or less successful adjustment to such stresses (Rowland, 1989). There has been a clear need for clinical psychologists and psychiatrists involved in cancer care to concentrate on patients who have been identified as having clinical signs of psychological disruption as a result of cancer and its treatment. This has left a vitally important role for nurses to work with patients in their care who may not fall into this category, but who all have immense need for emotional and psychological support.

An influential work by Benner and Wrubel (1989), two American nurses, offers a model for nurses to work with patients in facilitating coping, and is seen in the context of the caring role of the nurse. The authors cite Fagin and Diers' (1983) description of nursing:

Nursing is a metaphor for intimacy. Nurses are involved in the most private parts of people's lives, and they cannot hide behind technology or a veil of omniscience as other practitioners or technicians do. Nurses do for others publicly what other healthy persons do for themselves behind closed doors. Nurses, as trusted peers, are there to hear secrets, especially the ones born of vulnerability. Nurses are treasured when these interchanges are successful, but most often people do not wish to remember their vulnerability or loss of control, and nurses are indelibly identified with those terrible personal times. (p. 257)

It is the skilled use of these intimate moments which make cancer nurses a vital link in the chain of communication and support for patients.

Benner and Wrubel (1989) advocate a phenomenological rather than a normative model for coping in which illness is seen as a lived experience inseparable from body, mind, external world and previous experience. In this approach there is no 'ideal' coping style or mental health, rather individuals are seen as living through an experience of illness in which caring allows health professionals to connect with that individual's experience and facilitate their pathway through it. O'Connor *et al.* (1990) in a study of interview data from 30 patients with cancers of the breast, lung and colon, who were within 6 months of diagnosis, identified six major themes in patients search for meaning after a cancer diagnosis. These included seeking an understanding of the personal significance of the cancer diagnosis; looking at the consequences of a cancer diagnosis; reviewing life; restructuring and revaluing of attitudes towards self, life and others; learning to live with cancer; and hope. Facilitating patients both with coping and to find such meaning represents nurses' function in cancer care.

Nurses' role in facilitating patients and their families to adjust and adapt to life with cancer is varied, and can be seen to operate at a number of levels. All nurses working in cancer care roles operate within the model of support described above. There are in addition nurses who have taken this role further and work at a sophisticated level with patients in a variety of contexts. Clinical nurse specialists in breast and stoma care offer counselling and advice to patients and their families with regard to their specific treatments and problems, and in helping them to adapt to the impact of, for example, mastectomy, reconstructive breast surgery or the formation of a stoma. Other nurses have developed innovative roles in psychological support, providing an important intermediary between ward nurses and psychologists and psychiatrists. Further roles exist in palliative care, addressing psychosexual concerns, paediatric care and family support, and research nurses focus on the particular need for support among patients undergoing treatment in the context of a clinical trial. Nursing's unique position in combining an intense personal involvement with patients and their families, and in being at the sharp end of the administration of treatment and in providing physical care, places nurses at the centre of the fundamentally important role of supporting patients.

17.2.2 ADMINISTERING CANCER TREATMENTS AND PROVIDING SUPPORTIVE CARE TO PATIENTS DURING INTENSIVE CANCER TREATMENT PROGRAMMES

Nurses have advanced skills in the administration of cancer chemotherapy, and in monitoring the side-effects of these and in working with patients undergoing other treatments. Cancer nurses have been working on projects to develop optimum methods of administering cancer chemotherapy and other therapies, in ensuring safety in its administration and in managing side-effects. For example, Long and Ovaska (1992) report a comparative study of the incidence of infection amongst patients with venous access ports using a commercially prepared package with a nurse developed procedure; and Pritchard and Mallett (1992) have undertaken significant work in attempting to identify optimum procedures for a variety of nursing tasks including the administration of intravenous therapy.

A study under way at the Royal Marsden Hospital is recording the conversation which occurs between nurses and patients during the administration of chemotherapy for ovarian cancer. This study is important because it is not only the method of administration that is important but the kind of education and support patients receive during treatment that will determine the overall quality of care (Dennison, 1993).

Not only are cancer nurses preoccupied with the process of treatment administration, but also the effects of treatment on patients and in minimizing side-effects. The management of nausea and vomiting induced by cytotoxic drugs has received most attention since it is the most frequently experienced problem (Grant and Padilla, 1983). Chemotherapy induced vomiting can affect compliance with the treatment regimen, and may on occasions be so severe that a patient will withdraw from treatment. The role of the cancer nurse is to prevent and or control nausea and vomiting (Peters, 1989). This can be achieved through:

1. Prophylactic use of antiemetics.
2. The active use of established antiemetic regimens designed for use with different cytotoxic combinations.
3. Anticipating and managing delayed onset of nausea and vomiting between treatment cycles.
4. Advising patients on nutritional intake so that optimal nutritional status is maintained during treatment, aiding subsequent recovery and the experience of symptoms such as chemotherapy induced fatigue.
5. Working to prevent and manage anticipatory nausea and vomiting.

Nurses have also been active in identifying methods of preventing and managing stomatitis and alopecia induced by cancer therapy. A number of studies have been reported comparing different oral care regimens (e.g. Kenny, 1990). An interesting study has been undertaken in which a nurse examined the usefulness of employing an innovative preventative strategy for stomatitis induced by 5-fluoruracil (5-FU). The patients hold ice chips in their mouths for 5 minutes prior to administration of 5-FU and for a further 30 minutes, and this was found to significantly reduce the incidence of stomatitis when compared with patients who did not use ice chips (Dose, 1992). Nurses have been rationalizing the situations in which preventative measures for chemotherapy induced alopecia should be used, the drugs for which techniques such as scalp cooling are effective and in making careful assessment of the emotional impact hair loss is likely to have for an individual (Tierney, 1987).

17.2.3 MANAGING THE PROBLEMS CAUSED BY CANCER AND ITS TREATMENT

Cancer causes a wide range of problems for patients and their families, therefore patients have many needs for care and support at all stages of the disease process. These problems may be physical, psychological, social or financial. Holmes and Dickerson (1987) found that amongst a group of 72 patients in an oncology unit, more than one-third were distressed by such symptoms as their appearance, tiredness, inability to concentrate, feeling miserable, loss of mobility, inability to sleep, loss of appetite and constipation. Eleven per cent were distressed by pain and 6% by nausea or diarrhoea. A recent study of 28 patients undergoing initial treatment and 32 patients being treated for recurrence found that fatigue was the most troublesome symptom amongst both groups of patients (Munkres *et al.*, 1994). Lewis (1984) has reviewed research on the impact of cancer on the family and identified 11 separate issues caused by a family member having cancer, these are:

1. Emotional strain.
2. The physical demands of caring for a family member.
3. Uncertainty over the patient's health, and the likely outcome of the disease.
4. Fear of the patient dying.
5. Alterations in roles for different family members, and in family lifestyle.
6. Financial pressures.
7. Concerns over how to physically comfort the patient.
8. Inadequacy of supportive services for families.
9. Existential concerns raised for family members.
10. Negative effects on sexual relationships.

11. Non-convergent needs of family members.

Nurses are frequently the first and most intense point of contact with the health care professions for patients and their families, and consequently work to assess patients' needs for care, support or intervention for the problems identified. This also means acting as co-ordinator of patient care so that they are appropriately referred to other members of the multidisciplinary team for assistance with particular problems.

17.2.4 FACILITATING REHABILITATION TO NORMAL LIFE FOLLOWING CANCER TREATMENT

With the increasing numbers of individuals successfully treated for their disease, and an ever increasing group of patients living for many years with their cancer effectively controlled, rehabilitation has been integrated into cancer treatment programmes. Cancer rehabilitation is a dynamic health orientated process designed to promote maximum levels of functioning in individuals with cancer related health problems (Watson, 1990). This process is relevant to all health carers, and is a philosophy of care, which begins at diagnosis, not merely on the completion of treatment. Such rehabilitation needs should be addressed by an interdisciplinary team (Wells, 1990). Dietz (1981) describes four categories of rehabilitation:

1. Preventative – rehabilitation measures designed to improve physical functioning and reduce morbidity and disability.
2. Restorative – measures to control or eliminate residual cancer disability for patients who are cured of the disease.
3. Supportive – to lessen disability amongst individuals with ongoing disease.
4. Palliative – to maximize life quality amongst those with advanced disease.

A number of cancer rehabilitation programmes have been set up in the UK and the USA and comprise interdisciplinary teams focusing on the assessment of health problems resulting from the disease, offering therapeutic interventions, and follow-up (Watson, 1990). Nurses are recognized to be members of such rehabilitation teams. Anderson (1989) identified an important rehabilitation role for nurses regardless of whether they are a member of a formally designated rehabilitation team. This includes assessment, developing formal and informal patient education programmes, acting as a counsellor to address issues such as disease meaning, body image and sexuality, active planning for discharge, and acting in the key role of co-ordinator of the multidisciplinary team to ensure the rehabilitation needs of patients are addressed.

17.2.5 PROVIDING SUPPORT AND SYMPTOM MANAGEMENT FOR INDIVIDUALS WITH RECURRENT AND ADVANCED DISEASE

The care of patients with advanced disease has been increasingly recognized as a vital aspect of cancer nursing care, so much so that palliative care has become recognized as a speciality in its own right, and nurses are working in a variety of roles with patients with advanced cancer. These range from staff nurses working in hospice and continuing care units, to clinical nurse specialists in palliative care working in hospice, hospital and community settings, and nurse consultants in specific aspects of palliative care. In all of these situations nurses have developed expertise and experience in managing the symptoms and needs of advanced cancer patients and their families. This involves offering expert advice on the management of symptoms to general practitioners and community nursing services, teaching other health carers to care for patients' needs, and where necessary providing psychological support to patients and their families in adjusting to advanced disease and in offering bereavement support following the death of the patient

(Bunn, 1988). Bergen (1992) has demonstrated the value of palliative care nurses as members of a team of carers in meeting the needs of patients dying of cancer when considered within a framework of quality assurance. Dicks (1989) has outlined the contribution of nursing to palliative care and has highlighted that this is in the assessment of the deficiency of self-care brought about by the disease, its treatment and patients' reactions to these with the aim of promoting independence or, where this is impossible, adaptation to the limits of advancing disease.

Great emphasis has been given in the research literature to the needs of those patients who are in the terminal stages of their disease. Much less attention has been given to patients at or around the time of recurrence. This is a devastating moment for patients and their families and requires great sensitivity on the part of health carers. Currently there is something of a divide between provision and understanding for those with end stage disease compared with those patients who have more recently been identified as having on-going disease. Increasingly palliative care nurses are recognizing the needs of patients with recurrence, and have begun to attempt to identify these at an early stage so that interventions can be tailored to the specific problems of such patients.

17.2.6   MANAGING CANCER CARE SERVICES TO ENSURE OPTIMAL CARE DELIVERY

Nurses hold key management positions in cancer care services, and find themselves having to balance the many conflicting demands of limited resources, the need to employ highly qualified staff, to identify and set standards for the service, and ensure that quality care is delivered and is appropriate to meet the needs of patients at an optimal level. In today's health care environment when all health care services are having to compete for finite health budgets it is becoming increasingly important for nurses to be accom-

plished political lobbyists, and to continue to demand representation on committees and bodies determining health strategies and allocating resources at local and government levels.

There are many examples of cancer nurses internationally who have played a significant role in raising awareness of the needs of patients with cancer and ensuring that cancer care services are recognized and supported. Such nurses have frequently been highly influential to nursing and health care as a whole, and reflect the high calibre of nurses that the speciality of cancer care attracts. One example of such influence can be seen in the development of palliative cancer care services in the UK, where the development and success of the community palliative care nurse role has reversed the trend towards expanding the number of inpatient hospice services.

Nurses are also leading the way in establishing quality assurance and audit programmes, so that standards of care can be set and the quality of care delivered and evaluated (Luthert and Robinson, 1993). In the future innovative nursing roles in cancer care are likely to develop, and these will further extend nursing practice into for example the independent, collaborative nurse practitioner (Anthes, 1992), and the research practitioner (Wilson-Barnett *et al.*, 1990).

17.2.7   RESEARCHING AND EVALUATING NURSING PRACTICE IN CANCER CARE

Nursing research in cancer care is evolving rapidly and has moved from the situation where occasionally an outsider to the nursing profession was interested enough in an area important to nursing practice to study it, e.g. Field's (1989) sociological work on nurses and dying cancer patients and the study of Maguire *et al.* (1980) of a nurse counsellor for women with breast cancer. Cancer nursing research is also moving away from the situation where the only nurses involved in research are those working as data collectors and protocol managers for medical research. Nurses as advanced practitioners are increasingly undertaking research relevant to their own role and practice, and to their client group's nursing needs, and are also working in collaborative projects with cancer scientists, doctors and other health care professionals. This development in research activity by cancer nurses means that it is now possible to identify the particular orientation of cancer nursing research. Studies focus on the impact, physical, social or psychological, of cancer on individuals, and are beginning to identify and evaluate supportive strategies in the management of patient's problems. Key areas for cancer nursing research have been identified by a group of British nurses and include:

1. Patient problems, systematic methods of assessment, and studies related to the management of these.
2. The experiences and needs of patients, survivors, close relatives and significant others.
3. Methods of facilitating coping and adjusting to cancer (Corner, 1993).

Work is also under way to secure funding for nursing research initiatives, and to create environments in which such research can be stimulated and supported.

Research studies have been undertaken by nurses and are beginning to form a body of knowledge for nursing practice in a number of areas. Areas of focus for such studies include:

1. Nurses' attitudes toward cancer and the effect these have on the care patients receive.
2. Communication and psychological support for patients with cancer and their families.
3. Health behaviour and cancer prevention.
4. The administration and effects of cancer treatment.

5. The prevalence of cancer symptoms and problems.
6. The development and evaluation of assessment tools for research and practice.
7. Intervention studies for clinical problems.
8 The impact of cancer care on nurses.

In both Britain and the USA it is possible to identify emerging programmes of nursing research in cancer care, and centres where a substantial amount of research is being undertaken evaluating new practices and interventions for clinical problems, using innovative research approaches. One example of such a centre is the Royal Marsden Hospital/Institute of Cancer Research, where in the section of nursing a research-practitioner role is being developed and evaluated. This has as its aim the integration of academic research and nursing practice, which in nursing has hitherto been very difficult to ally together. Lecturers within the Unit have developed research studies which engage them directly in practice which they in turn are evaluating. For example, a recently commenced study is evaluating a nursing clinic for lung cancer patients with dyspnoea, using non-pharmacological interventions for this difficult symptom based on breathing retraining techniques identified for use with chronic pulmonary disease patients; relaxation; anxiety reduction; and discussion of the meaning of dyspnoea to the patient. Another study is exploring issues of sexuality and intimacy amongst women and their partners following treatment for cervical cancer using in-depth interviews. Findings from this interview study are being used to develop a multidisciplinary intervention strategy for women to assist them with problems identified, which will then be evaluated using a case study approach.

17.3   CONCLUSIONS

Clearly the scope of cancer nursing is immense. Nurses with expertise in the care of patients with cancer contribute at every stage along the disease continuum and are important members in a central position in the multidisciplinary team. Increasingly research is being undertaken which is demonstrating the effectiveness an informed and committed nurse can have on the experience of cancer both to the sufferer and to the family. Nurses are also undertaking studies which are evaluating new approaches to the management of the needs and problems of patients with cancer and innovative strategies of care are being evaluated. Thus the developing field of nursing research in cancer care widens the scope of cancer nursing considerably and suggests an exciting future ahead.

REFERENCES

Anderson, J.L. (1989) The nurses' role in cancer rehabilitation, review of the literature. *Cancer Nursing*, **12**, 85–94.

Anthes, J. (1992) Independent nursing practice – a new direction in Australia, in Bailey C.D. (ed.) Cancer *Nursing, Changing Frontiers*. Proceedings of Seventh International Conference on Cancer Nursing (ed. C.D. Bailey). Rapid Communications, Oxford, pp. 160–3.

Bennen, P. and Wrubel, J. (1989) *The Primacy of Caring; Stress and Coping in Health and Illness*, Addison Wesley, California.

Bergen, A. (1992) Evaluating nursing care of the terminally ill in the community: a case study approach. *International Journal of Nursing Studies*, **29**, 81–93.

Bond, S. (1978) Processes of communication about cancer in a radiotherapy department. Unpublished PhD thesis, University of Edinburgh.

Bunn, F. (1988) An exploratory study of the role of the Macmillan Nurse. Unpublished BSc dissertation, King's College, University of London.

Cancer Relief Macmillan Fund (1988) Public Attitudes and Knowledge of Cancer in the UK. Unpublished Research Report.

Contanch, P.H. (1983) Relaxation training for control of nausea and vomiting in patients receiving chemotherapy. *Cancer Nursing*, **6**, 277–83.

Corner, J. (1988) Assessing nurses' attitudes to cancer: a critical review of the literature. *Journal of Advanced Nursing*, **13**, 640–8.

Corner, J. (1991) Cancer nursing research. *Nursing Times*, **87**, 42–4.

Corner, J. (1993) Building a framework for nursing research in cancer care. *European Journal of Cancer Care*, (in press).

Corner, J. and Wilson-Barnett, J. (1992) The newly registered nurse and the cancer patient: an educational evaluation. *International Journal of Nursing Studies*, **29**, 177–90.

Dennison, S. (1993) an exploration into the verbal communication that occurs between the nurse and the patient whilst the nurse is delivering intravenous cancer chemotherapy. Unpublished MSc dissertation, Surrey University.

Dicks, B. (1989) Palliative care – the influence of nursing. *Palliative Medicine*, **3**, (3).

Dietz, J.H. (1981) *Rehabilitation Oncology*, John Wiley, New York.

Donovan, M.I. and Girton, S.E. (1984) *Cancer Care Nursing*, 2nd edn, Appleton Century Crofts, Norwalk, Connecticut.

Dose, A.M. (1992) Crytherapy for prevention of 5-fluorouracil induced mucositis, in *Cancer Nursing Changing Frontiers* (ed. C.D. Bailey), Proceedings of the Seventh International Conference on Cancer Nursing. Rapid Communications, Oxford, pp. 95–7.

Easson, E.C. (1967) Cancer and the problem of pessimism. *Journal for Clinicians*, **1**, 7–14.

Eddy, D.M. and Eddy, J.F. (1984) *Patient Delay in the Detection of Cancer*. Proceedings of American Cancer Society, Fourth National Conference on Human Values and Cancer, American Cancer Society, New York.

Fagin, C. and Diers, D. (1983) Nursing as metaphor: occasional notes. *New England Journal of Medicine*, **309**, 116. (Cited by Benner, P. and Wrubel, J. (1989) *The Primacy of Caring, Stress and Coping in Health and Illness*, Addison Wesley, California.)

Faithfull, S. (1991) Patients' experiences following cranial radiotherapy: a study of somnolence syndrome. *Journal of Advanced Nursing*, **16**, 939–46.

Field, D. (1989) *Nursing the Dying*, Routledge, London.

Grant, M.M. and Padilla, G.V. (1983) An overview of cancer nursing research, *Oncology Nursing Forum*, **10**, 58–69.

Holland, J.C. and Rowland, J.H. (eds) (1989). *Handbook of Psychooncology*, Oxford University Press, New York.

Holmes, S. and Dickersen, J. (1987) The quality of life: design and evaluation of a self-assessment instrument for use with cancer patients. *International Journal of Nursing Studies*, **24**, 15–24.

Kenny, S.A. (1990) Effect of two oral care protocols on the incidence of stomatitis in haematology patients. *Cancer Nursing*, **13**, 345–53.

Lewis, F.M. (1984) The impact of cancer on the family: a critical analysis of research literature. *Patient Education and Counselling*, 269–89.

Leininger, M.M. (1981) *Caring: an essential human need*, C.B. Stack, Thorofare, New Jersey.

Long, M.C. and Ovaska, M. (1992) Comparative study of nursing protocols for known access parts. *Cancer Nursing*, **15**, 18–21.

Luthert, J.M. and Robinson, L. (eds) (1993) *The Royal Marsden Hospital Manual of Standards of Care*, Blackwell Scientific Publications London.

McIntosh, J. (1977) *Communication and Awareness on a Cancer Ward*, Croom Helm, New York.

Maguire, F.P., Tait, A., Brooke, M. *et al.* (1980) The effects of counselling on the psychiatric morbidity associated with mastectomy. *British Medical Journal* **28**, 1454–6.

Munkres, A., Oberst, M. and Hughes, S.H. (1992) Appraisal of illness, symptom distress, self-care burden, and mood states in patients receiving chemotherapy for initial and recurrent cancer. *Oncology Nursing Forum*, **19**, 1201–9.

O'Connor, A.P., Wicker, B.A. and Germinor B.B. (1990) Understanding the cancer patient's search for meaning. *Cancer Nursing*, **13**, 167–75.

Peters, C.A. (1989) Myths of antiemetic administration. *Cancer Nursing*, **12**, 102–6.

Pritchard, A.P. and Mallett, J. (eds) (1992) *The Royal Marsden Hospital Manual of Clinical Nursing Procedures*, Blackwell Scientific Publications, London.

Roach, M.S. (1984) *Caring: The Human Mode of Being: Implications for Nursing. Perspectives in Caring, Monograph 1*, University of Toronto, Faculty of Nursing.

Rowland, J.H. (1989) Interpersonal resources: coping, in *Handbook of Psychooncology*, (eds. J.C. Holland and J.H. Rowland), Oxford University Press, New York, pp. 44–71.

Siehl, S. (1982) The clinical nurse specialist in oncology. *Nursing Clinics of North America*, **17**, 753–61.

Sontag, S. (1979) *Illness as Metaphor*, Allen Lane, London.

Storr, S. (1988) The clinical nurse specialist: from outside looking in. *Journal of Advanced Nursing*, **13**, 265–72.

Tierney, A.J. (1987) Preventing chemotherapy induced alopecia in cancer patients: is scalp cooling worthwhile? *Journal of Advanced Nursing*, **12**, 303–10.

UKCC (1991) The report of the Post-registration Education and Practice Project. United Kingdom Central Council for Nursing, Midwifery and Health Visiting, London.

Watson, M., Denton, S., Baum, M. and Greer, S. (1988) Counselling breast cancer patients: a specialist nurse service. *Counselling Psychology Quarterly*, **1**, 23–32.

Watson, P.G. (1990) Cancer rehabilitation, the evolution of a concept. *Cancer Nursing*, **13**, 2–12.

Wells, R. (1990) Rehabilitation: making the most of time. *Oncology Nursing Forum*, **17**, 503.

Wilson-Barnett, J., Corner, J. and DeCarle, B. (1990) Integrating nursing research and practice – the role of the researcher as teacher. *Journal of Advanced Nursing*, **15**, 621–25.

Yarbro, C.H. (1991) The history of cancer nursing, in *Cancer Nursing a Comprehensive Textbook*, (eds S.B. Baird, R. McCorkle and M. Grant), W.B. Saunders, Philadelphia, pp. 10–20.

Yasko, J.M. (1991) Role implementation in cancer nursing, in *Cancer Nursing a Comprehensive Textbook*, (eds S.B. Baird, R. McCorkle and M. Grant), W.B. Saunders, Philadelphia, pp. 21–30.

PART TWO

A SYSTEMATIC REVIEW OF ONCOLOGY

HODGKIN'S DISEASE

Alan Horwich

18.1 INTRODUCTION

Hodgkin's disease has frequently provided a focus for academic oncology units, presenting as it does particular challenges to those involved with diagnostic radiology, radiotherapy and medical oncology. It is a highly curable neoplasm with common presentation in the young adult age range, and was first described by Thomas Hodgkin in 1832. Though the cell of origin remains obscure, the presence of characteristic binuclear cells was described by Sternberg and by Reed at the beginning of this century.

The tumour is both highly radiosensitive and highly chemosensitive and each of these modalities can be curative alone. A particular challenge to modern oncology is the correct deployment of combined modality therapy.

18.2 INCIDENCE

In England and Wales the incidence in males is approximately 4 per 100 000 and in females 3 per 100 000. This represents approximately 1% of cancers registered in developed countries per annum, approximately half the incidence of non-Hodgkin's lymphomas. It is even more uncommon as a cause of cancer deaths, accounting for only 2 of the 273 cancer deaths per 100 000 men per annum recorded for England and Wales in the 1970s. The disease is more common in Denmark, Sweden, New Zealand and Norway, with a young adult age peak of between 4 and 5 per 100 000, than in the underdeveloped countries such as Colombia and Nigeria where the incidence is only approximately 1.5 per 100 000. There is some evidence that the age incidence pattern is associated with local economic conditions and there is also an association with social class (Hooven *et al.*, 1975; Henderson, *et al.*, 1979). Epidemiological observations are consistent with the idea that Hodgkin's disease may develop as a rare consequence of a common infection, especially when infection is delayed until adolescence or young adulthood (Gutensohn Mueller and Cole, 1977). There have been reports of case clusters, especially based on a number of cases observed in a school in Albany, New York (Vianna *et al.*, 1972). However, the significance of these is unclear.

18.3 AETIOLOGY

The prime candidate for an infectious aetiological agent in Hodgkin's disease has been the Epstein–Barr virus (EBV). This virus infects about 90% of the world population. Childhood infection is common and leads to a life-long carrier state but delayed primary infection is associated with the disease of infectious mononucleosis. The virus has the ability to immortalize B-lymphocytes *in vitro*. It is thought to replicate in oropharyngeal epithelium and to remain latent in B-lymphocytes *in vivo*. The function of some of its protein products have been characterized. For example, the latent membrane protein (LMP) 2 is needed for immortalization of B-lymphocyte and the LMP1 is oncogenic in fibroblasts.

The virus has been closely associated with two other human malignant diseases, namely Burkitt's lymphoma and nasopharyngeal carcinoma.

There is an excess risk of Hodgkin's disease among patients who have had infectious mononucleosis and additionally patients with Hodgkin's disease have a higher antibody titre to the EBV viral capsular antigen. Components of the EBV genome are found in about 20% of patients with Hodgkin's disease located in the Reed–Sternberg cells. The site of integration is monoclonal, implying infection before malignant proliferation. In this setting the cells express a high concentration of the LMP1 viral product.

In contrast to non-Hodgkin's lymphomas there is no striking increase in Hodgkin's disease in patients with pre-existing immunological abnormality, and additionally Hodgkin's disease does not seem to be a consequence of cytotoxic therapies for other cancers.

18.4 PATHOLOGY

Hodgkin's disease is usually classified using a system described by Lukes and Butler modified at the Rye Conference in 1966 (Lukes and Butler, 1966). The four categories are as follows:

1. **Lymphocyte predominant Hodgkin's disease (LP)**. This is uncommon and may be diffuse or nodular. Reed–Sternberg cells are uncommon, though other abnormal large polyploid cells may be present.
2. **Mixed cellularity Hodgkin's disease (MC)**. These tumours do not have sclerotic bands and Reed–Sternberg cells are quite common. The mixed cellular picture includes histiocytes, eosinophils, plasma cells, lymphocytes and neutrophils.
3. **Nodular sclerosis (NS)**. This subtype is characterized by bands of collagenous connective tissue containing nodules of both malignant and reactive cells. Some

authors have found a worse prognosis when the cellular content is lymphocyte depleted (Bennett *et al.*, 1983).

4. **Lymphocyte depleted Hodgkin's disease (LD)**. There are two subtypes of this, diffuse fibrosis and reticular. Reed–Sternberg cells are usually common.

In the Royal Marsden Hospital 5% of cases were LP, 52% NS, 29% MC and 14% LD. Of these four groups lymphocyte predominant Hodgkin's disease has a good prognosis whereas lymphocyte depleted Hodgkin's disease carries a much higher risk of recurrence.

The cell of origin of Hodgkin's disease and of the Reed–Sternberg cell has been the subject of intense research, including immunohistological or gene rearrangement studies; it has appeared that a small proportion of Hodgkin's disease is either related to the B-cell or T-cell lineage, but most cases demonstrate the characteristics of neither. Immunohistologically these cells are stained by the monoclonal antibody Ki-1; this stains almost all types of Hodgkin's disease and also some non-Hodgkin's lymphomas.

The different histological patterns correlate with stage at presentation, with the majority of LP presenting in stage I or II, whereas only about one-fifth of LD Hodgkin's disease presents in these stages (Desforges *et al.*, 1979). It may be that the individual histological subtypes do not influence prognosis independent of stage. Bennett *et al.* (1983) divided NS Hodgkin's disease into two types, grades I and II depending upon the cellular pattern. Those with LD or numerous pleomorphic Hodgkin's cells were placed in grade II and the remainder in grade I. In patients stratified in clinical stages I and II there was a significantly worse prognosis for patients with grade II NS Hodgkin's disease.

18.5 PRESENTATION

The usual presentation is with painless lymph node enlargement sometimes associated with systemic symptoms of sweats, fever, weight loss or occasionally generalized pruritus or alcohol-induced pain. The commonest nodal site is cervical, especially in the supra-clavicular region (60%); less common are axillary nodes (20%), inguinofemoral nodes (15%) spleen (10%) or liver (7%) (Kennedy *et al.*, 1985). The lymphoid tissue of Waldeyer's ring may be involved, especially when there is upper cervical lymphadenopathy. Splenomegaly may occur in the absence of splenic infiltration. In advanced or recurrent disease almost any sites of the body may be involved; typical sites are bone where there may be either sclerotic or mixed appearance on plain X-ray, lung where involvement may range from diffuse infiltrations to round 'cannon ball' lesions, pleura associated with an effusion, and epidural masses causing neuro-logical impairment. Bone marrow infiltration is uncommon unless there is other evidence of stage III or IV Hodgkin's disease, or there are systemic symptoms. Mediastinal nodal disease may become extremely large and be associated with respiratory compromise, superior vena caval obstruction and pericardial effusion.

Though nodes involved by Hodgkin's disease are described as typically 'rubbery' in texture and though they may be associated with alcohol-induced pain, excision biopsy is required for a firm diagnosis.

18.6 INVESTIGATION AND STAGING

18.6.1 INVESTIGATION

Routine blood tests should include a full haematological profile, together with renal and liver function tests. The presentation erythrocyte sedimentation rate (ESR) has been correlated with prognosis (Tubiana *et al.*, 1984), as have a low haemoglobin and a low lymphocyte count. Mild abnormalities of liver enzymes do not correlate well with pathologi-cal evidence of liver infiltration.

Chest X-ray may reveal enlarged mediasti-nal or hilar lymph nodes and also may

suggest lung disease. There is no doubt that CT scanning of the thorax is more sensitive when the mediastinum is involved. A plain chest X-ray is used to distinguish the adverse prognostic definition of bulky mediastinal mass which is usually applied to a mass which is greater than a third of the transtho-racic diameter at the T6 vertebral body level. The infradiaphragmatic lymph nodes can be demonstrated also by CT scanning of abdomen and pelvis and this carries some ad-vantages over lymphography, not only in terms of patient acceptability but also because it images well the upper para-aortic region and may show gross involvement of liver or spleen. It should, however, be realized that there is no sensitive imaging modality for the detection of Hodgkin's disease in the spleen. The rarity of bone involvement at presenta-tion would argue against routine bone scan-ning; however, symptomatic patients should have plain X-rays of the relevant bone and also bone scan.

Gallium-67 localizes to affected nodes in 80–90% of patients (Johnson *et al.*, 1977). It is also taken up in non-malignant conditions such as sarcoid, pyogenic infection and other inflammatory processes. High dose gallium improves the sensitivity (Anderson *et al.*, 1983). This technique is used especially in monitoring response to treatment and in the evaluation of a mass residual after treatment (Karimjee *et al.*, 1992).

MRI has been extensively investigated in Hodgkin's disease and also has some value in the evaluation of a residual mass. It is also es-pecially useful in evaluating neurological lesions.

18.6.2 STAGING LAPAROTOMY

In the past when localization of all sites of Hodgkin's disease was critical for the delin-eation of radiation fields, the staging of Hodgkin's disease was further refined by the performance of a staging laparotomy during which para-aortic lymph node biopsy and splenectomy were performed for histological assessment of intra-abdominal spread. This technique showed that about one-third of patients presenting with clinical stage I or II Hodgkin's disease had occult involvement of the spleen and about 3% had occult involvement of the liver. The spleen is involved in approximately the same proportion of infra-diaphragmatic presentations, though in these patients there is a strong correlation between radiological evidence of para-aortic disease and splenic involvement (Barrett *et al.*, 1981). Staging laparotomy is now rarely performed in the UK for the following reasons :

1. Even when the laparotomy is negative, if the patient is treated with mantle radiotherapy the abdomen is the commonest site of recurrence.
2. Other prognostic factors have enabled the decision to be made about using combination chemotherapy.
3. Staging laparotomy is a major operation, and there is concern over the long term health hazards of splenectomy, including risk of infection and leukaemogenesis.

The era of staging laparotomy provided considerable information about the natural history of Hodgkin's disease and in particular allowed construction of models predicting abdominal involvement risk based on other clinical presentation factors (Table 18.1).

The Ann Arbor staging classification is used for Hodgkin's disease (Carbone *et al.*, 1971) and is shown in Table 18.2. The stage number has a prefix indicating whether the staging is based on clinical and radiological investigations (Clinical Stage – Key CS) or on staging laparotomy (Pathological Stage – PS). The number also has a suffix which indicates whether one of the following symptoms is absent (A) or present (B). These symptoms are unexplained weight loss of more than 10% of the original body weight, profuse night sweats and recurrent fever greater than 38°C. With the original classification, local extension from an involved node was not felt to be an adverse feature and it was therefore noted by the suffix (e) rather than changing the staging to stage IV. Diffuse extranodal involvement or multiple sites within the extranodal organ indicate stage IV. Further refinements of the Ann Arbor staging classification are the indication of the number of involved sites and also of splenic involvement, and the division of stage III into two groups based on the extent of nodal involvement (Desser *et al.*, 1977).

18.7 PROGNOSTIC FACTORS

A range of prognostic factors has been analysed and the following are some of those found to indicate an adverse prognosis; older

Table 18.1 Staging laparotomy: examples of use of prognostic index

Stage	Factor	No. observed	% Laparotomy positive observed
IA	F <50 LP/NS	236	11
	M <50 MC/LD	276	36
IIA	F LP/NS 2/3 areas Med +	650	20
	M MC/LD 2/3 areas Med +	98	50
IB + IIB	F Med + No EN	229	20
	M Med – No EN	134	51

Med +/– = Mediastinum involved/not involved
Source: the International Data Base on Hodgkin's Disease

Table 18.2   The Ann Arbor staging classification

Stage I	Involvement of a single lymph node region (I) or single extralymphatic site (IE)
Stage II	Involvement of two or more lymph node regions on the same side of the diaphragm (II), which may also include the spleen (IIS), localized extralymphatic involvement (IIE), or both (IISE), if confined to the same side of the diaphragm
Stage III	Involvement of lymph node regions on both sides of the diaphragm (III), which may also include the spleen (IIIS), localized extralymphatic involvement (IIIE), or both (IIISE)
Stage IV	Diffuse or disseminated involvement of extralymphatic site (e.g. bone marrow, liver or multiple pulmonary metastases)

age, MC or LD histology, raised ESR, multiple sites of involvement and a positive laparotomy. As shown in Table 18.1 prognostic factors can be used to identify the probability of staging laparotomy identifying widespread disease. Alternatively as shown in Table 18.3 the analysis can be of survival. The definition of adverse prognosis can define the need for more aggressive initial therapies. Thus in early stage Hodgkin's disease a prognostic factor analysis may help define the indications for combined chemotherapy and radiation and in advanced disease it can provide the indications for high dose chemotherapy. For example, Table 18.4 reveals the results of a multifactorial prognostic factor analysis in early Hodgkin's disease (Horwich *et al.*, 1986). This shows one way of stratifying prognosis in early stage Hodgkin's disease and other prognostic factor analyses have tended to use similar criteria (Sutcliffe *et al.*, 1985). Prognostic factor analysis can also be used to predict recurrence after radiotherapy alone, rather than to predict overall survival. In this setting factors such as bulky mediastinal disease or total number of nodal sites appear especially important (Verger *et al.*, 1988). Similarly it may be considered that an important determinant of the use of initial chemotherapy would be the possibility of successful salvage in those patients who subsequently relapsed. In practice, however, this group is difficult to identify at the outset since the major determinants of successful salvage

in this setting are the disease free interval and the extent of disease at relapse (Roach *et al.*, 1990).

18.8   TREATMENT

18.8.1   RADIOTHERAPY IN EARLY HODGKIN'S DISEASE

Standard radiotherapeutic treatment techniques in early Hodgkin's disease are based on the concept of subclinical disease spread to adjacent lymph node areas from more obviously enlarged nodes (Gilbert, 1939). This has provided the basis for extended radiation field techniques (Peters, 1950). The development of linear accelerators allowed large field techniques to ensure the homogeneous irradiation of lymph node chains (Kaplan, 1962). The mantle field is illustrated in Figure 18.1(a) and with the patient positioned with neck extended the field extends from the mastoid process superiorily to the level of the lower border of the T10 vertebral body inferiorily. The technique leads to irradiation of bilateral cervical and supraclavicular and axillary nodes together with mediastinal nodes, and should be planned using a supine simulator film since the mediastinal contour is posture dependent. The usual technique incorporates parallel opposed anterior and posterior portals shaped by the use of individually designed lung blocks.

Table 18.3   Analysis of prognosis in 238 adults with clinical stage I or II Hodgkin's disease (The Royal Marsden Hospital 1963–79)

Factor	Level	5 year % survival	
Age	< 40 years	86	
	40–59 years	82	$P < 0.001^*$
	≥ 60 years	70	
Sex	Male	81	$P = 0.06$
	Female	88	
Histology	Lymphocyte depleted	44	
	Mixed cellularity	82	$P = 0.007^+$
	Lymphocyte predominant	85	
	Nodular sclerosing	85	
Symptoms	A	86	$P = 0.03$
	B	75	
Number of involved sites‡	1	88	
	2	86	$P = 0.1^*$
	3	84	
	> 3	75	
Mediastinum‡	Not involved	83	
	< 1/3	92	$P > 0.1^{*\S}$
	≥ 1/3	77	
Peripheral node diameter‡	≥ 5 cm	81	$P > 0.1$
	< 5 cm	87	
Erythrocyte sedimentation rate‡	< 40 mm/hour	90	$P = 0.03$
	≥ 40 mm/hour	77	

*Test for trend.
+Heterogeneity test.
‡Based on 194 patients treated during 1970–79.
§≥ 1/3 significantly worse than < 1/3 ($P = 0.03$).

The corresponding field to treat infra-diaphagmatic nodes is called 'inverted-Y' field and treats the para-aortic and bilateral pelvic lymph nodes. If there has been no splenectomy the upper part of the field extends to the left lateral upper abdominal wall to include the spleen and splenic hilar nodes. Similarly, this is treated by anterior and posterior extended fields with lead shaping. Where both mantle and inverted-Y fields are employed the arrangement is called total nodal irradiation (TNI). Alternatively for some very good prognosis presentations or in the context of combined chemotherapy and radiotherapy for early Hodgkin's disease, the field is sometime restricted to encompass only enlarged lymph nodes and this is called 'involved field' (IF) irradiation.

Hodgkin's disease is highly radiosensitive and even large masses can be successfully treated with moderate doses of radiotherapy. In-field recurrence is uncommon at doses over 30 Gy given in daily fractions of 1.5–2 Gy, 5 days per week and the standard prescriptions are to doses between 35 and 40 Gy (Carmel and Kaplan, 1976; Hanks *et al.*,

Table 18.4 Prognosis of clinical stage I and II Hodgkin's disease (The Royal Marsden Hospital)

	Definition of group	Predicated 5 year survival
(A) One of	Age > 60 years Lymphocyte depleted histology > 3 sites Mediastinal/thoracic ratio > 1/3 Systemic symptoms	78%
(B) Two of	Erythrocyte sedimentation rate > 40 Male sex 3 sites Mixed cellularity histology	84%
(C)	Neither A nor B	92%

1982; Tubiana, *et al.*, 1984). In general these doses are well tolerated; however, there is a particular problem in the irradiation of bulky mediastinal masses, since even these doses are beyond lung tolerance, and this stimulated development of the technique of split course shrinking field radiotherapy.

Since the construction of individual lead blocks and their positioning represents a complex planning process, it is usual to verify

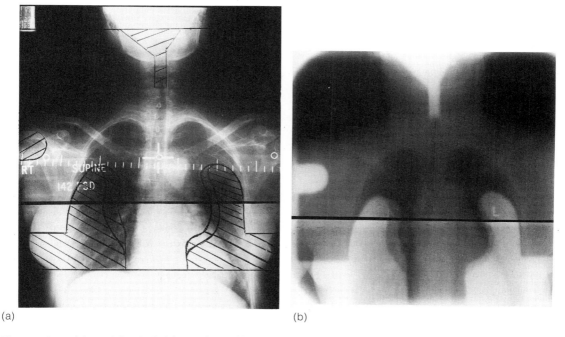

(a)   (b)

Figure 18.1 (a) Mantle field simulator film. The (L) buccal shield is small due to (L) cervical disease and the (L) humeral head is not shielded to avoid protecting (L) axillary nodes. The lung blocks are of dual thickness to allow partial transmission of radiation to lung adjacent to the hilar regions as shown by the check film (b) taken on the treatment set.

an appropriate treatment set-up by exposing a radiograph at the start of the first treatment representing the set-up of that treatment (Figure 18.1(b). In some centres this quality assurance measure is repeated each week during treatment.

18.8.2 TOXICITY OF RADIOTHERAPY

Though the total dose of radiation is not high, the large volume of tissue irradiated may be associated with general symptoms of fatigue, nausea and weight loss. Additionally there may be some skin reaction with erythema or even desquamation in sites of maximum dose build-up such as the lateral aspects of the neck and the axilla. During the second half of therapy some patients develop oesophagitis or hoarseness of the voice. Hair loss occurs within the field; this is usually restricted to the lower occipital region of the scalp and the beard area. With standard radiation doses hair growth recovers.

Bone marrow function is suppressed within the field, but this rarely causes significant changes in peripheral blood counts when a single extended field is employed, though total nodal irradiation can lead to more prolonged suppression and if radiotherapy is used following chemotherapy both the extent of suppression and its duration may be hazardous. Inverted-Y field may appear associated with some gastrointestinal side-effects, such as colicky pain, flatulence and diarrhoea.

The risk of late complications of radiotherapy for Hodgkin's disease depends on dose and technique. The severity of radiation pneumonitis is very much influenced by volume of lung within the field. This complication becomes apparent 2–12 months following radiotherapy, when acute pneumonitis may be palliated with a combination of steroids and antibiotics. Even without symptoms of acute pneumonitis some patients would progress to a paramediastinal fibrosis, leading typically to a long term distortion of the chest X-ray appearances and a narrow appearing mediastinum.

There are two types of cardiac toxicity described, coronary artery fibrosis and myocardial fibrosis. Additionally pericarditis can occur. At conventional doses if equally weighted anterior and posterior mediastinal portals are employed daily, cardiac toxicity is extremely rare. Myocardial PET scanning using gallium-201 suggested a reduction in myocardial perfusion in two-thirds of patients treated with mediastinal radiotherapy (Maunoury *et al.*, 1992). Upper gastrointestinal toxicity from radiotherapy occurs predominately in patients who have had a staging laparotomy (Hayat, 1984).

Because of the low doses of radiotherapy spinal cord toxicity is uncommon, though considerable caution must be exercised when matching adjacent extended fields to avoid a localized area of overdose, which might cause transverse myelitis. However, a common neurological side-effect of treatment is a syndrome resembling Lhermittes. This can occur several months after completion of radiotherapy and may last several months more, but it does not progress to transverse myelitis. Major skeletal toxicity can occur following moderate doses of radiation in the patient who has not completed bone growth.

18.8.3 RADIOTHERAPY RESULTS

Overall 10 year survival probabilities following radical radiotherapy for stage I and II Hodgkin's disease are of the order of 90% (Hellman and Mauch, 1982; Hoppe *et al.*, 1982; Verger *et al.*, 1988; Tubiana, *et al.*, 1989).

18.9 TREATMENT WITH CHEMOTHERAPY

The activity of single agent or two drug combinations in Hodgkin's disease was known for some two to three decades, before the drug combination of mustine, vincristine, procarbazine and prednisolone (MOPP) was developed by DeVita and colleagues and

Table 18.5 Combination regimens for Hodgkin's disease

MOPP	Mustine hydrochloride	6 mg/m^2	i.v. on days 1 and 8
	Vincristine	1.4 mg/m^2	i.v. on days 1 and 8
	Procarbazine	100 mg/m^2	Orally daily on days 1–14 incl.
	Prednisolone	40 mg	Orally daily on days 1–14 incl.
	Cycle = 28 days		
MVPP	Mustine hydrochloride	6 mg/m^2	i.v. on days 1 and 8
	Vinblastine	6 mg/m^2	i.v. on days 1 and 8
	Procarbazine	100 mg/m^2	Orally daily on days 1–14 incl.
	Prednisolone	40 mg	Orally daily on days 1–14 incl.
	Cycle = 42 days		
ChIVPP	Chlorambucil	6 mg/m^2	Orally daily on days 1–14 incl.
	Vinblastine	6 mg/m^2	i.v. on days 1 and 8
	Procarbazine	100 mg/m^2	Orally daily on days 1–14 incl.
	Prednisolone	40 mg	Orally daily on days 1–14 incl.
	Cycle = 28 days		
ABVD	Adriamycin	25 mg/m^2	i.v. on days 1 and 15
	Bleomycin	10 u/m^2	i.v. on days 1 and 15
	Vinblastine	6 mg/m^2	i.v. on days 1 and 15
	DTIC	375 mg/m^2	i.v. on days 1 and 15
	Cycle = 28 days		

proved to be curative in a large proportion of patients (DeVita *et al.*, 1970). The first report indicated that 81% of 43 previously untreated patients had complete remission, and in a follow-up report on 198 patients, 55% of all treated patients remained in remission for more than 5 years.

Major developments since MOPP have included firstly, an attempt to reduce its toxicity by the substitution of nitrogen mustard by chlorambucil in the CLVPP regimen (chlorambucil, vinblastine, procarbazine and prednisolone) (Nicholson *et al.*, 1970; Dady *et al.*, 1982) and secondly, a completely distinct and highly active combination of adriamycin, bleomycin, vinblastine and DTIC (ABVD) was devised (Bonadonna *et al.*, 1982) (Table 18.5). As shown in Table 18.6 these combinations have distinct side-effects. There is some variation in how these drugs are administered but in general MOPP is given to a total of 6 cycles with intravenous mustine and vincristine on days 1 and 8 of the cycle and with the oral medications on days 1 through 14.

ABVD on the other hand is given by injection once every 14 days. Optimal treatment is dependent on the ability to administer full dose chemotherapy according to the correct time schedule.

With most schedules based on these combinations the complete remission rate varies from 50 to 80% but somewhere between one-third and one-half of patients achieving a complete response subsequently relapse, usually within 5 years.

More recently the idea evolved that alternating non-cross-resistant chemotherapy schedules would improve survival, because of the earlier treatment of tumour stem cells resistant to the initial regimen. A large CALGB study randomized patients between MOPP chemotherapy, ABVD chemotherapy and the combination of MOPP alternating with ABVD (Canellos *et al.*, 1992). The results from this trial are shown in Table 18.7. Although MOPP chemotherapy appeared inferior it was noted that significantly reduced drug doses were administered in successive

Table 18.6   Chemotherapy toxicity

Regimen	Early	Late
ChIVPP	Bone marrow suppression	Leukaemogenesis
	Neuropathy	
ABVD	Bone marrow suppression	Cardiomyopathy
	Nausea and vomiting	
	Alopecia	
	Pneumonitis (if RT)	
VBM	Bone marrow suppression	?
	Pneumonitis (if RT)	

cycles of this chemotherapy. There remains no significant difference between ABVD and the alternating regimen. MOPP-like regimens have a different toxicity profile to ABVD, and in particular the CLVPP regimen represents a combination with minimal side-effects, the majority of patients suffering no nausea, vomiting or hair loss. However, the problems with MOPP-like regimens stem from the alkylating agents causing sterility and leukaemogenesis.

Fertility is discussed in Chapter 16. However, it is clear that the vast majority of men treated with MOPP or one of its variants will develop azoospermia. Induction of amenorrhoea in women is highly age dependent, being rare in patients treated under the age of 22 years and relatively common in patients treated over the age of 30 years (Chapman *et al.*, 1981). ABVD is said not be associated with infertility.

18.10   SECOND CANCERS

As shown in Table 18.8 the treatment of Hodgkin's disease is clearly associated with an increase of second cancers. These may be categorized as acute non-lymphatic leukaemias, non-Hodgkin's lymphomas or second tumours. The large International Database on Hodgkin's Disease (IDHD) has been able to link leukaemia with the use of alkylating agent combination chemotherapy with an even greater risk in patients also

Table 18.7   Results of CALGB chemotherapy trial in stages III and IV Hodgkin's disease

Regimen	Cycles (no.)	Patients (no.)	CR (%)	5 year failure free survival (%)	5 year survival (%)
MOPP	6–8	123	67	50	66
MOPP/ABVD	12	123	83	65	75
ABVD	6–8	115	82	61	73

CR, Complete remission; CALGB, Cancer and Leukaemia Group B.

Table 18.8 Hodgkin's disease: second cancers
IDHD[a]

Cancer	Males			Females		
	O[b]	O/E[c]	P	O	O/E	P
All	410	2.98	< 0.001	221	2.58	< 0.001
Leukaemia	102	28.58	< 0.001	56	25.66	< 0.001
Non-Hodgkin's lymphoma	79	35.55	<0.001	27	24.22	< 0.001

Significant excess of solid tumours of bronchus, skin (Normal), salivary gland, breast and, in men only, thyroid and intestine.
[a]IDHD – International Database on Hodgkin's Disease
[b]O – Observed
[c]E – Expected

having radiotherapy. For non-Hodgkin's lymphoma there is a close association with an original diagnosis of lymphocyte predominant Hodgkin's disease and recently it has been suggested that a considerable proportion of patients with LP Hodgkin's disease may in reality have a form of non-Hodgkin's lymphoma. The increased incidence of solid tumours has been linked to the use of wide field radiation; however, one large cohort study of lung cancer following Hodgkin's disease reported there to be a higher risk associated with the use of chemotherapy than with the use of radiotherapy (Kaldor *et al.*, 1992).

Other chemotherapy complications

Both MOPP and ABVD regimens cause bone marrow suppression and other common complications associated with MOPP include alopecia, thrombophlebitis and peripheral neuropathy. If mustine is replaced by chlorambucil it is rare for the patient to suffer significant nausea, thrombophlebitis or alopecia. With ABVD there is an increased risk of cardiac toxicity secondary to adriamycin and of lung toxicity secondary to bleomycin and both of these would be exacerbated by mediastinal radiotherapy.

18.11 COMBINED MODALITY THERAPY FOR HODGKIN'S DISEASE

As previously discussed the traditional treatment for localized Hodgkin's disease has been with extended field radiotherapy. However, whether or not the patient has had a staging laparotomy a common site of recurrence is within the abdomen and the appreciation that Hodgkin's disease was frequently more widespread than was at first suspected made it logical to evaluate combined modality therapy, adding combination chemotherapy to achieve spatial cooperation with localized irradiation by eradicating subclinical metastases. As shown in Table 18.9 the policy is certainly successful in reducing recurrence rates after initial treatment; however, there has very rarely been a survival difference demonstrated, and this is because of the ability of combination chemotherapy to salvage patients relapsing after initial radiation therapy.

Though in many respects, a reduction in the number of patients relapsing is a highly desirable subjugate endpoint for survival, there is concern about the additive toxicity of employing both modalities. This is being mitigated by a reduction in the total dose of each modality, e.g. the combination of 2–4 cycles of chemotherapy with involved field irradiation. A separate development has been the evolution of

Table 18.9 Randomized trials of combined modality therapy for early Hodgkin's disease

Reference	Patients	Therapy	Actuarial RFS	Survival differences
Hoppe *et al.*, 1982	PSI and II	TNI RT and MOPP	NSD (10 years)	NSD
Coltman and Dixon, 1982	PSI and II	EF IF and MOPP	68% (5 years) 81% (5 years)	NSD
Nissen and Nordentoft, 1982	PSI and II	TNI M and MOPP	70% (8 years) 90% (8 years)	NSD
Tubiana *et al.*, 1989	Clinical stages I and II	TNI TNI and MOPP	76% (4 years) 87% (4 years)	NSD
Pavlovsky *et al.*, 1988	Clinical stages I and II, F	CVPP CVPP and RT	76% (7 years) 70% (7 years)	NSD
	UnF	CVPP CVPP and RT	34% (7 years) 75% (7 years)	66% 84%
Anderson *et al.*, 1983	PSI and II	M M and MOPP	67% (10 years)	NSD

PS, pathological stage; UnF, unfavourable prognosis; F, favourable prognosis; TNI, total nodal irradiation; RT, radiotherapy; EF, extended field radiotherapy; IF, involved field radiotherapy; M, mantle field radiotherapy; MOPP, mustard, vincristine, prednisolone, procarbazine; CVPP, cyclophosphamide, vinblastine, prednisolone, procarbazine; NSD, no significant difference.

alternative drug regimens for Hodgkin's disease designed to reduce toxicity, and a good example of this is the combination of vinblastin, methotrexate and bleomycin (VBM) designed at Stanford University Medical School (Horning *et al.*, 1988). Patients with pathological stage IA, IIA or IIIA Hodgkin's disease were treated with involved field radiotherapy followed by 6 cycles of VBM and 95% of patients remained free from any evidence of progression. Since the combination had little adverse effect on either male or female fertility other studies of these agents are currently underway.

The major comparison of combined chemotherapy and radiotherapy with chemotherapy alone was performed by Pavlovsky *et al.* (1988). This was a randomized trial in stage I and II Hodgkin's disease of chemotherapy using cyclophosphamide, vinblastin, prednisone and procarbazine, versus the same combination followed by radiotherapy. There was little difference in either relapse free survival or survival in patients with a relatively good prognosis, however, for those with unfavourable presentations (Table 18.9) there was a large difference in actuarial relapse free survival (75% vs 34% at 7 years) and in survival (84% vs 66% at 10 years), favouring combined chemotherapy and radiotherapy.

Additionally chemotherapy alone has been used in early Hodgkin's disease and compared with radiotherapy. The Northern Italy trial (Cimino *et al.*, 1992) compared 6 cycles of MOPP with extended field radiotherapy. Forty-five patients were treated with radiotherapy and 44 with MOPP. Complete remission was achieved in all the patients having radiotherapy and in 40 of 44 patients having MOPP. Ten of 44 patients treated with MOPP died of Hodgkin's disease compared with only 2 of 45 in the radiotherapy group. The difference in survival was attributed to a difficulty in salvaging patients who had relapsed after initial MOPP therapy.

In conclusion combined modality therapy is widely employed for adverse presentations in

stages I and II and especially those presenting with systemic symptoms, bulky mediastinal disease or multiple sites of involvement. It is also widely used for clinical stage III Hodgkin's disease (Brada *et al.*, 1989) and is an experimental approach to stages IIIB and IV disease based on patterns of relapse after chemotherapy alone which tend to be in previously involved sites.

Stage IIIB and stage IV Hodgkin's disease

The main approach to treatment is with combination chemotherapy. As discussed above it would appear that ABVD chemotherapy is as effective as alternating combinations. Postchemotherapy irradiation has been employed at relatively low radiation dose levels and with excellent results (Prosnitz *et al.*, 1982; Vose *et al.*, 1991).

18.12 SALVAGE THERAPY

Patients failing initial chemotherapy for advanced Hodgkin's disease have a relatively poor prognosis (Fisher *et al.*, 1979). Patients having MOPP chemotherapy can be salvaged with ABVD especially if there was complete remission to initial therapy, a long disease free interval and no systemic symptoms (Santoro *et al.*, 1982). Patients with a limited extent of disease at relapse may benefit from radiotherapy (Brada *et al.*, 1992).

Patients failing two previous chemotherapy regimens have a worse prognosis and are candidates for investigation of high dose chemotherapy using haemopoietic stem cell support. A recent trial suggests that this approach, based on high doses of BCNU, etoposide, cytosine arabinoside and melphalan (BEAM) carries a better prognosis than if patients are treated with these agents at conventional dose levels (Linch *et al.*, 1993).

18.13 CONCLUSIONS

Hodgkin's disease presents a particular challenge to the oncologists, requiring as it does the appropriate deployment of surgery, chemotherapy and radiotherapy in the assessment and treatment of patients who present with a broad spectrum of disease severity. There is particular opportunity to tailor the treatment to the individual patient and their disease, in order to maximize the chances of cure and minimize the risk of severe morbidity. The relative rarity of this illness should encourage the treatment of patients within collaborative trials in order to improve management in the future, and the major current issues include the design of an appropriate chemotherapy regimen for initial combined modality therapy, the modification of chemotherapy and radiotherapy principles in the setting of combined modalities, the design of more effective combination drug regimens in advanced Hodgkin's disease and the development of safe salvage protocols for the patients who have failed initial therapy. It is clear that the relapse pattern of Hodgkin's disease may be slow and this together with the possibility of long term morbidity of treatment suggest the need for prolonged and careful follow-up of all patients.

REFERENCES

Anderson, K.C., Leonard, R.C.F. and Canellos, G.P. (1983) High dose gallium imaging in lymphoma. *American Journal of Medicine*, **75**, 327–31.

Barrett, A., Gregor, A., McElwain, T.J. and Peckham, M.J. (1981) Infradiaphragmatic presentation of Hodgkin's disease. *Clinical Radiology*, **32**, 221–4.

Bennett, M.H., MacLennan, K.A., Easterling, M.J. *et al.* (1983) The prognostic significance of cellular subtypes in nodular sclerosing Hodgkin's disease: an analysis of 271 non-laparotomised cases (BNLI Report No. 22). *Clinical Radiology*, **34**, 497–501.

Bonadonna, G., Santoro, A., Bonfante, V. and Valagussa, P. (1982) Cyclic delivery of MOPP and ABVD combinations in stage IV Hodgkin's disease: rationale, background studies, and recent results. *Cancer Treatment Report*, **66**, 881–7.

Brada, M., Ashley, S., Nicholls, J. *et al.* (1989) Stage III Hodgkin's disease – long-term results following chemotherapy, radiotherapy and combined modality therapy. *Radiotherapy and Oncology*, **14**, 185–98.

Brada, M., Eeles, R., Ashley, S. *et al.* (1992) Salvage radiotherapy in recurrent Hodgkin's disease. *Annals of Oncology*, **3**, 131–5.

Canellos, G.P., Anderson, J.R., Propert, K.J. *et al.* (1992) Chemotherapy of advanced Hodgkin's disease with MOPP, ABVD, or MOPP alternating with ABVD. *New England Journal of Medicine*, **327**, 1478–84.

Carbone, P.P., Kaplan, H.S., Musshoff, K. *et al.* (1971) Report of the committee on Hodgkin's disease staging classification. *Cancer Research*, **31**, 1860–1.

Carmel, R.J. and Kaplan, H.S. (1976) Mantle irradiation in Hodgkin's disease. An analysis of technique, tumour eradication and complications. *Cancer*, **37**, 2813–15.

Chapman, R.M., Sutcliffe, S.B. and Mapas, J.S. (1981) Male gonadal dysfunction in Hodgkin's disease. *Journal of the American Medical Association*, **245**, 1323–28.

Cimino, G., Biti, G.P., Cartoni, C. and Magrini, S.M. (1992) Chemotherapy versus radiotherapy in early-stage Hodgkin's disease: evidence of a more difficult rescue for patients relapsed after chemotherapy. *European Journal of Cancer*, **28A**, 1853–5.

Coltman, C.A., Jr and Dixon, D.O. (1982). Second malignancies complicating Hodgkin's disease a southwest oncology group ten year follow-up. *Cancer Treatment Report*, **66**, 1023–33.

Dady, P.J., McElwain, T.J., Austin, D.E. *et al.* (1982) Five years experience with ChIVPP: effective low-toxicity combination chemotherapy for Hodgkin's disease. *British Journal of Cancer*, **45**, 851–59.

DeVita, V.T., Serpick, A.A. and Carbone, P.P. (1970) Combination chemotherapy in the treatment of advanced Hodgkin's disease. *Annals of Internal Medicine*, **73**, 881–95.

Desforges, J.F., Rutherford, C.J. and Piro, A. (1979) Hodgkin's disease. *New England Journal of Medicine*, **301**, 1212–22.

Desser, R.K., Golomb, H.M., Ultmann, J.E. *et al.* (1977) Prognostic classification of Hodgkin's disease in pathologic stage III, based on anatomical considerations. *Blood*, **49**, 883–93.

Fisher, R., DeVita, V. and Hubbard, S.P. (1979) Prolonged disease free survival in Hodgkin's disease with MOPP reinduction after first relapse. *Annals of Internal Medicine*, **90**, 761–3.

Gilbert, R. (1939) Radiotherapy in Hodgkin's disease (malignant granulomatosis): anatomic and clinical foundations; governing principles; results. *American Journal of Roentgenology*, **41**, 198–241.

Gutensohn Mueller, N.E. and Cole, P. (1977) Epidemiology of Hodgkin's disease in the young. *International Journal of Cancer*, **19**, 595–604.

Hanks, R.E., Kinzie, J.J., Herring, D.F. and Kramer, S. (1982) Patterns of care outcome studies in Hodgkin's disease: results of the national practice and implications for management. *Cancer Treatment*, **66**, 805–8.

Hayat, M. (1984) Long-term follow-up of patients with clinical stages I, II Hodgkin's disease: comparison of initial splenectomy and spleen irradiation. Proceedings of the Second International Conference of Malignant Lymphoma, Lugano (Abstract 25).

Hellman, S. and Mauch, P. (1982) Role of radiation therapy in the treatment of Hodgkin's disease. *Cancer Treatment Report*, **66**, 915–23.

Henderson, B.E, Dworsky, R., Pike, M.C. *et al.* (1979) Risk factors for modular sclerosis and other types of Hodgkin's disease. *Cancer Research*, **39**, 4507–511.

Hoover, R., Mason, T.J., McKay, F.W. and Fraumeni, J.F.J. (1975) Geographic patterns of cancer mortality in the United States, in *Persons at High Risk of Cancer: an approach to cancer etiology and control*, (ed. J.F. Fraumeni Jr), Academic Press, New York, pp. 343–60).

Hoppe, R.T., Coleman, C.N., Cox, R.S. *et al.* (1982). The management of stage I-II Hodgkin's disease with irradiation alone or combined modality therapy: the Stanford experience. *Blood*, **59**, 455–65.

Horning, S.J., Hoppe, R.T., Hancock, S.L. and Rosenberg, S.A. (1988) Vinblastine, bleomycin and methotrexate: an effective adjuvant in favorable Hodgkin's disease. *Journal of Clinical Oncology*, **6**, 1822–31.

Horwich, A., Easton, D., Nogueira-Costa, R. *et al.* (1986). An analysis of prognostic factors in early stage Hodgkin's disease. *Radiotherapy and Oncology*, **7**, 95–106.

Johnson, G.S., Go, M.F. and Benua, R.S. (1977) Gallium-67 citrate imaging in Hodgkin's disease. Final report of Cooperative Group. *Journal of Nuclear Medicine*, **18**, 693–9.

Kaldor, J.M., Day, N.E., Bell, J. *et al.* (1992) Lung cancer following Hodgkin's disease: a case-control study. *International Journal of Cancer*, **52**, 677–81.

Kaplan, H.S. (1962) The radical radiotherapy of regionally localized Hodgkin's disease. *Radiology*, **78**, 553–61.

Karimjee, S., Brada, M., Husband, J. and McCready, V.R. (1992) A comparison of Gallium-67 single photon emission computed tomography and computed tomography in mediastinal Hodgkin's disease. *European Journal of Cancer*, **28A**, 1856–57.

Kennedy, C.L., Husband, J.E. and Bellamy, E.A. (1985) The accuracy of CT scanning prior to para-aortic lymphadenectomy in patients with bulky metastases from testicular teratoma. *British Journal of Urology*, **57**, 755–8.

Linch, D.C., Winfield, D., Goldstone, A.H. *et al.* (1993) Dose intensification with autologous bone-marrow transplantation in relapsed and resistant Hodgkin's disease: results of a BNLI randomised trial. *Lancet*, **341**, 1051–4.

Lukes, R.J. and Butler, J.J. (1966) The pathology and nomenclature of Hodgkin's disease. *Cancer Research*, **26**, 1063–83.

Maunoury, C., Pierga, J.Y., Valette, H. *et al.* (1992) Myocardial perfusion damage after mediastinal irradiation for Hodgkin's disease: a thallium-201 single photon emission tomography study. *European Journal of Nuclear Medicine*, **19**, 871–3.

Nicholson, W.M., Beard, M.E.J., Crowther, D. *et al.* (1970) Combination chemotherapy in generalized Hodgkin's disease. *British Medical Journal*, **3**, 7–10.

Nissen, N.I. and Nordentoft, A.M. (1982) Radiotherapy versus combined modality treatment of stage I and II Hodgkin's disease. *Cancer Treatment Report*, **66**, 799–803.

Pavlovsky, S., Maschio, M., Santarelli, M.T. *et al.* (1988) Randomized trial of chemotherapy versus chemotherapy plus radiotherapy for stage I–II Hodgkin's disease. *Journal of the National Cancer Institute*, **80**, 1466–73.

Peters, M.V. (1950) A study of survivals in Hodgkin's disease treated radiologically. *American Journal of Roentgenology*, **63**, 299–311.

Prosnitz, L.R., Farber, L.R., Kapp, D.S. *et al.* (1982) Combined modality therapy for advanced Hodgkin's disease: long term follow-up data. *Cancer Treatment Report*, **66**, 871–9.

Roach, M., Brophy, N. and Cox, R. (1990) Prognostic factors for patients relapsing after radiotherapy for early-stage Hodgkin's disease. *Journal of Clinical Oncology*, **8**, 623–9.

Santoro, A., Bonadonna, G., Bonfante, V. and Valagussa, P. (1982) Alternating drug combinations in the treatment of advanced Hodgkin's disease. *New England Journal of Medicine*, **306**, 770–5.

Sutcliffe, S.B., Gospodarowicz, M., Bergsagel, D.E. *et al.* (1985) Prognostic groups for management of localized Hodgkin's disease. *Journal of Clinical Oncology*, **3**, 393–401.

Tubiana, M., Henry-Amar, M., Carde, P. *et al.* (1989) Toward comprehensive management tailored to prognostic factors of patients with clinical stages I and II in Hodgkin's disease. The EORTC Lymphoma Group controlled clinical trials, 1964–1987. *Blood*, **73**, 47–56.

Tubiana, M., Henry-Amar, M., Hayat, M. *et al.* (1984) The EORTC treatment of early stages of Hodgkin's disease:

the role of radiotherapy. *International Journal of Radiation Oncology, Biology, Physics*, **10**, 197–210.

Verger, E., Easton, D., Brada, M. *et al.* (1988) Radiotherapy results in laparotomy staged early Hodgkin's disease. *Clinical Radiology*, **39**, 428–31.

Vianna, N.J., Greenwald, P., Brady, J. *et al.* (1972) Hodgkin's disease: cases with features of a community outbreak. *Annals of Internal Medicine*, **77**, 169–80.

Vose, J.M., Bierman, P.J., Anderson, J.R. *et al.* (1991) CHLVPP chemotherapy with involved-field irradiation for Hodgkin's disease: favorable results with acceptable toxicity. *Journal of Clinical Oncology*, **9**, 1421–5.

Martin J.S. Dyer

19.1 INTRODUCTION

The non-Hodgkin's lymphomas (NHL) are, as the negative description implies, an extremely diverse collection of tumours. They comprise the solid tumours of 'mature', antigen receptor bearing lymphocytes of both B- and T-cell lineages as well as the rare tumours of histiocytes. Their phenotypic diversity is reflected in their biological diversity: some patients may survive for many months or even years with little or no therapy, whilst others with rapidly progressive, chemotherapy resistant disease may survive only a few weeks.

Over the past decade, the new genetics and in particular the molecular analysis of the common recurrent chromosomal translocations has defined several molecular events of importance in the pathogenesis and progression of NHL. It is now possible to understand the biological heterogeneity of NHL in terms of mutation, deregulated expression and/or loss of function of several crucial genes. These advances have both diagnostic and possible therapeutic implications and will form the primary focus of this short chapter.

The interested reader is referred to Magrath (1990a), an excellent textbook.

19.2 FIRST STEPS

The clinical manifestations of the NHL are protean. Precise diagnosis and therapy depend on adequate biopsy material and accurate staging. Histological examination of biopsied lymph node forms the basis of diagnosis, although this should now be supplemented routinely with immunological, cytogenetic and molecular genetic analyses (see below).

The basic distinction to be drawn is between those tumours which retain a follicular growth pattern, resembling normal germinal centres and which are generally low grade tumours, and those which do not (generally high grade tumours).

19.2.1 FOLLICULAR NHL

These NHL need to be differentiated from 'reactive' follicular hyperplasia, which may not be trivial. Follicular NHL are invariably of the B-cell lineage. More than 80% have the translocation t(14;18)(q32.3;q21.3) which deregulates expression of the BCL-2 gene. They generally follow a waxing and waning clinical course. Most are widely disseminated at presentation. The slow growth of these tumours often allows therapy to be deferred until clinically indicated, even in young patients. Control and even remission of follicular NHL is often possible with oral alkylating agents (chlorambucil) but the majority of patients continue to relapse with time. Rare, spontaneous remissions have also been well documented. These NHL are ideal targets for experimental therapies with antibodies or other biological agents.

Two further points should be considered:

1. Follicular NHL may depend on stimulation by T cells for continued proliferation *in vivo* (Umetsu *et al.*, 1990).

2. Follicular NHL transform to high grade lymphomas or even acute leukaemias at a variable rate. Such transformation is associated with survival of less than a year.

19.2.2   DIFFUSE NHL

These have a far more aggressive clinical course and require intensive therapy. Nevertheless many present with genuinely localized disease and up to 50% are potentially curable with combination chemotherapy. For those who relapse or who fail to achieve remission the outlook remains grim and the value of 'salvage' chemotherapy is debatable. Palliation with steroids, either high or low dose, can often be achieved.

Eighty per cent of cases are of the B-cell lineage, 15% of the T-cell lineage, with only rare cases truly representing histiocytic malignancies.

19.2.3   CLINICAL STAGING

Staging of the NHL is performed as for Hodgkin's disease using the Ann Arbor scheme. Essential staging studies are:

1. History and physical examination
2. ENT examination
3. Chest X-ray
4. (Thoracic) Abdominal/pelvic CT scan
5. ECG
6. Urea and electrocytes/LFTs + calcium
7. LDH/uric acid/albumin
8. FBC
9. Bone marrow aspirate and trephine.

19.3   EPIDEMIOLOGY AND AETIOLOGY

There are approximately 4500 new cases of NHL per annum in the UK. Most occur in the elderly in whom intensive high dose chemotherapy is inappropriate. (Figure 19.1) In contrast to the peak incidence of B-cell and T-cell precursor acute lymphoblastic leukaemia (ALL) in childhood, paediatric NHL (of

mature T/B cells) is rare and represents a different biological spectrum of disease from NHL of adults (Ribeiro *et al.*, 1992). The increasing incidence with age is accounted for predominantly by the increase in the number of cases of follicular NHL. For reasons which are unknown follicular NHL is genuinely rare in the Orient and in developing countries.

The pathogenesis of NHL remains unknown. A viral component has been recognized in three situations:

1. Epstein–Barr virus (EBV) infection in endemic Burkitt's lymphoma in equatorial Africa (Magrath, 1990b).
2. HTLV-1 retrovirus in adult T-cell lymphoma/leukaemia (ATLL) seen principally in South Western Japan and the Caribbean basin (Kuefler and Bunn, 1986).
3. NHL arising as a consequence of prolonged immunosuppression either following transplant (Cleary and Sklar, 1984) or HIV infection/AIDS (Ballerini *et al.*, 1993).

The last group has been projected to comprise up to 20% of NHL cases in the USA. These NHL are almost invariably B-cell neoplasms and arise on a 'background' of chronic polyclonal B-cell proliferation. AIDS NHLs are aggressive malignancies, many of which are identical to Burkitt's lymphoma and have a particularly poor prognosis.

None of these viruses appear to transform cells directly *in vivo*. For example, only about 1 in 1000 individuals infected with HTLV-1 will go on to develop ATLL; other unknown factors are necessary.

Evidence for a viral aetiology of other NHLs is lacking.

19.4   CLASSIFICATION

The purposes of disease classification are to bring together similar cases to define common pathogenic mechanisms and disease specific therapies. In the ALLs, the combination of immunophenotypic, cytogenetic and molecular genetic analyses has allowed the

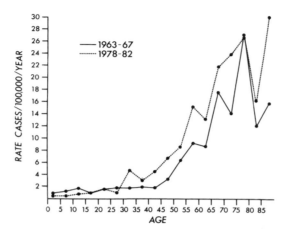

Figure 19.1 Age distribution of NHL in the UK.———, 1963–67; ......, 1978–82. Data from Barnes *et al.* (1986) with permission.

identification of particular subgroups of disease associated with a poor prognosis and allowed for the rational and effective introduction of alternative therapies such as allogenic bone marrow transplantation in first remission.

In comparison, the definition of comparable prognostic subgroups in NHL remains in its infancy. Classification of the NHLs, particularly in the UK, remains rooted in histological examination of fixed tumour biopsy sections; formalin fixation precludes detailed immunophenotypic and genetic analyses. Systematic application of the techniques of the 'new biology' has however begun to define new subtypes of disease, and should eventually provide for a system of classification of comparable biological significance to that seen in ALL.

19.4.1 HISTOLOGICAL CLASSIFICATION

Classification of the NHL by histological examination alone has produced a plethora of schemes of varying complexity. None of these are satisfactory. 'The Working Formulation', the result of an international study comparing the six major classification schemes extant in 1982, is shown in Table 19.1. Whilst these

groupings are to a degree necessarily subjective and also many cases fall outside the recognized patterns, such schemes do form a useful 'framework', and expert histopathological opinion of optimally preserved biopsy material remains (and will remain) the cornerstone of diagnosis in NHL.

19.4.2 IMMUNOLOGICAL CLASSIFICATION

The development of monoclonal antibodies (MAb) against leucocyte differentiation antigens has allowed not only objective assessment of lineage (B-cell vs T-cell vs histiocyte), but also in B-cell NHL the assessment of clonality through demonstration of restricted expression of immunoglobulin (Ig) κ or λ light chain expression. A list of some of the MAb useful in the diagnosis of B-cell NHL is shown in Table 19.2. Therapeutic attempts have been made with many of these MAbs. Similarly, the functions of many of these antigens are now becoming known: this may allow for the development of other novel targeted therapies.

When considering NHL diagnosis, most MAb will only function either on cell suspensions or freshly frozen tissue: formalin fixation destroys the antigenic determinants

Table 19.1 A working formulation of NHL for clinical use: recommendations of an expert international panel

LOW GRADE

A Small lymphocytic consistent with CLL
  plasmacytoid
B FOLLICULAR: predominantly small cleaved
  cell
C FOLLICULAR: mixed small cleaved and
  large cell

INTERMEDIATE GRADE

D FOLLICULAR: predominantly large cell
E DIFFUSE: small cleaved cell
  (MANTLE-ZONE
  LYMPHOMA)
F DIFFUSE: mixed small and large cell
G DIFFUSE: **large cell**
  cleaved cell
  non-cleaved cell

HIGH GRADE

H DIFFUSE: **large cell, immunoblastic**
  plasmacytoid
  clear cell
  epitheliod cell component
I DIFFUSE: **lymphoblastic**
  convoluted cell
  non-convoluted cell
J DIFFUSE: **small non-cleaved cell**
  Burkitt's lymphoma
  follicular areas

MISCELLANEOUS: COMPOSITE
  MYCOSIS FUNGOIDES
  HISTIOCYTIC
  EXTRAMEDULLARY
    PLASMACYTOMA
  UNCLASSIFIABLE
  OTHER

From Rosenberg *et al.*, 1982 with permission. Note that the Working Formulation distinguishes between low, intermediate and high grade NHL, whereas nearly all clinical studies discriminate only between low and high grade disease. For these practical purposes Working Formulation groups D and E are generally included amongst low grade diseases with F and G being included amongst the high grade.

recognized by MAb. However, it may prove possible to produce MAb against formalin resistant determinants of some antigens. Secondly, NHL may for reasons which are unclear preferentially lose expression of differentiation antigens. T-cell NHL seem particularly susceptible in this regard and this may hinder diagnosis (Picker *et al.*, 1987).

A very readable, concise guide to the expression and function of the leucocyte differentiation antigens may be found in *The Leucocyte Antigen Facts Book* (Barclay *et al.*, 1993).

19.4.3 CYTOGENETIC AND MOLECULAR CYTOGENETIC CLASSIFICATION OF NHL (REVIEWED IN OFFIT, 1992)

A further development has been the finding of recurrent chromosomal abnormalities in the NHL. A list of some of these abnormalities is shown in Table 19.3 and an example of a transformed lymphoblastic lymphoma with t(14;18)(q32.3;q21.3) and multiple other chromosomal abnormalities is shown in Figure 19.2. In B-NHL, these translocations are specifically targeted to the Ig heavy and light chain chromosome loci, whereas in the T-NHL, the T-cell receptor (TCR) genes are similarly targeted. Such translocations may represent errors in the process of somatic recombination in which functional Ig and TCR genes are created.

Translocations are not specific for a specific histological subgroup. Translocations involving MYC on chromosome 8q24.1 are seen not only in Burkitt's lymphoma but also in other B-cell and rarely T-cell NHLs. Most NHLs with MYC translocations pursue a rapidly progressive course requiring intensive combination chemotherapy, and acquisition of MYC translocation has been shown to be directly associated with transformation from low grade to high grade NHL (de Jong *et al.*, 1988).

Nevertheless, a subgroup of B-NHL with t(8;14)(q24.1;q32.3) as the sole abnormality has been shown to follow an indolent clinical course. These data indicate that it is not the activation/deregulation of a single gene which determines biological behaviour but rather the concerted effects of several events

Table 19.2   Antibodies useful in the diagnosis of B-NHL

Antibody/antigen	Expression	Functions	NHL therapy
CD45	All haemopoietic cells Different isoforms expressed on different cell types (CD45RO on T-NHL)	Unknown: Phospho-tyrosine phosphatase	No
CDw52 (Campath-1)	All lymphoid cells/NHL except myeloma	Unknown	Yes
CD19	All B-cells/B-NHL BCP-ALL	B-cell signal transduction	Yes
CD37	Mature B-cells	Unknown	No
CD5	T-cells, B-cell subset B-CLL Mantle-zone B-NHL	Ligand for CD72 (a B-cell antigen)	Yes
CD10	B-cell/T-cell precursors Germline centre B-cells Epithelia BCP-ALL, follicular B-NHL	Neutral endopeptidase	Yes
Anti-immunoglobulin (anti-idiotypic)	Mature B-cells (clone specific)	Antigen receptor	Yes

Table 19.3   Cytogenetic classification of B-NHL

Deregulated gene/(chromosome)	Translocation	Distribution
MYC/8q24.1	t(8;14)(q24.1;q32.3) or t(8;22)(q24.1;q11) or t(2;8)(p11;q24.1)	All Burkitt's lymphoma 50–80% transformed low-grade B-NHL (secondary event) Rare low-grade B-NHL (primary event) Rare T-NHL
Cyclin D1/11q13 (BCL-1)	t(11;14)(q13;q32.3)	80% mantle-zone lymphoma 30% splenic lymphoma with villous lymphocytes Rare B-CLL, myeloma B-PLL
BCL-2/18q21.3	t(14;18)(q32.3;q21.3)	85% follicular B-NHL 30% diffuse B-NHL Rare acute leukaemias
BCL-6/3q27.1 Unknown Unknown/9p13.3	t(3;14)(q27;q32.3) t(2;5)(p23;q35) t(9;14)(p13;q32.3)	Diffuse B-NHL CD30+ anaplastic B-NHL (also T-cell NHL) Plasmacytoid B-NHL

Note: Some of the common chromosomal translocations detected in B-NHL. Note that the immunoglobulin heavy chain locus is located at 14q32.3 and is a frequently targeted site as are the immunoglobulin light chain loci at 2p11 (Ig kappa) and 22q11 (Ig lambda).

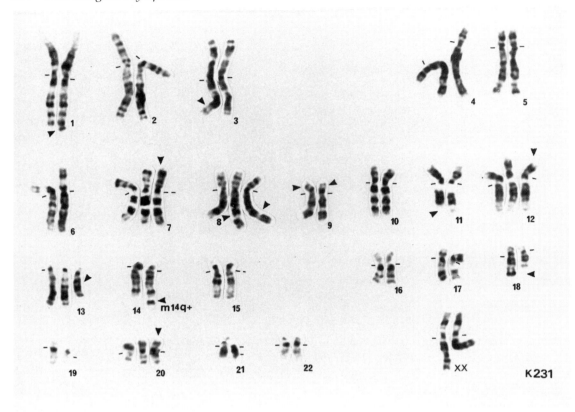

Figure 19.2 Karyotype of acute leukaemia arising as 'blast crisis' of follicular B-NHL showing t(14;18) and variant MYC translocation t(8;9) along with multiple other abnormalities. Concurrent activation of both BCL-2 and MYC are crucial events in such transformation.

including concurrent activation of synergistic oncogenes (such as BCL-2 and C-MYC; Vaux *et al.*, 1988) as well as loss of tumour suppressor gene function (Gaidano *et al.*, 1991).

19.5 THE BCL-2 PARADIGM

The identification of genes involved in the pathogenesis of NHL has numerous direct clinical applications, best illustrated with reference to the BCL-2 gene. For a review of this fascinating gene see Korsmeyer (1992).

The translocation t(14;18)(q32.3;q21.3) which juxtaposes the BCL-2 gene with the IGH locus occurs in 85% of follicular B-NHL,

30% of diffuse B-NHL as well as rare cases of acute leukaemia. In B-NHL the translocation breakpoints in the BCL-2 gene occur predominantly in two clusters in the 3′ portion of the gene: the translocation does not disrupt the gene but rather results in deregulated expression.

The clustering of breakpoints occurs not only in the BCL-2 gene but also in the IGH locus and has allowed the development of polymerase chain reaction (PCR) strategies to detect the t(14;18)(q32.3;q21.3) at a frequency of 1 NHL cell in 10^5 normal cells. Moreover, the use of PCR allows the use of formalin fixed biopsy material which cannot be used for other molecular genetic techniques such as Southern blotting.

Application of molecular genetic techniques for the detection of the t(14;18) (q32.3;q21.3) has shown that:

1. Diffuse B-NHLs with the translocation have a worse prognosis than those without (Offit *et al.*, 1989).
2. The presence of residual B-NHL cells in harvested bone marrow may contribute to eventual relapse (Gribben *et al.*, 1991).

Furthermore, the BCL-2/IGH hybrid mRNA produced as a consequence of the t(14;18)(q32.3;q21.3) may possibly serve as a target for therapy with antisense oligonucleotides (Reed *et al.*, 1990).

19.6 THERAPY

The choice of therapy with NHL depends on the age and general condition of the patient, as well as the histological subtype and site, bulk and spread of disease. Approaches to therapy can be divided along the lines of low and high grade diseases.

19.6.1 LOW GRADE DISEASE

Nearly all of these patients will have disseminated disease at the time of diagnosis. Control and palliation may be obtained with oral chlorambucil with or without prednisolone, or alternatively intravenous cyclophosphamide with vincristine and prednisolone (CVP) may be used. However in many, it is feasible simply to observe; treatment should be instituted when clinically indicated. About 30% of patients with low grade NHL become long term survivors: most of these are patients who present with localized disease in whom excision biopsy followed by local radiotherapy may be sufficient. For patients who present with disseminated disease, most die with either progressive or transformed disease. Trans-

formation to high grade disease is associated with a particularly poor prognosis.

A more vigorous approach to therapy is often employed in the younger patient with low grade disease, although whether this is ultimately of more benefit is open to question. New adenosine analogues such as 2′ chlorodeoxyadenosine may have a role to play in certain subgroups of B-NHL (Beutler, 1992). The relatively slow growth of these tumours, along with the ease of biopsy, has permitted experimental therapy with a wide range of so-called 'biological' therapies involving either recombinant cytokines such as interleukin-2, the interferons or monoclonal antibodies. Most of these approaches have not been successful but antibodies capable of either perturbing the immune system such as anti-idiotypic antibodies (Levy and Miller, 1990) or antibodies capable of redirecting natural effector mechanisms (Hale *et al.*, 1988) may prove more successful. Some NHL seem particularly susceptible to MAb therapy: polyclonal B-cell lymphoproliferative conditions appear to be sensitive to a cocktail of CD21 and CD24 MAbs (Fischer *et al.*, 1991). This subject has recently been reviewed (Grossbard *et al.*, 1992).

19.6.2 HIGH GRADE DISEASE

The majority of patients with high grade disease have apparently localized disease which is sensitive to combination chemotherapy and most attain remission. The most commonly used protocol comprises cyclophosphamide, hydroxydaunorubicin, vincristine and predinosolone (CHOP) adapted from the C-MOPP protocol used in Hodgkin's disease (DeVita *et al.*, 1975). Table 19.4 shows

Table 19.4 CHOP protocol: 21 day cycle

Cyclophosphamide	750 mg/m²	i.v.	Day 1
Adriamycin	50 mg/m²	i.v.	Day 1
Vincristine	1.4 mg/m²	i.v.	Day 1
Prednisolone	100 mg	p.o.	Days 1–5

the standard CHOP protocol. Results with CHOP do not appear to be significantly bettered by the use of multi-drug combinations such as MACOP-B, particularly if full doses of all components of CHOP are given.

With these approaches up to 50% of patients with high grade disease may achieve long term disease free survival. Problems arise with the patient who either fails to attain remission with first-line therapy or whose remission is only short-lived. Although many patients still have 'chemotherapy sensitive' disease, responses with second-line 'salvage' chemotherapy are generally only transient, and a review of 398 patients thus treated showed only 3% in continuous remission at 2 years.

Escalation of therapy in those patients, with reinfusion of autologous harvested bone marrow (autologous bone marrow transplantation or ABMT) has therefore been attempted. This approach is clearly limited by the age/condition of the patient and by the presence of residual tumour cells in the harvested marrow which may contribute to lymphomatous relapse. An important prognostic factor is the responsiveness of the NHL to chemotherapy at standard dosage prior to transplant: as might be expected patients with resistant disease fare badly.

Given the patient selection involved in ABMT it is difficult to draw any general conclusions about the role of this procedure in NHL. To assess its value directly, in the UK, the British National Lymphoma Investigation (BNLI) group are presently comparing in a randomized trial the effects of ABMT in first remission in high grade NHL; after attaining remission patients are being randomized to either stopping all therapy or to proceeding directly to ABMT. Only through such large multicentre studies will be the role of ABMT emerge.

19.7 CONCLUSIONS

Although conventional chemotherapy has made great progress in the treatment of the NHLs, most patients still die of their disease.

The 'new biology' is beginning to shed light on the nature of the genes whose deregulation and loss of function lead to malignancy. The challenge to both clinicians and scientists alike is to translate this improved understanding into improved diagnosis and therapy.

REFERENCES

Ballerini, P., Gaidano, G., Gong, J.Z. *et al.* (1993) Multiple genetic lesions in acquired immunodeficiency syndrome-related non-Hodgkin's lymphoma. *Blood*, **81**, 166–76.

Barclay, A.N., Birkeland, M.L., Brown, M.H. *et al.* (1993) *The Leucocyte Antigen Facts Book*, Academic Press, London.

Barnes, N., Cartwright, R.A., O'Brien, C. *et al.* (1986) Rising incidence of lymphoid malignancies. *British Journal of Cancer*, **53**, 393–8.

Beutler, E. (1992) Cladribine (2-chlorodeoxyadenosine). *Lancet*, **340**, 952–4.

Cleary, M.L. and Sklar, J. (1984) Lymphoproliferative disorders in cardiac transplant patients are multiclonal lymphomas. *Lancet*, **ii**, 489–93.

De Jong, D., Votedijk, B.M.H., Beverstock, G.C. *et al.* (1988) Activation of the C-MYC oncogene in a precursor B-cell blast crisis of follicular lymphoma, presenting as composite lymphoma. *New England Journal of Medicine*, **128**, 181–201.

DeVita, V.T., Canellos, G.P., Chabner, B. *et al.* (1975) Advanced diffuse histiocytic lymphoma, a potentially curable disease: results with combination chemotherapy. *Lancet*, **i**, 248–50.

Fischer, A., Blanche, S., Le Bidois, J. *et al.* (1991) Anti-B-cell monoclonal antibodies in the treatment of severe B-cell lymphoproliferative syndrome following bone marrow and organ transplantation. *New England Journal of Medicine*, **324**, 1451–56.

Gaidano, G., Ballerini, P., Gong, J.Z. *et al.* (1991) p53 mutations in human lymphoid malignancies: association with Burkitt lymphoma and chronic lymphocytic leukemia. *Proceedings of the National Academy of Sciences, USA*, **88**, 5413–17.

Gribben, J.G., Freedman A.S., Neuberg, A. *et al.* (1991) Immunologic purging of marrow assessed by PCR before autologous bone marrow transplantation for B-cell lymphoma. *New England Journal of Medicine*, **325**, 1525–33.

Grossbard, M.L., Press, O.W., Appelbaum, F.R. *et al.* (1992) Monoclonal antibody-based therapies of leukemia and lymphoma. *Blood*, **80**, 863–78.

Hale, G., Dyer, M.J.S., Clark, M.R. *et al.* (1988) Remission induction in non-Hodgkin lymphoma with reshaped monoclonal antibody CAMPATH-1H. *Lancet*, **ii**, 1394–400.

Korsemeyer, S.J. (1992) BCL-2 initiates a new category of oncogenes: regulators of cell death. *Blood*, **80**, 879–86.

Kuefler, P.R. and Bunn, P.A. (1986) Adult T cell leukemia/lymphoma. *Clinics in Haematology*, **15**, 695–726.

Levy, R., and Miller, R.A. (1990) Therapy of lymphoma directed at idiotypes. *Journal of the National Cancer Institute Monographs*, **10**, 61–8.

Magrath, I.T. (ed.) (1990a) *The Non-Hodgkin's Lymphomas*, Edward Arnold, London.

Magrath, I.T. (1990b) The pathogenesis of Burkitt's lymphoma. *Advances in Cancer Research*, **55**, 133–270.

Offit, K., Koduru, P.R.K., Hollis, R. *et al.* (1989) 18q21 rearrangement in diffuse large cell lymphoma: incidence and clinical significance. *British Journal of Haematology*, **72**, 178–83.

Offit, K. (1992) Chromosome analysis in the management of patients with non-Hodgkin's lymphoma. *Leukemia and Lymphoma*, **7**, 275–82.

Picker, L.J., Weiss, L.M. Madeiros, L.J. *et al.* (1987) Immunophenotypic criteria for the diagnosis of non-Hodgkin's lymphoma. *American Journal of Pathology*, **128**, 181–201.

Reed, J.C., Stein, C., Subasinghe, C. *et al.* (1990) Antisense-mediated inhibition of BCL-2 expression and leukemic cell growth and survival: comparisons of phosphodiester and phosphorothioate oligonucleotides. *Cancer Research*, **50**, 6565–70.

Ribeiro, R.C., Pui, C-H., Murphy, S.B. *et al.* (1992) Childhood malignant non-Hodgkin lymphomas of uncommon histology. *Leukemia*, **8**, 761–5.

Rosenberg, S.A. and members of the non-Hodgkin's lymphoma Pathologic Classification Project (1982) National Cancer Institute sponsored study of the classification of non-Hodgkin's lymphomas. Summary and description of a working formulation for clinical usage. *Cancer*, **49**, 2122–35.

Umetsu, D.T., Esserman L., Donlow, T.A. *et al.* (1990) Induction of proliferation of human follicular lymphoma cells by cognate interaction with CD4+ T-cell clones. *Journal of Immunology*, **144**, 2550–7.

Vaux, D.D., Cory, S. and Adams, J.M. (1988) The BCL-2 gene promotes haemopoietic cell survival and cooperates with C-MYC to immortalise pre B-cells. *Nature*, **335**, 440–3.

ACUTE LEUKAEMIAS

Jayesh Mehta and Ray Powles

20.1 INTRODUCTION

Acute leukaemia is a neoplastic disease of the blood characterized by abnormal clonal proliferation and accumulation of immature blood precursors. Depending upon the cell lineage involved primarily, acute leukaemia is classified as acute myelogenous leukaemia (AML) or acute lymphoblastic leukaemia (ALL).

20.2 AETIOLOGY

While the exact cause of leukaemia is not known in most patients, a number of predisposing factors have been identified. Acute leukaemia occurs with increased frequency in congenital diseases such as Down, Fanconi, Klinefelter, Wiskott–Aldrich and Bloom syndromes.

Environmental factors implicated in leukaemogenesis include ionizing radiation, aromatic hydrocarbons such as benzene, and certain antimalignancy drugs (mainly alkylating agents and plant alkaloids). Leukaemia associated with prior drug therapy is almost always of myeloid origin and is being seen with increasing frequency as treatment regimens for malignancies (especially Hodgkin's disease) become more aggressive and successful, and more patients become long term survivors. Aplastic anaemia is a stem cell disorder and a number of patients treated with therapeutic modalities other than bone marrow transplantation (BMT) develop myelodysplasia and AML a few years later.

AML has been described following drug-induced aplastic anaemia after therapy with chloramphenicol and phenylbutazone.

A number of retroviruses are leukaemogenic in animal models, but the only human leukaemia associated with a viral infection is adult T-cell leukaemia resulting from infection with the human T-cell leukaemia virus I.

Neoplastic haematological stem cell diseases such as chronic myeloproliferative disorders or myelodysplastic syndromes often transform into an aggressive process that resembles acute leukaemia ('secondary leukaemia' as against 'primary leukaemia' that arises *de novo* without any preceding haematological disease or cytotoxic chemotherapy) after a variable period of time. Chronic myeloproliferative diseases transform into AML more frequently than ALL, whereas myelodysplastic syndromes terminate into AML.

20.3 INCIDENCE

The incidence of acute leukaemia in the UK is approximately 9 per 100 000 population. There are two peaks of incidence of acute leukaemia; in children aged 5–14 years and in adults aged 55–75 years. Both types of acute leukaemia are slightly more common in males. ALL is primarily a disease of children and young adults, whereas AML occurs at all ages. The incidence of AML increases with advancing age.

20.4 PATHOPHYSIOLOGY

Leukaemia arises as a result of malignant transformation of a single haematopoietic progenitor followed by expansion of the malignant clone. Studies of women heterozygous for glucose-6-phosphate dehydrogenase isoenzymes has shown that all malignant cells produce the same isoenzyme and the leukaemic transformation is clonal.

AML is characterized by defective maturation of the myeloid cell line beyond the myeloblast or promyelocyte stage, and ALL beyond the lymphoblast stage. Leukaemic cell accumulate in the body due to excessive proliferation and failure of terminal differentiation. The malignant cells circulate in the blood and infiltrate various organs of the body.

Failure of marrow function, partly due to infiltration by malignant cells and partly by other mechanisms such as production of inhibitors of haematopoiesis by the leukaemic cells, results in anaemia, neutropenia and thrombocytopenia.

Childhood ALL occasionally starts with pancytopenia and a hypoplastic marrow which shows no evidence of leukaemia initially. Typical ALL then evolves over the next few weeks or months.

Unlike solid tumours, leukaemia is a disseminated systemic disease at presentation. However, infiltration of organ parenchyma is uncommon. It may occur late in the course of relapsed or resistant disease. Extramedullary disease is usually commoner at relapse than at presentation.

20.5 CLASSIFICATION

It is important to distinguish between ALL and AML because the natural history, prognosis and therapy of the two are different. ALL and AML can often be differentiated from examination of marrow or blood films stained with one of the Romanowsky stains. Lymphoblasts are 10–15 μm in diameter with

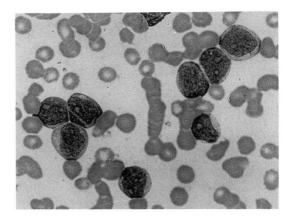

Figure 20.1 Peripheral blood in acute myeloid leukaemia (M1). Note prominent nucleoli and lack of cytoplasmic granulation. Courtesy of Dr J. Luckit.

a thin rim of a granular cytoplasm and a round or convoluted nucleus. Myeloblasts are larger (12–20 μm in diameter) with a lower nuclear–cytoplasmic ratio, discrete nuclear chromatin and multiple nucleoli (Figure 20.1). The presence of Auer rods or abnormal granules in the cytoplasm is diagnostic of AML (Figure 20.2). Characteristic abnormalities of the erythroid lineage may be seen with certain subtypes of AML (Figure 20.3), and prominent cytoplasmic vacuolation with B-cell ALL (Figure 20.4).

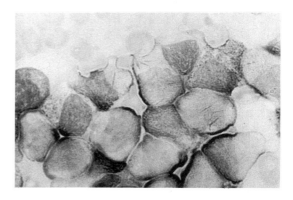

Figure 20.2 Bone marrow in acute promyelocytic leukaemia (M3). Note multiple Auer rods. Courtesy of Dr J. Treleaven.

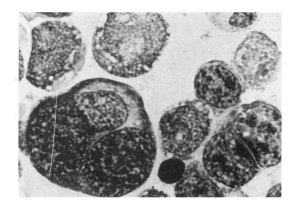

Figure 20.3 Bone marrow in acute erythroleukaemia (M6). Note multinucleate megaloblasts. Courtesy of Dr J. Treleaven.

The most widely used classification of the acute leukaemias is the one proposed by the French-American-British cooperative group (Bennett *et al.*, 1985a, b; Bain, 1990; Catovsky *et al.*, 1991) based on morphology and cytochemistry (Table 20.1). While the subclassification of AML and ALL into further subtypes is to some extent arbitrary and without significant therapeutic implication, certain subtypes exhibit unique characteristics and prognostic variations.

Morphological criteria are often insufficient to classify the disease and cytochemical studies on the peripheral blood or bone marrow may

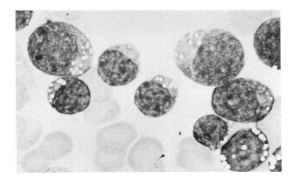

Figure 20.4 Peripheral blood in B-cell acute lymphoblastic leukaemia (L3). Note prominent cytoplasmic vacuolation. Courtesy of Dr J. Treleaven.

help. The phenotype of the leukaemic cell can be further defined by immunological and enzymatic studies. The presence of nuclear terminal deoxynucleotidyl transferase (TdT) activity in most of the leukaemic cells strongly supports the diagnosis of ALL.

Between 50% and 60% of adult and 80% of childhood ALL cases lack the surface characteristics of T or B cells but express an antigen known as common ALL antigen (CALLA). Five percent of ALL cases show surface expression of immunoglobulin and belong to the B-cell lineage. These correspond to the FAB L3 subtype. T-ALL cells have receptors for unsensitized sheep erythrocytes allowing E rosette formation.

20.6 INVESTIGATIONS

The basic investigations required to diagnose and classify acute leukaemia, and monitor the course of the disease and response to therapy are shown in Table 20.2. Most cases can be diagnosed on examination of the peripheral blood film alone, but BM examination is mandatory in all cases to classify the disease properly and to assess cellularity. Chromosomal karyotype of the malignant clone is often predictive of the nature of the disease and its response to therapy (Woods *et al.*, 1985; Pui *et al.*, 1990). The relationship of the karyotype to prognosis of certain types of acute leukaemia is shown in Table 20.3.

Most of these investigations have to be repeated at regular intervals to monitor the clinical situation and course of the disease, and assess the response to therapy.

20.7 CLINICAL FEATURES

Most of the clinical features are attributable to pancytopenia, or to infiltration of various organs of the body by leukaemic cells, or to metabolic disturbances resulting from a high tumour burden.

When the disease has evolved relatively slowly, the presenting complaints may be

Table 20.1 The FAB classification of acute leukaemia

FAB type	Morphology	Cytochemistry
Acute myelogenous leukaemia		
M0	Acute leukaemia with minimal evidence of myeloid differentiation	SBB–. MPO–. PAS–. MPO+ immunologically or ultrastructurally
M1	Acute myeloid leukaemia without maturation. Very undifferentiated cells with occasional cytoplasmic granules or Auer rods (Figure 20.1)	SBB+. MPO+. PAS–
M2	Acute myeloid leukaemia with maturation Differentiation beyond the promyelocyte stage clearly evident. Numerous Auer rods.	SBB+. MPO+. PAS–
M3	Acute promyelocytic leukaemia. Hypergranular promyelocytes predominate. Some cells contain multiple Auer rods in bundles (Figure 20.2)	SBB+. MPO+. PAS–
M3V	Variant form of promyelocytic leukaemia. Cells show fine granules or are agranular. Nuclei are reniform, bilobed, multilobed or convoluted	SBB+,. MPO+. PAS–
M4	Acute myelomonocytic leukaemia. Both granulocytic and monocytic precursors seen	SBB+. MPO+. NSE+. Some cells PAS+
M5a	Acute monoblastic leukaemia. Large monoblasts with abundant basophilic cytoplasm which may be vacuolated predominate	MPO–. SBB±. PAS±. NSE+ with flouride inhibition
M5b	Acute monocytic leukaemia. Significant population of promonocytes and monocytes in addition to monoblasts	Same as M5a
M6	Acute erythroleukaemia. Megaloblastoid and multinucleated red cell precursors in addition to myeloblasts (Figure 20.3)	MPO+. SBB+. Red cell precursors PAS+ and acid phosphatase +
M7	Acute megakaryoblastic leukaemia. Pleomorphic appearance of cells. May show cytoplasmic budding or bizarre platelets. Factor VII related antigen, glycoprotein IIb, platelet factor 4 or platelet-derived growth factor expressed on the surface of the blasts	MPO–. SBB–. PAS±. NSE±. Platelet peroxidase+ ultrastructurally

Table 20.1   contd.

Acute lymphoblastic leukaemia

L1	The common type of leukaemia in children. The malignant cells are small and homogeneous with a high nuclear–cytoplasmic ratio, regular nuclei and inconspicuous nucleoli	SBB–. MPO–. PAS+. Acid phosphatase+ in T-ALL. Localized NSE+ in T-ALL
L2	Commoner in adults with larger and heterogeneous cells with a low nuclear – cytoplasmic ratio. Nuclei may be cleft with one or more prominent nucleoli	Same as L1
L3	The least common type accounting for less than 5% of all cases of ALL, is seen in both adults and children. The cells are of B-cell origin with large nuclei, prominent nucleoli and markedly vacuolated cytoplasm (Figure 20.4)	SBB–. MPO––. PAS–. Vacuoles oil red O+

MPO, myeloperoxidase; SBB, Sudan black B; PAS, Periodic acid-Schiff; NSE, non-specific esterase.
SBB or MPO are classified as positive when reactivity is seen in ≥ 3% of blasts.

dyspnoea on exertion, easy fatiguability and pallor due to anaemia. Bleeding due to thrombocytopenia with or without coagulation disturbances is a major problem. Disseminated intravascular coagulation is a feature of acute promyelocytic leukaemia. Petechiae and easy bruisability are common. With decreasing platelet counts gum bleeding and gastrointestinal haemorrhage occur. With very low platelet counts, there is a serious danger of intracerebral haemorrhage.

Infections are frequent with neutrophil counts of less than $0.5 \times 10^9/l$. The common sites of infection are the oral cavity, the perianal area, skin, urinary tract and lungs. Cytotoxic chemotherapy breaks down mucosal barriers and increases the chance of infections. Septicaemia often occurs from organisms colonizing the gastrointestinal tract. Gram-negative bacilli, Gram-positive cocci and fungi such as *Candida* species are common pathogens.

Generalized lymphadenopathy and organomegaly may be seen in ALL. Massive mediastinal lymphadenopathy is a particular feature of T-ALL. Meningeal infiltration is very common in B-ALL, and is much commoner in ALL than in AML. Testicular involvement may be seen in males with ALL.

Extramedullary infiltration in the form of gum hypertrophy and skin lesions is a feature of the monocytic and myelomonocytic subtypes of AML. Meningeal infiltration in cases of AML is usually associated with the monocytic subtypes.

20.8   ASSESSMENT OF PROGNOSIS

A number of features at presentation signify a poor overall risk, either in terms of probability of achievement of complete remission or in terms of duration of the remission. Advanced age and presence of infection at diagnosis make adequate therapy difficult. Morbidity and mortality as a result of the aggressive nature of the therapy are particularly high in the elderly. However, advanced age is not an adverse prognostic factor once remission has been achieved.

In ALL poor prognostic factors (Hoelzer *et al.*, 1988; Henze *et al.*, 1991) include male sex, age less than 2 or greater than 10 years,

Table 20.2   Investigations at presentation

I.   For diagnosis, classification and prognosis

Peripheral blood
  Complete blood count
  Differential count
  Cytochemistry
  Karyotype
  Immunophenotype
  Serum lysozyme
  Serum LDH

Bone marrow
  Differential count
  Cytochemistry
  Karyotype
  Immunophenotype
  Immunofluorescence studies for TdT
  Trephine biopsy to assess cellularity and fibrosis

Other
  Cytological examination of the cerebrospinal
    fluid
  Urine lysozyme (elevated in M4 and M5)

II.   To guide therapy

Blood grouping: patient and family
HLA typing: patient and family
CMV serology
Coagulation studies
Surveillance cultures (blood, urine, stool, throat,
  perineum)
Chest radiograph
Serum chemistry: electrolytes, uric acid, renal
  function, liver function
Urine examination

Table 20.3   Chromosomal abnormalities associated with acute leukaemia

FAB subtype	Karyotype	Relative prognosis
AML		
M2	t(8;21)	Good
M3	t(15;17)	Good
M4 with eosinophilia	inv 16 or -16	Good
Various (therapy-related AML)	- 5, -7, 5q-, 7q-	Poor
ALL		
L1 or L2	Hyperdiploidy	Good
L1 or L2	6q-	Good
L3	t(8;14)	Poor
L1 or L2	Ph[1][t(9;22)]	Poor
Biphenotypic		
L2 or M4	t(4;11)	Poor

and FAB subtypes M6 and M7 (Creutzig *et al.*, 1990). High serum lactate dehydrogenase (LDH) levels are associated with a poor prognosis (Kantarjian *et al.*, 1988).

Certain karyotype abnormalities are associated with a relatively better or worse prognosis as shown in Table 20.3. Secondary acute leukaemia evolving from a pre-existing haematological disease usually responds poorly to therapy.

leucocyte count greater than $20 \times 10^9/l$, B-cell phenotype (L3), presence of the Ph[1] chromosome, meningeal involvement, and the presence of myeloid markers on the surface (biphenotypic disease). The association of high leucocyte counts with T-cell phenotype is responsible for the poor prognosis of T-ALL. Testicular relapse accounts for poorer outcome for males.

In AML poor prognostic factors include prior radiation or cytotoxic drug therapy (secondary leukaemia), high leucocyte count,

20.9   MANAGEMENT

In general, acute leukaemias are very responsive to cytotoxic chemotherapy with a high proportion achieving complete remission. The disease and its intensive therapy are both associated with a number of life-threatening complications which require expert multidisciplinary medical and nursing care in a setting with essentially unlimited facilities for investigations and supportive management. Management is therefore best left to specialized units with experience in the care of such patients.

Specific treatment should begin as soon as possible in ALL because the disease is steadily progressive and the prognosis is related to the total body burden of malignant cells. Some cases of AML, especially those arising from a preceding myelodysplastic phase, do not require immediate therapy.

20.9.1 SUPPORTIVE THERAPY

Before specific chemotherapy to induce a remission is begun, the patient's general condition must be stabilized as much as possible without inordinately delaying treatment. Supportive management as outlined below may be required before the patient is fit to receive chemotherapy.

(a) Transfusions

A platelet count of less than $10 \times 10^9/l$ greatly increases the risk of serious bleeding. Bleeding can occur at higher counts if there is fever or infection or if the rate of fall of platelets has been fast. Prophylactic platelet transfusions to maintain the platelet count above $20 \times 10^9/l$ reduces the risk of serious haemorrhage considerably. Packed cells should be transfused to keep the haemoglobin around 100 g/l, but only when the leucocyte count is not high. A high haematocrit with a high leucocyte count could predispose to leukostasis and cerebrovascular accidents. A haemoglobin of 100–120 g/l is desirable in patients with low platelet counts and who are refractory to platelet transfusions because a given level of platelets is more protective at a higher haematocrit due to increased platelet–vessel wall interactions. Anovulatory agents should be administered to menstruating women to avoid uterine bleeding during thrombocytopenia.

Patients with evidence of DIC require heparinization (10 000–20 000 U/d) and fresh-frozen plasma and cryoprecipitate. Patients with acute promyelocytic leukaemia should be prophylactically heparinized before chemotherapy is begun. Heparinization is not necessary when these patients are treated with the differentiating agent all-*trans* retinoic acid.

Occasionally, surgery may be necessary in patients prior to or during therapy. It is essential to maintain the platelet count above $50 \times 10^9/l$ to prevent bleeding and promote healing.

It is important to use cytomegalovirus (CMV)-negative blood products for patients who are CMV-negative or have not yet been screened because CMV-positivity greatly increases the risk of CMV disease during subsequent allogeneic BMT.

(b) Infections

Since therapy of acute leukaemia is associated with a considerable period of neutropenia which places the patient at risk of serious infections, patients are nursed in single rooms with strict reverse isolation or in rooms with high-efficiency particulate air filtration. Standard prophylactic measures include chlorhexidine mouthwashes, amphotericin lozenges and nystatin suspension. Total gut decontamination with co-trimoxazole or oral neomycin, and prophylactic systemic antimicrobial agents are not universally employed.

A febrile neutropenic patient must be treated with broad-spectrum antimicrobial agents at the full doses immediately after clinical assessment and cultures without awaiting results. The usual combination is one of an aminoglycoside and an anti-*Pseudomonas* penicillin with or without a cephalosporin. Therapy is modified depending upon culture results. Antifungal agents may have to be added if fever persists after 4–5 days of therapy. Antibiotics are usually continued until the neutrophil count increases to more than 0.5–$1 \times 10^9/l$. Geographical patterns of occurrence of infectious diseases also must be considered (Mehta, 1987).

A patient with acute leukaemia who is infected at diagnosis presents a difficult problem. A patient with circulating neutrophils is usually not started on myelosuppressive therapy because disappearance of the circulating neutrophils impairs the ability to overcome the infection significantly. A patient with no neutrophils due to complete effacement of the marrow by leukaemia may benefit from cytotoxic chemotherapy together with antibiotics.

The myelosuppression following induction chemotherapy is severe and may be prolonged, especially with AML. This may predispose the patient to serious infections. Recombinant growth factors such as granulocyte colony-stimulating factor (G-CSF) or granulocyte–macrophage colony-stimulating factor (GM-CSF) can be used to shorten the period of neutropenia. This is useful in neutropenic patients with life-threatening infections that are poorly responsive to antimicrobial agents but their role in decreasing the rate of infections remains to be determined (Powles *et al.*, 1990). The role of granulocyte transfusions in neutropenic patients with life-threatening infections remains controversial, especially with the availability of growth factors.

The incidence of herpetic infections (stomatitis and zoster) during induction therapy is high enough to warrant prophylactic use of acyclovir.

(c)   Leukostasis

The stickiness of the malignant cells predisposes patients with AML and a high white count (over $100 \times 10^9/l$) to leukostasis and intracerebral haemorrhage. The risk can be significantly reduced by immediate cranial irradiation (a single fraction of 6 Gy), or oral hydroxyurea $3 \, g/m^2$ per day for 2 days, or by leukapheresis. Leukapheresis is standard on presentation at some centres, to reduce the tumour burden and to harvest adequate malignant cells for cryopreservation for future studies.

(d)   Fluid and electrolyte balance

Hyperkalaemia and hyperuricaemia may result in the early phases of therapy due to massive cell destruction and precipitate cardiac abnormalities and renal failure. Allopurinol (300 mg) should be started prior to chemotherapy. A high fluid intake should be ensured and renal function and electrolytes carefully monitored.

20.9.2   CHEMOTHERAPY

(a)   ALL

More than half of children with ALL can be cured but the number of adults and children with high risk disease becoming long term survivors with conventional chemotherapy still remains small. The phases in the therapy of ALL are induction of remission, consolidation, central nervous system prophylaxis, and maintenance.

Induction of remission

Weekly vincristine (VCR, 1.4 mg/m²) for 4 weeks and daily prednisolone (40 mg/m²) for 4 weeks are the two basic drugs used for remission induction. Most aggressive modern protocols however also include 1–3 doses of an anthracycline agent such as daunorubicin or doxorubicin (45 mg/m²) and 10 doses of L-asparaginase (4000–6000 U/m²). The addition of these drugs has a beneficial effect on the duration of the remission achieved (Hoelzer *et al.*, 1984; Balis, 1988).

Consolidation

Once complete remission (CR) has been achieved, additional courses of the initially successful drugs in combination with other agents are administered to reduce the clinically undetectable mass of leukaemic cells even further. Some of the other drugs utilized are cytosine arabinoside (ARA-C), etoposide, teniposide and cyclophosphamide.

Central nervous system prophylaxis

The meninges constitute a sanctuary site from which leukaemic cells are not effectively eliminated by conventional chemotherapy. Leukaemic cells invade the meninges after penetrating the walls of the veins. Destruction of arachnoid trabeculae leads to contamination of cerebrospinal fluid. The cells then proliferate and reach the brain parenchyma after destroying the pia-glial membrane.

Combined cranial irradiation (24 Gy) and intrathecal methotrexate (MTX) reduce the risk of CNS relapse to approximately 5%. Cranial irradiation results in complete though reversible alopecia. Abrupt onset of drowsiness, lethargy and irritability lasting a week or two, known as the somnolence syndrome, can occur 3–6 weeks after cranial irradiation. While there is little evidence to suggest that childhood cranial irradiation results in any significant retardation of intellectual development, some patients may fall behind on numerical skills. Leukoencephalopathy is a serious complication resulting from white matter degeneration and necrosis associated with intrathecal MTX, therapy after cranial irradiation. The irradiation alters the blood–brain barrier which allows diffusion of the drug into the parenchyma.

In view of the complications of irradiation, some centres have explored the use of intermediate or high dose MTX (1 g/m^2) with leucovorin rescue at regular intervals with intrathecal MTX as a substitute for irradiation. Some of the most aggressive protocols for therapy of B-ALL or adult ALL employ intraventricular delivery of chemotherapy through indwelling Ommaya reservoirs for prophylaxis or therapy of meningeal leukaemia. Combination intrathecal chemotherapy with ARA-C, MTX and hydrocortisone is employed to treat meningeal disease.

Maintenance

Following completion of the first three phases of therapy, oral maintenance chemotherapy is required for a period of 2–3 years with daily 6-mercaptopurine (6-MP, 75 mg/m^2) and weekly MTX (20 mg/m^2), without which the majority of patients relapse within a few months. It is essential to give full dose maintenance therapy as adequacy of the dose has an impact on remission duration. A third drug such as cyclophosphamide may be added in poor prognosis patients with some benefit. Another strategy is to add periodic intensification pulses of VCR and prednisolone.

6-MP suppresses lymphopoiesis and increases susceptibility to viral infections such as measles, varicella and herpes zoster. *Pneumocystis carinii* pneumonia is a serious complication that can be prevented by cotrimoxazole prophylaxis (two tablets twice a day thrice a week) during the course of the maintenance therapy.

(b) AML

The aim of combination chemotherapy in AML is to produce severe marrow hypoplasia that allows regeneration of normal bone marrow. The mainstay of therapy is a combination of an anthracycline antibiotic (daunorubicin, doxorubicin or idarubicin) and ARA-C (Champlin and Gale, 1987). A third drug such as etoposide or 6-thioguanine is often added.

A commonly used induction regimen is daunorubicin 50 mg/m^2 for 1–3 days and ARA-C 100 mg/m^2 twice a day for 7–10 days, with or without 6-thioguanine 100 mg/m^2 twice a day for 7–10 days. This regimen is repeated every 2–3 weeks until complete remission. There is some evidence to suggest that idarubicin is superior to daunorubicin and that high dose ARA-C has a favourable impact on duration of remission. A very aggressive 5 day induction regimen is: idarubicin 5 mg/m^2 daily, ARA-C 2 g/m^2

twice a day and etoposide 100 mg/m² twice a day (Mehta *et al.*, 1992).

Complete remission (less than 5% blasts in a normocellular bone marrow with normal blood counts, and resolution of all organomegaly and evidence of extramedullary disease) can be achieved in 60–80% of patients. However, up to 10⁹ malignant cells may remain in the body at the time of achievement of CR and further consolidation therapy is essential. This consists of two to three courses of chemotherapy with the same drugs employed during induction of different drugs. There is no evidence to suggest that prolonged maintenance therapy after consolidation therapy is of any benefit in prolonging the duration of the remission (Preisler *et al.*, 1987), and most strategies of treatment revolve around intensive short term consolidation.

The outlook of patients who show little or no response to the first cycle of therapy, or have significant amount of disease after two cycles, is extremely poor. A small proportion of patients with primary resistant disease can be salvaged by allogeneic BMT if a suitable donor is available (Biggs *et al.*, 1992). Anthracyclines cause irreversible cardiotoxicity at a cumulative dose of 400–450 mg/m². Therapeutic options in resistant and refractory patients who have been heavily pretreated become limited (Gore *et al.*, 1989).

The use of GM-CSF during induction therapy is being explored to synchronize cell cycles of the malignant clone to improve response to chemotherapy and to reduce the duration of neutropenia (Bettelheim *et al.*, 1991). The chromosome 17 breakpoint due to the characteristic t(15;17) translocation in acute promyelocytic leukaemia consistently involves the gene for retinoic acid receptor-α This results in an exquisitive response of this form of leukaemia to the differentiating agent all-*trans* retinoic acid with a high proportion of complete remissions and insignificant complications (Warrell, 1992). The best dosage schedule and its place in combination with standard chemotherapy are being investigated because when used by itself, resistance develops rapidly and relapse occurs within a few months.

20.9.3   BONE MARROW TRANSPLANTATION

BMT overcomes dose limiting myelotoxicity and allows escalation in the dose of chemoradiotherapy to supralethal levels which, while completely destroying malignant cells, also destroys normal marrow cells (Appelbaum *et al.*, 1988). Immunologically mediated graft-versus-leukaemia reactions associated with allogeneic BMT contribute significantly to the control of minimal residual disease (Mehta, 1993).

The usual donor is an HLA-matched sibling. Autologous BMT (ABMT) is an alternative if a matched sibling donor is not available. There is some evidence to suggest that purging the autologous marrow *in vitro* prior to transplant with 4-hydroperoxy-cyclophosphamide or mafosfamide decreases relapse, but engraftment is significantly delayed with prolonged pancytopenia after transplantation. Matched unrelated donors are being increasingly utilized when ABMT is of limited value. The indications for BMT are different for different types of leukaemia (Santos, 1989; Ramsay and Kersey, 1990). Table 20.4 shows comparative survival in acute leukaemia with BMT and conventional chemotherapy.

Newer post-transplantation strategies employed to enhance the therapeutic efficacy of ABMT include maintenance chemotherapy for 2 years in ALL, and immunotherapy with interleukin 2 (IL-2) with or without interferon-α.

Autologous peripheral blood stem cell transplantation (PBSCT) using stem cells obtained by leukapheresis during recovery from chemotherapy induced myelosuppression or after mobilization with G-CSF or GM-CSF are increasingly being utilized to provide rescue after high dose chemoradiotherapy; either in addition to or instead of marrow.

Table 20.4 Long-term disease-free survival after conventional chemotherapy and bone marrow transplantation in acute leukaemia

Disease	Allograft (%)	Autograft (%)	Chemotherapy (%)
ALL			
CR1	30–60	20–60	10–70[*]
Rel1/CR2	20–40	10–30	<10–30
Rel2 or beyond	10–30	<10	<10
Primary refractory disease	10–20	0	0
AML			
CR1	30–70	20–50	<10–40[+]
Rel1/CR2	20–40	10–30	<10
Rel2 or beyond	10–30	<10	0
Primary refractory disease	10–20	0	0

[*]The wide range reflects good prognosis childhood disease at one end of the spectrum and poor prognosis disease such as Ph+ ALL at the other
[+]The lower figure applies to high-risk disease such as secondary AML and the higher to good-risk disease such as acute promyelocytic leukaemia in some series.

The potential advantages are decreased relapse due to decreased contamination of the harvested product with malignant cells and some immunological reaction against minimal residual disease due to the large number of immunocompetent cells infused along with the stem cells. Haematopoietic recovery is significantly faster after PBSCT than after BMT.

20.9.4 IMMUNOTHERAPY

IL-2 activates endogenous natural killer cells to activated killer cells. There is evidence to suggest that these cells contribute to control of minimal residual disease (Reittie *et al.*, 1989). IL-2 has been tried in AML beyond the first CR to see if it prolonged the duration of the second CR (Maraninchi *et al.*, 1991). It has also been administered after ABMT with or without other immunomodulatory agents such as interferon-α to reduce the incidence of relapse. Linomide is a novel immunomodulatory agent which acts by increasing the endogenous production of IL-2.

20.10 RELAPSE

Approximately 80% of children with ALL who complete 3 years of maintenance chemotherapy become long term survivors. The greatest number of relapses occur within the first year after cessation of maintenance chemotherapy. Relapses 4–5 years after completion of maintenance are unusual. The outlook of conventionally treated adult ALL is much poorer, with approximately 20% of patients becoming long term survivors. Relapse in adult ALL has been described as long as 8 years after completion of maintenance therapy. Relapse after cessation of maintenance chemotherapy is usually chemosensitive and can be treated, but relapse on maintenance chemotherapy is usually poorly responsive to therapy.

Up to 80% of patients with AML achieve CR but relapse rates are high and long term survival can be expected in only 15–20% of patients. Certain chemotherapy protocols have been reported to yield 40% long term survival in selected subgroups of patients (Burke *et al.*, 1989). The outcome of acute leukaemia that relapses after BMT is almost always extremely poor with poor response of the disease and severe toxicity (Gore *et al.*, 1989).

Appropriate management of multiply relapsed or resistant disease where a curative intent is inappropriate consists of oral 6-MP or etoposide to achieve reasonable cyto-reduction with analgesics and supportive therapy. The role of oral idarubicin in this setting is being explored (Davis *et al.*, 1991).

20.11   LONG TERM EFFECTS

Most children treated for leukaemia grow and develop normally (Voorhess *et al.*, 1986). Girls reach puberty normally, menstruate, and a number have borne normal children. Secondary AML after therapy of ALL is now being seen due to widespread use of plant alkaloids (etoposide and teniposide) in the therapy of ALL. BMT is associated with a significant number of long term adverse effects including secondary malignancies, and endocrine and pulmonary complications. These are mostly secondary to the use of total body irradiation in BMT.

REFERENCES

Appelbaum, F.R., Fisher, L.D. and Thomas, E.D. (1988) Chemotherapy v marrow transplantation for adults with acute nonlymphocytic leukemia: a five-year follow-up. *Blood*, **72**, 179–84.

Bain, B.J. (1990) *Leukaemia Diagnosis: A Guide to the FAB Classification*, Gower Medical Publishing, London

Balis, F.M. (1988) Pharmacologic considerations in the treatment of acute lymphoblastic leukemia. *Pediatric Clinics of North America*, **35**, 835–51.

Bennett, J.M., Catovsky, D., Daniel, M.T. *et al.* (1985a) Proposed revised criteria for the classification of acute myeloid leukemia. *Annals of Internal Medicine*, **103**, 620–5.

Bennett, J.M., Catovsky, D., Daniel, M.T. *et al.* (1985b) Criteria for the diagnosis of acute leukemia of megakaryocyte lineage (M7). *Annals of Internal Medicine*, **103**, 460–2.

Bettelheim, P., Valent, P., Andreeff, M. *et al.* (1991) Recombinant human granulocyte-macrophage colony-stimulating factor in combination with standard induction chemotherapy in de novo acute myeloid leukemia. *Blood*, **77**, 700–11.

Biggs, J.C., Horowitz, M.M., Gale, R.P. *et al.* (1992) Bone marrow transplants may cure patients with acute leukemia never achieving remission with chemotherapy. *Blood*, **80**, 1090–3.

Burke, P.J., Karp, J.E., Geller R.B. and Vaughan, W.P. (1989) Cures of leukemia with aggressive postremission treatment: an update of timed sequential therapy (Ac-D-Ac). *Leukemia*, **3**, 692–4.0.0163.

Catovsky, D., Matutes, E., Buccheri, V. *et al.* (1991) A classification of acute leukemia for the 1990s. *Annals of Hematology*, **62**, 16–21.

Champlin, R. and Gale, R.P. (1987) Acute myelogenous leukemia: recent advances in therapy *Blood*, **69**, 1551–62.

Creutzig, U., Ritter, J. and Schellong, G. (1990) Identification of two risk groups in childhood acute myelogenous leukemia after therapy intensification in study AML-BFM-83 as compared with study AML-BFM-78. AML-BFM Study Group. *Blood*, **75**, 1932–40.

Davis, C.L., Rohatiner, A.Z., Amess, J.A. and Lister, T.A. (1991) Oral idarubicin as a palliative agent in leukemia. *Hematologic Oncology*, **9**, 59–60.

Gore, M., Powles, R., Lakhani, A. *et al.* (1989) Treatment of relapsed and refractory acute leukemia with high-dose cytosine arabinoside and etoposide. *Cancer Chemotherapy and Pharmacology*, **23**, 373–6.

Henze, G., Fengler, R., Hartmann, R. *et al.* (1991) Six-year experience with a comprehensive approach to the treatment of recurrent childhood acute lymphoblastic leukemia (ALL-REZ BFM 85). A relapse study of the BFM group. *Blood*, **78**, 1166–72.

Hoelzer, D., Thiel, E., Loffler, H. *et al.* (1984) Intensified therapy in acute lymphoblastic and acute undifferentiated leukemia in adults. *Blood*, **64**, 38–47.

Hoelzer, D., Thiel, E., Loffler, H. *et al.* (1988) Prognostic factors in a multicenter study for treatment of acute lymphoblastic leukemia in adults. *Blood*, **71**, 123–31.

Kantarjian, H.M., Walters, R.S., Smith, T.L. *et al.* (1988) Identification of risk groups for development of central nervous system leukemia in adults with acute lymphocytic leukemia. *Blood*, **72**, 1784–9.

Maraninchi, D., Blaise, D., Viens, P. *et al.* (1991) High-dose recombinant interleukin-2 and acute myeloid leukemias in relapse. *Blood*, **78**, 2182–7.

Mehta, B.C. (1987) Geographical variations in blood disease: India, in *Oxford Textbook of Medicine*, 2nd edn, (eds D.J. Weatherall, J.G.G. Ledingham and D.A. Warrell), Oxford Scientific Publications, Oxford, pp. 19.270–19.273.

Mehta, J. (1993) Graft-versus-leukemia reactions in clinical bone marrow transplantation. *Leukemia and Lymphoma*, **10**, 427–32.

Mehta, J., Powles, R., Treleavan, J. *et al.* (1992) Idarubicin (IDR), high-dose ARA-C and VP-16 for induction of remission in untreated primary AML under 50 years. *Blood*, **80**, (Suppl 1), 113a.

Powles, R., Smith, C., Milan, S. *et al.* (1990) Human recombinant GM–CSF in allogeneic bone-marrow transplantation for leukemia: double-blind, placebo-controlled trial. *Lancet*, **336**, 1417–20.

Preisler, H., Davis, R.B., Kirshner, J. *et al.* (1987) Comparison of three remission induction regimens and two postinduction strategies for the treatment of acute nonlymphocytic leukemia: a Cancer and Leukemia Group B Study. *Blood*, **69**, 1441–9.

Pui, C.H., Crist, W.M. and Look, A.T. (1990) Biology and clinical significance of cytogenetic abnormalities in childhood acute lymphoblastic leukemia. *Blood*, **76**, 1449–63.

Ramsay, N.K., Kersey, J.H. (1990) Indications for marrow transplantation in acute lymphoblastic leukemia. *Blood*, **75**, 815–8.

Reittie, J.E., Gottlieb, D., Heslop, H.E. *et al.* (1989) Endogenously generated activated killer cells circulate after autologous and allogeneic marrow transplantation but not after chemotherapy. *Blood*, **73**, 1351–8.

Santos, G.W. (1989) Marrow transplantation in acute nonlymphocytic leukemia. *Blood*, **74**, 901–8.

Voorhess, M.L., Brecher, M.L., Glicksman, A.S. *et al.* (1986) Hypothalamic-pituitary function of children with acute lymphocytic leukemia after three forms of central nervous system prophylaxis. A retrospective study. *Cancer*, **57**, 1287–91.

Warrell, R.P. Jr (1992) All *trans*-retinoic acid: what is it good for? *Journal of Clinical Oncology*, **10**, 1659–61.

Woods, W.G., Nesbit, M.E., Buckley, J. *et al.* (1985) Correlation of chromosome abnormalities with patient characteristics, histologic subtype, and induction success in children with acute non-lymphocytic leukemia. *Journal of Clinical Oncology*, **3**, 3–11.

CHRONIC LEUKAEMIAS

Jane Mercieca, Estella Matutes and Daniel Catovsky

21.1 INTRODUCTION

The term chronic leukaemia has been used historically to describe the leukaemias arising from morphologically mature-looking cells (resembling normal blood leucocytes) that run a relatively long and protracted clinical course measured in months or years. The prototypes of these are chronic lymphocytic leukaemia (CLL) and chronic granulocytic leukaemia (CGL) affecting, respectively, lymphocytes and granulocytes. The contrast has been made with the acute leukaemias which are proliferations of blast (immature) cells and which, before the era of effective treatment, had a survival measured in weeks or months. Paradoxically, the number of acute leukaemias which are curable by modern therapy has been increasing whilst although improvements have occurred, cures in the chronic leukaemias are still rare.

21.2 CHRONIC LYMPHOID LEUKAEMIAS

The chronic lymphoid leukaemias are an heterogeneous group of disorders resulting from the clonal expansion of mature lymphocytes (Catovsky and Foa, 1990). Previously most of these disorders were grouped together with chronic lymphocytic leukaemia (CLL). In recent years, however, the development of monoclonal antibodies has enabled an objective classification of these disorders according to their B- or T-cell lineage and their stage of cellular maturation. As a result of these advances, together with closer analysis of morphological detail and histological patterns of infiltration, a number of discrete syndromes have emerged and the FAB group have proposed a classification of the chronic lymphoid leukaemias (Table 21.1) (Bennett *et al.*, 1989). The accurate classification of these diseases is important because of the different prognostic and therapeutic implications between disease entities.

21.3 CHRONIC B-CELL LEUKAEMIAS

21.3.1 CHRONIC LYMPHOCYTIC LEUKAEMIA

(a) Epidemiology

B-cell chronic lymphocytic leukaemia (CLL) is one of the commonest leukaemias in Western countries, accounting for about 25% of all leukaemias seen in clinical practice. It is, however, uncommon in the Far East, comprising only 2.5% of all leukaemias there. CLL is chiefly a disease of the elderly with a peak incidence between the ages of 60 and 80, and is extremely rare below the age of 30; it is twice as common in males. The incidence of familial leukaemia is greater in CLL than in other leukaemias but no consistent HLA linkage or other genetic factors have been identified. The cause of CLL is unknown and no relationship has been found between the incidence of the disease and environmental factors.

Table 21.1 FAB proposal for the classification of the chronic lymphoid leukaemias

Leukaemias of mature B cells

A. Primary leukaemias

1.	Chronic lymphocytic leukaemia – common	CLL
2.	Chronic lymphocytic leukaemia – mixed	CLL/PL
3.	Prolymphocytic leukaemia (B-cell type)	B-PLL
4.	Hairy cell leukaemia	HCL
5.	Hairy cell leukaemia variant	HCL-V
6.	Plasma cell leukaemia	PCL

B. Leukaemic phase of non-Hodgkin's lymphoma

1.	Splenic lymphoma with villous lymphocytes	SLVL
2.	Follicular lymphoma	FL
3.	Intermediate or mantle cell lymphoma	MCL
4.	Lymphoplasmacytic lymphoma*	LPL

Leukaemias of mature T cells

A. Primary leukaemias

1.	Large granular lymphocytic leukaemia	LGL leukaemia
2.	T-cell prolymphocytic leukaemia	T-PLL

B. Leukaemia/lymphoma syndromes

1.	Adult T-cell leukaemia/lymphoma	ATLL
2.	Sezary syndrome	SS
3.	Peripheral T-cell non-Hodgkin's lymphoma	T-NHL

Modified from Bennett *et al.*, 1989, with permission.
* Includes Waldenstrom's macroglobulinaemia.

(b) Clinical features

Approximately one-quarter of patients present with asymptomatic lymphocytosis revealed from an incidental blood count. Others may present because of painless lymphadenopathy, symptoms or anaemia or a severe chest infection.

Lymphadenopathy which is symmetrical and non-tender is the most frequent abnormality on physical examination, found in up to 80% of patients. The cervical, axillary and inguinal regions are commonly involved and lymph node enlargement may also be demonstrated in the mediastinum on chest X-ray and in the abdomen by ultrasound or CT scan. Splenomegaly of variable degree is found in up to two-thirds of patients; hepatomegaly is less common. Systemic symptoms such as fever, sweating and weight loss are unusual but may occur with bulky abdominal disease. Infection and transformation to a high grade lymphoma (Richter's syndrome) should also be considered as possible causes of B symptoms.

Infections are common, particularly in advanced disease, and are a major cause of morbidity and mortality. Upper respiratory tract infections are the most frequent and there is also an increased incidence of herpes zoster. The susceptibility of infections is multifactorial, resulting from a combination of hypogammaglobulinaemia, defects in T-cell mediated immunity and neutropenia.

Autoimmune haemolytic anaemia (AIHA) and thrombocytopenia (ITP) are well recognized complications of CLL. Although the Coombs' test may be positive in 5–10% of patients, only half have evidence of haemolysis. The incidence of ITP is about 2%. The association of both AIHA and ITP (Evans' syndrome) is less common but well recognized. One or other complication may be manifested in the same patient at different times.

Patients with CLL have an increased frequency of second malignancies with an increase of 9% compared with 2% in patients with other primary tumours; skin, gastrointestinal tract, lung and prostate are the commonest sites.

(c) Diagnosis/laboratory findings

The diagnostic criteria for B-CLL utilized in the current staging systems are the presence of a persistent lymphocytosis of $> 10 \times 10^9/l$ with lymphocytic infiltration of the bone marrow of at least 40%. With lower lymphocyte counts ($5–10 \times 10^9/l$) additional criteria such as surface marker studies are required to confirm the diagnosis.

Careful examination of a peripheral blood film is the most important diagnostic procedure. Morphologically, the lymphocytes are small with scanty cytoplasm, clumped nuclear chromatin and an inconspicuous nucleolus. The presence of smear/smudge cells which correlates with the level of WBC is often of diagnostic value. In some cases, however, there may be considerable morphological heterogeneity. A proportion of larger nucleolated lymphocytes (prolymphocytes) may be seen, though usually less than 10%.

CLL results from the clonal proliferation of a CD5 positive B cell. These cells have been found in the mantle zone of normal lymph nodes and have been implicated in autoimmunity, although in AIHA and ITP associated with CLL the antibodies are polyclonal and are not produced by these B cells. B-CLL has a characteristic immunophenotype which distinguishes it from other B-lymphoproliferative disorders. The cells express weak cell surface immunoglobulin (SmIg) of a single light chain isotype (kappa or lambda) and express B-cell antigens CD19, CD20, CD37, as well as CD5 (a B and T marker) and CD23. The CLL cells are negative for FMC7 and express weakly membrane CD22 (Table 21.2).

Anaemia and thrombocytopenia are poor prognostic features only if due to marrow infiltration but not if they are immune mediated or secondary to iron, B12 or folate

Table 21.2 Membrane markers in chronic B-cell leukaemias

Marker	CLL	B-PLL	HCL	SLVL	FL	MCL
SmIg	++*	++	++	++	++	+
CD5	++	−/+	−	−	−/+	+
CD23	++	−	−	−/+	−	−/+
FMC7/CD22	−/+*	++	++	++	++	++
CD19/20/37**	++	++	++	++	++	++
CD10	−	−	−	−/+	+	−/+
HC2/B-ly-7	−	−	++***	−/+	−	−
CD25	−	−/+	++.	−/+	−	−

For definition of abbreviations, see Table 21.1.
* Weak expression.
** Pan-B markers.
*** Negative in HCL variant.
−/+, Positive in less than 50% of cases; +, positive in 50–75% of cases; ++, positive in > 75% of cases.

deficiency. It is therefore important to identify the cause and treat appropriately before staging.

The bone marrow aspirate will characteristically show a lymphocytic infiltrate of > 40% with cells showing the same morphological features as those seen in the peripheral blood. The trephine biopsy is a more important investigation as it allows a more accurate assessment of the haemopoietic reserve and also shows the pattern of lymphocytic infiltration, which is of prognostic significance. Four histological patterns of infiltration are recognized: nodular, interstitial, mixed nodular and interstitial and diffuse. Diffuse or packed infiltration is associated with advanced disease and poor prognosis.

Cytogenetic analysis reveals a clonal abnormality in about half the cases. The commonest abnormality is trisomy 12 seen in 15–20% of cases. Structural abnormalities of chromosomes 13 and 14 are also a frequent finding. Patients with chromosome abnormalities (apart from those involving 13q) have a poorer survival than those with a normal karyotype. Those with complex abnormalities have the worst prognosis overall (Juliusson *et al.*, 1990).

(d) Course and prognosis

The clinical course of CLL is very variable with some patients surviving for many years without treatment and eventually dying of unrelated conditions, while others may have a rapidly progressive course, dying within a short time from either disease. Various staging systems have been developed to define the different prognostic groups. The two most widely used are those of Rai *et al.* (1975) and, more recently, Binet adopted by the International Workshop on Chronic Lymphocytic Leukaemia (1981) (Table 21.3). These have been shown to correlate with survival but do not distinguish stable patients from those who are progressing. A number of additional clinical and laboratory features have been found to be of prognostic significance independent of clinical stage. Factors associated with an adverse prognosis include: a short lymphocyte doubling time (> 12 months), an increased number of

Table 21.3 Staging systems for CLL

Rai classification (Rai *et al.*, 1975)

0	Lymphocytosis only
I	Lymphocytosis plus lymphadenopathy
II	Lymphocytosis plus splenomegaly and/or hepatomegaly
III	Lymphocytosis plus anaemia (Hb < 11 g/dl)
IV	Lymphocytosis plus thrombocytopenia (platelets < 100×10^9/l)

International Working Party classification (Binet *et al.*, 1981)

Stage	Organ enlargement*	Haemoglobin (g/dl)	Platelets ($\times 10^9$/l)
A	0, 1 or 2 areas	> 10	> 100
B	3, 4 or 5 areas		
C		< 10 and/or	< 100

* Involved areas include cervical, axillary or inguinal nodes, spleen or liver.

prolymphocytes (> 10%), a diffuse pattern of bone marrow infiltration, cytogenetic abnormalities, male sex and age over 70 years (Catovsky *et al.*, 1989).

In newly diagnosed CLL patients it is important to allow a period of observation to be able to assess the activity of the disease. Most stage A patients have stable disease at the time of diagnosis and may not require early treatment. However, some form of therapy is usually required after a variable period of time in those who progress. The decision to begin treatment is based on clinical indications (see below).

In a proportion of patients with advanced disease there is transformation of the cell clone to a more aggressive type of disease. Prolymphocytoid transformation is the commonest form, occurring in up to 30% of cases with a progressive rise in the proportion of prolymphocytes seen in the peripheral blood. Patients with 10–55% prolymphocytes have features intermediate between CLL and B-PLL and are designated CLL/PL. Clinically these patients have a more aggressive course that is less responsive to conventional therapy and is associated with rising lymphocyte counts and splenomegaly. Immunoblastic transformation, or Richter's syndrome, the development of a large cell lymphoma in a patient with CLL, has been reported to occur in 3–5% of CLL patients. Fever, weight loss and localized lymphadenopathy, especially intra-abdominal, are typical features. Some patients benefit from CHOP chemotherapy but the prognosis is generally poor with most patients dying within 6 months. Studies using DNA analysis indicate that in 50% of cases transformation arises from a different clone to that of the CLL.

(e) Treatment

As present treatment for CLL is not curative it is necessary to decide on the optimal time to start therapy as well as which treatment to give. Data from the MRC (Catovsky *et al.*, 1991) and French trials (French Cooperative Group on Chronic Lymphocytic Leukaemia, 1990) have shown that treatment of early disease (stage A) is harmful, due mainly to disease progression following a clinical response in some patients. Treatment should therefore be delayed until there is evidence of clinical progression. Furthermore, in 50% of stage A patients the main causes of death are not CLL related; thus, specific CLL treatment is unlikely to alter this. The majority of patients will eventually require therapy and this should be considered when there is evidence of bone marrow failure (stage C) with a downward trend in haemoglobin and platelet counts, progressive lymphadenopathy and/or hepatosplenomegaly or a rapidly rising lymphocyte count (doubling time < 12 months).

(f) Chemotherapy

For many years the alkylating agent chlorambucil has been the mainstay of treatment for CLL, either alone or in combination with prednisolone. This may be given as continuous low dose 0.1 mg/kg daily or intermittently at a higher dose, 10 mg/m² × 6 days every 4 weeks. Responses occur in about 70% of patients but are rarely complete and most of the responding patients will eventually relapse and may be resistant to further treatment with alkylating agents. There is no evidence that the addition of prednisolone, either with chlorambucil or with oncovin and cyclophosphamide, as in COP, improves results in CLL. However, corticosteroids may be useful as initial treatment for the first few weeks in patients with stage C disease by improving bone marrow function.

The role of anthracyclines in CLL is still unresolved. The French CLL 80 trial showed a statistically significant survival difference in stage C patients between CHOP (51% 5 year survival) and COP (18% 5 year survival) (French Cooperative Group on Chronic Lymphocytic Leukaemia, 1989). Other groups using anthracycline-containing combinations have shown a higher response rate with more complete remissions but no survival advantage compared to alkylating agents only. There are a number of ongoing trials examining the role of anthracyclines which should resolve this issue, e.g. the MRC CLL3 trial which compares chlorambucil alone (10 mg/m² a day × 6 days) with chlorambucil at the same dose plus epirubicin (50 mg/m² I.V. day 1); either treatment is repeated every 4 weeks.

The availability of new lymphocytotoxic agents, namely the purine nucleoside analogues fludarabine, 2′ deoxycoformycin (DCF) and 2-chlorodeoxyadenosine (2-CdA), has recently aroused interest by offering the potential to improve the response to treatment and ultimately also improve the survival. These drugs are structurally very similar and all interfere with the purine degradation pathway although their exact mechanism of action differs.

The largest clinical experience in the treatment of CLL has been with fludarabine which appears to be the most promising of these agents. Studies at MD Anderson Hospital by Keating *et al.* (1991) in 78 previously treated

patients given fludarabine at a dose of 25–30 mg/m² × 5 days every 4 weeks gave an overall response rate of 56%. Complete remission (CR) was achieved in 15%. In patients receiving fludarabine as first line therapy the overall response rate was 80% with 37% CR. The addition of prednisolone did not confer any advantages. The response rate for fludarabine in previously untreated patients is the highest reported for any single agent in the treatment of CLL. It is too early to evaluate the durability of these responses and their potential for improving survival. However, the fact that a substantial number of patients achieve a CR raises the possibility of conducting autologous bone marrow transplantation. The median time to relapse in responders is 21 months. The experience at the Royal Marsden Hospital has been similar with 50% good responses (CR+PR) in previously treated, mostly refractory CLL (Figure 21.1).

2′ Deoxycoformycin has been very successful in the treatment of hairy cell leukaemia and also has activity in CLL. It has been used primarily in patients with advanced and

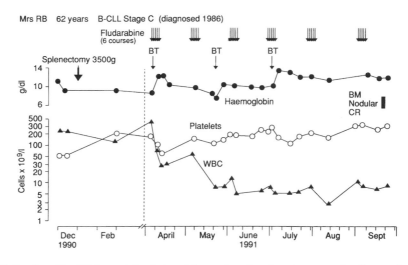

Figure 21.1 Patient with CLL resistant to chlorambucil who improved after splenectomy and subsequently achieved a good partial remission with fludarabine.

refractory disease in whom partial remissions have been obtained in about 25% of patients. 2-CdA, which is also highly active in hairy cell leukaemia, has been used in CLL with a response rate of 48% in refractory patients (Piro *et al.*, 1988). It has also been used successfully in some patients resistant to fludarabine (Juliusson *et al.*, 1992).

Figure 21.1 shows that other forms of treatment may be useful including **splenectomy** for patients with hypersplenism, refractory AIHA or ITP and patients with a large residual spleen and poor response to treatment (Coad *et al.*, 1993). **Splenic irradiation** is as effective as chlorambucil and may relieve symptoms related to splenomegaly. **Apheresis** may be useful as an interim measure in patients with an extremely high lymphocyte count due to refractory disease or, rarely, at presentation prior to other therapy. **Allogeneic bone marrow transplantation** has been performed in a few centres for younger patients with advanced and progressive disease. **Intravenous immunoglobulin infusions** have been shown to reduce the incidence of bacterial infections but did not improve survival and should be considered for selected patients with repeated bacterial infection. Treatment of autoimmune complications (AIHA or ITP) is the same as for other patients with these disorders, starting with prednisolone and often followed by danazol, azathioprine or continuous cyclophosphamide.

21.3.2   B-CELL PROLYMPHOCYTIC LEUKAEMIA

Prolymphocytic leukaemia (B-PLL) differs from CLL both morphologically and clinically. Patients characteristically present with a large spleen, little or no lymphadenopathy and a marked lymphocytosis (usually $> 100 \times 10^9/l$). The diagnostic feature is the presence of $> 55\%$ prolymphocytes in the peripheral blood. The cells are uniform in appearance and are larger than those of CLL with a prominent central nucleolus but relatively condensed nuclear chromatin. The immunophenotype of the cells differs from CLL in that the cells express high density SmIg, FMC7 and CD22 and usually lack CD5 (Table 21.1).

Patients with B-PLL tend to have a more aggressive clinical course and are less responsive to treatment. Good responses have been achieved using CHOP and fludarabine. Splenectomy or splenic irradiation are useful in selected patients and are often part of the overall treatment strategy.

21.3.3   HAIRY CELL LEUKAEMIA

Hairy cell leukaemia (HCL) accounts for approximately 2% of all leukaemias. It predominantly affects middle-aged males, with a median age of onset of about 50 years and a male : female ratio of 4 : 1. The aetiology remains unknown.

(a)   Clinical and laboratory features

Presenting symptoms result from the low blood counts and splenomegaly is the most frequent physical finding with a palpable spleen in 70% of patients. The liver is also enlarged in half the cases but peripheral lymphadenopathy is rare. The blood counts reveals varying degrees of cytopenia as a result of bone marrow failure and/or splenic sequestration. Hairy cells are present in the peripheral blood but their proportion is variable and in some cases few are seen. Profound monocytopenia is a characteristic feature of HCL and has been implicated in the pathogenesis of atypical infections which may occur. Large abdominal nodes have been reported by us in patients with longstanding disease (Mercieca *et al.*, 1992) but may be found at diagnosis in about 20% of cases. For this reason abdominal CT scan should be part of the initial investigation of HCL.

(b) Diagnosis

Hairy cells are best seen on peripheral blood films. They are large cells with abundant cytoplasm and characteristic villous projections; the nucleus is eccentric and round or indented in shape. Bone marrow aspirates are difficult to obtain as a result of increased reticulin fibres. A bone marrow trephine biopsy is an essential investigation and usually shows a diffuse or patchy infiltration by hairy cells in characteristic loose arrangement. Hairy cells have a unique immunophenotype and express strongly CD11c, CD25, HC2 and B-ly-7 in addition to other B-cell markers (monoclonal SmIg, CD19, CD20) (Table 21.2).

(c) Treatment

Most patients will eventually require treatment for progressive pancytopenia or splenomegaly. Recent advances in treatment have considerably improved the outlook for patients and most will have a near-normal life expectancy (Saven and Piro, 1992).

With the advent of effective chemotherapeutic agents, splenectomy, once the mainstay of treatment, is now less frequently performed and is reserved for patients with massive spleens disproportionate to the degree of bone marrow involvement. Alpha-interferon was the first agent shown to have substantial activity in HCL. Doses of 3 mega units three to five times a week are commonly used. The overall response rate is about 85% but with few CRs. Best results are obtained if treatment is continued for at least 1 to 2 years. On stopping, most patients will eventually relapse with a median duration of remission of 15 months after stopping treatment. Clinical remission is maintained on continuation of interferon.

The purine analogues DCF (Pentostatin) and 2-CdA are extremely effective in HCL (Dearden and Catovsky, 1990; Piro *et al.*, 1990), inducing a high frequency of complete remissions which appear to be durable (over 4 years in patients treated with DCF). DCF is given at a dose of 4 mg/m^2 every 2 weeks and treatment is usually completed in 4–6 months. 2-CdA is given as a continuous infusion at a dose of 0.1 mg/kg/day for 7 days with complete remission rates of 75–85% after a single course. It is likely that these agents will have an increasing role in the management of this condition.

21.3.4 HAIRY CELL LEUKAEMIA VARIANT

A group of HCL patients present with high WBC (> 50×10^9/l) and splenomegaly. The cells have prominent nucleoli and lack some of the hairy cell antigens such as HC2 and CD25. These patients respond less well to the treatment used in HCL but the disease has, otherwise, a protracted clinical course (Sainati *et al.*, 1990).

21.4 LEUKAEMIC PHASE OF NON-HODGKIN'S LYMPHOMA (B-CELL TYPE)

21.4.1 SPLENIC LYMPHOMA WITH CIRCULATING 'VILLOUS' LYMPHOCYTES (SLVL)

This disorder is primarily a splenic lymphoma with a variable degree of lymphocytosis and has often been confused in the past with both CLL and HCL (Mulligan *et al.*, 1991). Dominant splenomegaly with little or no lymphadenopathy are the typical clinical findings. The lymphocytes are slightly larger than those of CLL with short villi, usually in a polar distribution, a small nucleolus and often some lymphoplasmacytic cells. The bone marrow is easily aspirable and there may be little involvement early in the disease; the bone marrow biopsy shows a nodular or mixed nodular and interstitial pattern of infiltration. The

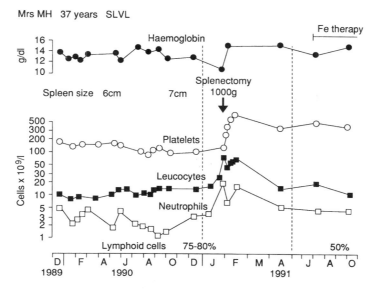

Figure 21.2 Haematology chart of patient with SLVL whose counts improved after splenectomy.

pattern of splenic infiltration is primarily in the white pulp, in contrast to HCL where there is only red pulp involvement. Two-thirds of patients have a small monoclonal band, usually IgM. The membrane phenotype is similar to that of other NHLs and distinct from HCL and CLL (Table 21.2). SLVL has a benign clinical course. When treatment is required splenectomy (Figure 21.2) appears to be the treatment of choice; chemotherapy with single alkylating agents may be useful in some patients. Transformation to a large cell NHL may be seen in 5% of cases. Autoimmune haemolytic anaemia is rare but well documented.

21.4.2 FOLLICULAR LYMPHOMA

Most patients with follicular lymphoma have some degree of bone marrow involvement (often paratrabecular infiltration) at presentation and some may also have a lymphocytosis. Histologically it corresponds to Working Formulation B and C and clinically resembles CLL with lymphadenopathy and splenomegaly. The circulating lymphocytes are very small and often have a deep nuclear cleft. Membrane markers are helpful in distinguishing these cells from CLL (Table 21.2). Patients presenting with high WBC and bulky disease have a more aggressive clinical course and often require combination chemotherapy with anthracyclines, e.g. CHOP. Fludarabine (25 mg/m^2 × 5 days every month) is also effective in these cases with a 65% response rate in our experience.

21.4.3 MANTLE CELL LYMPHOMA

This disease has previously been described as intermediate NHL and encompasses diffuse centrocytic in the Kiel classification; it corresponds to group D in the Working Formulation. Some of these patients evolve with leukaemia. The lymphocytes seen in the peripheral blood are pleomorphic; most are medium to large size with a moderate amount of cytoplasm and irregular, often moderately clefted nuclei. As in CLL the cells are CD5+ but differ in several other markers (Table 21.2). Treatment is often CHOP and/or other combinations used for high grade NHL;

single agent chemotherapy, including fludarabine, is ineffective. The overall prognosis is significantly worse than that of follicular lymphoma and SLVL.

21.4.4 LARGE CELL LYMPHOMA

A leukaemic phase is an uncommon complication of large cell lymphoma of B-cell type and may be difficult to diagnose on morphological grounds alone. The cells are large, blastic and often resemble acute leukaemia, especially monocytic leukaemia. In most cases the cells are centroblasts (Kiel classification); treatment is for high grade NHL.

21.5 T-CELL LEUKAEMIAS

In the Western world chronic T-cell leukaemias are much rarer than their B-cell counterparts, accounting for less than 10% of the chronic lymphoid leukaemias. Considerable confusion has surrounded the definition of T-cell CLL as this term has been used to describe several different T-cell disorders now recognized as distinct entities. All these T-cell disorders arise from post-thymic (mature) T lymphocytes which are TdT- and CD1a- (Catovsky and Foa, 1990; Matutes and Catovsky, 1991).

21.5.1 LARGE GRANULAR LYMPHOCYTE (LGL) LEUKAEMIA

The benign nature of this condition and, until recently, the lack of clonal markers for T-cells have, in the past, resulted in uncertainty as to the leukaemic nature of this disease (Loughran and Starkebaum, 1987).

(a) Clinical and laboratory features

The diagnosis should be suspected in cases with a persistent (> 6 months) T-cell lymphocytosis and it is usually possible to establish this using simple clinical and laboratory guidelines, as follows:

1. Lymphocytosis $> 5 \times 10^9/l$ persisting for 6 months or longer without an obvious cause.
2. 80% or more granular T-lymphocytes in the peripheral blood.
3. Neutropenia or other cytopenia in the absence of heavy bone marrow infiltration.
4. Predominance of a discrete T-cell subset by membrane marker analysis. Clonality is demonstrated by T-cell receptor rearrangement in most cases.

Symptoms result from the cytopenias with neutropenia and recurrent infections the most frequent. The pathogenesis of the cytopenias is likely to be cell-mediated suppression of normal haemopoiesis by the T-lymphocytes. Moderate splenomegaly is the most common clinical finding. In about 30% of patients there is serological and/or clinical evidence of rheumatoid arthritis but the exact relationship between LGL leukaemia and Felty's syndrome is unclear. The WBC is usually only moderately raised ($5-25 \times 10^9/l$) and the lymphocytes have abundant cytoplasm with prominent azurophilic granules. Despite the relatively uniform morphology the membrane phenotype is heterogeneous. The most common phenotype is CD3+, CD4–, CD8+, CD16–, CD56+. These lymphocytes have cytotoxic or suppressor function.

(b) Treatment

Many patients do not require therapy. Splenectomy is of limited value in correcting the cytopenias and the neutropenia rarely improves. Some patients respond to alkylating agents and/or prednisolone; cyclosporin A and deoxycoformycin have also been successful in some patients.

21.5.2 T-PROLYMPHOCYTIC LEUKAEMIA (T-PLL)

T-PLL (Matutes *et al.*, 1991) is characterized by very high lymphocyte counts (> $100 \times 10^9/l$)

and splenomegaly; generalized lymphadeno-pathy and skin involvement are also often seen. In half the cases the morphology of the cells is similar to that seen in B-PLL. In about 20% the cells are smaller and without a prominent nucleolus. Nuclear irregularities and basophilic cytoplasm are also common features. The most frequent phenotype is CD4+ CD8– but in a third of cases the cells co-express CD4 and CD8 or are CD4– CD8+.

T-PLL is an aggressive disease with a median survival of 7 months. Responses have been obtained with the combination CHOP and deoxycoformycin is a useful agent with responses in about 50% of patients, including some CRs. The humanized monoclonal antibody Campath-1H also seems to show activity in this disease.

21.5.3 ADULT T-CELL LEUKAEMIA/LYMPHOMA (ATLL)

ATLL has a distinct geographical distribution affecting the Southwest islands of Japan, the Caribbean basin and some areas of South America. These is evidence that the disease is caused by the human retrovirus HTLV-I which is integrated into the DNA of the leukaemic cells. Most patients have a leukaemic picture at presentation and are usually suffering from the acute form of the disease, but in 10% it is the chronic or smouldering form. A quarter of patients have lymphomatous disease with little or no blood involvement. The main clinical manifestations of ATLL are hyper-calcaemia, generalized lymphadenopathy, hepatosplenomegaly and skin lesions. The acute form of the disease has a median survival of 6 months. Good responses have been documented with a number of combinations used in high grade NHL but remissions are usually of short duration. DCF is moderately effective in some patients.

21.5.4 SEZARY SYNDROME

Sezary syndrome is primarily a cutaneous T-cell lymphoma with circulating malignant T cells in the peripheral blood. These cells are of two types: the large Sezary cell and the smaller Lutzner cell which can be seen in two-thirds of cases. The characteristic feature of these cells is the convoluted or cerebriform nucleus which is well demonstrated by electron microscopy. The main clinical feature is the skin involvement and biopsies demonstrate the classical epidermotrophism of the T cells. Lymphadenopathy is also commonly seen and occasionally hepatosplenomegaly. Treatment may be directed primarily at the skin using phototherapy with ultraviolet (PUVA) or topical steroids. For more advanced disease systemic chemotherapy may be required and we have had success using DCF with a response rate of 55%, including some very prolonged complete remissions.

21.6 CHRONIC MYELOID LEUKAEMIAS

The term chronic myeloid leukaemia (CML) may be used as a generic term for a group of related conditions that involve proliferation of the myeloid elements of the bone marrow, chiefly granulocytes and megakaryocytes and sometimes also monocytes. It is also commonly used to describe the classical form of the disease. The CMLs can be classified as follows:

1. Chronic granulocytic leukaemia (CGL) (Ph positive, BCR positive)
2. Chronic granulocytic leukaemia (CGL) (Ph negative, BCR positive)
3. Atypical chronic myeloid leukaemia (CML) (Ph negative, BCR negative)
4. Juvenile CML
5. Chronic neutrophilic leukaemia
6. Eosinophilic leukaemia
7. Chronic myelomonocytic leukaemia.

21.6.1 CHRONIC GRANULOCYTIC LEUKAEMIA (CGL)

(a) Epidemiology

Chronic granulocytic leukaemia comprises < 20% of all the leukaemias and occurs with an annual incidence of about one case per 100 000 of the population worldwide. Patients most often present in the fifth and sixth decades of life and there is a slight male predominance (ratio 1.4 : 1). In most cases there are no known predisposing factors, although the incidence of CGL was significantly increased in the atomic bomb survivors in Japan.

(b)   Pathogenesis

CGL is an acquired abnormality arising in a single pluripotential stem cell, giving rise to a clone with a growth advantage over normal cells. This stem cell replicates excessively and produces vast numbers of more differentiated progeny so that at the time of diagnosis the total granulocyte mass is increased by 5- to 30-fold. Detailed cytogenetic and molecular studies have provided valuable insights into the nature and pathogenesis of this disease.

In 1960 the Philadelphia (Ph) chromosome was discovered in myeloid cells from patients with CGL (Nowell and Hungerford, 1960) and was later identified as a reciprocal translocation between chromosomes 9 and 22, designated t(9;22) (Rowley, 1973). The Ph chromosome is found in 90–95% of patients with typical CGL. As a result of the translocation the ABL gene from chromosome 9 comes into close juxtaposition to part of the BCR gene on chromosome 22 forming a hybrid BCR-ABL gene. The resulting gene product is a protein of 210 kDa with tyrosine kinase activity that is expressed in the leukaemic cells. It is not known precisely how this protein is involved in the pathogenesis of CGL, but it is likely that it interferes with the control mechanisms for proliferation of haemopoietic stem cells.

(c)   Clinical features

The most common presentation is with lethargy and other symptoms of anaemia. Some patients present with abdominal swelling or discomfort as a result of splenomegaly and, not infrequently, symp-toms of hypermetabolism including weight loss and sweating which may mimic thyrotoxicosis. As more routine blood tests are performed an increasing number of patients are asymptomatic at the time of diagnosis. More unusual symptoms are priapism and visual symptoms in patients with extreme leucocytosis and hyperviscosity and gout or renal impairment due to hyperuricaemia from excessive purine breakdown.

Splenomegaly is the principal physical sign, present in 80–90% of patients. The liver is also enlarged in about 50% and occasionally patients at diagnosis may have generalized lymphadenopathy which does not necessarily indicate transformation.

(d)   Laboratory findings

The appearances of the peripheral blood are diagnostic. At diagnosis the leucocyte count is usually between $50 \times 10^9/l$ and $300 \times 10^9/l$. However, in occasional patients it may be less than $50 \times 10^9/l$ or greater than $500 \times 10^9/l$. The differential leucocyte count shows the full spectrum of granulocytic cells from blasts to mature neutrophils with a predominance of myelocytes and neutrophils; blasts constitute less than 5% of the differential count. There is invariably a basophilia and eosinophils are usually also increased. Patients with WBC $> 150 \times 10^9/l$ will usually be anaemic; platelets are usually moderately elevated $(400–700 \times 10^9/l)$.

Bone marrow examination is useful to obtain material for cytogenetic analysis and to determine the degree of marrow fibrosis. It may also sometimes reveal an impending blast crisis not yet apparent in the peripheral blood. The features are of a densely hypercellular marrow with increased granulopoiesis, normal maturation, increased numbers of megakaryocytes and reduced erythropoiesis.

Other characteristic laboratory findings are a low neutrophil alkaline phosphatase, elevated B12 and B12 binding proteins due to increased production of transcobalamin I by myeloid cells and a raised urate level.

(e) Course and prognosis

In the majority of patients CGL is a biphasic or triphasic disease. The initial chronic phase lasts for a variable period of time; the median duration is 3.5 years but in some patients may be over 10 years. The disease may then change abruptly to an acute transformation but, more often, there is a gradual acceleration that ultimately progresses to transformation. Various clinical and laboratory features have been analysed in an attempt to predict survival and several prognostic scoring systems have been described (Sokal *et al.*, 1984; Kantarjian *et al.*, 1990; The Italian Cooperative Study Group, 1991). Features generally associated with a worse prognosis include large spleens, high leucocyte counts, anaemia and a high requirement for cytotoxic drugs to control the WBC.

The patient may be asymptomatic when the disease begins to accelerate but there are various features associated with this phase.

Blast transformation is defined by the presence of more than 30% blasts or blasts plus promyelocytes in the blood and/or bone marrow. Symptoms such as fever, sweats, weight loss or bone pain may be present. Other possible manifestations include lymphadenopathy, splenic pain and subcutaneous nodules.

(f) Treatment

There are a number of therapeutic options in the management of CGL (Goldman, 1990). The only curative treatment at present is allogeneic bone marrow transplantation and this is the treatment of choice for younger patients with HLA compatible siblings. Conventional treatment with busulphan or hydroxyurea provides good symptomatic control but does not appear to prolong survival. Interferon-alpha is also an effective treatment and some studies have shown a survival benefit in responders, but treatment is not tolerated by some patients. Other, newer forms of treatment such as volunteer donor allografts (McGlave *et al.*, 1990) and autografts (Butturini *et al.*, 1990) are also promising.

(g) Management of the chronic phase

Busulphan, an alkylating agent derivative, was the mainstay of treatment until recently. Its effects are principally upon relatively early precursor cells and therefore changes in the blood count may be delayed and persist longer than with other treatments. For this reason blood counts need to be monitored closely and the drug stopped as the leucocyte count approaches normal. Busulphan may be administered either continuously at low dosage (2–8 mg) or as a single higher dose (1–1.5 mg/kg) every 4–8 weeks. The most serious adverse effect is severe marrow hypoplasia which may be irreversible and fatal. Other side-effects include pulmonary fibrosis, sterility and pigmentation. For these reasons hydroxyurea has become the favoured treatment for CGL in chronic phase in recent years. Hydroxyurea is a ribonucleotide reductase inhibitor that blocks DNA synthesis. It gives rapid control of the leucocyte count and there is fairly rapid reversal of the drug's effects on cessation of therapy; treatment therefore needs to be given continuously. The starting dose is usually 2 g/day; dosage is adjusted once the leucocyte count falls to a suitable maintenance dose (usually 1–1.5 g/day). Treatment is generally well tolerated but occasionally causes nausea and skin rashes.

Alpha-interferon (IFN) has been the most significant chemotherapeutic advance in the treatment of CGL in recent years. IFN given at a minimum dose of 3 mega units daily induces a complete haematological response in 70–80% of patients and a cytogenetic response with reduction in the number of Ph-positive dividing cells in up to 25%

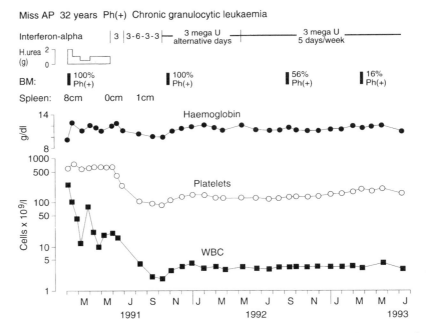

Figure 21.3   Patient with CGL, Ph positive, entered into the MRC CGL 3 trial. Haematological control was achieved with hydroxyurea and has been well controlled subsequently with alpha-interferon only. The gradual reduction of Ph-positive metaphases in the bone marrow samples over a 2 year period should be noted.

(Figure 21.3) (Talpaz *et al.*, 1987). Complete suppression of the Ph-positive clone may occur which may be sustained in a minority, some of whom have no evidence of BCR/ABL transcripts by PCR (Talpaz *et al.*, 1991). The Houston group responsible for these initial studies of IFN in CGL have concluded that IFN prolongs life by 2 years in haematological responders and has an even greater benefit in those with a cytogenetic response. Results of randomized studies have not been conclusive in this respect; the survival results of the UK MRC CGL 3 trial are not yet available but the cytogenetic and haematological responses have been confirmed (Figure 21.3).

IFN causes a number of side-effects, some of which will resolve after a few weeks on treatment, particularly the 'flu-like' symptoms. Other effects are anorexia, weight loss, mood changes, alopecia and abnormal liver enzymes. About 20% of patients may be unable to tolerate long term treatment.

(h)   Bone marrow transplantation

Allogeneic BMT can cure patients with CGL and should be performed in the chronic phase as results are poor in more advanced stages. The leukaemia free survival is 40–60%. However, lack of an HLA-compatible sibling and the numbers of older patients limit the applicability of this treatment to about 10% of patients.

Progress has been made in using HLA matched volunteer donors for patients without an HLA compatible sibling. At present there is about a 20% chance of finding a compatible donor for a Caucasian patient. The results are inferior to using a sibling donor marrow because of an increased incidence of graft-versus-host disease. Leukaemia free survival at 2 years is about 40%.

Autologous BMT using peripheral blood stem cells after high dose chemotherapy have yielded some promising preliminary results. In the future it may be possible to select out Ph-negative stem cells so that complete remission would be possible.

(i) Management of the accelerated phase

Control may be achieved in the short term by adding or changing cytotoxic drugs. In patients with refractory splenomegaly splenectomy may be useful.

(j) Management of blastic transformation

The blast cells should be immunophenotyped and classified as myeloid or lymphoid so that appropriate treatment may be given. Myeloid transformation is often treated with the same drugs as used in primary AML. In most patients chemotherapy results in a decrease in the number of blasts; this is often followed by a prolonged period of pancytopenia which may be fatal. Generally, the blasts reappear but in about 20% of patients chronic phase haemopoiesis may be restored for a short period.

Using similar treatment to that for adult ALL, there is a 50% response rate in patients with lymphoblastic transformation. The blasts have a B-cell precursor phenotype (TdT+, CALLA+ or −, CD19+). Most of the responding patients will re-establish chronic phase haemopoiesis and some will have long periods free of symptoms before relapsing.

21.6.2 Ph-POSITIVE ACUTE LYMPHOBLASTIC LEUKAEMIA

About 20% of adults and 2–3% of children who present with ALL have a Ph chromosome due to t(9;22). There are usually no features suggestive for CGL. The presence of the Ph chromosome in ALL confers a poor prog-

nosis and patients should be treated appropriately. Occasional patients in remission have haemopoiesis typical or CGL chronic phase.

21.6.3 Ph-NEGATIVE CHRONIC MYELOID LEUKAEMIA AND ATYPICAL CML

Ten per cent of patients with clinical and laboratory features similar to Ph-positive CGL lack the Ph chromosome. Recently molecular genetic studies have revealed the BCR rearrangement in about half of these patients. By haematological, molecular and clinical criteria these cases could also be designated CGL. In those that lack this rearrangement there are subtle but distinct differences from classical CGL and they are designated atypical CML. The atypical features include a lower leucocyte count without the predominance of myelocytes, absence of basophilia or eosinophilia and thrombocytopenia (Galton, 1992). A relative monocytosis and dysplastic changes in the neutrophils are also features of atypical CML. Clinically patients are older with a greater male predominance and less marked splenomegaly. Some cases may be difficult to distinguish from chronic myelomonocytic leukaemia (CMML). Treatment is generally with cytotoxic agents as used in CGL but the response to treatment and prognosis are poorer.

21.6.4 JUVENILE CHRONIC MYELOID LEUKAEMIA

This is a rare disorder usually occurring in children under 5 years of age and should be clearly distinguished from true CGL in childhood. The child may present with fever, sweating, weight loss or various septic lesions. Hepatosplenomegaly, lymphadenopathy and rashes are the usual clinical findings. The blood picture is different from that seen in CGL with immature granulocytes, monocytosis and thrombocytopenia with no basophilia or eosinophilia. A characteristic feature is a raised level of fetal haemoglobin. Cytogenetic studies are normal. Response to treatment, usually with drugs used in acute myeloid leukaemia, is generally poor.

21.6.5 EOSINOPHILIC LEUKAEMIA

This is a very rare condition which may, in some cases, be difficult to distinguish from the hypereosinophilic syndrome (HES). Features suggestive of eosinophilic leukaemia include the presence of immature abnormal-looking eosinophils and cytogenetic abnormalities but not the Ph chromosome. Other signs and symptoms include sweats, weight loss and splenomegaly. Cardiac abnormalities may be present and are due to the direct toxic effect of eosinophil cationic proteins also seen in HES. Patients may respond to a variety of drugs including hydroxyurea, vincristine and prednisolone. The condition may remain stable for some years but will ultimately transform to a blastic phase which is very resistant to treatment.

21.6.6 CHRONIC NEUTROPHILIC LEUKAEMIA

This is also extremely rare. The only consistent abnormality is of a raised neutrophil count and the diagnosis can only be made when all other causes have been excluded. Neutrophil alkaline phosphatase is high, in contrast to CGL, and the Ph chromosome is negative. Treatment is only necessary if the patient is symptomatic.

21.6.7 CHRONIC MYELOMONOCYTIC LEUKAEMIA

Chronic myelomonocytic leukaemia has been included in the FAB classification of the myelodysplastic syndromes. The diagnostic feature is the presence of increased numbers of monocytes in the peripheral blood and various dysplastic features are also often seen. Patients with high WBC (and $> 5 \times 10^9/l$ monocytes) have more features of myeloproliferative disease than myelodysplasia. Patients are usually elderly and may present with symptoms of anaemia or weight loss. Other features include moderate splenomegaly and high serum lysozyme levels. The disease often runs an indolent course requiring little treatment but it usually transforms to a more acute phase which is not very responsive to treatment.

REFERENCES

Bennett, J.M., Catovsky, D., Daniel, M.T. *et al.* The French-American-British Cooperative Group (1989) Proposals for the classification of chronic (mature) B and T lymphoid leukaemias. *Journal of Clinical Pathology*, **42**, 567–84.

Binet, J.L., Auquier, A., Dighiero, G. *et al.* (1989) A new prognostic classification of chronic lymphocytic leukaemia derived from a multivariate survival analysis. *Cancer*, **48**, 198–206.

Butturini, A., Keating, A., Goldman, J. and Gale, R.P. (1990) Autotransplants in chronic myelogenous leukaemia: strategies and results. *Lancet*, **335**, 1255–8.

Catovsky, D. and Foa, R. (1990) *The Lymphoid Leukaemias*, Butterworth, Oxford.

Catovsky, D., Fooks, J., Richards, S. for the MRC Working Party on Leukaemia in Adults (1989) Prognostic factors in chronic lymphocytic leukaemia: the importance of age, sex and response to treatment in survival. *British Journal of Haematology*, **72**, 141–9.

Catovsky, D., Richards, S., Fooks, J. and Hamblin, T.C. (1991) CLL trials in the United Kingdom. The Medical Research Council trials 1, 2 and 3. *Leukaemia and Lymphoma*, **5**, (Suppl), 105–12.

Coad, J.E., Matutes, E. and Catovsky, D. (1993) Splenectomy in lymphoproliferative disorders: a report on 70 cases and review of the literature. *Leukaemia and Lymphoma*, **10**, 245–64.

Dearden, C. and Catovsky, D. (1990), Treatment of hairy cell leukaemia with 2'-deoxycoformycin. *Leukaemia and Lymphoma*, **1**, 179–85.

French Cooperative Group on Chronic Lymphocytic Leukaemia (1989) Long-tern results of the CHOP regimen in stage C chronic lymphocytic leukaemia. *British Journal of Haematology*, **73**, 334–40.

French Cooperative Group on Chronic Lymphocytic Leukaemia (1990) Natural history of stage A chronic lymphocytic leukaemia. *British Journal of Haematology*, **76**, 45–57.

Galton, D.A.G. (1992) Haematological differences between chronic granulocytic leukaemia, atypical chronic myeloid leukaemia and chronic myelomonocytic leukaemia. *Leukaemia and Lymphoma*, **7**, 343–50.

Goldman, J.M. (1990) Options for the management of chronic myeloid leukaemia – (1990). *Leukaemia and Lymphoma*, **3**, 159–64.

International Workshop on Chronic Lymphocytic Leukaemia (1981) Chronic lymphocytic leukaemia: proposals for a revised prognostic staging system. *British Journal of Haematology*, **48**, 365–7.

The Italian Cooperative Study Group on Chronic Myeloid Leukaemia (1991) Confirmation and improvement of Sokal's prognostic classification of Ph+ chronic myeloid leukaemia: the value of early evaluation of the course of the disease. *Annals of Haematology*, **63**, 307–14.

Juliusson, G., Elmhorn-Rosenborg, A. and Liliemark, J. (1992) Response to 2-chlorodeoxyadenosine in patients with B-cell chronic lymphocytic leukaemia resistant to fludarabine. *New England Journal of Medicine*, **327**, 1056–61.

Juliusson, G., Oscier, D.G., Fitchett, M. *et al.* (1990) Prognostic subgroups in B-cell chronic lymphocytic leukaemia defined by specific chromosomal abnormalities. *New England Journal of Medicine*, **323**, 720–4.

Kantarjian, H.M., Keating, M.J., Smith, T.L., Talpaz, M. and McCredie, K.B. (1990) Proposal for a simple synthesis prognostic staging system in chronic myelogenous leukaemia. *American Journal of Medicine*, **88**, 1–7.

Keating, M.J., Kantarjian, H., O'Brien, S. *et al.* (1991) New agents and strategies in CLL treatment. *Leukaemia and Lymphoma*, (Suppl), 139–42.

Loughran, T.P. and Starkebaum, G. (1987) Large granular lymphocyte leukaemia. Report of 38 cases and review of the literature. *Medicine*, **66**, 397–403.

Matutes, E., Brito-Babapulle, V., Swansbury, J. *et al.* (1991) Clinical and laboratory features of 78 cases of T-prolymphocytic leukaemia. *Blood*, **78**, 3269–74.

Matutes, E. and Catovsky, D. (1991) Mature T-cell leukaemias and leukaemia/lymphoma syndromes. Review of our experience in 175 cases. *Leukaemia and Lymphoma*, **4**, 81–91.

McGlave, P.B., Beatty, P., Ash, R. and Hows, J.M. (1990) Therapy for chronic myelogenous leukaemia with unrelated donor bone marrow transplantation: results in 102 cases. *Blood*, **75**, 1728–32.

Mercieca, J., Matutes, E., Moskovic, E. *et al.* (1992) Massive abdominal lymphadenopathy in hairy cell leukaemia: a report of 12 cases. *British Journal of Haematology*, **82**, 547–54.

Mulligan, S.P., Matutes, E., Dearden, C. and Catovsky, D. (1991) Splenic lymphoma with villous lymphocytes: natural history and response to therapy in 50 cases. *British Journal of Haematology*, **78**, 206–9.

Nowell, P.C. and Hungerford, D.A. (1960) A minute chromosome in human chronic granulocytic leukaemia. *Journal of the National Cancer Institute*, **25**, 85–109.

Piro, L.D., Carrera, C.J., Beutler, E. and Carson, D.A. (1988) 2-Chlorodeoxyadenosine: an effective new agent for the treatment of chronic lymphocytic leukaemia. *Blood*, **72**, 1069–73.

Piro, L.D., Carrera, C.J., Carson, D.A. and Beutler, E. (1990) Lasting remissions in hairy-cell leukaemia induced by a single infusion of 2-chlorodeoxyadenosine. *New England Journal of Medicine*, **322**, 1117–21.

Rai, K.R., Sawtisky, A., Cronkite, E. *et al.* (1975) Clinical staging of chronic lymphocytic leukaemia. *Blood*, **46**, 219–34.

Rowley, J.D. (1973) A new consistent chromosome abnormality in chronic myelogenous leukaemia indentified by quinacrine fluorescence and giemsa staining. *Nature*, **243**, 290–3.

Sainati, L., Matutes, E., Mulligan, S. *et al.* (1990) A variant form of hairy cell leukaemia resistant to alpha-interferon: clinical and phenotypic characteristics of 17 patients. *Blood*, **76**, 157–62.

Saven, A. and Piro, L.D. (1992) Treatment of hairy cell leukaemia. *Blood*, **79**, 1111–20.

Sokal, J.E., Cox, E.B., Baccarani, M. *et al.* and the Italian Cooperative CML Study Group (1984) Prognostic discrimination in 'good-risk' chronic granulocytic leukaemia. *Blood*, **63**, 789–99.

Talpaz, M., Kantarjian, H.M., McCredie, K.B. *et al.* (1987) Clinical investigation of human alpha interferon in chronic myelogenous leukaemia. *Blood*, **69**, 1280–8.

Talpaz, M., Kantarjian, H., Kurzrock, R. *et al.* (1991) Interferon-alpha produces sustained cytogenetic responses in chronic myelogenous leukaemia. *Annals of Internal Medicine*, **114**, 532–8.

MYELOMA

Sue E. Height and Jennifer G. Treleaven

22.1 INTRODUCTION

Multiple myeloma accounts for 10% of haematological malignancy and 1% of all malignant disease. It is characterized by a neoplastic proliferation of a clone of plasma cells which produce a monoclonal protein (M protein).

The median age of onset is 70 years and it is extremely rare under the age of 40. Known risk factors include exposure to radiation either a single high dose such as associated with the atom bomb or chronic low dose exposure. Agricultural workers who are exposed to pesticides also have a higher incidence than the general population. There is an unexplained excess of cases amongst the black population and rare familial occurrences.

22.2 PRESENTING FEATURES

The common presenting features in myeloma are bone pain, pathological fractures, fatigue, infections, symptoms of hypercalcaemia and renal impairment (Kyle, 1975), and an estimated 90% of patients are symptomatic at diagnosis. However, since this large series was published there is evidence that many patients are now being diagnosed earlier in the course of the disease and this may have implications when current survival data are compared with earlier data (Riccardi *et al.*, 1991).

22.3 PATHOGENESIS

Normal bone marrow plasma cells are terminally differentiated and do not actively proliferate. Circulating plasmablasts are detectable in normal peripheral blood and constitute 0.5–1.0% of the mononuclear cell population (MacLennan and Chan, 1991). It is thought that they originate from lymphoid follicles in Peyers' patches, lymph nodes and the spleen and migrate to the bone marrow. One hypothesis suggests that the marrow may be 'seeded' in different sites by circulating plasmablasts which then give rise to plasma cells. Monoclonal circulating B cells at various stages of differentiation from late B cells to plasma cells have been demonstrated in myeloma, although their exact pattern of migration is not known (Jensen *et al.*, 1991). They can be induced to differentiate into terminal plasma cells *in vitro* in the presence of IL-6 and IL-3. This provides a possible model of how myeloma evolves in multiple sites in the marrow although the molecular basis of malignant transformation in the myeloma cell is not known. A circulating pre-plasma cell clonogenic population may disseminate the disease to multiple sites in the marrow where the marrow microenvironment provides the necessary growth and differentiation factors for myeloma cell development.

Cytokines have been implicated in the pathogenesis of the disease and a complex network of stimulatory and inhibitory growth factors has been studied. IL-6 is produced by marrow stromal cells and myeloma cells and appears to be an important growth factor and differentiating agent for myeloma cells *in vitro*. The positive feedback of IL-6 on myeloma cells may lead to increased production and a cascade effect. An overproduction of IL-6 has been found in 37% of patients (Bataille *et al.*, 1989) and correlated with a more aggressive disease and poorer prognosis. Monoclonal anti-IL-6 has been used to treat patients with plasma cell leukaemia (Klein-*et al.*, 1991) but this an experimental approach.

IL-6 is also an osteoclast activator in conjunction with IL1-β and TNF and may be important in the development of lytic bone lesions. The inhibition of erythropoeisis by TNF may contribute to the anaemia which is sometimes disproportionate to the level of marrow involvement, although other possible mechanisms should always be borne in mind including occult bleeding, folate deficiency and chemotherapy-induced marrow suppression.

There is synergy between the stimulator cytokines GM-CSF, G-CSF, IL-3 and IL-5 *in vitro*, whereas interferon-α and interferon-γ are inhibitory and this has been exploited by the use of interferon-α in treatment.

The commonest cytogenetic abnormalities found in myeloma involve chromosomes 1 and 14 but are not specific for the disease. Increased levels of bcl-2 protein have been found in patients with myeloma including those who do not have a demonstrable cytogenetic abnormality at this locus.

22.4 DIAGNOSIS

The diagnosis of multiple myeloma depends on the demonstration of at least two of the following;

1. The presence of an M protein or monoclonal band in the serum or urine.
2. Bone marrow infiltration by atypical plasma cells (> than 10%).
3. The presence of osteolytic lesions.

22.4.1 M PROTEIN

Serum protein electrophoresis is performed as a screening procedure in cases of suspected myeloma and usually demonstrates the presence of a monoclonal band (90% of patients), or rarely, a biclonal band (3% of patients). The electrophoretic pattern may occasionally appear normal if the paraprotein is only present in small amounts. However, immunoparesis is usually apparent with reduced amounts of normal immunoglobulins.

Immunoelectrophoresis and immunofixation using monospecific antisera to the various isotypes are performed to determine the heavy and light chain isotype. The frequency of the different types is as follows: IgG 55%, IgA 26%, κ or λ light chain only 19%, IgD 1–2%. IgE and non-secretory myeloma are very rare, κ chains are found approximately twice as frequently as λ chains, except in IgD myeloma where the ratio is reversed.

Light chains (Bence Jones proteins) are not usually detectable in the serum due to renal tubular metabolism and they are not detected by urine dipsticks. This can cause diagnostic difficulty in cases of light chain disease when no heavy chain component is produced by the myeloma cells. To identify and quantitate light chains a 24 hour urine collection, immunoelectrophoresis or immunofixation are necessary. Very rarely (< 1%), a non-secretory type of myeloma is found where no paraprotein is produced but is detectable within the plasma cells themselves.

22.4.2 BONE MARROW ASPIRATE

The bone marrow aspirate demonstrates at least 10% plasma cells with atypical features such as bizarre forms with nuclear : cytoplasmic asynchrony and multinucleate plasma cells (Figures 22.1, 22.2). In some cases more primitive plasmablasts may be present. However, bone marrow infiltration may be patchy and a negative aspirate in the presence of other diagnostic criteria may indicate the need to repeat the marrow. Trephine biopsy may give a more accurate indication of the degree of infiltration (Terpstra *et al.*, 1992).

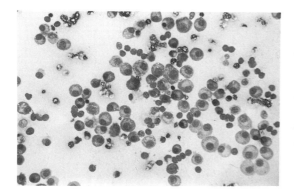

Figure 22.1 Plasma cells which are characterized by eccentric nuclei, perinuclear halo and basophilic cytoplasm.

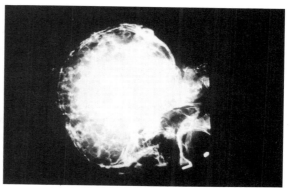

Figure 22.3 Multiple lytic lesions in the skull.

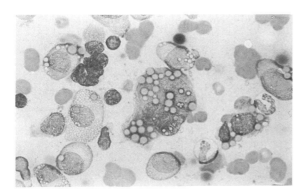

Figure 22.2 Atypical plasma cells with cyto-plasmic inclusions (Russell bodies).

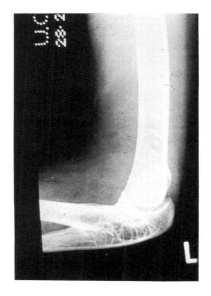

Figure 22.4 Lytic lesions in the ulna.

Immunostaining of the marrow may confirm the clonality of the plasma cell infiltrate by demonstrating heavy and light chain restriction. In the normal marrow the ratio of $\kappa : \lambda$ plasma cells is $2 : 1$ and disturbance of this ratio may provide supportive evidence for clonality.

22.4.3 SKELETAL LESIONS

Lytic lesions, generalized osteoporosis and pathological fractures in myeloma result from uncoupling of bone resorption and synthesis (Figures 21.3, 21.4). Excessive bony resorption

is pathologically related to increased numbers of atypical osteoclasts in the vicinity of myeloma cells within the bone marrow. At an advanced stage of the disease there is concurrent inhibition by TNF, IL-6 and IL-1β of normal bone formation by osteoblast and this contributes to the accelerated rate of bone loss in lytic lesions. In the rare patients who lack lytic lesions or have osteosclerotic lesions, the rate of bone resorption is also increased but is matched by normal or increased bone synthesis.

Although bone scans are usually abnormal in myeloma, they often underestimate the extent of skeletal involvement by up to 50% (Frank *et al.*, 1982) due to the osteolytic nature of the lesions. The primary investigation remains the skeletal survey to demonstrate the axial skeleton and skull. Involvement of the extremities by myeloma is extremely rare and therefore the survey does not routinely include the lower arm or leg. Vertebral lesions may be best demonstrated by CT scanning or MRI. Even in the absence of symptoms extensive disease of the marrow may be detected (Moulopoulos *et al.*, 1992).

There are several conditions which must be distinguished from myeloma; these include benign monoclonal gammopathy of unknown significance (MGUS), solitary myeloma, extramedullary plasmacytoma and plasma cell leukaemia.

22.4.4 MGUS

The diagnostic criteria for MGUS include the presence of a serum M band < 2.5 g/l with no detectable light chains in the urine, plasma cells of less than 10% in the bone marrow with no atypical forms, and the absence of osteolytic lesions. Although many patients remain stable for years with no treatment, 24% evolve into myeloma or related disorders (median time from initial diagnosis is 10 years) and so they must be followed up indefinitely. The most useful parameter to monitor is the paraprotein level.

22.4.5 SOLITARY MYELOMA

This is rare condition characterized by only a single site of bony involvement and often no detectable M band in the serum. It tends to occur in younger patients and although it responds to local radiotherapy it may recur or evolve into myeloma. The prognosis is better than for myeloma.

22.4.6 EXTRAMEDULLARY PLASMACYTOMA

This is a soft tissue mass consisting of plasma cells and may occur at any site where immunoglobulin-producing cells are located such as the gastrointestinal tract or respiratory tract, and may be single or multiple. Spread to bone may occur but it does not usually involve the marrow. Local treatment with surgery and radiotherapy is usually effective for isolated lesions and chemotherapy is indicated in cases where dissemination has occurred. Extramedullary plasmacytoma may also occur in advanced myeloma.

22.4.7 PLASMA CELL LEUKAEMIA

This is diagnosed as a primary disease when the peripheral blood contains either 20% circulating plasma cells or a total count of $2 \times 10^9/l$. The immunophenotype of these cells is CD38+, cytoplasmic Ig+ but they are often negative for other B-cell markers. Hypercalcaemia, renal failure and bony lesions are often present at diagnosis. This disease has a particularly poor prognosis and the median survival is 10 months.

22.5 STAGING AND PROGNOSIS

The staging system of Salmon and Durie (Durie and Salmon, 1975) is the most widely used (Table 22.1), although other methods of assessing prognosis have since been devised.

22.5.1 β_2 MICROGLOBULIN

β_2 microglobulin is the light chain of the HLA type I antigens present on cell membranes and is shed into the blood as a result of membrane turnover. It is renally excreted without metabolism and accumulates in renal impairment. β_2 microglobulin is detected by radioimmunoassay and levels rise with age, but normally do not exceed 2 mg/l. In myeloma the level varies in relation to tumour mass and renal impairment, and alone is the

Table 22.1 The Salmon and Durie staging system (Durie and Salmon, 1975, reproduced with permission)

		Cell mass ($\times 10^{12} m^2$)
Stage I	All of the following Hb > 10 g/dl Ca^{++} < 2.65 μmol/l Normal X-rays or solitary plasmacytoma only Low levels of M protein (IgG < 50 g/l, IgA < 30g/l) Urinary Bence Jones protein < 4 g/24 hours	< 0.6 low
Stage II	Fitting neither Stage I or III	0.6–1.20 intermediate
Stage III	One or more of the following Hb < 8.5 g/dl Ca^{++} > 2.65 μmol/l Lytic bone lesions M Protein (IgG > 70 g/l, IgA > 50 g/l) Urinary Bence Jones protein > 12g/24 hours	> 1.20 high

A, serum creatinine < 170 μmol/l; B, serum creatinine > 170 μmol/l.

single most important prognostic indicator (Cuzick *et al.*, 1985). The β_2 microglobulin level at diagnosis, uncorrected for renal failure, discriminates between patients with β_2 microglobulin levels of < 4 g/l of whom half will survive more than 3 years, whilst of those with β_2 microglobulin of > 20 g/l only one-fifth will survive 3 years. In addition, it has prognostic value in patients who have been treated and are in plateau phase with no measurable M protein (approximately 10% of patients); a stable β_2 microglobulin indicating continued plateau phase whilst a rising β_2 microglobulin reflects disease progression. However, the β_2 microglobulin is not raised in a few patients with aggressive disease and this limits its general applicability.

22.5.2 C-REACTIVE PROTEIN (CRP)

IL-6 stimulates CRP synthesis and inhibits albumin synthesis by the liver. There appears to be a direct relationship between CRP and IL-6 levels in myeloma and serum CRP may indicate disease activity. In a recent study, patients with high CRP levels (> 6 mg/l) had high tumour mass, low serum albumin and high labelling indices and showed a direct correlation with patient survival. However, there was no direct relationship between CRP and β_2 microglobulin which appeared to retain its independent prognostic value. A simple system incorporating CRP and β_2 microglobulin has been proposed (Bataille *et al.*, 1992)

22.5.3 PLASMA-CELL LABELLING INDEX

Uptake of tritiated thymidine by plasma cells in a bone marrow aspirate sample is measured to assess the number of cells actively synthesizing DNA and the calculated percentage is the labelling index (LI). An alternative method uses a monoclonal antibody to 5-bromo-2-deoxyuridine to measure DNA synthesis.

There is a broad correlation between the LI and survival but not with tumour mass, and this may be because the LI reflects the growth rate of the tumour. Patients with a low LI (< 0.8%) are likely to have a stable condition but require monitoring. According to the Salmon and Durie system, the group of patients with high tumour mass (stage III) who had a LI of < 1% had a median survival of 30.5 months compared with those with a high LI (> 3%) who had a median survival of only 5.3 months.

22.6   TREATMENT AND ASSESSMENT OF RESPONSE

Before effective treatment for myeloma was introduced in the 1960s the median survival was 7 months. Even with combination chemotherapy the median survival is only 36 months and newer regimens include dose escalation in the form of high dose therapy and biological agents to improve the response rate and survival.

The assessment of response to treatment of myeloma is problematical. Complete remission (CR) may be defined as the absence of detectable M protein in the serum, no light chains in the urine and less than 5% plasma cells in the bone marrow with no abnormal forms seen. However, many patients do not attain CR and the definition of partial remission (PR) is reduction by 50% or more of the paraprotein level or reduction in the myeloma cell infiltrate by greater than 50% in Bence Jones myeloma or non-secretory myeloma.

In patients who respond to treatment the Bence Jones protein falls to 50% of presentation levels by 2 months, whereas the M protein falls to 50% of pretreatment levels by 3 months. Therefore, 3 months from the start of treatment is the optimal time to evaluate treatment response and identify patients who have resistant disease by the persistence of Bence Jones protein and M protein (McLaughlin and Alexanian, 1982). Paradoxically, patients with a very rapid response to chemotherapy tend to have a poor prognosis, presumably because of the high proliferative capacity of their tumour (Boccadero *et al.*, 1987). Serial measurement of the M protein may appear to be the simplest way of monitoring patients but there are potential problems. The disappearance of detectable M protein may indicate initial response to treatment but in some patients subsequent disease progression is not marked by a reappearance of the original M protein but by new bony lesions. Also, the kinetics of M proteins may vary according to their subtype.

Most patients who experience a response to induction therapy eventually reach a plateau phase and no further response is seen despite continued treatment. This stable phase may last many months but is temporary and is inevitably followed by relapse. No survival benefit has been demonstrated in patients who continue on chemotherapy during this plateau phase (Belch *et al.*, 1988; Kildahl-Anderson *et al.*, 1988), and indeed it increases the risk of development of myelodysplasia or secondary acute myeloid leukaemia (AML). It is now standard policy to discontinue chemotherapy at plateau and continue monitoring of the patient. However, there is benefit from commencing interferon-α as maintenance treatment during this phase.

The first effective chemotherapy for myeloma consisted of the combination of oral melphalan (9 mg/m^2) and prednisolone (100 mg) for four consecutive days with the repetition of the course every 4–6 weeks (Alexanian *et al.*, 1969). Variability in response was noted and was attributed to variable absorption of orally administered melphalan; this now seems to be less important than intrinsic cellular resistance to the drug in certain cases (Fernberg *et al.*, 1990). The main limitation of melphalan is unpredictable renal and bone marrow toxicity in the presence of renal impairment.

Treatment with high dose steroids as a single agent has been investigated in a recent study using dexamethasone for previously untreated patients. The response rate of 43% with dexamethasone was less than that expected with VAD but it implied a major contribution of dexamethasone to the effectiveness of steroid-containing regimens (Alexanian *et al.*, 1992). In addition, there were fewer serious complications of treatment as compared with VAD (4% vs 27%)

and the authors advocate this approach as initial treatment for patients with pancytopenia and hypercalcaemia or those requiring simultaneous radiotherapy for a pathological fracture.

Steroids appear to block mRNA expression of IL-6 in myeloma cells (Ishikawa *et al.*, 1990). Marrow stromal cells are also an important site of production of IL-6 in myeloma and they too may be affected by steroids.

22.6.1 COMBINATION CHEMOTHERAPY

The introduction of alternating, non-cross-resistant combinations of drugs to circumvent drug resistance led to the development of the standard regimens currently used in myeloma (Table 22.2).

The Vth MRC trial demonstrated a significant survival advantage of patients randomized to receive ABCM (adriamycin, BCNU, cyclophosphamide and melphalan) as first line therapy over intermittent melphalan (median survival 24 months and 32 months respectively, MacLennan *et al.*, 1992). This study also demonstrated that more patients reached plateau phase with ABCM (61% vs 49% with melphalan.)

The choice of induction therapy depends on several factors. The presence of acute or chronic renal failure precludes the use of melphalan as an initial agent since its haematological and renal toxicity are exacerbated in an unpredictable manner. Regimens containing non-renally excreted drugs, e.g. VAD or VAMP, are preferable in these patients. There may be other advantages in avoiding the use of melphalan as an induction agent in young patients who may undergo a transplant procedure, since it may be used as a conditioning agent at high dose.

The multidrug resistance gene (mdr-1) which codes for the membrane p-glycoprotein responsible for resistance to the vinca alkaloids, epidophyllotoxins and anthracyclines has been extensively studied in myeloma. Cells with the mdr-1 phenotype may survive initial chemotherapy and regrowth of this population may be responsible for relapse and subsequent resistance to therapy employing the same agents as used for induction.

Table 22.2 Chemotherapy regimens

Cyclo-VAMP
Vincristine   0.4 mg by continuous i.v. infusion into large vein daily for 4 days (total dose 1.6 mg)
Adriamycin   9 mg/m² continuous i.v. infusion into large vein daily for 4 days (total dose 36 mg/m²)
Methylprednisolone   1.5 g p.o. or i.v. daily for 4 days, 1 g i.v. day 5, 500 mg day 6
Cyclophosphamide   500 mg i.v. days 1, 8 and 15

VAD
Vincristine   0.4 mg/m² daily by continuous i.v. infusion for 4 days
Doxorubicin   9 mg/m² daily by continuous i.v. infusion for 4 days
Dexamethasone   40 mg daily p.o. for four days starting day 1 (and days 9 and 17 of alternate cycles)

ABCM   given on a 6-week cycle with dosage adjustment needed for FBC, renal, hepatic impairment
Adriamycin   30 mg/m² i.v. day 1
BCNU   30 mg/m² i.v. day 1
Melphalan   6 mg/m²/day p.o. for days 22,23,24 and 25
Cyclophosphamide   100 mg/m²/day p.o. for days 22,23,24 and 25

Low dose cyclophosphamide
Cyclophosphamide 500 mg i.v. once a week

Methods of overcoming resistance including calcium antagonists, cyclosporin and amiodarone have been used.

22.6.2 HIGH DOSE THERAPY

High dose melphalan (140 mg/m^2) was used without marrow rescue as initial treatment at the Royal Marsden and resulted in a 27% CR rate in previously untreated patients and a 66% PR rate in previously treated patients. However, the median duration of response was only 18 months and there was no definite evidence of a plateau in relapse free survival (Selby *et al.*, 1987). These results prompted the introduction of treatment to clear the marrow prior to high dose melphalan with autologous marrow rescue (Gore *et al.*, 1989), and this resulted in a CR rate of 50%.

At the Royal Marsden Hospital all new patients, those refractory to other treatments and relapsed patients under the age of 65 with good performance status, currently receive cyclo-VAMP every 3 weeks to CR or plateau. This is followed by consolidation therapy with high dose melphalan with dosage adjustment for marrow infiltration and EDTA clearance. Patients with poor renal function (EDTA clearance < 30 ml/min) may receive high dose busulphan as an alternative. Marrow rescue is performed by autologous peripheral blood stem cell (APBSC) harvest using G-CSF prior to collection or autologous bone marrow harvested in remission. Patients commence α-interferon following recovery of the blood count in an attempt to try to reduce the incidence of post-transplant relapse.

Elderly patients or those who are not fit for cyclo-VAMP receive oral melphalan and prednisolone every 3 weeks, or alternatively low dose cyclophosphamide.

Autografting offers a high dose procedure to a large number of patients. The optimum time seems to be when the patient is still responsive to treatment and in a relatively good clinical state. Treatment related mor-

tality in experienced hands is less than 5% and the use of peripheral stem cell harvests may further reduce morbidity. One risk factor which has been identified is amyloidosis.

The major disadvantage of autologous transplantation is that myeloma cells may be re-infused with the harvested marrow and various purging strategies have been developed. Molecular studies of minimal residual disease applied to both marrow harvests and peripheral stem cells may help to resolve this question (Billadeau *et al.*, 1992). Autografting does not confer a graft-versus-myeloma effect as seen in allogeneic BMT and this may be associated with post-transplant relapses. However, no formal comparison of autografting and conventional chemotherapy has been made.

Allografting is an option for only 7% of patients with myeloma due to the constraints of age (only 25% are under the age of 50) and the availability of an HLA matched sibling donor. The transplant related mortality in the long term is of the order of 40–50%. The European Bone Marrow Transplant Registry review of 90 patients undergoing allogenic transplantation (Gahrton *et al.*, 1991) showed that the group who were still responsive to treatment, had stage I disease and had only received first line treatment did better than those who were stage II or III, had unresponsive disease and had received three or more types of therapy. The long term survival was better in those who were in CR after engraftment and those with mild (grade I) rather than severe graft-versus-host disease. This study concluded that allogeneic transplantation may be a reasonable treatment for patients with a suitable donor who have failed first line treatment, or those with poor prognostic disease at diagnosis including IgD myeloma, stage III disease or high β_2 microglobulin.

22.6.3 α-INTERFERON

α-Interferon has been shown to maintain the plateau phase, the duration of response and increase survival in patients who received α-interferon as maintenance when compared with those who did not (Mandelli *et al.*, 1990). The mechanism of action of α-interferon may be to increase and maintain the proportion of cells in G_0. The standard dose is between 3 and 5×10^6 IU/m^2 administered subcutaneously three times per week. There does not appear to be a dose–response curve in its therapeutic effect; however, side-effects which limit the tolerated dose do seem to be dose related. The most important toxicities include leucopenia, thrombocytopenia, fever, fatigue, weight loss and malaise. It may also elevate the β_2 microglobulin (Tienhaara *et al.*, 1991). A transient elevation of AST is seen in up to 10% of patients, some develop rashes or neurological complications including seizures. Patients commencing interferon must be warned of possible side-effects although these ameliorate over the first few weeks of treatment. Monitoring of the FBC is essential. α-Interferon has been shown to be of some benefit during chemotherapy in a minority of patients (Oken *et al.*, 1989) and may be useful in up to 20% of relapsed patients. It does not appear to be particularly effective as a single agent in induction.

22.7 SYMPTOMATIC TREATMENT

Pain control and palliation of symptoms remain a key part of myeloma management. Lytic lesions in a long bone which appear to be involving the cortex may require prophylactic pinning to prevent pathological fracture. When fractures do occur they usually require pinning, local radiotherapy and adequate analgesia.

Hemibody irradiation may be indicated as a palliative procedure in selected patients. It has been found to produce rapid relief from multiple painful sites in 80–90% of patients and also may reduce both the M protein and degree of bone marrow involvement. Adequate hydration prior to hemibody irra-

diation and the use of prophylactic antiemetic are important. Side-effects include mucositis, diarrhoea and some loss of taste and oropharyngeal dryness (Jaffe *et al.*, 1979). Radiation pneumonitis is a serious complication which occurs up to 6 months following upper hemibody irradiation. It is dose related and has a higher incidence in those patients who have received previous mediastinal or lung irradiation (Fryer *et al.*, 1978) or the drugs BCNU, melphalan or cyclophosphamide. A period of pancytopenia lasting for up to 6 weeks usually follows hemibody irradiation and this may limit its usefulness in patients with poor marrow reserve due to extensive marrow involvement or pretreatment. The need for transfusions and the risk of neutropenic sepsis leading to hospital admission may have to be considered very carefully in terms of possible risk and benefit for patients whose quality of life may already be severely compromised.

22.8 COMPLICATIONS

22.8.1 RENAL IMPAIRMENT

Evidence of renal impairment is present in up to 50% of patients with myeloma at diagnosis and may be the presenting feature. Several factors may contribute and include the intrinsic renal lesions associated with Bence Jones proteins, hypercalcaemia, dehydration, sepsis, hyperuricaemia and the use of non-steroidal anti-inflammatory drugs.

Bence Jones protein monomers or dimers (molecular weight 22 000 or 44 000 respectively) enter the glomerulus where they are deposited and are directly toxic to the renal tubule. There are three types of lesion which may be distinguished by their immunohistological and ultrastructural detail and to some extent they are dependent on the type of Bence Jones protein and its inherent properties.

The commonest lesion, myeloma kidney, is due to deposition of intraluminal Bence Jones protein as insoluble tubular casts which cause tubular atrophy and a giant cell reaction. Light chain deposition disease is associated with κ Bence Jones protein and damage to the basement membrane. Amyloidosis appears to be particularly related to the deposition of a specific subgroup of λ chains as basement membrane precipitates of fibrils which stain with Congo Red and show green birefringence under polarization microscopy (Solomon, 1986). Myeloma kidney and light chain deposition disease are more commonly associated with acute renal failure than amyloidosis.

Patients with acute renal failure at presentation may require dialysis as an interim measure and in approximately 50% of patients even severe acute renal failure is reversible. Good prognostic features for recovery of renal function include an abrupt fall in glomerular filtration rate before presentation, the demonstration of normal sized kidneys, little evidence of tubular damage on renal biopsy and the presence of correctable factors such as sepsis or dehydration. If renal impairment is reversible then the overall prognosis is that of the underlying disease and its response to treatment. However, long-term support may be necessary for those who do not respond to correction of reversible factors. The prognosis for these patients is poor and there is a correlation between creatinine and high tumour mass (*Lancet* Editorial, 1988)

The fourth MRC trial (Cooper, *et al.*, 1984) demonstrated the benefit of active rehydration at presentation and maintenance of a fluid intake of at least 3 litres a day in patients with myeloma. Chemotherapy regimens containing melphalan must be avoided in renal impairment because of unpredictable renal and haematological toxicity.

22.8.2   CORD COMPRESSION

Cord compression is an emergency and requires immediate attention. An urgent CT, MRI or myelogram should be arranged to confirm the clinical diagnosis, and high dose dexamethasone 4 mg po/iv qds commenced immediately. Bony impingement on the cord, particularly in the cervical region, requires an urgent neurosurgical opinion. If imaging demonstrates a soft tissue mass compressing the cord, local radiotherapy and steroids are appropriate. However, the patient requires close monitoring and if further deterioration occurs neurosurgical advice should be sought. Physiotherapy should be commenced as soon as possible.

22.8.3   HYPERVISCOSITY

The hyperviscosity syndrome is characterized by blurred vision, headache, spontaneous bruising and bleeding and is particularly associated with IgA myeloma. Urgent plasmapheresis is indicated to reduce the level of paraprotein until effective chemotherapy can be given.

22.8.4   HYPERCALCAEMIA

Hypercalcaemia is a common finding at presentation and most patients respond to rehydration and steroids. Chemotherapy to control the underlying disease is essential and for patients who do not respond to these measures the use of intravenous biphosphonates should be considered once dehydration has been corrected. Clodronate is a potent inhibitor of osteoclast activity which does not impair bone mineralization and may be appropriate for long term oral administration.

22.8.5   INFECTIONS

Patients with myeloma are at increased risk of infections due to hypogammaglobulinaemia and the immunosuppressive effects of treatment. Bacterial pulmonary infections are common during the first few months of treatment and the MRC has recently been evaluating the possible benefit of intravenous immunoglobulin during this phase. Herpes zoster and oropharyngeal candidiasis are also common problems in patients with myeloma.

REFERENCES

Alexanian, R., Haut, A., Khan, A.U. *et al.* (1969) Treatment for multiple myeloma: combination chemotherapy with different melphalan dose regimens. *Journal of the American Medical Association*, **208**, 1680–5.

Alexanian, R., Dimopoulos, M.A., Delasalle, K. and Barlogie, B. (1992) Primary dexamethasone treatment of multiple myeloma. *Blood*, **80**, 887–90.

Bataille, R., Boccadoro, M., Klein, B. *et al.* (1992) C-reactive protein and β_2 microglobulin produce a simple and powerful myeloma staging system. *Blood*, **80**, 733–7.

Bataille, R., Jourdan, M., Zhang, X.G. and Klein, B. (1989) Serum levels of interleukin-6 – a potent myeloma cell growth factor, as a reflection of disease severity in plasma cell dyscrasia. *Journal of Clinical Investigation*, **84**, 2008–11.

Belch, A., Shelley, W., Bergsagel, D. *et al.*, (1988). A randomised trial of maintenance versus no maintenance melphalan and prednisolone in responding multiple myeloma patients. *British Journal of Cancer*, **57**, 94–9.

Billadeau, D., Quam, L., Thomas, W. *et al.* (1992) Detection and quantitation of malignant cells in the peripheral blood of multiple myeloma patients. *Blood*, **80**, 1818–24.

Boccadero, M., Massaia, M., Dianzani, U. and Pileri, A. (1987) Multiple myeloma: biological and clinical significance of bone marrow plasma cell labelling index. *Haematologica*, **72**, 171–5.

Cooper, E.H., Forbes, M.A. and Crockson, R.A. (1984) Proximal renal tubular function in myeloma: observations in the fourth Medical Research Council trial. *Journal of Clinical Pathology*, **37**, 852–8.

Cuzick, J., Cooper, E.H. and MacLennan, I.C.M. (1985) The prognostic value of serum $\beta2$ microglobulin compared with other presentation features in myelomatosis (a report to the Medical Research Council's Working Party on leukaemia in adults). *British Journal of Cancer*, **52**, 1–6.

Durie, B.G.M. and Salmon, S.E. (1975) A clinical staging system for multiple myeloma: correlation of measured myeloma cell mass with presenting clinical features, response to treatment and survival. *Cancer*, **36**, 842–54.

Editorial (1988) Renal involvement in myeloma. *Lancet*, 1202–3.

Fernberg, J.O., Johansson, B., Lewensohn R. and Mellstedt, H. (1990) Oral dosage of melphalan and response to treatment in multiple myeloma. *European Journal of Cancer*, **26**, 393–6.

Frank, J.W., Le Besque, S., and Buchanan, R.B. (1982). The value of bone imagery in multiple myeloma. *European Journal of Nuclear Midicine*, **7**, 502–5.

Fryer, C.J.H. Fitzpatrick, P.J., Rider, W.D. and Poon, P. (1978) Radiation pneumonitis: experience following a large single fraction of radiation. *International Journal of Radiation Oncology, Biology and Physics*, **4**, 931–6.

Gahrton, G., Tura, S., Ljungman, P. *et al.* (1991) Allogenic bone marrow transplantation in multiple myeloma. *New England Journal of Medicine*, **325**, 1267–72.

Gore, M.E., Selby, P.J., Viner, C. *et al.* (1989) Intensive treatment of multiple myeloma and criteria for complete remission. *Lancet*, **ii**, 879–82.

Ishikawa, H., Tanaka, H., Iwato, K. *et al.* (1990) Effect of glucocorticoids on the biologic activities of myeloma cells; inhibition of Interleukin 1β osteoclast activating factor-induced bone resorption. *Blood*, **75**, 715–20.

Jaffe, J.P., Bosch, A. and Raich, P.C. (1979) Sequential hemi-body radiotherapy in advanced multiple myeloma. *Cancer*, **32**, 124–8.

Jensen, G.S., Mant, M.J., Belch, A.J. *et al.*, (1991) Selective expression of CD45 isoforms defines CALLA+ monoclonal B lineage cells in peripheral blood from myeloma patients as late stage B cells, *Blood*, **78**, 711–19.

Kildahl-Anderson, O., Bjark, P., Bondevik, A. *et al.* (1988) Multiple myeloma in central and Northern Norway 1981–1982: a follow-up study of a randomised clinical trial of 5-drug combination chemotherapy versus standard therapy. *European Journal of Haematology*, **41**, 47–51.

Klein, B., Wijdenes, J., Zhang, X, *et al.* (1991) Murine anti-interleukin-6 monoclonal antibody therapy for a patient with plasma cell leukaemia. *Blood*, **78**, 1198–204.

Kyle, R. (1975) Multiple myeloma: review of 869 cases. *Mayo Clinic Proceedings*, **50**, 29–40.

McLaughlin, P. and Alexanian, R. (1982) Myeloma protein kinetics following chemotherapy. *Blood*, **60**, 851–5.

MacLennan, I.C.M. and Chan, E.Y.T. (1991) The origin of bone marrow plasma cells, in *Epidemiology and Biology of Multiple Myeloma*, (eds G.I. Obrams and M. Potter), Springer-Verlag, Berlin, p. 129.

MacLennan, I.C.M., Chapman, C., Dunn, J. and Kelly, K. (1992) Combined chemotherapy with ABCM versus melphalan for treatment of myelomatosis. *Lancet*, **339**, 200–5.

Mandelli, F., Avvisati, G., Amadori, S. *et al.* (1990) Maintenance treatment with recombinant interferon alfa-2 in patients with multiple myeloma responding to conventional induction chemotherapy. *New England Journal of Medicine*, **322**, 1430–4.

Medical Research Council Working Party on Leukaemia in Adults (1984) Analysis and management of renal failure in fourth MRC myelomatosis trial. (1984) *British Medical Journal*, **288**, 1411–16.

Moulopoulos, L.A., Varma, D.G., Dimonpoulos, M.A. *et al.* (1992) Multiple myeloma; spinal MR imaging in patients with untreated newly diagnosed disease. *Radiology*, **185**, 833–40.

Oken, M.M., Kyle, R.A., Greipp, P.R. *et al.* (1989) Complete Remission (CR) induction with VBMCP and Interferon (rIFNa2) in multiple myeloma: a 3 year follow up. *Proceedings of the American Society of Clinical Oncology*, **8**, 272.

Riccardi, A., Gobbi, P.G., Ucci, G. *et al.* (1991) Changing clinical presentation of multiple myeloma. *European Journal of Cancer*, **27**, 1401–5.

Selby, P.J., McElwain, T.J., Nandi, A.C. *et al.* (1987) Multiple myeloma treatment with high dose intravenous melphalan. *British Journal of Haematology*, **66**, 55–62.

Solomon, A. (1986) Clinical implications of monoclonal light chains. *Seminars in Oncology*, **13**, 341–9.

Terpstra, W.E., Lokhorst, H.M., Blomjous, F. *et al.* (1992) Comparison of plasma cell infiltration in bone marrow biopsies and aspirates in patients with multiple myeloma. *British Journal of Haematology*, **82**, 46–9.

Tienhaara, A., Remes, K. and Pelliniemi, T.T, (1991) Alpha interferon raises serum β_2 microglobulin in patients with multiple myeloma. *British Journal of Haematology*, **77**, 335.

TUMOURS OF THE UTERINE CERVIX AND CORPUS UTERI

Peter R. Blake

23.1 INTRODUCTION

Invasive cancer of the genital tract accounts for approximately 15 000 cases of cancer in females in the UK per annum. This is second only to breast cancer of which there are approximately 25 000 cases per annum. The treatment of gynaecological cancer involves the gynaecologist, radiotherapist and medical oncologist as well as the nursing professions, physiotherapist, occupational therapist and specialists in counselling and terminal care.

Whilst increased use of screening programmes has altered the proportion of patients seen with pre-invasive and invasive neoplasia of the cervix, resulting in an overall drop in the incidence of invasive disease, there is a rising incidence in some subgroups of women and, in addition, there is a rising incidence of both ovarian and endometrial cancer. Gynaecological cancer is, therefore, an area where there are epidemiological, diagnostic and therapeutic changes taking place at the same time.

23.2 ANATOMY

The female reproductive organs lie within the pelvis and comprise the vulva, vagina, uterus, fallopian tubes and ovaries. They are represented in Figure 23.1(a) and (b). The uterus comprises the corpus, which is the upper part of the uterine body, and the cervix, which is the lower one-third which enters into the vagina. The relationship to other structures in the pelvis is, therefore, that the uterus lies above and in continuity with the vagina. Anteriorly it is related to the bladder, the peritoneum and the abdominal cavity, and posteriorly it is related to the rectum, pouch of Douglas, peritoneum and abdominal cavity. Laterally the uterus abuts the parametrial tissues, the broad ligaments and the fallopian tubes and ovaries. The ureter runs close to the lateral margin of the cervix. Tumours of the upper two-thirds of the uterus, the 'body' of the uterus, and of the lower third, the cervix, will be discussed separately.

23.3 MALIGNANT DISEASE OF THE CERVIX

Whilst the incidence of invasive cervical cancer in the UK is only about 4000 cases per annum, cervical cancer is the second most common female malignancy after breast cancer worldwide. The incidence varies widely from one country to another and between cultures within the same country. In Columbia, Central America, there is a 5.5% life-time risk of developing invasive carcinoma of the cervix, whilst in England and Wales this risk is 1.25% and in Spain and Israel the risk is only 0.5%.

Invasive squamous carcinoma of the cervix is often preceded by cervical intra-epithelial neoplasia. This pre-invasive disease is commonly asymptomatic and may be detected by cytological examination of cells taken from the cervix at cervical smear and studied using the Papanicolau stain. The ease and reliability of this technique has resulted in the

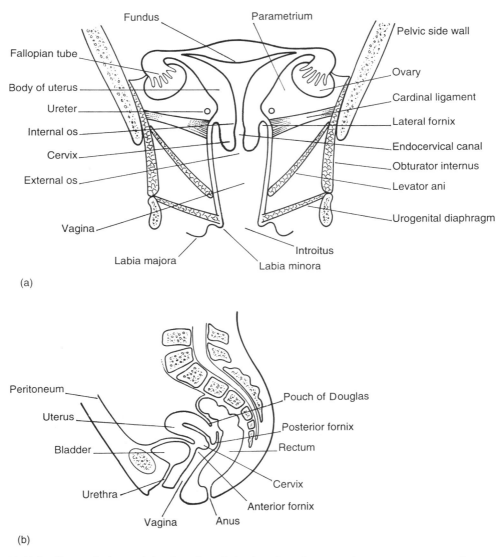

Figure 23.1(a) Coronal view of the female pelvis showing the reproductive organs in relation to the pelvic side wall and supporting structures. **(b)** Lateral view of the female pelvis showing the relationship of the uterus to the bladder, rectum and peritoneum.

establishment of many screening programmes for pre-invasive and early invasive cervical neoplasia. In some areas such as British Columbia, Iceland and Finland a well organized programme with a high compliance rate, has resulted in a large proportion of cases of cervical neoplasia being found in the early, curable stages and has, therefore, reduced the incidence of invasive disease and mortality. In other countries, such as the UK, a less marked decrease in mortality has been seen due to a poorer compliance rate and, in the past, a less well organized service.

Cervical intra-epithelial neoplasia has its peak incidence in woman between the ages of 25 and 40, whilst the peak age for invasive carcinoma is approximately 10 years later. There is some evidence suggesting that patients developing invasive carcinoma at an early age have a worse prognosis than older women, the disease following a more accelerated and aggressive course (Dattoli *et al.*, 1989).

23.3.1 AETIOLOGY

There are several aetiological factors associated with carcinoma of the cervix, but the most marked of these is sexual behaviour of both the woman and her partner.

(a) The female factor

There appears to be an aetiological link between sexual intercourse and the development of cervical neoplasia. Two aspects of sexual behaviour, the age at first intercourse and the number of sexual partners, have been studied extensively. There is a higher incidence of both pre-invasive cervical intra-epithelial neoplasia and of invasive disease in girls who commence regular intercourse in their teens compared with those who do not commence sexual activity until a later age. This suggests that the adolescent cervix is more vulnerable to potential oncogenic agents. In addition, the number of sexual partners appears to be important, with some studies having found a history of six or more sexual partners to be a significant risk factor.

Both low socioeconomic status and multiparity are associated with a higher incidence of cervical neoplasia, but neither of these risk factors can probably be considered to be independent of age at first intercourse.

(b) The male factor

Whilst the influence of the sexual histories of the women's partners has been less extensively studied than the sexual histories of the women themselves, there has been noted, in some studies, to be an association between cervical neoplasia and a history in the male partner of having multiple other sexual partners.

These observations would support the suggestion that there is a transmissible agent involved in cervical neoplasia.

(c) Contraception

A lower incidence of cervical neoplasia has been found in women using barrier methods of contraception than in those using the oral contraceptive pill. Whilst this is further evidence of there being a transmissible agent in the aetiology of cervical neoplasia, it is not clear whether oral contraceptives themselves are involved in the development of cervical cancer.

(d) Smoking

Smoking produces changes in the DNA of cervical squamous cells and, in addition, decreases the population of Langerhan's cells responsible for cell mediated immunity in the cervix. Both these findings could indicate an important role for smoking in the development of cervical neoplasia, both by direct carcinogenesis and by rendering the cervix more vulnerable to infection by a transmissible agent. (Trevathan *et al.*, 1983).

(e) Transmissible infective agents

Most research in this area has concentrated in recent years on the roles of viruses and, in particular, the herpes and papilloma viruses. Whilst herpes simplex virus type 2 (HSV2) was shown to be weakly oncogenic in the laboratory, analysis of many cervical tumours has failed to show any HSV2 DNA, and it seems unlikely that this virus is involved in carcinogenesis.

Human papilloma viruses, however, have attracted more attention in recent years and it seems that there may be a possible link between certain types of papilloma virus and cervical neoplasia. Over 70 types of HPV have now been isolated and several of these infect the lower female genital tract. HPV types 16 and 18 are found in genital wart disease and HPV types 16 and 18 have been particularly associated with cervical intra-epithelial neoplasia and invasive disease. Both these viruses have the ability to transform cells in culture and these transformed cells can give rise to tumours in immunocomprised mice. It is tempting, therefore, to think that it is these HPVs that are the transmissible agent involved in cervical neoplasia. However, as methods of detecting these viruses by the polymerase chain reaction have improved, the viruses can be found in small quantities in many normal women as well as in women with cervical neoplasia. In particular, it appears that normal women may well be infected with the virus and then eradicate it without any neoplasia developing (Munoz *et al.*, 1988).

The role of HPV is still not clear, but it may be involved in neoplasia in association with other factors by interacting with the tumour suppressor gene p53 (Tidy and Wrede, 1992).

(f) Site of action of the transmissible agent

The majority of neoplasias of the cervix arise at the squamocolumnar junction, an area known as the 'transformation zone', where columnar epithelium undergoes the metaplastic process of becoming squamous epithelium (Figure 23.2). This transformation zone is larger in puberty, pregnancy and when taking the oral contraceptive pill. If this area of the cervix is seen as the 'target' on which a transmissible agent could work, then this could go some way to explain why sexual intercourse in puberty is a risk factor. The importance of multiparity and the use of the oral contraceptive pill in cervical neoplasia could also be explained.

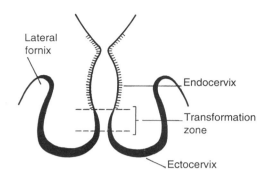

Figure 23.2 The 'transformation zone' on the cervix, where the columnar epithelium of the endocervix meets the squamous epithelium of the ectocervix.

23.3.2 CONCLUSIONS ABOUT THE EPIDEMIOLOGY AND AETIOLOGY OF CERVICAL NEOPLASIA

Epidemiological data show an association between cervical cancer and sexual behaviour. A sexually transmissible agent might be involved in this process as may other agents such as smoking. The cervix may be rendered more vulnerable to such an agent in certain times of life, particularly puberty but, as yet, it cannot be declared for certain that HPV has a causal role in cervical neoplasia until more evidence has accrued.

23.3.3 PATHOLOGY

(a) Anatomy of the cervix

The cervix is the circular fibromuscular lower part of the uterus. It is continuous with the vagina below and with the body of the uterus above. It is related to the cardinal ligaments laterally, the uterovesical ligaments anteriorly and the uterosacral ligaments posteriorly. The ureters lie in close proximity at the lateral margins of the cervix (Figure 23.1). The endocervical canal connects the vagina with the uterine cavity and is lined by columnar epithelium, whilst the exocervix is covered by stratified squamous epithelium. The cervix and body of the uterus are small in childhood, enlarge during puberty and the reproductive years and then atrophy after the menopause. The junction between the columnar and squamous epithelium (the transformation zone) enlarges in puberty, pregnancy and when taking the oral contraceptive pill and it also changes in position, being usually just inside the external cervical os in young women, but rising up the endocervical canal after the menopause.

Lymphatic drainage

There is a relatively well defined pattern for the lymphatic drainage of the cervix with direct drainage to the internal, external and common iliac nodes. Other node groups which may be involved by direct lymphatic spread are the parametrial, obturator and presacral nodes. Spread to the para-aortic nodes is uncommon without pelvic node involvement and the supraclavicular nodes may be

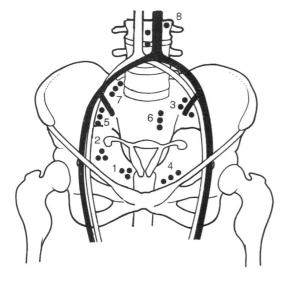

Figure 23.3 The lymphatic drainage of the cervix to: paracervical (1), parametrial (2), internal iliac (3), obturator (4), external iliac (5), presacral (6), common iliac (7) and the para-aortic (8) nodes.

involved subsequent to para-aortic node disease (Figure 23.3).

(b)   Spread of disease

Cervical carcinoma spreads predominantly by direct invasion and lymphatic permeation. Direct spread is superiorly into the body of the uterus and inferiorly into the vaginal mucosa. Laterally, the parametrial tissues and ligaments of the uterus may be involved and, rarely, the bladder anteriorly or rectum posteriorly can be invaded by advanced disease. Spread is usually direct, but seedlings from cervical cancer can occasionally be noted in the lower vagina. Blood-borne spread is unusual and is to the lungs, bone and liver.

(c)   Pathology of pre-invasive disease

Changes in the metaplastic process at the transformation zone may lead to dysplasia, which is known as cervical intra-epithelial neoplasia (CIN). The terms CIN1, CIN2 and CIN3 are used to describe increasing degrees of cellular dysplasia from mild to moderate to severe. It is known that CIN3 can develop into invasive carcinoma but, whilst it is known that a proportion of CIN1 and CIN2 will revert to normal epithelium, it is not known what proportion of CIN3 may revert and what proportion progress to invasive disease as ethical considerations dictate that all cases of CIN3 are treated.

(d)   Micro-invasive carcinoma of the cervix

Once the basement membrane beneath the epithelium is invaded the neoplastic process can no longer be termed pre-invasive and if this change is only visible microscopically, such disease is referred to as being micro-invasive. In the FIGO classification (FIGO, 1992) this is stage Ia, which is subdivided into stage Ia (i) and Ia (ii) (Table 23.1). When disease is more than 5 mm deep or wider

Table 23.1 Staging for carcinoma of the cervix (FIGO)

Stage	Features
0	Pre-invasive carcinoma (CIN)
Ia1	Preclinical carcinoma, minimal microinvasion: diagnosed by microscopy only
Ia2	Preclinical carcinoma, microinvasion < 5 mm deep and < 7 mm wide: diagnosed by microscopy only
Ib	Carcinoma more extensive than Ia2 but confined to the uterus (including body of uterus)
IIa	Carcinoma extending beyond the cervix into the upper two-thirds of the vagina
IIb	Carcinoma extending into the parametria but not reaching the pelvic side wall
IIIa	Carcinoma confined to the vagina and involving the lower third
IIIb	Carcinoma extending to the pelvic side wall or causing ureteric stenosis or obstruction
IVa	Carcinoma involving the mucosa of the bladder or rectum, or extending beyond the true pelvis
IVb	Blood-borne spread to distant organs

than 7 mm, it is no longer referred to as micro-invasive, but falls within the category of FIGO stage Ib.

(e) Invasive carcinoma of the cervix

Between 85% and 95% of cervical carcinomas are squamous, the remainder being predominantly adenocarcinomas, adenosquamous carcinomas or, very rarely, sarcomas, lymphomas and melanomas.

Squamous carcinoma

Most squamous carcinomas involve the exocervix and are visible on a speculum examination. Some, however, develop within the endocervical canal and may remain occult until reaching quite a large size (a barrel carcinoma). Visible tumours may be either exophytic or ulcerating with underlying infiltration of surrounding structures.

Commonly, tumours are graded as well differentiated (grade 1), moderately differentiated (grade 2) and poorly differentiated (grade 3). Squamous carcinomas may be divided into keratinizing, large cell nonkeratinizing, and small cell non-keratinizing. Rarely, tumours similar to oat cell carcinoma of the bronchus are seen and these have a similar poor prognosis. Occasionally squamous carcinomas having the appearance of condylomata acuminata are seen; these are called verrucous carcinomas.

Adenocarcinoma

Adenocarcinomas arise from the glandular epithelium lining the endocervical canal and the endocervical glands. Because of the much more irregular nature of the boundary between the epithelium and the underlying stroma, it is much more difficult in the case of adenocarcinoma to define an *in situ* stage equivalent to CIN3. However, pre-invasive forms of adenocarcinoma are being seen with increasing frequency and criteria are being developed to define these. Adenocarcinoma has often been thought to carry a worse prognosis than squamous carcinoma, but this is probably due to the later presentation of disease on the exocervix, leading to an increased bulk of tumour, stage for stage.

Adenosquamous carcinoma

An increasing number of squamous carcinomas are being reported as showing glandular elements. Whilst this may reflect a change in the incidence of adenosquamous carcinoma, it may also be a product of increasing use of histochemical stains for mucin production.

23.3.4 SCREENING AND TREATMENT OF PRE-INVASIVE NEOPLASIA OF THE CERVIX

Screening of the cervix is carried out by obtaining a sample of cells from the endocervix and the exocervix by scraping the surface with a spatula. The most commonly used spatula is Ayre's and is made of wood. The cells obtained on the spatula are spread onto a microscope slide and fixed quickly with alcohol prior to staining by the Papanicolau technique. Cells will be reported as being normal, inflammatory, showing mild atypia, mild dyskaryosis, moderate dyskaryosis, severe dyskaryosis or of being malignant or, finally, of being characteristic of invasive carcinoma. Cervical cytology can give rise to both false-negative and false-positive results and confirmation of cytological findings should be sought by colposcopy and biopsy.

(a) Colposcopy

This technique involves looking at the cervix with a low power microscope and can be carried out without the need for a general anaesthetic. By staining the cervix and upper vagina with acetic acid or iodine, areas of abnormal epithelium can be identified and biopsied precisely. In the case of extensive abnormalities, cone biopsy may be necessary.

(b) Treatment of cervical intra-epithelial neoplasia

CIN may be removed under colposcopic control by laser vaporization, radical diathermy or surgical excision. Excision can be by scalpel, cutting laser or hot wire loop. Excision is increasingly favoured over ablative methods as it allows more accurate histological assessment of the depth of invasion of an abnormality than is possible on biopsy alone.

23.3.5 SYMPTOMS AND SIGNS OF INVASIVE CARCINOMA OF THE CERVIX

The most common symptom of invasive cervical cancer is of bleeding which may be postcoital, intermenstrual or postmenopausal. Vaginal discharge is the second commonest symptom, with pain only occuring in advanced cases. Similarly, rectal bleeding and haematuria are symptoms of locally advanced disease. Examination of the patient should involve palpation of the abdomen to look for enlarged kidneys and an enlarged or irregular liver, palpable para-aortic nodes or an enlarged bladder. The inguinal and supraclavicular areas should be examined for metastatic lymph nodes. The vulva should be inspected and then the vagina and cervix examined using a speculum. If an abnormality is seen a smear or punch biopsy should be taken for diagnosis, and then the cervix should be examined bimanually to assess the size, shape and mobility of the uterus and any extension of tumour into surrounding tissues. Rectal examination gives additional information on posterior and parametrial spread.

23.3.6 INVESTIGATIONS

Investigations to assess the extent of disease must include an examination under anaesthetic, when both abdominal and pelvic examination will be carried out. In addition, a cystoscopy is necessary to rule out bladder involvement and, if there is any suspicion of posterior spread, proctoscopy and sigmoidoscopy should also be completed. The uterine cavity should be curetted following dilatation of the cervix and curettage of the endocervical canal. The cervix itself is biopsied if histological diagnosis has not already been made by punch biopsy.

A full blood count, serum electrolytes and renal and liver function tests will give an indication as to whether or not there is renal impairment or liver metastases. Further examination of the renal tract can be by Intravenous Urogram (IVU) or ultrasound scan and a chest X-ray can demonstrate metastatic disease. Pelvic and para-aortic nodes can be imaged by lymphography, CT scanning, ultrasound scanning or MRI. Most commonly these days a CT scan will be used to assess the state of the liver, renal tract, para-aortic and pelvic lymph nodes and direct spread within the pelvis.

23.3.7 CLINICAL STAGING

The most widely used staging system is that of FIGO (International Federation of Gynaecology and Obstetrics). This is listed in Table 23.1. Apart from micro-invasive disease, which is defined histologically, the system depends largely on clinical examination under anaesthetic. Findings of cystoscopy, proctoscopy, chest X-ray and IVU can all be used in determining FIGO stage, but other imaging techniques do not alter tumour staging. Whilst the FIGO system does divide cervical tumours into prognostic groups, it still fails to take tumour volume into consideration, with the exception of micro-invasive disease. Tumour volume is probably one of the most important prognostic factors and yet a wide range of volumes can occur in any one FIGO stage (Magee *et al.*, 1991). Therefore, in addition to recording FIGO stage it is also important to record nodal status as determined by CT scan, lymphogram or ultrasound examination, and also tumour bulk as measured at the time of examination under anaesthetic.

Nodal status has a profound effect on survival. Those patients having stage Ib carcinoma of the cervix with positive pelvic nodes have a 5 year survival only half that of those with negative pelvic nodes. It is very unusual for patients with involved para-aortic nodes to survive 5 years as this is commonly a marker of widespread dissemination (Shingleton and Orr, 1987).

23.3.8 TREATMENT

(a) Micro-invasive disease FIGO stage Ia

Cone biopsy, completely excising a CIN3 lesion, should be adequate treatment for young women, providing that the depth of invasion is less than 3 mm with no marked lymphatic vessel involvement. If a cone biopsy cannot completely encompass a lesion, then simple hysterectomy should be undertaken with conservation of the ovaries. If the lesion invades further than 3 mm, or if there is lymphatic invasion, then the risk of involved lymph nodes rises and radical hysterectomy and lymphadenectomy is the treatment of choice for young women or radiotherapy for those unfit for radical surgery.

(b) Invasive cervical cancer

The treatment of invasive cervical cancer will depend on the stage of disease, the size of the tumour and the fitness of the patient. It can incorporate chemotherapy, radiotherapy and surgery. The treatment strategy for individual patients should be arrived at after discussion between specialists in all three disciplines.

23.3.9 SURGERY

Surgery is the treatment of choice for young patients with small volume stage Ib disease in whom there is a low risk of nodal metastases. Involved nodes should not have been visualized on imaging, should be thought to be highly unlikely because of the small volume of the tumour or because there are good prognostic factors, such as good differentiation and the absence of lymphatic vessel invasion.

Surgery for invasive cervical carcinoma should include a radical hysterectomy and a pelvic lymphadenectomy. This is often colloquially called a 'Wertheim's' hysterectomy, although this is a misnomer. A long vaginal cuff should be taken as a routine in this operation, but in a young woman with a squamous carcinoma it should be possible to conserve the ovaries and avoid the menopause. Advantages of surgery over radiotherapy, in young women, include the avoidance of further shrinkage of the vagina after treatment, and the maintenance of pliability and lubrication of the vaginal mucosa. In addition, the very small risk of late induction of a second malignancy is avoided.

23.3.10 RADIOTHERAPY

For older women, or women with more bulky tumours, radiotherapy is the treatment of choice as the results of treatment are equal to those of surgery and the treatment is better tolerated. However, there is morbidity in terms of fibrosis in the normal tissues causing some reduction in the size of the vagina and its pliability and lubrication. Women with a high risk of nodal involvement because of large volume disease, poor differentiation or lymphatic vessel involvement should also be treated by radiotherapy.

Carcinoma of the cervix is treated by a combination of both external and intracavitary radiotherapy. In some centres stage Ib tumours are treated by intracavitary radiotherapy alone, provided that the tumours are not bulky. Commonly, a maximum diameter of 4 cm would be regarded as the upper limit of size for a tumour to be treated by intracavitary brachytherapy alone. More bulky tumours, or those of higher stage, or with a high likelihood of pelvic lymph node involvement, should be treated by external beam radiotherapy to cover the lymph nodes draining the cervix. These include the external, internal and common iliac nodes.

The volume encompassed by external radiotherapy should include these nodes with the primary tumour. This will commonly be from the junction of the fourth and fifth lumbar vertebra to the bottom of the obturator foramina, and laterally to 1 cm outside the bony margin of the pelvis. If lymphography has been used to delineate the pelvic nodes, then the volume may be more individually designed with shielding of the upper corners to protect small bowel. This volume can be encompassed by either a parallel opposed pair or, if it is appropriate to try to spare the posterior half of the rectum in the absence of uterosacral ligament involvement, then either a four-field 'box' technique or a technique using three fields with an anterior and two wedged lateral fields can be used (Figure 23.4). Ideally a 5–8 MeV Linear Accelerator should be used, in view of the depth of the tumour volume below the surface of the lateral fields. Cobalt irradiation can be used, but may result in subcutaneous fibrosis in obese patients. Those patients with disease in the vaginal mucosa below the upper third

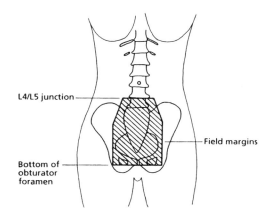

Figure 23.4 The anterior external beam radiotherapy field used to treat primary cervical cancer and the 'first station' lymph nodes.

should have the field extended to cover the full length of the vagina.

(a) Intracavitary brachytherapy for cervical cancer

Historically, cervical cancer was one of the first tumours to be treated by radiotherapy, when radium was inserted into the endocervical canal and upper vagina to irradiate local disease. Techniques were developed in several centres, notably Paris, Stockholm and Manchester, which allowed consistency in treatment and, therefore, enabled the effectiveness and morbidity of treatment to be measured. A technique commonly used these days is the 'Manchester' technique involving an intrauterine tube and two vaginal ovoids placed in the lateral vaginal fornices (Figure 23.5). The proportions of radioisotope, initially radium and more latterly caesium, within the intrauterine tube and the vaginal ovoids, were calculated to give a constant dose rate to a geometrical point 'A' when using different lengths of intrauterine tube and different sizes of vaginal ovoids. This constancy of dose rate when using applicators of different sizes is an important aspect of the Manchester system.

Active sources

The radioisotope used for intracavitary brachytherapy was initially radium which, because of its gaseous daughter product radon, is hazardous. This has, therefore, been replaced by caesium, but the hazards of handling active sources have largely led to the development of after-loading techniques minimizing source handling and staff exposure.

After-loading brachytherapy

The basis of after-loading brachytherapy is that applicators are placed within the cervix and vaginal fornices and that the radioisotope is only introduced into these when the applicators are correctly positioned, check radiographs have been taken and the patient is comfortable and in a protected environment. The sources may then be inserted either manually or by remote control. Manual methods are common and have the advantage of being cheap, but do not entirely protect staff as the sources have to be inserted by staff and cannot be removed for short periods while attending to a patient's needs. Remote systems have the advantage of complete protection of staff, but have the disadvantage of cost and the necessity for interlocking mechanisms. These ensure that the correct source has been inserted into the correct applicator for the programmed length of time.

Remote after-loading systems allow the dose-rate of brachytherapy to be increased. Classically, the dose-rate with the Manchester system was approximately 50 cGy/hour to

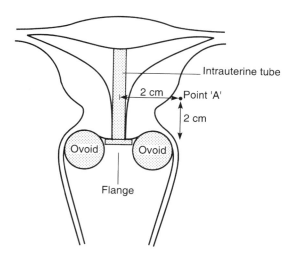

Figure 23.5 The 'Manchester sytem' of an intrauterine tube and two 'ovoid' applicators in the lateral fornices of the vagina for the treatment of cervical cancer. Manchester point 'A' lies 2 cm lateral to the axis of the intrauterine tube and 2 cm above the flange of the intrauterine tube.

Point 'A'. With modern engineering methods, caesium pellets can be produced which will allow a dose rate of between 150 and 200 cGy/hour to Point 'A'. Many systems now use sources that allow a higher than standard dose-rate to be delivered. This has the advantage of reducing treatment time, but does have radiobiological consequences necessitating a small reduction in dose (Brenner and Hall, 1991).

If the concept of increasing dose-rate is taken further, then high dose-rate brachytherapy, delivering doses at rates in excess of 1 Gy/min to Point A, gives the opportunity of very short treatment times. This allows complete geometrical stability of the applicator during the treatment and the possibility of a high patient throughout. However, there is considerably less time for repair of radiation damage in the normal tissues in a high dose-rate treatment and, therefore, such treatments have to be fractionated over several days, as opposed to the continuous treatment given by a low dose-rate brachytherapy implant. Early clinical results show no difference between treatment at low dose-rate and high dose-rate (Fu and Philips, 1990), although mathematical modelling indicates that there is an increased risk of late normal tissue damage from fractionated high dose-rate brachytherapy compared to a continuous low dose-rate insertion, unless the dose is reduced.

(b) The integration of external beam and intracavitary brachytherapy

Brachytherapy, used alone for the treatment of cervical cancer, is commonly given as two fractions when utilizing the Manchester system. At standard radium dose-rates this involves two insertions, each lasting 3 days, spaced 1 week apart. This allows a period of time between the first and second insertion for the tumour to shrink and for vaginal hygiene to be attended to. If treatment is to be with external beam therapy also, then brachytherapy can either precede or succeed the external beam therapy.

Classically, intracavitary brachytherapy to central disease was carried out prior to external beam therapy, which was given to treat the nodes on the pelvic side wall. A dose was given from the brachytherapy that would be in excess of the tolerance dose to central pelvic tissues if the external beam therapy, intended to top up the dose to the pelvic side walls, was given to the whole pelvis. Therefore, some central shielding was needed in the external beam field to protect those tissues that had received a high brachytherapy dose, in particular the rectum and bladder.

Whilst this programme of treatment has existed for many years, there can be problems in locating the central shield, particularly in cases where the intracavitary sources have been pulled markedly away from the midline by tumour. Mispositioning of a shield over these sources could lead to relative underdosing on one side and overdosing on the other, which would have consequences both for recurrence and for complications of treatment.

Increasingly, external beam therapy is used prior to intracavitary brachytherapy and the brachytherapy dose is reduced, so as to avoid the need for any central shielding in the external beam fields. Typically, a dose of 45–50 Gy would be given over 4.5–5.5 weeks in 1.8 Gy or 2 Gy fractions to the pelvis as described earlier. An intracavitary insertion would then be undertaken to give a further 25–30 Gy to Point A at standard dose-rate. If higher than standard dose-rates were used, then a lower dose would be delivered. Parametrial boosts may then be used to give a further 5 Gy to bulky disease within the parametria or involved nodes on the pelvic side walls.

The dose to the rectum from the intracavitary insertion should not exceed two-thirds of the dose given to Point A and care must be taken, when using rigid applicators, that the uterus is not forcibly pushed posteriorly in the pelvis against the sigmoid colon or small bowel. Equally, an overly curved, rigid intrauterine tube could overdose the dome of the bladder whilst sparing the bowel. A curvature of 20–30° is probably suitable in most cases, depending on the patient's anatomy.

23.3.11 CHEMOTHERAPY FOR CARCINOMA OF THE CERVIX

Carcinoma of the cervix is not a highly chemosensitive tumour. Response rates to single agents have seldom been reported in excess of 40% and the most effective drugs appear to be cisplatin and ifosfamide. Currently, trials are underway into the role of these drugs, alone and in combination with others, for recurrent disease and in the neo-adjuvant setting prior to radiotherapy for advanced, bulky disease (Hoskin and Blake, 1991). Responses are seen to combination chemotherapy regimens including these drugs, and the best response rate is seen in primary untreated disease. However, the response rate in metastatic disease is lower and in recurrent disease, within an irradiated area, is very low indeed. Therefore, the results of clinical trials are still awaited to prove the true benefit in survival brought about by these drugs, although they can be used judiciously for palliation of advanced and metastatic disease.

23.3.12 SPECIAL SITUATIONS

(a) Non-squamous carcinoma of the cervix

Adenocarcinoma and mixed carcinomas of the cervix have traditionally had a poor prognosis. However, tumour bulk is probably the most important prognostic factor and adenocarcinomas are frequently larger than squamous carcinomas, stage for stage, due to their origin being within the endocervical canal and their consequent late detection. Therefore, bulk for

bulk, they probably fare no worse than squamous carcinomas. Small cell carcinoma of the cervix behaves like small cell carcinoma at any other site. It is ideally treated with chemotherapy followed by radiotherapy to the sites of bulk disease and usually has a poor prognosis.

(b) The incidental finding of cervical cancer

Occasionally invasive cervical cancer is found in the specimen following a simple hysterectomy. If the depth of invasion indicates a risk of lymphatic spread, then postoperative pelvic radiotheraphy should be prescribed and, if the cuff of vagina is inadequate, or the margins of excision not clear, then vault radiotheraphy also should be delivered. With this technique the results of treatment are not worse than radical surgery or radical radiotherapy alone.

(c) Cervical carcinoma during pregnancy

This difficult situation arises uncommonly and treatment depends on the wishes of the parents as well as on the stage of disease. Treatment would be similar to that for non-pregnant patients in the first and second trimester of pregnancy, with treatment preceded by abortion or hysterotomy. Caesarean section should precede treatment in the third trimester when there is the chance of producing a viable child.

(d) Haemorrhage

Carcinoma of the cervix can present with severe haemorrhage which should be treated in the first instance by firm vaginal packing, bed rest and a blood transfusion. Urgent external beam radiotherapy may well produce haemostasis within 24–48 hours but, very occasionally, an intracavitary insertion is needed and, in intractable cases, arterial embolization or ligation should be considered.

(e) Recurrent carcinoma of the cervix

Recurrent carcinoma of the cervix within an irradiated area has been referred to earlier in considering chemotherapy. It carries a very poor prognosis. However, recurrence following radical surgery can be treated by radiotherapy and, on occasions, long term remission and apparent cure is achieved. Nevertheless, this can commonly be at the expense of late treatment side-effects.

Occasionally, recurrence after radical radiotherapy, if central, can be treated by either posterior, anterior or total pelvic exenteration involving diversion of the urinary and gastrointestinal tracts. Selection of patients for this procedure must include both the physical and psychological assessment of the patients' ability to cope with the resulting stomas.

23.3.13 RESULTS OF TREATMENT

Approximately 50% of patients with carcinoma of the cervix can be cured of their disease (Table 23.2). Most recurrences occur within the first 3 years and 5 year survival rates are a good measure of the effectiveness of therapy. More than 90% of patients with small stage I tumours, with uninvolved lymph nodes, can be cured of their disease but results remain disappointing for stage III and IV tumours, with 5 year survival rates of only approximately 30% and 10% respectively.

23.3.14 CONCLUSIONS

Cytological screening programmes and colposcopy should reduce the incidence of invasive carcinoma of the cervix and appear to have done so in some populations of older women. However, overall there is an increasing incidence of pre-invasive neoplasia of the cervix and, in young women, there is also an increasing incidence of invasive disease. A transmissible agent, most probably the human papilloma virus, is implicated in the aetiology

Table 23.2 Results of treatment of cervical carcinoma

Stage	% of total	5 years survival (%)
I	35	76
II	34	55
III	26	30
IV	4	7

Modified from FIGO, 1988.

of cervical cancer but is unlikely to be the only causative agent. Treatment of early disease with both radiotherapy and surgery is equally effective, but for more advanced tumours radiotherapy is preferable. Chemotherapy still does not have a defined role in the treatment of cancer of the cervix and is currently under study as neoadjuvant treatment for advanced cervical cancer and for recurrent disease.

23.4 TUMOURS OF THE BODY OF THE UTERUS

The vast majority of tumours of the body of the uterus are carcinomas of the endometrium; however, the uterus can also be the site of sarcomas, namely malignant mixed müllerian tumours, leiomyosarcomas and endometrial stromal sarcomas and also the site of gestational trophoblastic tumours.

23.4.1 CARCINOMA OF THE ENDOMETRIUM

Carcinoma of the endometrium occurs predominantly in postmenopausal women and 80% of these will have already passed the menopause. The median age is 60 years with less than 5% of all tumours occurring in women under the age of 40. The incidence varies widely worldwide and is highest in areas of low birth rate, the greatest incidence being amongst white Americans. In England and Wales there are 4000 new cases per year registered, similar to the number of registrations for invasive carcinoma of the cervix and just less than that for carcinoma of the ovary. However, whilst ovarian cancer carries a mortality rate of 85% and cervical cancer 50%, the mortality rate of endometrial cancer is much better at only 30%.

Endometrial cancer presents often at an early stage because the predominant symptom is of postmenopausal bleeding, a symptom which is seldom ignored by the patient. Seventy-five per cent of patients have tumours confined to the body of the uterus at the time that diagnosis is made. The main risk factor for developing endometrial cancer is excessive oestrogen stimulation of the endometrium without the opposing effects of progestogens. Extra-ovarian oestrogens may be given exogenously as hormone replacement therapy, or may be produced endogenously either by aromatization of androgens, particularly in body fat, or from oestrogen producing tumours, such as ovarian granulosa cell tumours. Because of the production of oestrogens in fat, it is not surprising that this tumour is most common in women who are overweight and postmenopausal (Follson *et al.*, 1989). A small percentage of carcinomas of the endometrium are associated with an endometrioid carcinoma of the ovary and these two tumours can appear to be separate rather than metastases from either primary. This raises the possibility that a common aetiological factor may induce this particular histological type of carcinoma in both ovary and endometrium. Unopposed exogenous oestrogens should not be given without either a cyclical break in therapy or the addition, on a cyclical basis, of progestogens for any woman who still has a uterus (Jelovsek *et al.*, 1980).

Tamoxifen, which is increasingly used in the prophylaxis of breast cancer in high risk families, has weak oestrogenic effects and may cause hyperplasia of the endometrium and, possibly, endometrial carcinoma. However, data is insufficient to confirm this yet.

Diabetes can be associated with endometrial cancer even in the absence of obesity.

(a) Anatomy of the body of the uterus

The body of the uterus is a pear-shaped organ which is hollow and muscular. It is in continuity with the fallopian tubes at the cornua superiorly and with the cervix and vagina inferiorly (Figure 23.1(a),(b). The length of the uterine cavity is approximately 5 cm, as is the width of the fundus. However, the size of the uterine cavity can vary considerably throughout a woman's life, being small in childhood, at its largest in the reproductive years and becoming small again after the menopause.

The outer surface of the body of the uterus is covered by peritoneum continuous with the broad ligaments laterally. These contain the fallopian tubes and are attached to the ovary by the mesovarium. Inferiorly, the uterus is in continuity with the cervix at the internal os. The parametria, on either side of the upper part of the cervix, are thickened to form the cardinal ligaments that run to the pelvic side wall, and with the uterosacral ligaments posteriorly, support the uterus. The wall of the uterus has an inner lining of endometrium and then a muscular layer of myometrium. The thickness of the wall varies throughout life, being at its thickest in the child-bearing years.

Histologically the endometrium is a simple cuboidal epithelium containing glandular elements that develop under oestrogen stimulation during the reproductive years. The endometrium proliferates under oestrogenic stimulation before ovulation. When progestogen levels rise in the secretory phase of the cycle after ovulation, the endometrium is shed as the menses or period. These hormones are produced by the ovary, which is itself under the control of the pituitary gland through the gonadotrophins, follicle-stimulating hormone (FSH) and luteinizing hormone (LH).

(b) Spread of disease

Endometrial carcinoma may spread directly through the endometrial cavity, along the fallopian tubes to the ovaries or through the internal os into the endocervical canal and upper vagina. More frequently, it invades the myometrium, occasionally infiltrating the full thickness of the muscle layer and penetrating the serosa overlying the uterus or the parametria laterally. Occasionally, spread of disease can be so marked within the pelvis that it is impossible to distinguish the tumour from ovarian carcinoma.

Blood-borne spread is uncommon, but when it does occur is to the lung and bone.

Lymphatic drainage

Lymphatic spread of disease is to both the pelvic and para-aortic nodes and para-aortic involvement can be direct, as there is a lymphatic pathway from the upper part of the uterus joining those of the fallopian tube and ovary, which drain directly to the para-aortic nodes.

(c) Pathology

Endometrial carcinomas arise as raised areas, which may be papillary, and are most commonly situated in the upper part of the endometrial cavity. Occasionally, they may form polyps and these can be extruded through the cervix. Most commonly, endometrial carcinoma is an adenocarcinoma which is graded as well, moderately or poorly differentiated or anaplastic. The most common type is the endometrioid adenocarcinoma and up to 25% of these may contain benign squamous changes. These latter tumours are known as adenoacanthomas. Occasionally, squamous carcinoma is seen in the endometrium and this carries a poor prognosis. Papillary adenocarcinomas and clear cell carcinomas also have a worse prognosis than the endo-metrioid adenocarcinomas, but are fortunately less frequent. In cases where the tumour involves both the cervix and the body of the uterus, and when a definite site of origin cannot be determined, it is usual to call an adenocarcinoma an endometrial cancer and a squamous carcinoma a cervical cancer.

(d) Symptoms and signs

Most women present with an episode of post-menopausal bleeding and seek urgent advice. Younger women may have intermenstrual or postcoital bleeding and those with advanced disease may suffer pain or vaginal discharge. A diagnosis of senile vaginitis in a post-menopausal woman, having had vaginal spotting, should not be made without full examination and a diagnostic curettage if an obvious source of bleeding cannot be found in the vagina.

(e) Investigations

The most important investigation for the diagnosis of endometrial cancer is the diagnostic curettage. In addition, investigations should include those not only to assess possible spread of disease, but also the medical condition of the patient, as these women are frequently overweight and hypertensive.

Hysteroscopy will allow inspection of the uterine cavity and the tumour may well be visible. However, subepithelial spread will not necessarily be detected.

In diagnostic curettage, the cervix is inspected and then the endocervical canal curetted before the uterine body. Curettings from the body are sent to the pathologists separately from those from the endocervical canal. For there to be true cervical involvement endocervical glands must be seen to be occupied by tumour (FIGO IIa) or stromal invasion must be seen (FIGO IIb). Stage II disease has a poorer prognosis than stage I disease as there is an approximately three times greater risk of pelvic nodes being involved.

Hysterectomy

Once a diagnosis of endometrial cancer has been made, the great majority of patients will undergo hysterectomy and bilateral salpingo-oophorectomy. Only a small minority who are medically or psychologically unfit will be referred for radical radiotherapy on the basis of a diagnosis made at curettage only.

Staging

Staging involves the inspection of the resected uterus and adnexae. The FIGO system is most commonly used, which takes account of the degree of spread of disease and the depth of myometrial invasion (Figure 23.6).

(f) Prognostic factors

Extent and grade of disease

The prognosis of endometrial cancer depends particularly upon whether or not pelvic nodes are involved. The larger the volume of tumour, the higher the risk of lymph node involvement. Consequently, there is a close link between prognosis and stage. However, even within stage I disease tumour bulk is of prognostic importance, and the depth of myometrial invasion is an indicator of the risk of there being lymph node metastases in the pelvic and para-aortic regions. In addition, involvement of the lower segment of the uterus and increasing tumour grade are also important and the more deeply invasive tumours tend to be of a worse histological grade than those that are only superficial (Table 23.3) (Boronow *et al.*, 1984; Creasman *et al.*, 1987).

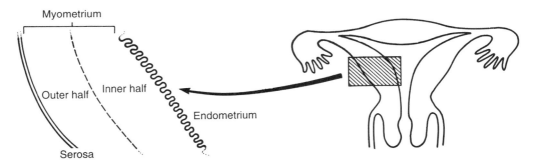

Figure 23.6 A section of the wall of the uterus showing the endometrium, myometrium and serosa. Tumours of the endometrium are staged as follows:

Ia   the endometrium only
Ib   the uterine body; invasion < half myometrium
Ic   the uterine body; invasion > half myometrium
IIa the uterus, with endocervical gland involvement
IIb the uterus, with stromal invasion of the cervix
IIIa the uterus and adnexae with involvement of the serosa or positive ascites or peritoneal washings
IIIb the uterus and adnexae with vaginal involvement either direct or metastatic
IIIc the uterus and adnexae with pelvic or para-aortic node involvement
IVa carcinoma involving the bladder or the rectum
IVb distant metastases or involvement of other abdominal organs or inguinal lymph nodes.

Table 23.3 Correlation of tumour grade with depth of myometrial invasion

	Grade		
Myometrial invasion	*1*	*2*	*3*
None (Ia)	58	52	38
< 50% (Ib)	30	28	16
> 50% (Ic)	12	20	46

Values given are in percentages.

(g) Treatment

Surgery

The primary treatment for patients with stage I endometrial cancer, which will be 75% of patients, is total abdominal hysterectomy (TAH) and bilateral salpingo-oophorectomy (BSO). A radical hysterectomy does not improve survival further for patients with stage I disease and many would be unfit for such a procedure. Only occasionally are patients seen who are unfit for TAH and BSO. At the time of operation, the peritoneal cavity must be inspected and washings taken for cytology. The liver, omentum, uterine adnexae and retroperitoneal nodes should be examined carefully for evidence of tumour infiltration. In many cases, spread to the cervix is not detected until there is histological assessment of the resected uterus and, therefore, where stage II disease is occult clinically, the surgical treatment remains the same as for stage I.

For those cases where tumour is known to be stage II prior to operation there are two courses that can be followed. As the pelvic lymph nodes are at increased risk of involvement, it is important that these be treated and, therefore, the surgical option would be radical hysterectomy and lymphadenectomy. However, as many of these patients would be unfit for such a procedure, an alternative is to give external beam radiotherapy to the pelvis, to treat the pelvic nodes, and follow this with a simple hysterectomy. Patients diagnosed clinically as having stage III or IV disease are not suitable for treatment by surgery; radiotherapy should be given, on an individualized basis, with or without chemotherapy or hormonal therapy. Less than 30% of patients with disease of stage III and IV will survive 5 years.

Radiotherapy

Radiotherapy may be given as:

1. An adjuvant to surgery
2. Radical treatment
3. For palliation

Adjuvant radiotherapy for stage I carcinoma of the endometrium There is evidence to show that after local surgery alone there will be a recurrence rate at the vaginal vault of approximately 7% (Piver, 1982). This can be virtually eliminated by radiotherapy. In the past, such radiotherapy was given by preoperative intracavitary insertion, but this had the disadvantage of extra anaesthesia for the insertion in addition to that needed for the TAH and BSO. It also entailed a delay in performing the definitive surgery. In addition, because of the effect of the radiotherapy on the tumour, interpretation of the pathological specimens could be difficult. It has been shown that patients receiving radiotherapy after surgery do just as well as patients receiving it beforehand, without the need for extra anaesthesia or delay (Joslin *et al.*, 1977). This order of treatment also allows the pathological specimen to be studied to provide both a depth of tumour invasion and a grade of tumour. This allows those who have little risk of recurrence to be excluded from further treatment, and those at greater risk of having pelvic nodal disease to receive external beam radiotherapy in addition to vault irradiation.

Clinicians vary in their criteria for determining whether or not external beam radiotherapy is required. It is generally accepted that well and moderately differentiated tumours, that do not invade the myometrium, do not require external beam radiotherapy. In addition, the risk of vault recurrence is very low with these tumours and only those patients with disease in the lower third of the uterine cavity would require intravaginal irradiation. However, clinicians do not agree on whether or not tumours involving the inner or outer half of the myometrium require external beam radiotherapy or whether all patients with poorly differentiated tumours should have external beam treatment. A suggested regimen is included in Table 23.4. For those patients undergoing vault irradiation only, a dose of 60 Gy on the surface of the mucosa given as a single insertion at standard dose-rate would suffice. For those in whom it was felt that external beam radiotherapy was also required, 45 Gy given in 20–25 fractions, as a parallel opposed pair of 'box' treatment using three or four fields, would be followed by a vault insertion to give a further 20–25 Gy to the vaginal mucosa.

Whilst it is clear that intravaginal vault irradiation decreases the likelihood of recurrence, it is not so well proven that external beam radiotherapy prolongs survival. However, it does reduce the incidence of recurrence in the pelvis and the distressing side-effects that local disease causes.

Radical radiotherapy For those patients unfit for surgery with stage I or stage II disease and for patients with stage III disease, radiotherapy can be considered as a radical treatment. For patients with stage I disease and good prognostic indicators, intracavitary therapy alone can be carried out using a system either of multiple small ovoids inserted into the uterine cavity (Heyman's capsules), or an intrauterine tube or tubes. Heyman's capsules require considerable skill to arrange them within the uterine cavity sufficiently well to give a good dose distribution to the tumour, endometrium and myometrium. However, in some centres expertise has been developed in the use of these applicators and after-loading versions have now replaced those previously loaded with 'live' caesium sources. Intrauterine tubes have been developed to follow the lateral walls of the uterus in an attempt to produce a treatment volume of the same 'pear-shape' as the body of the uterus. Differentially loaded central intrauterine tubes have been used to try to achieve the same dose distribution (Kauppila *et al.*, 1987). However, because of the uncertainty involved in giving a high dose to such an irregular volume, many clinicians would give external beam radiotherapy to the uterus prior to the intracavitary insertion for stage I, II and III disease. The field used to cover this disease would be from the mid-sacroiliac joint to the bottom of the obturator foramina and, therefore, would cover the primary draining nodes of the body of the uterus. The para-aortic nodes would only be irradiated if there was

Table 23.4 Suggested postoperative radiotherapy protocol for stage I endometrial carcinoma

Depth of myometrial invasion	Tumour grade	Treatment
No invasion	G1 and G2	None unless tumour is in lower third of uterine cavity – if so, vaginal irradiation
< 50% (Ib)	G1 and G2	Vaginal irradiation
> 50% (Ic)	G1 and G2	External beam pelvic irradiation plus vaginal irradiation
All depths	G3	External beam pelvic irradiation plus vaginal irradiation

definite evidence of disease within the pelvic nodes, as this treatment is poorly tolerated in this generally elderly group of patients. A dose of 45 Gy in 25 fractions over 5 weeks would be typical for stage I disease, but 50 Gy may well be given for more advanced stages. The intracavitary insertion would aim to take the body of the uterus to a total dose of 65–70 Gy.

Palliative radiotherapy Patients with advanced stage III or IV disease will have individualized treatment and, in general, could only be considered for palliation. An exception to this are those patients with stage IIIa tumours, who have no evidence of disease beyond the serosa overlying the uterus and negative peritoneal washings. These patients will largely be treated as if they had had poor prognosis stage I disease with both external beam and intracavitary radiotherapy.

Hormonal therapy

Progestogens Response rates of 15–30% have been reported when using progestogens to treat recurrent carcinoma of the endometrium. Generally slow growing tumours that recur late after primary treatment respond more commonly than those that are either refractory to treatment or recur soon after it has been completed. Patients with well differentiated tumours, who are more likely to have positive oestrogen or progestogen receptor status within the tumour, have a response rate of up to 50% and, in the past, progestogens have been used as an adjuvant to therapy, even before surgery has been completed. However, the value of progestogens has never been proven and they carry a morbidity by virtue of their side-effects on the cardiovascular system. Progestogens can cause an increased incidence of fluid retention and heart failure in this elderly population and can give rise to thrombo-embolic

disease also. A large international study has been conducted to try to elucidate the role of progestogens as an adjuvant to surgery and radiotherapy for carcinoma of the endometrium, but is still to report its results (Kneale *et al.*, 1988). Many centres now adopt the policy of only using progestogens when there is assessable disease. When prescribed, a dose of 200– 400 mg per day of medroxyprogesterone acetate would be appropriate.

Tamoxifen Patients who have had previous evidence of tumour responsive to progestogens may also respond to tamoxifen and, very occasionally, non-progestogen sensitive tumours may also show some response. Because of this, tamoxifen has been used as second line therapy after progestogens and also in combination with those drugs.

Luteinizing hormone releasing hormone (LHRH) analogues These analogues are still in the trial stage, but have been shown to control disease refractory to progestogens. Their mode of action is uncertain as these patients are already postmenopausal and have naturally low concentrations of LH.

Chemotherapy Chemotherapy has generally not been a useful form of treatment in patients with endometrial carcinoma because of the age and fitness of the population with this tumour. Doxorubicin (adriamycin) has been considered to be an effective agent, but is cardiotoxic and unsuitable in the presence of heart disease, a common problem in this group of patients. Mitozantrone and cisplatin are currently being assessed. Partial response rates of 20–35% have been reported, but complete responses are rare.

(h) Results

Endometrial cancer has been considered to have a good prognosis, but this is largely due to the preponderance of early stage disease in the women presenting with this condition. Stage for stage, the survival is the same as for other gynaecological malignancies. Survival rates that are quoted are seldom disease specific and this elderly population frequently die from coexisting medical problems (Table 23.5).

Table 23.5 Results of treatment of carcinoma of the endometrium

Stage	% of total	5 year survival
I	74.0	72.0
II	13.5	56.0
III	6.0	31.5
IV	3.0	10.5

Modified from FIGO, 1988.

(i) Conclusions

Carcinoma of the endometrium occurs mainly in postmenopausal women and oestrogens play a part in its causation. It usually presents when still at an early stage and the primary treatment is surgery. Radiotherapy has a role in reducing the pelvic recurrence rate in early cases and providing palliation for advanced disease. Hormonal manipulation can be useful in the management of advanced and recurrent tumour, but its role as an adjuvant remains unproven.

23.4.2   UTERINE SARCOMAS

Uterine sarcomas occur very rarely and account for only 4% of all malignant uterine tumours. They are generally staged as stage I, II, III or IV, as are endometrial carcinomas, but without the substaging criteria. There are three types of uterine sarcoma:

1. Endometrial stromal sarcoma
2. Leiomyosarcomas
3. Malignant mixed müllerian (mixed mesodermal) tumours

(a)   Endometrial stromal sarcoma

These tumours are seen in a slightly younger age group (40–55 years) than other uterine sarcomas and are divided histologically into low grade and high grade tumours depending on whether there are less than or more than 10 mitoses per 10 high power fields (HPF). The low grade tumour, also known as endolymphatic stromal myosis, resembles normal endometrial stroma and is characterized by infiltration of the endometrium between muscle fibres and invasion of the lymphatic spaces. This tumour is usually an incidental finding at hysterectomy, but may occasionally cause abnormal vaginal bleeding. If these tumours do recur or metastasize to the lung, then they may respond to treatment with progestogens. High grade endometrial stromal sarcomas carry a poor prognosis and are often necrotic and cause vaginal bleeding and discharge. The disease is difficult to control both locally and when metastatic (Fekete and Vellios, 1984).

(b)   Leiomyosarcomas

Benign smooth muscle tumours of the uterus are very common and only 2–3% of all smooth muscle tumours are malignant. Only a tiny proportion (5–10%) of leiomyosarcomas arise in existing leiomyomas (fibroids), although they may arise in a uterus already affected by benign leiomyomas. These tumours have a tendency to spread directly to the abdominal cavity, via the lymphatics to lymph nodes and to metastasize in the blood stream to the lung. The prognosis of high grade tumours is equally poor to that of endometrial stromal sarcoma.

(c)   Malignant mixed müllerian tumours

These tumours are also known as mixed mesodermal tumours and are the most common uterine sarcoma, accounting for approximately 60–70% of the total. They occur most frequently between the ages of 60 and 70 and may distend the uterus and protrude through the cervical os. They contain both malignant epithelial and malignant stromal elements in varying proportions, the epithelial element usually being an endometrioid carcinoma which is poorly differentiated. The stromal element may be homologous, and composed of malignant cells derived from types that are normally found in the uterus, such as leiomyosarcoma, fibrosarcoma and endometrial stromal sarcoma, in which case they are still frequently reported as 'carcinosarcomas'. If the elements are not related to normal uterine tissue, as with rhabdomyosarcoma, osteosarcoma and chondrosarcoma, the tumour is described as heterologous. Occasionally, tumours are seen in which only the stromal element is malignant, these are known as adenosarcomas. As a rule, they are of low grade malignancy.

(d) Treatment and results

Uterine sarcomas fare badly whatever the histological nature and whatever the type of treatment. Postoperative radiotherapy may reduce the incidence of local pelvic recurrence, but has not been shown to prolong survival (Hornback *et al.*, 1986). Chemotherapy is seldom effective and should be regarded as experimental.

REFERENCES

Boronow, R.C., Morrow, C.P., Creasman, W.T. *et al.* (1984) Surgical staging in endometrial cancer: clinical–pathological findings of a prospective study. *Obstetrics and Gynecology*, **63** 835–32.

Brenner, D.J. and Hall, E.J. (1991) Fractionated high dose-rate versus low dose-rate regimen for intracavity brachytherapy of the cervix.1. General consideration based on radiobiology. *British Journal of Radiology*, **64**, 133–41.

Creasman, W.T., Morrow, C.P., Bundy, B.L. *et al.* (1987) Sugical-pathologic spread patterns of endometrial cancer (a GOG study). *Cancer*, **60**, 2035–41.

Dattoli, M.J., Gretz, H.F., Beller, U. *et al.* (1989) Analysis of multiple prognostic factors in patients with stage 1b cervical cancer: age as a major determinant. *International Journal of Radiation Oncology Biology and Physics*, **17**, 41–7.

Fekete, P.S. and Vellios, F. (1984) The clinical and histologic spectrum of endometrial stromal neoplasms: a report of 41 cases. *International Journal of Gynaecologic Pathology*, **3**, 198–212.

FIGO (1992) in *T.N.M. Atlas*, 3rd edn, 2nd revision, UICC, Springer-Verlag, Heidelberg, p. 196.

Follson, A.R., Kaye, S.A., Potter and J.D. and Prineas, R.J. (1989) Association of incident carcinoma of the endometrium with body weight and fat distribution in older women: early findings of the Iowa Women's Health Study. *Cancer Research*, **49**, 6828–31.

Fu, K. and Philips, T. (1990) High dose-rate versus low-rate intracavity brachytherapy for carcinoma of the cervix. *International Journal of Radiation Biology Oncology and Physics*, **19**, 791–6.

Hornback, N.B., Omura, G. and Major F.S. (1986) Observations on the use of adjuvant radiation therapy in patients with stage I and II uterine sarcoma. *International Journal of Radiation Oncology Biology and Physics*, **12**, 2127–30.

Hoskin, P.J. and Blake, P.R. (1991) Cisplatin, methotrexate and bleomycin (P.M.B.) for carcinoma of the cervix: the influence of presentation and previous treatment upon response. *International Journal of Gynaecological Cancer*, **1**, 75–80.

Jelovsek, F.R., Hammond, C.B., Woodard, B.H. *et al.* (1980) Risk of exogenous estrogen therapy and endometrial cancer. *American Journal of Obstetrics and Gynecology*, **137**, 85–91.

Joslin, C.A., Vaishampayan, G.V. and Mallik, A. (1977) The treatment of early cancer of the corpus uteri. *British Journal of Radiology*, **50**, 38–45

Kauppila, A., Sipila, P. and Koivula, A. (1987) Intracavitary irradiation of endometrial cancer of large uteri with 2-phase afterloading technique. *British Journal of Radiology*, **60**, 1093–7.

Kneale, B.L., Quinn, M.A. and Rennie, G.C. (1988) A randomised trial of progestogens in the primary treatment of endometrial carcinoma (letter). *British Journal of Obstetrics and Gynaecology*, **95**, 828.

Magee, B.J., Logue, J.P., Swindell, R. and McHugh, D. (1991). Tumour size as a prognostic factor in carcinoma of the cervix: assessment by transrectal ultrasound. *British Journal of Radiology*, **64**, 812–15.

Munoz, N., Bosch, X. and Kaldor, J.M. (1988) Does human papillomavirus cause cervical cancer? The state of the epidemiological evidence. *British Journal of Cancer*, **57**, 1–5.

Piver, M.S. (1992) Diagnosis and treatment of endometrial adenocarcinoma, in *Clinical Topics in Cancer: diagnosis and treatment*, (ed R.T. Silver), LeJacq, New York, pp. 378–395.

Shingleton, H.M. and Orr, J.W. (1987) *Cancer of the Cervix*, Churchill Livingstone, Edinburgh, p. 191.

Tidy, J.A. and Wrede, D. (1992) Tumour suppressor genes: new pathways in gynaecological cancer. *International Journal of Cancer*, **2**, 1–8.

Trevathan, E., Layde, P., Webster, L.A. *et al.* (1983) Cigarette smoking and dysplasia and carcinoma in situ of the uterine cervix. *Journal of American Medical Society*, **250**, 499–502.

OVARIAN CANCER

24

Eve Wiltshaw

Cancer of the ovary is a malignancy of the industrialized countries and within these countries it is the affluent who are most at risk. Unfortunately, because of the site of the ovaries within a large cavity, diagnosis is often delayed until the tumour has spread widely within the abdomen and pelvis. Perhaps because of this the prognosis is said to be the worst of all the gynaecological cancers and overall 5 year survival is still quoted at around 25–30%.

Thus the quest for earlier diagnosis and better methods of treatment have been the subject of intense study and discussion in recent years.

24.1 INCIDENCE, AETIOLOGY AND EPIDEMIOLOGY

In 1985 there were just over 5000 new cases of ovarian cancer in a UK population of 29 041 million women (approximate incidence of 14 per 100 000 women). This compares with an incidence of 21 in Scandinavia and 3 per 100 000 in Japan. The reasons for these differences remain uncertain but have a close correlation with reproduction and the use of hormones. The two consistent observations are the more pregnancies the less the risk and that oral contraceptives protect against ovarian cancer. Late menarche and early menopause also reduce the risk. These observations suggest that excessive ovulation over a lifetime may play an important part in the aetiology of the disease.

The evidence suggests that lifestyle is important whereas ethnic origin is not, since ethnic groups which have emigrated later take on the incidence of their adopted country rather than that of their origin.

Other aetiological factors which have been suggested are asbestos exposure, the use of talc on the perineum as well as high fat diet, excess consumption of coffee and the use of stilboestrol for menopausal symptoms. The evidence however is weak at the present time.

A few patients are at much higher risk of ovarian cancer due to genetic factors. Women whose mother or sister died of this tumour have a 20 fold increase of developing the disease over their lifetime and if two close relatives have been affected then the risk increases to approximately 40% at aged 40 years.

24.2 PATHOLOGY

The majority of ovarian cancers develop from the surface epithelium, and at the Norwegian Radium Hospital 94% of 1137 cases seen during the years 1968–73 were of this type, while 6% belonged to the group developing from the germinal or granulosa-theca cells. Within the common epithelial tumours there are a group usually called borderline tumours or tumours of low malignant potential. Although small in number they are of special interest and importance since their prognosis is so much better than the truly invasive tumours and their management is therefore different.

Analysis of 7095 cases from Stockholm (Kottmeier *et al.*, 1982) showed that borderline

Table 24.1   Distribution of histological type in 7095 cases of epithelial cancer (1976–82)

Histological type	%
Carcinoma	
Serous	44.2
Mucinous	11.8
Endometrioid	14.5
Mesonephroid (clear cell)	4.3
Unclassified or Undifferentiated	20.0
Borderline	
Serous	2.9
Mucinous	2.2
Other	0.1
	100

From Kottmeier *et al.*, 1982.

tumours amounted to 5.2% of epithelial lesions and that there were four main classes of epithelial invasive cancer. Table 24.1 shows the type and distribution with a clear majority being serous.

There are four major types of epithelial tumour: serous, mucinous, endometrioid and clear cell. Each can exist in a benign form, may show a histological appearance classed as borderline malignancy or can be frankly malignant. It is thought that serous and endometrioid tumours are derived from undifferentiated cells retaining a potential to develop along a tubal pathway and an endocervical route respectively. Endometrial pathways result in endometrioid tumours whilst clear cell tumours are thought now to originate from müllerian tissue in the majority of cases (Fox, 1990). The diagnosis of undifferentiated (or unclassified) tumours varies considerably but usually amounts to between 5% and 20% of all ovarian adenocarcinomas.

All neoplasms are graded by degree of differentiation (well, moderately and poorly) where again subjectivity is to some degree responsible for variations in the numbers diagnosed in each subgroup.

Borderline tumours have been clearly defined histologically by the Ovarian Tumour Panel of the Royal College of Obstetricians and Gynaecologists (1983) as tumours 'in which the epithelial component shows some, or all, of the characteristics of malignancy but in which there is no stromal invasion'. The lack of invasion by these tumours probably accounts for their frequent curability by surgery and the corresponding fact that most are diagnosed at an early stage in contrast to invasive carcinomas.

24.3   PRESENTATION AND SPREAD

Ovarian tumours are generally diagnosed late, simply because of their silent nature during initial growth. When symptoms do occur their nature depends largely on the size and position of tumour tissue. Thus a large single ovarian mass may cause lower abdominal swelling and frequency of micturition, whilst a smaller primary tumour with multiple secondary spread on the abdominal peritoneal surfaces may produce recurrent abdominal colic associated with incomplete bowel obstruction. Table 24.2 shows that the commonest symptoms are abdominal pain and swelling and it is very rare for an asymptomatic patient to be diagnosed. Abnormal bleeding is surprisingly uncommon and is more often associated with a histology of granulosa cell tumour than epithelial cancer

Table 24.2   Ovarian cancer: symptoms at the time of diagnosis (based on over 2000 patients from several series)

Symptom	% of total
Abdominal pain	50.8
Abdominal swelling	49.5
Gastrointestinal	21.6
Weight loss	17.5
Abnormal bleeding	17.1
Urinary	16.4
Pelvic pressure	5.0
Backache	4.9
Mass	2.8
None	0.4

From Coppleson, 1981.

or with direct involvement of the endometrium with tumour.

Ovarian cancer can present at any age but is uncommon under 30 years and the age distribution varies for different histological types. Figure 24.1 shows the age at presentation for epithelial cancers, germ cell tumours and granulosa cell tumours for patients seen at the Royal Marsden Hospital. The most important presenting sign is the presence of a pelvic mass on physical examination. Indeed in postmenopausal women the ovaries cease to be palpable and if an ovary can be felt at that time of life, it should be considered suspicious of neoplasm and should be investigated further.

Spread of ovarian cancer is mainly by exfoliation of cells from the surface of the tumour into the peritoneal cavity where implants then arise on the peritoneal surfaces of the abdominopelvic cavity. The cells tend to follow the circulatory path of intraperitoneal fluid and thus early implants will be formed in the paracolic gutters, undersurface of the right hemidiaphragm and then on the bowel mesentery and in the omentum. The tumour may also spread by local invasion of the pelvic side wall, the fallopian tube and the appendix.

Spread via lymphatics often occurs in later stages of the disease, especially to the para-aortic nodes, the diaphragmatic lymphatics and later to the mediastinal nodes.

Lastly, haematogenous spread seems to be a late phenomenon, except when the tumour is exceptionally invasive. When blood-borne metastasis does occur lung and liver are the organs most usually involved. Involvement of the pleura with a malignant effusion may be due to haematological spread or direct invasion through the diaphragm.

24.4 INVESTIGATION AND DIAGNOSIS

When ovarian cancer is suspected investigation to make the diagnosis and to describe the extent of the disease should be orderly and efficient in time and use of appropriate tests.

Because of the very various initial symptoms patients are often seen first by general or gastrointestinal physicians or surgeons but appropriate tests can rapidly resolve the diagnosis in most cases. First if a pelvic examination reveals a mass then the next appropriate test is either an ultrasound examination or a CT scan of the abdomen and pelvis. There are advantages and disadvantages to both these investigations and to do both is the ideal. Together they will show the extent and site of the pelvic mass, the presence of peritoneal deposits and ascites, omental involvement and intrahepatic and/or hepatic capsular lesions. Nodal disease in retroperitoneal tissues and pleural effusion may also be seen.

It is important that bowel contrast be given so that large bowel tumour can be

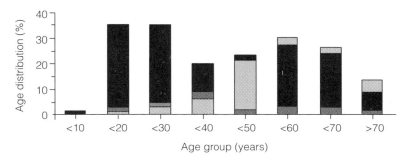

Figure 24.1 Age distribution of ovarian cancer: selected histologies. ⬚, Epithelial (*n* = 1416); ■, germ cell (*n* = 92); ▨, granulosa (*n* = 77).

differentiated from a primary ovarian mass. A cervical smear should be done also to exclude a primary in the cervix. At the same time blood tumour markers should be looked for. CA 125 is the best tumour marker for ovarian cancer and is raised in approximately 80% of cases. In young women it is essential to exclude a germ cell tumour before surgery is done. Blood alpha fetoprotein (AFP) and beta human chorionic gonadotrophin (βHCG) levels should be measured in all patients under the age of 30 years. One or both will be raised in the majority of germ cell tumours but only rarely in dysgerminoma.

The final investigation for a diagnosis is surgery and, except in very advanced cases, a full laparotomy is required in order to remove as much tumour as possible, as well as to acquire histological material. In very late stage disease where surgical cure is not possible laparoscopy may be preferable with biopsy of tumour and cytology of any ascitic fluid providing the basis for histological classification.

24.5   STAGING

The management and outcome of ovarian cancer depends a great deal on the stage of disease at diagnosis. Stage is, of course, an indication of the extent of tumour spread and there is an internationally accepted definition of each stage which has been provided by the International Federation of Gynaecology and Obstetrics (FIGO). The stages are designated I–IV and are shown in Table 24.3. The stage is determined by the surgical and histological findings but in some cases, e.g. stage IV, CT and chest X-ray appearances may add to the accuracy of the staging.

24.6   MANAGEMENT OF EPITHELIAL OVARIAN TUMOURS

24.6.1   SURGERY

Surgical removal of ovarian cancer remains the mainstay for most cases of ovarian malig-

nancy and laparotomy is also essential for accurate staging. Where malignancy is expected the incision should be midline or paramedian and an abdominal (not the Pfannensteil) approach so that the whole cavity can be inspected and biopsied. If there is ascites this should be drained and fluid sent for cytology. If there is no overt ascites, then 50–160 ml of saline should be instilled and the cavity washing examined cytologically.

After inspection of the extent of the tumour the ovarian mass should be removed intact if possible and a frozen section performed. If malignancy is confirmed and the tumour or tumours appear to be surgically removable, then a bilateral salpingo-oophorectomy (BSO) and total abdominal hysterectomy (TAH) should be performed, together with a subcolic omentectomy. A search should be made for peritoneal metastases, particularly in the paracolic gutters and on the liver surface and surface of the right hemidiaphragm. Any suspicious areas must be biopsied and some advocate biopsy of these areas even if the tissue appears normal. Any enlarged or abnormal retroperitoneal nodes should be sampled. The findings from this meticulous search for tumour will then allow the stage of disease to be accurately defined.

Occasionally in a young woman who wishes to keep her fertility potential a unilateral salpingo-oophorectomy may be performed. If she turns out to have stage Ia well differentiated carcinoma then this procedure could be sufficient for cure. However, the risks must be discussed with the patient before or after the laparotomy so that she fully understands her position.

Where all visible tumour is not removed by a TAH and BSO together with omentectomy some surgeons go on to try to excise all the peritoneal deposits including removal of pieces of bowel. This somewhat heroic surgery has been advocated because it is known that those patients in whom complete removal is possible do better than those with incomplete clearance. However, it has not

Table 24.3 FIGO staging (1987) for primary ovarian carcinoma

Stage I	Growth limited to the ovaries
Ia	Growth limited to one ovary: no surface tumour, capsule intact
Ib	Growth limited to both ovaries: no surface tumour, capsule intact
Ic	Tumour either stage Ia or Ib but with surface tumour or ruptured capsule or with ascites or cytological washings showing malignant cells
Stage II	Growth limited to the pelvis
IIa	Extension and/or metastasis to the uterus and/or tubes
IIb	Extension to other pelvic tissues
IIc	Tumour either stage IIa or IIb but with surface tumour or capsule rupture or with ascites (as in Ic)
Stage III	Tumour outside the pelvis in the form of peritoneal implants and/or involved retroperitoneal or inguinal nodes or omental tumour
IIIa	Tumour grossly limited to the pelvis but with microscopic peritoneal disease only
IIIb	Tumour with peritoneal nodules all < 2 cm in size and no positive nodes
IIIc	Abdominal implants > 2 cm in size and/or involved retroperitoneal or inguinal nodes
Stage IV	Tumour which has extended beyond the abdominopelvic cavity and retroperitoneal tissues usually by blood-borne spread, e.g. intrahepatic metastases and malignant pleural effusion

Table 24.4 Epithelial ovarian cancer stage and histology: The Royal Marsden Experience 1980–89

Histology	Stage I	II	III	IV	Total (no.)
Serous	14%	12%	55%	19%	496
Mucinous	46%	7%	34%	13%	143
Endometrioid	37%	17%	40%	6%	118
Clear cell	39%	20%	32%	9%	54
Adenocarcinoma	7%	16%	52%	25%	230
Total (no.)	220	138	503	180	1041
% of total	21%	13%	49%	17%	100%

been shown that extensive surgery for widespread disease is better than less radical surgery by a direct randomized study. Many believe that where removal is complete the tumour is naturally less invasive and it is the nature of the tumour rather than the skill and diligence of the surgeon which matters in regard to prognosis. Our own unit does not recommend radical removal of peritoneal disease except where a single area of bowel obstruction is likely or one or two large masses which might cause symptoms are present but easily excised.

The relationship between stage and histological type is shown in Table 24.4, which reveals that only 21% of patients will have surgically curable disease (i.e. stage I) at diagnosis and a similar percentage (17%) have stage IV when first seen.

24.6.2 POSTOPERATIVE MANAGEMENT

Historically all patients have been treated with postoperative therapy in the belief that survival could be improved over and above that obtained by surgery alone. The postoperative therapies that have applied include pelvic radiotherapy, abdominopelvic radiotherapy, intraperitoneal radiation with radioactive isotopes, such as ^{198}Au or ^{32}P, or chemotherapy with cytotoxic drugs.

Recently radiotherapy has been largely abandoned, partly because ovarian carcinoma is now recognized to be a tumour usually involving the whole abdominopelvic cavity and because of the impracticality of giving a sterilizing dose of radiation to such a large area without producing unacceptable toxicity. However, in stages of disease where minimal tumour is present postoperatively no large scale randomized study has been done to compare external beam abdominopelvic irradiation with a modern chemotherapeutic regimen, or indeed with no treatment and the value, if any, of radiotherapy here remains uncertain.

Postoperative chemotherapy is now the treatment of choice and it has been established that to date first line chemotherapy should contain a platinum compound, although the controversy over the use of high dose platinum single agent therapy versus a combination of drugs still goes on.

However, before deciding what chemotherapy to use it is necessary to enquire where it is of value and whether all patients need postoperative treatment.

24.6.3 STAGE I

If ovarian adenocarcinoma can be diagnosed before it has spread to other organs, then theoretically it should be curable by surgery.

Many papers have shown that there is near 100% survival for patients with well differentiated tumours confined to one ovary and with no tumour on the ovarian surface (stage Ia grade 1 histology). In these cases chemotherapy is not indicated and surgery itself may be confined to a unilateral removal of the affected ovary and its fallopian tube (USO). However in all other cases of stage I disease, most investigators advocate postoperative treatment, despite the lack of evidence for efficacy. Large clinical trials have never been done to show whether treatment is worthwhile and smaller trials have usually compared an alkylating agent versus some form of radiation therapy with negative results. Platinum chemotherapy has not been investigated adequately in this area to date.

The policy at the Royal Marsden Hospital since 1979 has been to carefully watch all stage I patients after surgery and only to treat when recurrence occurs. It is worldwide experience that 30% of patients will relapse after surgery alone or with added radiotherapy and that poor prognostic features are surface tumour, poorly differentiated histology and tumour cells in the peritoneal fluid. Nevertheless some patients with these features appear to be cured by surgery alone.

Our own study has now accrued 175 patients stage Ia–c and the overall survival at 5 years is 84% and the disease free survival 72%. Patients are followed with CA 125 levels every 3 months and CT scans every 6 months for the first 2 years and on relapse are given single agent chemotherapy with cisplatin or carboplatin as for later stage disease. So far these patients are doing just as well as patients treated elsewhere and our study has now led to a very interesting trial being run by the MRC comparing combination chemotherapy with no postoperative treatment. The results of our study show that while 32 patients have recurred, only 16 have died of ovarian cancer, while a further 16 patients have died of other causes. These figures are as good as those reported by Young *et al.* (1990) in two small randomized studies comparing treatments for stages I and II disease (Figure 24.2).

24.6.4 STAGES II–IV

Once ovarian cancer has spread to the pelvis or elsewhere the prognosis greatly worsens and surgery must be supplemented by postoperative chemotherapy. The questions now are what is appropriate chemotherapy, how much and for how long and what are its problems and benefits? Overall survival of the Royal Marsden series is shown in Figure 24.3.

Chemotherapy was first shown to be of benefit in late stage ovarian cancer in the 1960s and following the early papers many studies confirmed that single alkylating agents mainly given by mouth produced response rates of 30–50%, although the regressions were measured by very crude methods. Unfortunately, the responses rarely lasted more than 6 months and survival was also short.

Hopes for greater benefits were raised again when a combination of drugs appeared to improve the response rate and when cisplatin was found to produce responses in patients previously treated with other cytotoxic drugs, a situation not previously seen in ovarian cancer (Wiltshaw and Kroner, 1976). Since then it has become clear that single agent cisplatin is the most useful drug for the condition. Nevertheless, even metanalysis of

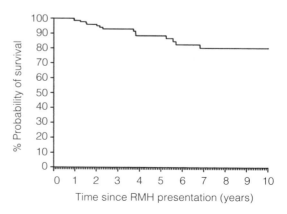

Figure 24.2 Overall survival: epithelial ovarian cancer. Stage I: no postoperative therapy. *n* = 175.

the relatively small trials in stages III and IV disease reported from Europe and the USA have not resolved the question, is single agent relatively high dose cisplatin (100 mg/m^2) as good as combination chemotherapy with cyclophosphamide plus or minus doxorubicin or hexamethyl melamine (Advanced Clinical Trialist Group, 1991)?

At the Royal Marsden Hospital it is our view that cisplatin alone given monthly at a dose of 100 mg/m^2 for five courses gives as good results as combination chemotherapy using cisplatin in lower doses (usually 50–75 mg/m^2). Certainly side-effects are less as well as toxicities. However, one has to say that this is not a popular view. The most commonly used treatment regimens at the present time are given in Table 24.5 and include the relatively new drug carboplatin. Carboplatin was introduced to overcome the more serious toxicities of cisplatin including renal, neurological and aural toxicity, whilst at the same time not reducing the original compound's efficacy. In this the drug has been very successful and studies so far suggest that given adequate doses carboplatin is just as efficacious as cisplatin in ovarian tumours. Table 24.5 shows the differences in toxicity but also the difference in the calculation of a proper dose. Most cytotoxic drug doses are based on the surface area of the patient but in the case of carboplatin, which is not really toxic at conventional doses, the amount required depends upon renal excretion rate which is not the case for cisplatin. Thus if there is renal impairment when carboplatin is administered lower doses will be needed. A simple formula has been devised by Calvert *et al.* (1989) for deriving the correct dose based on glomerular filtration rate (GFR) and area under the curve (AUC). Conventional doses of carboplatin in patients with a GFR of around 60 ml/min would be about 600 mg based on dosing of 400 mg/m^2 and this is equivalent to an AUC of 6 based on the Calvert formula (dose in mg = target AUC × (GFR + 25)).

The toxicities of the various regimens vary mostly in degree rather than in kind but carboplatin single agent treatment is the easiest on both patient and on staff. The drug does not require intravenous fluid support, nausea and vomiting can be overcome in most cases with modern antiemetic regimens including the 5HT3 inhibitors and renal, neurological and hearing toxicities are rare in patients who have had no exposure to other neurotoxic drugs (e.g. cisplatin or hexamethylmelamine).

The optimal dose of drugs used in ovarian cancer remains the subject of discussion. Since the paper by Levin and Hryniuk (1987) there has been a tendency for investigators to

Table 24.5 Commonly used chemotherapy regimens and their toxicities

	Regimen	Toxicity and side-effects						
		N&V	Alopecia	Neutro	Thrombo	Renal	Neuro	Oto
1	Cisplatin 100 mg/m^2 q 28 days × 5	+++	Rare	±	±	++	++	++
2	Cisplatin 50–75 mg/m^2 plus cyclophosphamide 75–100 mg/m^2 q, 28 days × 6–8	+++	+++	++	++	++	++	++
3	Carboplatin AUC6 or 400 mg/m^2 q 28 days × 6	++	Rare	+	++	Rare	Rare	Rare

The number of + signs represents the frequency of the side-effect or toxicity. Rare, <3% of cases.

increase the dose and frequency of chemotherapy in the belief that higher dose intensity will be matched by more responses and more survivors. However for the platinum compounds a study by Jodrell *et al.* (1992) strongly suggests that increased efficacy is not achieved by greater dosage above a certain fairly modest dose intensity.

At the present time an important study of carboplatin at AUC 12 versus AUC 6 is continuing in the Royal Marsden and other London Hospitals to try to resolve the question of higher dose benefits, if any. The advice at present is to give drugs at the highest safe dose as quickly as possible, allowing for recovery from toxicity, usually 3–4 weekly.

There are very few studies suggesting the best time limit for continuing cytotoxic drugs but six to eight courses are now commonly used. What studies have been done, including assessment of regression by laparotomy, suggest that all the benefits of chemotherapy will have been achieved by the first six treatments. This fits in well with the theory that resistance will develop if all tumour cells are not destroyed very quickly.

24.6.5 TREATMENT ASSESSMENT

It is very important that treatment is only continued in those patients who are or will shortly benefit from it. This seems obvious but many are subjected to further courses of therapy because assessment is not rigorous. All patients should be questioned about symptoms of disease and of toxicity before each new course is given, as well as being carefully examined. CA 125 is an excellent marker for measuring reduction in tumour after treatment and should be measured regularly if it was raised before chemotherapy began. Other follow-up measures should include abdominopelvic ultrasound or CT scanning which should be undertaken just before course 3 is administered and at the end of treatment. If all these measures suggest that a response is occurring or if no evidence of tumour growth is found in those patients previously without measurable disease, then treatment should proceed. However, if there is no measurable benefit after three courses of chemotherapy, it is very unlikely that improvement will occur by persisting with the chosen regimen and it should be abandoned. A full re-assessment should be made at the end of treatment including scanning to document the degree of response seen.

For some time it has been popular for cancer centres to advocate second surgery to assess response but this is of no benefit to the patient unless you can offer further useful treatment when resistance is evident. Up to now further therapy in this situation, including abdominopelvic or intraperitoneal radiotherapy or other chemotherapy, has not been helpful. It should be remembered also that complete regression, as measured by second look surgery together with negative histology, does not indicate cure and the practice is now losing favour. We would advocate second look surgery for those patients apparently without measurable disease at the end of chemotherapy only when a second line treatment may be used with good effect. Taxol and taxotere, new and apparently useful drugs, which are soon to come on the market may well be a case in point.

24.6.6 OUTCOME

Whilst chemotherapy has been made less toxic and safer it is still an unpleasant long term procedure and the benefits must be real to make it worthwhile. The treatment advocated here will result in approximately 60% showing measurable and significant regression of tumour, partial remission (PR) or complete regression (CR). There will be a further 20% of patients where response will not be measurable but the tumour shows no evidence of regrowth. These patients are not assessable (NA) and chemotherapy may or may not have been beneficial. About 20% of patients will not have responsive tumours.

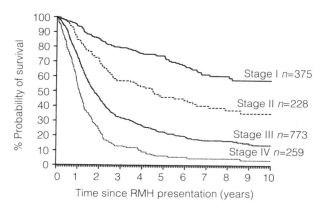

Figure 24.3   Overall survival: epithelial ovarian cancer.

The prognosis now depends on initial stage, degree of response, differentiation of tumour, rate of fall of CA 125 (the faster it falls the better the prognosis) and the amount of residual disease at the end of initial surgery.

Figure 24.3 shows the overall survival to be expected if the policies advocated here are followed. The curves shown are based on 1635 patients treated at the Royal Marsden Hospital since 1974 when cisplatin was introduced as first line therapy for stages III and IV disease. Some patients in this group were treated elsewhere with less than optimal chemotherapy and some with stage II disease were treated initially with radiotherapy and thus the outcomes shown might underestimate the benefits of the treatment advocated now.

24.6.7   TREATMENT FOR RELAPSE

Although there is no therapy generally available to treat patients with disease resistant to platinum compounds, some patients will respond again to cisplatin or carboplatin if they have responded well initially. A retrospective study at the Royal Marsden Hospital showed that after a 2 year period of remission, the response rate to a second exposure of platinum based chemotherapy at conventional dose will be of the order of 50%. For patients exposed 1 year previously that rate will drop to 17% and if exposed within 12 months, a second treatment is very unlikely to be beneficial (Gore *et al.*, 1989).

24.7   MANAGEMENT OF BORDERLINE EPITHELIAL TUMOURS

Surgery for borderline tumours, often called tumours of low malignant potential, should be similar to that of well differentiated invasive carcinomas. This is to say if the patient has stage I disease with tumour in only one ovary a USO is probably sufficient to cure most patients and no postoperative measures are needed. However, occasionally patients do present with later stage disease and a few stage I cases recur in the other ovary. These patients may develop a second frankly malignant tumour in the other ovary, although this is a rare phenomenon.

When such tumours arise in fertile young women decisions about the extent of surgery can be very difficult but if the tumour affects both ovaries the best advice would be a bilateral oophorectomy, together with a careful look for satellite nodules within the peritoneal tissues including the omentum.

If tumour recurs or has already spread outside one ovary postoperative treatment has not been clearly defined. Even stages III and IV disease do not necessarily carry a poor prognosis and in the case of serous tumours, some believe that the spread does not indicate metastases in the usual sense of the word. In the case of borderline mucinous tumours, spread can be associated with large amounts of mucoid ascites which causes serious distress to patients. In this case unfortunately present day chemotherapy has not been useful and the only relief for the patient is repeated laparotomies for the removal of the mucoid material (pseudomyxoma peritoneii). Serous tumours may well respond to chemotherapy as do true carcinomas but the effect on survival is uncertain.

The literature suggests that the 20 year survival for stage I disease may be as high as 90% and for stage III disease 70%. At the present time our own series of borderline cases stands at 64 cases of which none have died, despite the fact that 14% had stage II and 10% stage III disease at diagnosis. These patients should have careful follow-up, if possible at a cancer centre, where new therapy can be applied appropriately and more learnt about this rare group. Some characteristics of borderline tumours compared with frank carcinoma are shown in Table 24.6. A comprehensive review of borderline tumours is presented by Trimble and Trimble in *Cancer of the Ovary* (1993).

24.8 GRANULOSA CELL TUMOUR

Granulosa cell tumour is the commonest of the malignant gonadal stromal tumours but only accounts for some 3–9% of all ovarian neoplasms. Few of the other sex cord-stromal tumours (e.g. Sertoli–Leydig cell tumours) show malignant characteristics and are best treated by surgery.

Granulosa cell tumour sometimes occurs in young girls, usually 10–30 years old, and this adolescent type usually presents as stage I disease and is curable by conservative surgery (USO). However, the same tumour in older women is prone to recurrence, although these may occur as late as 20 years after diagnosis. Apart from stage at diagnosis the other best prognostic indicator seems to be the size of the primary tumour. In one series, tumours, larger than 15 cm had a 10 year survival of only 53%, while 100% of patients with smaller tumours were alive at 10 years (Fox *et al..*,1975). Thus in the older patient with a large tumour the treatment of choice is radical surgery (BSO, TAH and subcolic omentectomy). The value of postoperative radiotherapy and/or chemotherapy is unknown but often recurrence will eventually become apparent despite both adjuvant treatments.

It is probably best to postpone medical treatment until recurrence occurs, for while granulosa cell tumour seems to be sensitive to radiotherapy and cisplatin based chemotherapy, neither are curative and remissions are sometimes short lived. The recommended chemotherapy is a combination of cisplatin and cyclophosphamide given in the same way as for epithelial tumours (Table 24.5). Recently however a combination of cisplatin, bleomycin and either vinblastine (PVB) or etoposide (BEP) have been used in phase II trials. Both regimens appear to produce a high response rate and there have been long

Table 24.6 Some distinguishing features of borderline tumours

Characteristic	Cancer	Borderline tumours
Pathology	Stromal invasion	No stromal invasion
Age at diagnosis	Median 54 years	Median 45 years
Stage at diagnosis	20% Stage I	70% Stage I
Survival at 5 years	80% Stage I	100% Stage I

remissions (Colombo *et al.*, 1986). The regimens can be found in Section 24.9 but in the case of older women the toxicities are sometimes more severe than in young men and women treated for germ cell lesions. It is best for patients to be treated in a centre with experience of these regimens as toxicity can be lethal.

24.9 GERM CELL TUMOURS

Germ cell tumours (GSTs) in young women occur much less frequently than in men. In Western countries they constitute about 5% of all ovarian malignancies but are more frequent (15%) in oriental and black societies. Their proper management however is very important, first because the majority are curable and second because they usually occur in women under 30 years of age and often in teenagers. Because of their curability radical surgery should be avoided if at all possible. Similarly pelvic irradiation should only be used as a last resort. Happily the chemotherapy used rarely causes infertility and normal pregnancies may follow successful treatment.

A GST should always be suspected in woman under 30 years of age with a large ovarian mass, since in this age group epithelial cancers are rare (Fig. 24.1). Before surgery the tumour markers AFP and βHCG should be measured. If either are raised, then a presumptive diagnosis can be made. At laparotomy the primary tumour should be removed and assessment of tumour elsewhere in the abdominopelvic cavity must be carried out. However, the uterus and second ovary should be preserved.

Although the pathogenesis of GCTs is similar in the male and female, the different names given can often lead to confusion. The commonest GCTs are dysgerminoma (seminoma in males) endodermal sinus tumour usually associated with a high blood level of AFP and malignant teratoma. Often tumours are mixed.

In our own series of 92 cases, the proportion of the various histological types were dysgerminoma 28%, endodermal sinus tumour (EST) 25%, teratoma 38% and mixed tumours 8%.

Dysgerminoma spreads in the same way as seminoma, that is principally via the lymphatics. Thus for a left ovarian tumour progression is to the left para-aortic nodes followed by mediastinal involvement and occasionally as far as the supraclavicular nodes. Lung metastases come later. In the past management has consisted of radiotherapy to these nodal areas to prevent recurrence but this endangers fertility and may not cover all the areas already infiltrated by tumour. Today if dysgerminoma has spread beyond the ovary (stage II or more) single agent cisplatin or carboplatin as for epithelial ovarian cancer and given for 3–5 courses is usually curative.

For all other GCTs and for recurrent dysgerminoma combination chemotherapy after conservative surgery is recommended, even in stage I cases. Where tumour marker levels (AFP, HCG) are raised, then the rate of fall of the marker is an excellent indication of sensitivity of the tumour and of prognosis. Teratoma and EST unlike dysgerminoma spread initially intraperitoneally as does epithelial ovarian cancer. Later intrahepatic metastases and para-aortic nodal disease are more common than lung metastases. Treatment should be guided by marker levels and bulk of tumour as in testicular cancer and chemotherapy with the combination PEB or CEB (carboplatin, etoposide and bleomycin) should be continued for 2–3 courses after these levels have returned to normal (see Chapter 34 for details). A very good review of these interesting tumours and their management is given in *Textbook of Uncommon Cancer* (Williams *et al.*, (1988).

The outcome for GCT in girls and young women is an 80–85% survival at 5 years and few recurrences after 2 years.

24.10 ONGOING RESEARCH

The major areas for research at the present time are in early diagnosis and better anti-cancer drugs. Since most ovarian cancers are diagnosed after dissemination within the pelvis and abdomen the cure rate remains low and researchers are investigating the viability of screening all women for this condition. It looks as though CA 125 levels together with modern ultrasound examination over the pelvis will pick up the majority of ovarian tumours, but so far there has been an unacceptable level of unnecessary laparotomies in well women in research screening programmes. If this can be reduced further the introduction of screening nationally will probably only be constrained by costs.

Research is also quickening pace in those patients with a strong family history of either ovarian cancer or of ovarian, breast and colon malignancies. The gene or genes involved in very high risk cancer families will be able to pick out the women at excessively high risk where prophylactic oophorectomy may be indicated. A word of warning here however – prophylactic removal of the ovaries may not prevent a coelomic epithelial cancer appearing later.

New therapies for ovarian cancer have been appearing recently and the most well known are taxol and taxotere. Both drugs derive from the Pacific Yew; taxol from the bark and taxotere from the leaves. These are antimicrotubule agents which shift the dynamic equilibrium between tubulin dimers and microtubule towards polymerization, inducing excessively stable and non-functional microtubules. Early studies of taxol revealed serious toxicities described as acute hypersensitivity reactions but these problems have now been largely overcome. Claims here have been made that taxol produces responses in platinum resistant cases of ovarian cancer but how long any benefits from these responses can last have not yet been reported. A study is already under way of taxol plus cisplatin versus cisplatin and cyclophosphamide as first line treatment but it will take very large sample numbers to show whether taxol will increase the response and long term survival of epithelial ovarian cancer patients (Rowinsky *et al.*, 1991). Less is known about taxotere which has received much less publicity but this agent may in fact be more efficacious.

Lastly, a new generation of platinum compounds is being tested and the most promising of these seems to be JM216, a mixed ammine/amine platinum IV dicarboxylate, an oral compound which appears not to be entirely cross-resistant with cisplatin and carboplatin and which has little toxicity for the kidneys. This compound may also have a place in the management of colon cancer.

REFERENCES

Advanced Cancer Trialist Group (1991) Chemotherapy in advanced ovarian cancer: an overview of randomised clinical trials. *British Medical Journal*, **303**, 884–93.

Calvert, A.H., Newell, D.R., Gumbrell, L.A. *et al.* (1989) Carboplatin dosage: prospective evaluation of a simple formula based on renal function. *Journal of Clinical Oncology*, **7**, 1748–56.

Colombo, N., Sessa, C., Landoni, F. *et al.* (1986) Cisplatin, vinblastine and bleomycin combination chemotherapy in metastatic granulosa cell tumour of the ovary. *Obstetrics and Gynaecology*, **67**, 265–8.

Coppleson, M. (1981) *Gynecologic Oncology*, vol. 2, Churchill Livingstone, Edinburgh.

Fox, H. (1990) Pathology of Ovarian Cancer in *Clinical Gynaecological Oncology*, (eds J.H. Shepherd and J.M. Monaghan), Blackwell Scientific Publications, Oxford, p. 188.

Fox, H., Agrawal, K. and Langley, F.A. (1975) A clinico pathological study of 92 cases of granulosa cell tumour of the ovary with special reference to the factors influencing prognosis. *Cancer*, **35**, 231–41.

Gore, M., Fryatt, I., Wiltshaw, E. *et al.* (1989) Cisplatin/carboplatin cross resistance in ovarian cancer. *British Journal of Cancer*, **60**, 767–9.

Jodrell, D., Egorin, M.J., Canetta, R.M. *et al.* (1992) Relationship between carboplatin exposure and tumour response and toxicity in patients with ovarian cancer. *Journal of Clinical Oncology*, **10**, 520–8.

Kottmier, H.L., Kolstad, P., McGarrity, K. *et al.* (eds) (1982) *Annual Report on the Results of Treatment of Gynaecological Cancer*, vol. 18, Radium Hemmet, Stockholm.

Levin, L. and Hryniuk, W.M. (1987) Dose intensity of chemotherapy regimens in ovarian carcinoma. *Journal of Clinical Oncology*, **5**, 756–67.

Ovarian Tumour Panel of the Royal College of Obstetricians and Gynaecologists (1983) Ovarian epithelial tumours of borderline malignancy: pathological features and current status. *British Journal of Obstetrics and Gynaecology*, **90**, 743–50.

Rowinsky, E.K., Gilbert, K., McGuire, W.P. *et al.* (1991) Sequences of taxol and cisplatin: a phase I pharmacologic study. *Journal of Clinical Oncology*, **9**, 1692–703.

Trimble, E.L. and Trimble, C.L. (1993) Epithelial ovarian tumours of low malignant potential, in *Cancer of the Ovary*, (eds M. Markman and W.J. Hoskins), Raven Press, New York, pp. 415–29.

Williams, C.J. Krikorian, J.G. Green, M.R. and Raghavan, D. (1988) *Textbook of Uncommon Cancer*, John Wiley, Chichester.

Wiltshaw, E. and Kroner, T. (1976) Phase II study of cis-dichlorodiammine platinum (II) in advanced adenocarcinoma of the ovary. *Cancer Treatment Reports*, **60**, 55–60.

Young, R.C., Walton, L.A., Ellenberg, S.S. *et al.* (1990) Adjuvant therapy in stage I and stage II epithelial ovarian cancer. *New England Journal of Medicine*, **22**, 1021–7.

TROPHOBLASTIC DISEASES

25

Gordon J.S. Rustin

25.1 INTRODUCTION

Trophoblastic diseases are important to the oncologist for two reasons. First, choriocarcinoma is so curable if correctly treated that its diagnosis should never be missed. Secondly, many of the principles of management approach the ideal that we should aim for when managing more common tumours. The spectrum of trophoblastic diseases extends from benign hydatidiform moles (HM) which usually spontaneously resolve, to life threatening choriocarcinoma. The incidence of HM is between 0.5 and 2.5 per 1000 pregnancies. A woman who has had an HM has approximately a 1000 greater chance of developing choriocarcinoma than if she had a live birth. It is the less common choriocarcinoma developing after a non-molar pregnancy that poses the greater diagnostic problem.

25.2 TYPES AND PATHOLOGY OF GESTATIONAL TROPHOBLASTIC DISEASES (GTD)

This term includes the diseases detailed below as well as two conditions which are not followed by malignant sequelae. These are hydropic degeneration which is an aborted conceptus containing increased fluid content or liquefaction of placental villous stroma without undue trophoblastic hyperplasia; and placental site reaction which is the presence of trophoblastic cells and leucocytes in a placental bed.

25.2.1 COMPLETE HYDATIDIFORM MOLE (CHM)

CHM is an abnormal conceptus without an embryo/fetus, with gross hydropic swelling of the placental villi and usually pronounced trophoblastic hyperplasia, having both cytotrophoblastic and syncytial elements but no vascular elements. A classical mole resembles a bunch of grapes.

25.2.2 PARTIAL HYDATIDIFORM MOLE (PHM)

Histologically the main difference between complete and partial moles is the presence of some components of an embryo-fetus which may just be fetal blood vessels in the partial mole. Chroriocarcinoma develops less than one-tenth as often after partial than after complete moles which are also more common.

25.2.3 INVASIVE MOLE

This is as a tumour or tumour-like process invading the myometrium and characterized by trophoblastic hyperplasia and persistence of placental villous structures. It does not often progress to choriocarcinoma. It may metastasize, but does not exhibit progression of a true cancer and may regress spontaneously.

25.2.4 GESTATIONAL CHORIOCARCINOMA

This is a carcinoma arising from the trophoblastic epithelium that shows both cytotrophoblastic and syncytiotrophoblastic elements. It may arise from conceptions that give rise to a live birth, a stillbirth, an abortion at any stage, an ectopic pregnancy, or a HM or very rarely PHM. The lack of villous structures distinguishes choriocarcinoma morphologically from invasive mole. In most series over 50% of cases of choriocarcinoma are preceded by hydatidiform mole.

25.2.5   PLACENTAL SITE TROPHOBLASTIC TUMOUR

This tumour arises from the trophoblast of the placental bed and is composed mainly of cytotrophoblastic cells which accounts for the relatively low level of HCG associated with this condition. About one case of this tumour is seen for every 100 cases of invasive mole and choriocarcinoma. Complete surgical excision is the preferred treatment as they are not as chemosensitive as choriocarcinoma and may metastasize (Dessau *et al.*, 1990).

25.2.6   GESTATIONAL TROPHOBLASTIC TUMOURS

The reliance of persistently elevated HCG levels for diagnosis and frequent absence of tissue for histology makes it frequently impossible to differentiate between invasive mole and choriocarcinoma and the term gestational trophoblastic tumour (GTT) covers both disease states and placental site tumours.

25.3   EPIDEMIOLOGY

Many hospital based studies suggesting a very high evidence of HM in Asia, parts of Africa and South Central America may have been exaggerated due to an excess of complicated pregnancies attending hospitals (Bracken, 1987). Large differences in incidence in different racial groups have not been confirmed.

Studies from many countries show that the risk of HM increases progressively in women

aged over 40, reaching almost one-third of live births in those aged over 50. The risk is also slightly higher in pregnancies of those aged less than 15 years. A woman who has had a HM has a greater than 20 fold increased chance of having a further HM (Bagshawe *et al.*, 1986).

25.3.1   GENETICS

Complete HM appears to result from fertilization of a defective ovum from which the nucleus has been lost or inactivated. The chromosomal complement has been shown to arise by androgenesis (Lawler and Fisher, 1987); there are no maternal chromosomes although the mitochondrial DNA is of maternal origin. In most cases the paternal contribution stems from a duplication of a haploid sperm or, less often from two different sperm. The 10% of CHM that are heterozygous do not appear to have a higher chance of progressing to choriocarcinoma than the homozygous ones. On DNA fingerprinting a paternal band indicates the tissue as postgestational. If it is absent yet the tissue is histologically choriocarcinoma it arose by trophoblast differentiation of usually a bronchial or gastric carcinoma and is not curable by chemotherapy (Fisher *et al.*, 1992).

Genetic studies show PHM to be triploid with one maternal and two paternal chromosome sets thought to arise by dispermy. Twin pregnancies with a CHM and normal fetus occasionally occur and some of these pregnancies result in a live birth.

25.4   PRESENTATION

25.4.1   HYDATIDIFORM MOLE

The great majority of hydatidiform moles are removed or evacuated between 8 and 24 weeks of gestation with a peak around 14 weeks. Vaginal bleeding is the most common presenting symptom, with many women passing molar tissue mixed with blood clot per vagina. This blood loss can lead to considerable morbidity due to anaemia, especially in malnourished women. Acute life threatening uterine haemorrhage can occasionally occur. Excessive uterine enlargement, theca lutean cysts, toxaemia of pregnancy and hyperemesis gravidarum are frequently seen in these patients.

Symptoms due to uterine perforation, pelvic sepsis and disseminated intravascular coagulopathy can occasionally occur. Severe symptoms due to trophoblastic pulmonary embolization are sometimes seen to develop after evacuation but usually resolve with supportive care.

25.4.2 RISK OF MALIGNANCY

The major long term risk after molar pregnancy is the development of either invasive mole or choriocarcinoma. In the prechemotherapy era the risk of choriocarcinoma after HM was estimated to be less than 3%. The great majority of hydatidiform moles resolve spontaneously with fewer than 10% becoming invasive.

Factors which have been shown to be associated with an increased risk of malignant sequelae include: pre-evacuation HCG level > 100 000 iu/l, uterine size large for dates, large theca lutein cysts, maternal age > 40 years, medical induction, hysterectomy or hysterotomy, and oral contraceptives before HCG falls to undetectable levels (Stone and Bagshawe, 1979; Goldstein *et al.*, 1981).

25.4.3 INVASIVE MOLE AND CHORIOCARCINOMA

Invasive mole is seen in the early months following the evacuation of hydatidiform mole, and since most women know when they have had a mole it is only rarely recognized in the absence of such a history. Some centres diagnose invasive mole if the HCG level is still elevated at 8–10 weeks which gives an incidence of about 25%. Elevation at 6 months

gives an incidence of about 7%. The symptoms of invasive mole are due to the invasive trophoblast. These include, vaginal bleeding, amenorrhoea, infertility, abdominal pain and symptoms resulting from uterine perforation.

Although histology is the definitive way of differentiating invasive mole from choriocarcinoma, biopsy should be avoided because of the risk of severe haemorrhage. The symptoms may be identical but whilst all invasive moles are preceded by an HM only about 50% of choriocarcinomas have a history of prior molar pregnancy. The remainder follow a live birth, stillbirth, abortion or ectopic pregnancy, which may have occurred several years previously.

Choriocarcinoma can metastasize to virtually any part of the body. The commonest metastatic site is the lungs which in most cases are asymptomatic (Figure 25.1). Pleuritic pains and haemoptysis can occur due to the tumour invasion or following pulmonary infarction caused by tumour emboli. Dyspnoea is seen with more extensive metastases. Dyspnoea and signs of pulmonary

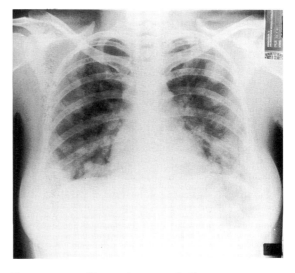

Figure 25.1 Classical cannon ball metastases in a woman with choriocarcinoma. Serum HCG should always be measured in a woman of reproductive age with such an X-ray.

hypertension can also result from the rare growth of choriocarcinoma in the pulmonary arterial bed (Seckl *et al.*, 1991), a diagnosis rarely considered.

The great vascularity of vaginal metastases makes them appear densely reddened. They bleed easily and may be missed without careful visual inspection. Cerebral metastases may present suddenly secondary to haemorrhage with headache, fits or loss of consciousness or related to the site of neurological damage. Liver metastases are usually now discovered incidentally on scans.

25.5 INVESTIGATIONS

25.5.1 HUMAN CHORIONIC GONADOTROPHIN (HCG)

HCG is a placental hormone that is secreted by the syncytiotrophoblast and serves to maintain corpus luteum function and preserve progesterone secretion during the early stages of gestation. Elevated serum levels are found if there are more than about 10^5 trophoblast tumour cells. The alpha subunit of HCG is nearly identical to the alpha units of thyroid stimulating hormone, follicle stimulating hormone (FSH) and luteinizing hormone (LH). The beta subunit shares many similarities with the beta subunits of other glycoprotein hormones, but the carboxyl terminal end contains unique amino acid sequences giving distinct antigenic characteristics. Unless immunoassays recognize antigens on the beta subunit, they may be influenced by LH levels.

Assays on urine are useful in the long term follow-up of patients although the background noise on urine assays tends to be higher than in serum so that values up to the equivalent of 30 iu/l may not be significant. Pregnancy tests will be positive in most patients with trophoblastic diseases but may miss some cases due to the lower sensitivity.

25.5.2 INVESTIGATIONS FOR DIAGNOSIS STAGING AND DETERMINING PROGNOSIS

(a) Hydatidiform mole

In a woman thought to be pregnant ultrasound scanning of the pelvis is the investigation most likely to confirm the presence of HM which produces a characteristic pattern of echoes that appear like a snowstorm. The presence of a live fetus must be excluded on ultrasound by carefully searching for a gestational sac and fetal heart. Large ovarian cysts are commonly visualized on the ultrasound and should be just observed. Evacuation and curettage is the only method by which tissue is usually available for histology. Biopsy of vaginal metastases should not be performed as this frequently leads to profuse bleeding which may be difficult to control due to the vascular nature of trophoblast. A full blood count is required to check for anaemia and 2 units of blood should be routinely cross matched prior to evacuation. T3 and T4 may be elevated due to a thyrotrophic effect of HCG and should be measured prior to surgery if there is any suspicion of thyrotoxicosis. A chest X-ray should be performed to exclude trophoblastic emboli or metastases of invasive mole or choriocarcinoma.

(b) Invasive mole and choriocarcinoma

To exclude a tumour deposit being choriocarcinoma, serum HCG requires to be measured. A normal level (< 2 iu/l) in the presence of clinically detectable disease excludes the diagnosis. An elevated level could be due to pregnancy, residual placental elements, ovarian germ cell tumour, placental site tumour, trophoblast differentiation in a carcinoma, most frequently gastric, or ectopic production from a variety of different tumours. Non-trophoblastic tumours are rarely associated with HCG levels > 1000 iu/l.

Histological confirmation of the diagnosis is not required if there is a history of a recent molar pregnancy, the HCG level is grossly elevated and the distribution of disease is typical of choriocarcinoma. In patients with grossly elevated levels of HCG and no molar history it is safer to treat them as having choriocarcinoma than risk biopsying a metastasis provided pregnancy has been excluded. Needle biopsies of the liver or other sites have resulted in fatal haemorrhagic consequences. Delays in starting therapy whilst recovering from surgical biopsies may allow tumour volume to greatly increase.

Clinical examination should include visual inspection of the vagina which may detect metastases. The only routine staging investigations required are posteroanterior and lateral chest X-ray and pelvic ultrasound. Cerebrospinal fluid (CSF) HCG should be measured if the patient fits into the high risk prognostic group (see below) or has lung metastases and is in the middle risk group. CSF levels of HCG that are more than one-sixtieth the serum level indicate the presence of brain metastases, though a normal ratio does not exclude them. A brain CT scan is only required if there is clinical suspicion of brain metastases or the HCG ratio is abnormal. MRI scans should be performed if despite suspicions of a cerebral metastasis the CT scan is normal, as MRI sometimes detects lesions missed on CT scan especially in the posterior fossa. MRI is the investigation of choice if spinal metastases are suspected. CT scans of the chest will detect metastases missed on chest X-ray but in our experience have not led to a change in management and are not routinely performed. Scans of the abdomen are only performed if there is clinical suspicion of disease there.

Prior to starting therapy a full blood count is required and renal and hepatic function must be assessed. Thyroid function should be measured in view of the association with thyrotoxicosis. The blood group of the patient and her partner responsible for the most recent or molar pregnancy is required for the prognostic score (see below).

25.5.3 STAGING

A new staging system has been proposed by the International Federation of Gynaecology and Obstetrics (Table 25.1).

Table 25.1   Staging of gestational trophoblastic tumours (FIGO, 1991)

			Risk factors (no.)*
I	a	Uterus	None
	b	Uterus	1
	c	Uterus	2
II	a	Extrauterine but	None
	b	limited to adnexa,	1
	c	vagina or broad ligament	2
III	a	Lungs with or without above	None
	b	Lungs with or without above	1
	c		2
IV	a	Other metastatic	None
	b	Other metastatic	1
	c	Other metastatic	2

*Risk Factors: HCG > 100 000 iu/ml; interval from antecedant pregnancy > 6 months.

25.5.4 INVESTIGATIONS FOR FOLLOW-UP

(a) Post mole

Following the diagnosis of a molar pregnancy follow-up is essential to detect those women who require chemotherapy for invasive mole or choriocarcinoma. Follow-up relies upon measurement of HCG in serum or urine, as a plateau or rise will indicate persistent or malignant trophoblast. In about 50% of patients the HCG level becomes undetectable by 7 weeks after evacuation. We stop follow-up in these women at 6 months as none of them have required chemotherapy (Bagshawe, *et al.*, 1986). A national follow-up service for HM patients has been in operation in the UK since 1972. Patients are registered centrally and then automatically sent boxes with prepaid returnable postage, containing tubes and a letter requesting that urine or serum samples be returned to one of three assay centres. It is recommended that HCG measurements be performed every 2 weeks until the limit of detection is reached, then monthly during the first year after evacuation and 3 monthly during the second year. It is advisable to confirm that the HCG is undetectable for 6 months before starting another pregnancy. It must be confirmed that the serum HCG has returned to normal after all further pregnancies because of the 2% chance of a further HM in a woman who has had an HM and the slightly increased risk of choriocarcinoma arising either from a subsequent mole or normal pregnancy.

(b) Post chemotherapy

Our policy is to continue HCG follow-up for life because of the potential of choriocarcinoma to recur after several years.

25.5.5 INVESTIGATIONS FOR MONITORING THERAPY

Serum HCG levels should be monitored at least weekly during therapy. HCG levels can sometimes rise during the early days of drug therapy even though the tumour is chemosensitive and is thought to be related to 'tumour lysis'. A plateau above the normal range may be due to cross-reaction of the assay with LH if the patient has become menopausal. However a plateau or rising level usually indicates drug resistance. Due to the accuracy of HCG monitoring repeat X-rays and scans are only required to confirm resolution of metastases or uterine or ovarian abnormalities at the end of treatment or to detect surgically resectable masses in patients with drug resistant disease.

25.6 TREATMENT

25.6.1 EVACUATION OF HM

Patients with clinical features and ultrasound suggestive of an HM should have any significant blood loss replaced and the uterus evacuated by suction evacuation. Even a large HM can be evacuated with little blood loss. The need for chemotherapy after evacuation of HM has been found to be two to three fold greater in patients who had undergone a medical induction, hysterectomy or hysterotomy compared with those whose HM had been evacuated by vacuum or surgical curettage or had aborted spontaneously. If bleeding is severe after uterine evacuation, use of ergometrine on one occasion is sometimes unavoidable. The single contraction produced by this agent appears to be less likely to produce embolization of trophoblast to distant sites than repeated contractions induced by oxytocin or prostaglandin. Many gynaecologists perform a second D&C if there is persistent uterine bleeding following the initial evacuation. Because curettage cannot gain access deep into the myometrium, further D&Cs will not remove invasive mole and are therefore of no value. We advise patients not to take oral contraceptives until HCG has reached the normal range after molar evacuation because they appear to increase the chance of requiring chemo-therapy.

25.6.2 PROPHYLACTIC CHEMOTHERAPY

Prophylactic chemotherapy, usually with actinomycin D 12 μg/kg for 5 days, has been advocated for those whose molar pregnancy is associated with high risk factors and for those patients in whom follow-up is likely to be difficult. There is a suggestion from non-randomized studies that those patients who received prophylaxis had a lesser chance of requiring subsequent chemotherapy than those patients not given prophylactic chemo-therapy. However it has been abandoned by certain centres because of unacceptable toxicity in women who had a high chance of never requiring chemotherapy.

(a) Selection of cases for chemotherapy

Chemotherapy may be given because of per-sistence or complications of invasive mole, because choriocarcinoma has been diagnosed or in some centres prophylactically to HM patients with the aim of preventing malignant sequelae. Most groups agree that treatment should be started if any of the following apply after a hydatidiform mole:

1. High level of HCG more than 4 weeks after evacuation (serum level > 20 000 iu/l: urine levels > 30 000 iu/l).
2. Progressively increasing HCG values at any time after evacuation.
3. Histological identification of chorio-carcinoma at any site or evidence of CNS, renal, hepatic or gastrointestinal metas-tases, or pulmonary metastases > 2 cm in diameter or > 3 in number.

Persistent uterine haemorrhage with an ele-vated HCG is an indication for therapy in most centres. The major risk in delaying treat-ment in the patient with very high levels of HCG is the development of uterine perfor-ation. The policy at the Charing Cross Hospital

with persistently elevated HCG levels has been to allow the HCG to remain detectable for up to 4–6 months after evacuation as spon-taneous disappearance of HCG can take that long. This results in less than 8% of molar patients requiring chemotherapy.

25.6.3 SURGERY

Apart from evacuation of an HM, as dis-cussed above surgery has only a limited role. Uterine perforation is best managed by local resection of tumour and uterine repair. Hysterectomy may be required for persistent heavy bleeding but this usually settles on chemotherapy. Angiographic embolization may be used to control bleeding if uterine preservation is desired.

Elective hysterectomy has been used in the hope of reducing the need for, or duration of, chemotherapy in patients not wishing to retain reproductive potential. Many such patients still however require a full course of chemotherapy. Surgical removal of drug resistant disease has a curative role in the rare patient in whom the disease is limited to resectable sites.

25.6.4 PROGNOSTIC FACTORS

Retrospective analysis has shown that various factors are related to survival. Not surpris-ingly patients with brain, gastrointestinal and liver metastases have a worse survival than patients with lung metastases. The level of HCG has a major bearing on survival, as does the interval from termination of prior preg-nancy to start of chemotherapy. Fatality rates varied from 3.1 per 100 cases in patients with an interval of less than 4 months to 63 per 100 cases in those with intervals greater than 25 months. The remission rate is lower in patients treated for choriocarcinoma asso-ciated with a term pregnancy compared to persistent trophoblastic tumour following HM, probably because of delayed diagnosis. A favourable but not statistically significant survival trend is seen in younger patients. As one would expect, prior therapy appears to predispose to drug resistance and worsens the survival. It is not clear why the mortality rate of patients with incompatible matings (A × O, O × A) has been found to be four times greater than compatible matings (A × A, O × O) and why patients with blood groups B and AB appear to have a poorer prognosis.

To try and stratify treatment according to these and other prognostic factors Bagshawe in 1976 prepared a scoring system in which a weighting applied for each factor and each was assumed to act as an independent variable where their effects were assumed to be additive. This system, which ascribes its patients to low, medium, or high risk groups according to their cumulative score, has been successfully used in several centres and over the years has been simplified. A system adopted by the World Health Organization is shown in Table 25.2. Between 1970 and 1992, of the 1372 patients treated for GTT at the Charing Cross Hospital, 279 fitted into the high risk group of whom 90 (32%) died; 240 fitted into the middle risk group of whom three (0.1%) died; and 853 fitted into the low risk group of whom two (0.002%) died from their gestational trophoblastic tumours.

25.6.5   CHEMOTHERAPY

Patients in whom chemotherapy is considered necessary require the care of a doctor well versed in the use of cytotoxic drugs; their dangers and the indications for dosage reduction are beyond the scope of this chapter. The three drugs with the most proven single agent activity against GTT are methotrexate, actinomycin D and etoposide. 6-Mercaptopurine, vincristine, cyclophosphamide, cisplatin and hydroxyurea also have proven activity. 5-Fluorouracil has been successfully used in China but not elsewhere. Primary drug resistance has only rarely been seen after methotrexate and actinomycin D and not so far after etoposide. Drug resistance developing during treatment is seen especially in patients with a high prognostic score (see above). The patient's prognostic group needs to be determined so that patients at higher risk of developing drug resistance are given combination chemotherapy as initial therapy.

Table 25.2   Scoring system based on prognostic factors

Prognostic factors	Score*			
	0	*1*	*2*	*4*
Age (years)	< 39	> 39		
Antecedent pregnancy	HM	Abortion	Term	
Interval[†]	4	4–6	7–12	>12
HCG (iu/l)	< 10^3	10^3– 10^4	10^4–10^5	>10^5
ABO groups (female × male)		O × A	B	
		A × O	AB	
Largest tumour, including uterine tumour (cm)		3– 5	> 5	
Site of metastases		Spleen	GI tract	Brain
		Kidney	Liver	
Metastases identified (no.)		1– 4	4–8	> 8
Prior chemotherapy			Single drug	2 or more

*the total score for a patient is obtained by adding the individual scores for each prognostic factor. Total score: < 4 = low risk; 5–7 = middle risk; > 8 = high risk.
[†]Interval: time (months) between end of antecedent pregnancy and start of chemotherapy.

Table 25.3 Low risk regimen

Day 1	MTX 50 mg i.m. at noon
Day 2	FA 6 mg i.m. at 6.0 p.m. or 30 hours later
Day 3	MTX 50 mg i.m. at noon
Day 4	FA 6 mg i.m. at 6.0 p.m.
Day 5	MTX 50 mg i.m. at noon
Day 6	FA 6 mg at 6.0 p.m.
Day 7	MTX 50 mg i.m. at noon
Day 8	FA 6 mg at 6.0 p.m.

Note: Courses are repeated after an interval of 6 days. Start each course on the same day of the week. FA, folinic acid; MTX, methotrexate.

(a) Low risk patients

There is general agreement that methotrexate followed by folinic acid is the preferred treatment for the low risk group, provided renal and hepatic function are normal. The most proven regimen is given over 8 days (Table 25.3). Provided patients drink at least 2 litres of fluid a day they are unlikely to develop mucositis. Apart from occasional cases of chemical pleurisy other side-effects are very uncommon. Of 347 low risk patients treated at Charing Cross Hospital between 1974 and 1986, all entered complete remission and only one died from intercurrent lymphoma (Bagshawe *et al.*, 1989). However, 69 (20%) had to change treatment because of drug resistance developing and 23 (6%) needed to change treatment because of drug induced toxicity. To prevent relapse courses of treatment should be repeated every 14 days and continue until the HCG level has been undetectable (< 2 iu/l) for about 6 weeks.

(b) Medium risk patients

The medium risk regimen of sequential single agents is maintained at the Charing Cross Hospital because it allows for clinical trial as a single agent of new drugs shown to be active in resistant patients. However as the current high risk regimen is of similar toxicity it is reasonable to split patients just into low and high risk groups. The medium risk regimen, which is continued for 8–10 weeks after HCG has become undetectable, is shown in Table 25.4.

Table 25.4 Medium risk patients – cycling regimen

A: Etoposide		100 mg/m^2 in 200 ml 150 mmol NaCl i.v. for 5 consecutive days
B: Day		
1	Hydroxyurea	500 mg p.o. 12 hourly for 2 doses
2	MTX	50 mg i.m. at noon
3	FA	6 mg i.m. at 6.0 p.m.
	6MP	75 mg p.o.
4	MTX	50 mg i.m. at noon
5	FA	6 mg i.m. at 6.0 p.m.
	6-MP	75 mg p.o.
6	MTX	50 mg i.m. at noon
7	FA	6 mg i.m. at 6.0 p.m.
	6-MP	75 mg p.o.
8	MTX	50 mg i.m. at noon
9	FA	6 mg i.m. at 6.0 p.m.
	6-MP	75 mg p.o.
C: Actinomycin D		0.5 mg daily (total dose) i.v. for 5 consecutive days

Note: Courses are given in the sequence ABACA with intervals usually of 6 drug free days between courses. FA, folinic acid; MTX, methotrexate; 6MP, 6-mercaptopurine.

(c)   High risk patients

Historical data showed that only 5/16 (31%) patients who were in this group but received single agent methotrexate survived (Bagshawe *et al.*, 1989). Several intensive multi drug regimens have been developed, including ones with the acronym CHAMOCA developed at the Charing Cross Hospital and MAC III used in Boston. Since 1979 patients in the high risk group at the Charing Cross Hospital have received a weekly alternating regimen called EMA/CO (Table 25.5, Figure 25.2). This regimen is given on the same day each week

Table 25.5   EMA/CO regimen for medium and high risk patients

Course 1 EMA:

Day 1	Actinomycin D 0.5 mg i.v. stat
	Etoposide 100 mg/m^2 i.v. in 200 ml N/S over 30 min
	Methotrexate 300 mg/m^2 i.v. 12 hour infusion
Day 2	Actinomycin D 0.5 mg i.v. stat
	Etoposide 100 mg/m^2 i.v. in 200 ml N/S over 30 min
	Folinic acid 15 mg p.o./i.m. b.d. for 4 doses starting 24 hours after the start of methotrexate
	5 day drug free interval to course 2

Course 2 CO:

Day 1	Vincristine 1.0 mg/m^2 i.v. stat (maximum 2.0 mg)
	Cyclophosphamide 600 mg/m^2 i.v. infusion over 20 min 6 day drug free interval and if no mucositis patients normally start each course on the same day of the week each time

Note: Intervals between courses should not be increased unless WBC< $1.5 \times 10^9/l$ and platelets are < $75 \times 10^9/l$ or mucositis develops. If mucositis develops, delay next course until it has healed. Continue alternating courses 1 and 2 until the patient is in complete HCG remission for 8+ weeks or there is evidence of drug resistance.

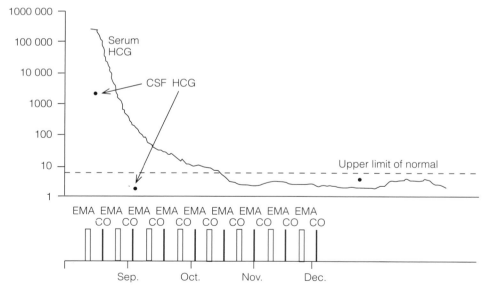

Figure 25.2   Graph of HCG levels of a 27-year-old woman who required high risk chemotherapy with EMA/CO for choriocarcinoma. She developed pleuritic chest pains 4 weeks after completing her third pregnancy and had greatly impaired lung perfusion by the time the diagnosis of choriocarcinoma in the pulmonary artery was made 5 months later.

unless the total white cell count falls below $1.5 \times 10^9/l$ or unless mucosal ulceration develops. Treatment is continued until the HCG level has been within the normal range for at least 8 weeks. Of 27 patients who received EMA/CO as initial therapy, 93% survived and one patient relapsed; of 20 who received EMA/CO after prior therapy, 74% survived and five patients relapsed (Newlands *et al.*, 1986). In patients who develop drug resistance, cisplatin 75 mg/m² and etoposide 100 mg/m² when substituted for the CO of EMA/CO can lead to a durable remission. In patients with extensive pulmonary metastases deaths may occur due to respiratory failure, which can be exacerbated by too aggressive initial therapy. Ventilation or high dose steroids have not been shown to be of any value in this situation, so extracorporeal membrane oxygenation is now being assessed.

(d) Central nervous system (CNS) metastases

Since 1980 we have used the EMA/CO regimen for these patients with the dose of methotrexate increased to 1 gm/m² and 12.5 mg of methotrexate given intrathecally with each course of CO. Of 18 patients who presented with CNS metastases, 13 (72%) are surviving disease free (Rustin *et al.*, 1989). Because of the vascular nature of these tumours and the 22% incidence of early deaths we now attempt early surgical excision to prevent intracerebral haemorrhage. Although radiotherapy has been used in other centres their reported results do not approach the 72% survival we obtained without radiotherapy.

25.7 LONG TERM SIDE-EFFECTS OF THERAPY

Patients are advised against subsequent pregnancy for a year after chemotherapy to avoid confusing a further pregnancy with relapse and to reduce the risk of delayed teratogenicity. A study of 445 long term survivors following chemotherapy showed that 86% of patients wishing to have a further pregnancy succeeded in having at least one live birth (Rustin *et al.*, 1984). The incidence of congenital abnormalities was not greater than expected. The incidence of second tumours has also been investigated. One case of myeloid leukaemia and one case of breast cancer were found in 457 long term survivors followed for a mean period of 7.8 years (Rustin *et al.*, 1983). The expected number for this group of women would have been 3.5 second tumours.

ACKNOWLEDGEMENTS

The author wishes to thank Professors K.D. Bagshawe and E.S. Newlands and his other colleagues at Charing Cross Hospital without whom this review would not have been possible. He is also indebted to the gynaecologists who have referred patients.

REFERENCES

Bagshawe, K.D. (1976) Risk and prognostic factors in trophoblastic neoplasia. *Cancer*, **38**, 1373–85.

Bagshawe, K.D., Dent, J. and Webb, J. (1986) Hydatidiform mole in England and Wales (1973–83). *Lancet*, **ii**, 673–7.

Bagshawe, K.D., Dent, J., Newlands, E.S. *et al.* (1989) The role of low-dose methotrexate and folinic acid in gestational trophoblastic tumours (GTT). *British Journal of Obstetrics and Gynaecology*, **96**, 795–802.

Bracken, M.B. (1987) Incidence and aetiology of hydatidiform mole: an epidemiological review. *British Journal of Obstetrics and Gynaecology*, **94**, 1123–35.

Dessau, R., Rustin, G.J.S., Dent, J., Paradinas, F.J. and Bagshawe, K.D. (1990) Surgery and chemotherapy in the management of placental site tumour. *Gynecologic Oncology*, **39**, 56–9.

Fisher, R.A., Newlands, E.S., Jeffreys, A.J. *et al.* (1992) Gestational and nongestational trophoblastic tumours distinguished by DNA analysis. *Cancer*, **69**, 839–45.

Goldstein, D.P., Berkowitz, R.S. and Bernstein, M.R. (1981) Management of molar pregnancy. *Journal of Reproductive Medicine*, **26**, 208–12.

Lawler, S.D. and Fisher, A. (1987) Genetic studies in hydatidiform mole with clinical correlations. *Placenta*, **8,** 77–88.

Newlands, E.S., Bagshawe, K.D., Begent, R.H.J. *et al.* (1986) Developments in chemotherapy for medium- and high risk patients with gestational trophoblastic tumours (1979–1984). *British Journal of Obstetrics and Gynaecology*, **93**, 63–9.

Rustin, G.J.S., Rustin, F., Dent, J. *et al.* (1983) No increase in second tumours after cytotoxic chemotherapy for gestational trophoblastic tumours. *New England Journal of Medicine*, **308**, 473–7.

Rustin, G.J.S., Booth, M., Dent, J. *et al.* (1984) Pregnancy after cytotoxic chemotherapy for gestational trophoblastic tumours. *British Medical Journal*, **288**, 103–6.

Rustin, G.J.S., Newlands, E.S., Begent, H.J. *et al.* (1989) Weekly alternating chemotherapy (EMA/CO) for treatment of central nervous system metastases of choriocarcinoma. *Journal of Clinical Oncology*, **7**, 900–3.

Seckl, M.J., Rustin, G.J.S., Newlands, E.S. *et al.* (1991) Pulmonary embolism, pulmonary hypertension, and choriocarcinoma. *Lancet*, **338**, 1313.

Stone, M. and Bagshawe, K.D. (1979) An analysis of the influences of maternal age, gestational age, contraceptive method, and the mode of primary treatment of patients with hydatidiform moles on the incidence of subsequent chemotherapy. *British Journal of Obstetrics and Gynaecology*, **86**, 782–92.

FURTHER READING

Goldstein, D.P. and Berkowitz, R.S., (1982), *Gestational Trophoblastic Neoplasms*, W.B. Saunders, Philadelphia, p. 143.

Rustin, G.J.S. and Bagshawe, K.D. (1984) Gestational Trophoblastic Tumours. Critical Review in *Oncology/Haematology* CRC Press, **3**, 103–42.

World Health Organization Scientific Group (1983) Gestational Trophoblastic Diseases. *WHO Technical Report Series 692* World Health Organization, Geneva.

SOFT TISSUE SARCOMAS

Meron E. Pitcher and J. Meirion Thomas

26.1 INTRODUCTION

Soft tissue sarcomas are rare, accounting for about 1% of all malignant tumours. The age adjusted incidence is 2 per 100 000 population with 1200 new cases diagnosed in the UK each year. Males and females are equally affected and all age groups are represented. If childhood sarcomas are excluded the peak incidence is in the fifth decade.

26.2 AETIOLOGY

In the majority of cases the cause of soft tissue sarcomas is unknown. Certain inherited disorders can predispose to their development. These include von Recklinghausen's neurofibromatosis (type 1) where the chance of developing a malignant peripheral nerve sheath tumour increases with age and severity of the disease (Sorenson *et al.*, 1986; Cohen and Rothner, 1989); the loss of a tumour suppressor gene on chromosome 17p has been implicated (Menon, *et al.*, 1990). Those with familial retinoblastoma have a 10–20% chance of developing second tumours, often sarcomas, later in life and this is thought to be due to inactivation or deletion of both alleles of the RBI tumour suppressor gene. Soft tissue sarcomas occur as part of the Li–Fraumeni syndrome where germline p53 mutations have been identified in association with familial polyposis, basal cell naevus syndrome and possibly tuberous sclerosis (Cooper and Stratton, 1991). Therapeutic irradiation can be associated with the development of sarcomas,

typically after a long latent period (Davidson *et al.*, 1986). Phenoxyacetic acid and chlorophenols used in the agriculture and timber industries may be responsible for some cases, although the evidence is tenuous (Wingreng *et al.*, 1990; Johnson *et al.*, 1990). Lymphangiosarcoma can occur in chronic lymphoedema after mastectomy (Stewart and Treves, 1948). Kaposi's sarcoma is seen in association with a human immunodeficiency virus infection, but the role of oncogenic viruses in other sarcomas remains uncertain.

26.3 PATHOLOGY

Macroscopically soft tissue sarcomas have a variable appearance. Most are firm and homogeneous; some are bony hard from calcification, others are fluctuant containing mucoid material (Hadju, 1979). All appear to have a well defined capsule from which the contents can be enucleated. This pseudocapsule is an integral part of the tumour consisting of compressed atrophic tissue and a reactive zone of oedematous neovascularized tissue containing infiltrating malignant cells which will almost inevitably give rise to local recurrence if enucleation is the only treatment. Local spread is along tissue planes, and satellite lesions, especially in high grade tumours, may be found some distance from the main tumour. Only late in the course of the disease does it cross fascial boundaries (Enneking *et al.*, 1981).

Microscopically sarcomas have no known dysplastic precursor or *in situ* component

Table 26.1   Histology of sarcomas seen at the Royal Marsden Hospital: October 1989 to September 1992

	No.	*%*
Malignant fibrous histiocytoma	65	21
Leiomyosarcoma	57	18
Liposarcoma	51	17
Synovial sarcoma	38	12
NOS*/Unclassifiable	34	11
Peripheral nerve sheath tumour	18	5
Dermatofibrosarcoma	9	
Soft tissue chondrosarcoma	5	
Haemangio/lymphangiosarcoma	5	
Rhabdomyosarcoma	5	
Soft tissue Ewing's	4	
Clear cell sarcoma	4	
Alveolar soft part sarcoma	4	
Embryonal rhabdomyosarcoma	2	
Haemangiopericytoma	2	
Primitive neuroectodermal tumour	2	
Fibrosarcoma	1	
Epithelioid sarcoma	1	
Total	307	

* Not otherwise specified.

(Fisher, 1992). A wide variety of histological appearances is seen as the tumour can differentiate towards a particular adult or embryonal cell type. In the 3 years October 1989 to September 1992 inclusive, the histology of sarcomas seen at the Royal Marsden Hospital for treatment are shown in Table 26.1.

Immunohistochemistry and electron microscopy, as well as light microscopic appearances of spindle, round, epithelioid or pleomorphic cells can help differentiate histological types. Consistent karyotypic abnormalities have been reported in different types of sarcomas (and in other tumours) and this may provide help in diagnosis as well as adding to understanding of molecular pathology. Histological grading is well related to overall survival. The type of differentiation, mitotic counts, cellularity and pleomorphism and a degree of necrosis may all contribute, but as yet there is no uniform grading system and intratumour variation can be a problem. A three tier grading system is used at the Royal Marsden Hospital. Certain histological types such as dermatofibrosarcoma protuberans and well differentiated liposarcoma are always of low grade and rarely metastasize. Others such as Ewing's sarcoma and rhabdomyosarcoma are always aggressive (Fisher, 1992).

Prognosis is worse for larger tumours (greater than 5 cm), those which are deep to the deep fascia, and in sites where wide excision may be impossible (e.g. the retroperitoneum or head and neck). The lungs are the most common site of metastases. Bony metastases are less frequent. Lymph node metastases are uncommon (2.6% in a series of 1772 from Memorial Sloan Kettering; Fong *et al.*, 1993) but are more frequently seen in angiosarcoma, embryonal rhabdomyosarcoma and epithelioid sarcoma; although the prognosis is poor, Fong *et al.* reported nine of 35 patients surviving more than 3 years after radical lymphadenectomy.

26.4 PRESENTATION

Between October 1989 and September 1992, 424 patients with soft tissue tumours were referred to the surgical division of the Sarcoma Unit at the Royal Marsden Hospital. Table 26.2 shows the ultimate diagnosis. A majority of patients complain of a swelling which has been increasing in size over several months (Figure 26.1). Symptoms of pain or impaired function are usually absent. Rarely the first symptom is of nerve compression, with paraesthesia or referred pain in the case of pelvic sarcomas (Ball *et al.*, 1991). The lower limb is the commonest site, comprising 56% of our 3 year series of primary soft tissue sarcomas (Table 26.3).

Clinical examination should establish the tumour size and anatomical site. In the limbs

Table 26.3 Site incidence of primary soft tissue sarcomas at the Royal Marsden Hospital: October 1989 to September 1992

	No.	*%*
Lower limb	125	56.2
Upper limb	40	17.9
Retroperitoneal/visceral	32	14.3
Trunk	17	7.6
Head and neck	9	4.0
	223	100

flexing neighbouring joints will relax the muscles in the compartment affected to assess mobility or fixation. Associated erythema and heat, suggesting cutaneous infiltration should be noted. Peripheral limb swelling may be due to venous occlusion, muscle wasting due to disuse, nerve compression or infiltration. Peripheral ischaemia is rarely, if ever, due to tumour but must be accurately noted as wide tumour resection may involve sacrifice of much collateral blood supply. Stigmata of neurofibromatosis such as axillary freckling and *café au lait* spots should be sought.

26.5 INVESTIGATION

CT scanning of the primary tumour provides valuable anatomical information, determines which muscles groups are involved and allows field planning for later radiotherapy

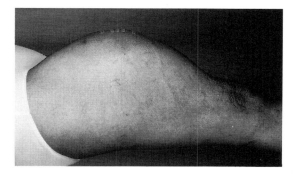

Figure 26.1 Soft tissue sarcoma of right quadriceps.

Table 26.2 Soft tissue tumours referred to the Royal Marsden Hospital: October 1989 to September 1992

	No.	*%*
Primary soft tissue sarcoma	223	52.6
Recurrent soft tissue sarcoma	84	19.8
Benign soft tissue tumour	84	19.8
Non soft tissue sarcoma malignancy*	22	5.2
Metastatic disease	11	2.6
	424	100

* See Table 26.4.

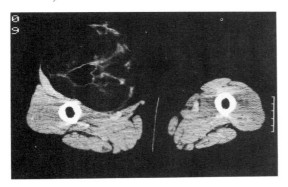

Figure 26.2 CT scan showing sarcoma of right quadriceps. (Same patient as in Figure 26.1.)

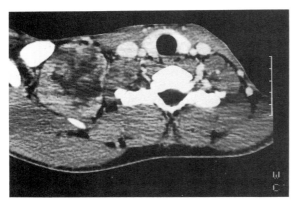

Figure 26.3 Sarcoma of right side of neck with central necrosis.

(Figures 26.2, 26.3). Relationship to arteries, veins and nerves can readily be seen, especially in the lower limb (Davidson *et al.*, 1987). With intravenous contrast outlining vessels more clearly, angiography is seldom required. In those with tumours of the pelvic girdle CT can accurately predict inoperability (Watkins and Thomas, 1987). In patients with retroperitoneal sarcomas, CT will give an indication of the number of organs involved which determines resectability and ultimate prognosis (Alvarenga *et al.*, 1991).

CT is usually accurate at diagnosing recurrence but in the presence of previous surgery and radiotherapy post-treatment changes may be difficult to distinguish from tumour. MRI can be helpful under these circumstances.

As the lungs are the most common site for metastatic disease a pulmonary CT should be performed at presentation. If this is equivocal then it can be repeated after a short interval of time to clarify the situation.

26.5.1 BIOPSY

Tissue diagnosis is essential, as a number of other conditions, both benign and malignant, can be clinically indistinguishable from soft tissue sarcoma. Those we saw seen at the Royal Marsden Hospital in a 3 year period are shown in Table 26.4. Tissue diagnosis is also essential for the planning of treatment, as some sarcomas (e.g. rhabdomyosarcoma, soft tissue Ewing's) are treated by chemotherapy

Table 26.4 Soft tissue tumours, other than soft tissue sarcomas, seen at the Royal Marsden Hospital: October 1989 to September 1992

	No.
Benign soft tissue tumours	
Fibromatosis	22
Lipoma	16
Neurofibroma	8
Arteriovenous malformation	6
Nodular fasciitis	5
Myxoma	5
Myositis ossificans	3
Osteomyelitis	3
Non-specific myositis	2
Other	14
Total	84
Non-soft tissue sarcomatous malignancy	
Bony chondrosarcoma	7
Lymphoma	6
Bony Ewing's	4
Carcinoma	3
Osteosarcoma	1
Carcinoma	1
Adamantinoma	1
Total	22

rather than surgery in the first instance. Fine needle aspiration cytology can be helpful (Kissin *et al.*, 1987) but we have found tru-cut (core biopsy) performed under local anaesthetic in the clinic to be more satisfactory. The subtype and grade of tumour can be correctly specified in more than 80% of samples (Kissin *et al.*, 1986; Ball *et al.*, 1990a).

Open biopsy is only necessary if a diagnosis cannot be established by repeated core biopsy. This may occur in very necrotic tumours or those which are extremely fibrotic and acellular like fibromatosis (Ball *et al.*, 1990a). The siting of the incision should not compromise the subsequent definitive operation. Vertical incisions in the long axis of the limb can be incorporated in the subsequent resection. Adequate representative tissue should be taken with minimal disturbance of tissue planes and avoidance of haematoma. A useful technique is to use a trochar and cannula through a stab incision in the capsule (Westbury, 1987). Open biopsy can be complicated by tumour infection or by wound breakdown and tumour fungation (Figure 26.4), so should only be performed when core biopsy fails.

26.5.2 STAGING

There are a number of staging systems in use for soft tissue sarcoma (Suit *et al.*, 1985). They incorporate size of the primary tumour, histological grade and the presence of metastases. The most common staging system used is shown in Table 26.5.

26.6 PROGNOSTIC FACTORS

The outcome of treatment of soft tissue sarcomas is dependent on many factors, both biological and therapeutic, but the most important are the grade of the tumour and its resectability. Histological grade of the tumour remains the most significant determinant of prognosis (Leibel *et al.*, 1985; Markhede *et al.*, 1982); about 50% of high grade tumours will metastasize but low grade tumours rarely do. The difference in survival according to histological subtype is a direct influence of tumour grade. Necrosis within the tumour is often an indication of its aggressiveness and is an adverse factor (Costa *et al.*, 1984). At present, assessment of DNA ploidy and cell proliferation do not offer a significant improvement in predicting the behaviour of sarcomas. Larger tumours have a worse prognosis, as do those with deep fixation (Serpell *et al.*, 1991). In a series from the Royal Marsden Hospital (Robinson *et al.*, 1990) those greater than 15 cm had a worse prognosis; other series have reported tumours larger than 5 cm (Suit *et al.*, 1985) or 10 cm (Collin *et al.* 1987a; Stotter *et al.*, 1990) having a worse outcome. Age greater than 53, proximal anatomical site and regional lymph node metastases have also been described as poor prognostic features (Collin *et al.*, 1987a).

The rate of local recurrence relates to the adequacy of local treatment. Wide or radical surgery with radical radiotherapy affords the best local control (Stotter *et al.*, 1990). Recurrence rates are highest if surgical margins are incomplete (Collin *et al.*, 1987b). Previous local recurrence, high grade of tumour, and older age may be relevant factors. Whether local recurrence *per se* is a poor prognostic indicator for survival remains controversial.

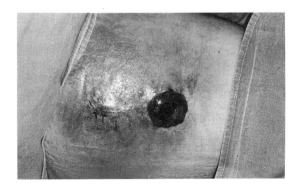

Figure 26.4 Tumour fungation through incisional biopsy wound.

Table 26.5 Staging system for soft tissue sarcoma

Stage I		
IA	(G1, T1, N0, M0)	
	Grade 1 tumour <5 cm in diameter with no regional lymph node or distal metastasis	
IB	(G1, T2, N0, M0)	
	Grade 1 tumour >5 cm in diameter with no regional lymph node or distant metastasis	
Stage II		
IIA	(G2, T1, N0, M0)	
	Grade 2 tumour <5 cm in diameter with no regional lymph node or distant metastasis	
IIB	(G2, T2, N0, M0)	
	Grade 2 tumour >5 cm in diameter with no regional lymph node or distant metastasis	
Stage III		
IIIA	(G3, T1, N0, M0)	
	Grade 3 tumour <5 cm in diameter with no regional lymph node or distant metastasis	
IIIB	(G3, T2, N0, M0)	
	Grade 3 tumour ≥5 cm in diameter with no regional lymph node or distant metastasis	
Stage IV		
IVA	(G1–3, T1–2, N1, M0)	
	Tumour of any grade or size with histologically verified metastasis to regional lymph nodes, but no distant metastasis	
IVB	(G1–3, T1–2, N0–1, M1)	
	Clinically diagnosed distant metastasis	

From Suit *et al.*, 1988.

Site is also important as it has a major impact on resectability. Retroperitoneal tumours often involve multiple organs or major vascular structures and cannot be completely or widely excised (Alvarenga *et al.*, 1991). In addition the total dose of radiotherapy normally used in the treatment of sarcoma would exceed the tolerance of many surrounding organs such as gut, kidney, liver and spinal cord. Head and neck sarcomas can rarely be widely excised, for anatomical reasons, and again the scope for adequate radiotherapy may be limited; the main cause of death is local tumour (Eeles *et al.*, 1990). Gynaecological sarcomas are discussed in Chapter 23.

26.7 MANAGEMENT

The aim in primary treatment of soft tissue sarcoma is cure of local disease with the least possible functional impairment. The lowest recurrence rates for low grade tumours may be achieved by adequate surgery alone but for high grade tumours this must be supplemented with adequate radiotherapy. About one half of limb and limb girdle sarcomas are of low or intermediate grade and of the high grade tumours about half will metastasize. Unfortunately there is no adjuvant chemotherapy to prevent this. Because few patients with metastatic disease can be salvaged, and given the small recurrence rate, about 70% of patients with limb and limb girdle sarcomas will not recur after adequate primary treatment. Enneking *et al.* (1981) classified operations for sarcoma (of the thigh) into four categories:

1. **Radical excision.** This removes the entire anatomical compartment containing the tumour, within its fascial envelope.
2. **Wide excision.** The tumour is resected with a layer or margin of healthy tissue.
3. **Marginal excision.** Meaning enucleation (or local excision) of the tumour from within the pseudo-capsule and includes those resections where tumour is exposed over any part of its surface.

4. **Intracapsular excision.** Intracapsular excision is simply a debulking procedure where macroscopic disease is left behind.

Following surgery alone overall recurrence rates are 90% with marginal excision, 40% after wide excision and 20% following radical excision (Lindberg *et al.*, 1981). Although this classification has not been bettered, there are several anomalies. Sarcomas do not always arise within a defined compartment and are frequently extra- or inter-compartmental. In this situation, depending on the site and size of the tumour, the degree of clearance can be variable. We prefer to think of surgical resections as either being adequate or inadequate; generally speaking Enneking's radical and wide definitions can be regarded as adequate.

26.7.1 LIMBS AND LIMB GIRDLES

This is the most common site of soft tissue sarcomas. In the proximal part of the limb wide resection of muscle or a complete muscle group is compatible with remarkably good function. The tumour is frequently applied to a major artery, nerve or to bone. These structures rarely need to be sacrificed and adventitia, perineurium and periosteum respectively provide an adequate plane of clearance. Occasionally the outer table of bone can be resected with the tumour; for example with large or proximal adductor tumours we routinely resect the outer table of body of pubis which enhances clearance and greatly facilitates the dissection. A satisfactory tumour clearance can often be obtained without compartmental resection, especially in the quadriceps compartment, where retention of one innervated head of muscle improves knee stability. More distally, especially in the upper limb, wide excision can result in significant impairment, and tendon transfer or joint stabilization may need to be considered. Skin and soft tissue defects frequently result after resection of sarcomas, particularly postirradiation recurrent

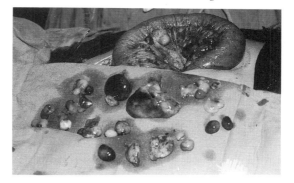

Figure 26.5 Transperitoneal metastases from retroperitoneal sarcoma.

sarcoma. In our series of 307 sarcomas, 26 (8.5%) required such reconstruction usually by myocutaneous transposition but less commonly by free tissue transfer and microvascular anastomosis (Figure 26.6).

Amputation is rarely required as primary treatment for previously untreated sarcoma. In our series of 223 such patients only two amputations were performed. One had a hindquarter amputation for extensive lymphangio- sarcoma secondary to longstanding lymphoedema; the other developed an uncontrollable infection of a bulky tumour at the knee following open incision biopsy before referral to our unit and there was no option but to advise an above-knee amputation. In the 84 patients referred with recurrent disease, amputation was performed in four (5%).

We perform radical or wide excision where possible but a marginal excision with radiotherapy is preferred to amputation, although a slightly higher incidence of local recurrence can be expected. However because there is no convincing evidence that local recurrence is a risk factor for dissemination, a small number of patients who recur can be treated secondarily by amputation. Radiotherapy reduces the local recurrence rate, and is used in all those with high grade tumours, those with marginal resections and those who have recurred after previous surgery. Our practice is to use it postoperatively once the wound has healed, in single daily fractions of 2 Gy to a total of 60 Gy over 6 weeks. Lindberg *et al.* (1981) reported 229 adults treated by macroscopic tumour excision (with 2–3 cm margin) and postoperative radiotherapy with a local recurrence rate of 20%. Even lower rates have been reported by Leibel *et al.* (1982) and Karakousis *et al.* (1986). The 5 year actuarial local recurrence rate at the Royal Marsden Hospital is 13% (Robinson *et al.*, 1990). For extremity sarcomas the overall survival is reported to be approximately 60–70% (Leibel *et al.*, 1982; Markhede *et al.*, 1982; Karakousis, 1986).

Some units recommend preoperative irradiation on the basis that it reduces tumour bulk to make surgery easier, sterilizes satellite lesions and reduces the risk of contamination of the wound by viable tumour cells. Retrospective analysis (Suit, 1989) suggests little difference in rates of local control. As preoperative radiation significantly increases wound morbidity, we use it for tumours with limited mobility or which look only marginally resectable on CT scan. Brachytherapy (interstitial radiotherapy) has been used and satisfactorily reduces the rates of local recurrence but with a high wound complication rate (Brennan *et al.*, 1991).

Local recurrence in previously irradiated tissue provides a surgical challenge because adequate skin and soft tissue cover may not be available. In the past amputation was frequently performed for this reason alone. For proximal limb sarcomas several myocutaneous flaps are available such as the inferiorly based rectus abdominous flap for proximal thigh defects and the latissimus dorsi flap for defects around the pectoral girdle, arm and chest wall. The advent of free tissue transfer by microvascular anastomosis has enabled increased limb salvage in more distal sarcomas, on occasions even when joints have been involved.

26.7.2 RETROPERITONEUM

Retroperitoneal sarcomas comprise 16% of our series. Most present as an abdominal mass, are otherwise asymptomatic and can achieve a

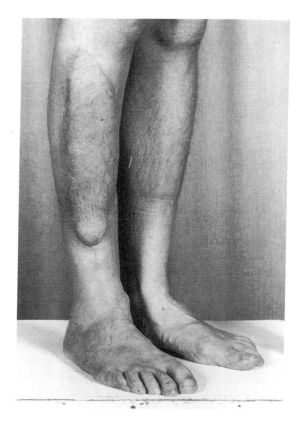

Figure 26.6   Free rectus abdominis flap following wide excision of synovial sarcoma.

massive size. They are frequently misdiagnosed as other intra-abdominal pathology and too often laparotomy is the first investigation. Ideally CT or MRI scan should be performed and resectability assessed. The first resection provides the best chance of local clearance of disease; transperitoneal dissemination can be induced by breaching the tumour capsule (Figure 26.5).

Unfortunately, of the patients that come to laparotomy, gross tumour clearance can only be achieved in about 25%. (The terms radical and wide are not used with reference to retroperitoneal sarcomas). Even in the 25% of patients where gross tumour clearance is achieved, local recurrence subsequently occurs in 80% (Alvarenga *et al.*, 1991). The cure rate in retroperitoneal sarcoma is therefore less than 5%. The reasons for this are that adequate surgical excision can rarely be achieved and radiotherapy is contraindicated or limited by the tolerance of surrounding vital structures. Intraoperative radiation therapy has been used after resection with some success (Willett *et al.,* 1991) but a large tumour bed is a contraindication. Occasionally spacers can be used to displace and protect vital structures during postoperative irradiation (Ball *et al.,* 1990b). Generally speaking the only long term survivors, often at the expense of multiple laparotomies, are patients with low grade tumours. For these reasons we do not advise patients with recurrent retroperitoneal sarcoma to have further laparotomies until symptoms appear.

26.7.3 TRUNK

Sarcomas of abdominal and chest wall are relatively uncommon, comprising 8% of our series. Wide resection may entail full thickness excision of abdominal or chest wall; to protect the viscera and to prevent herniation the resultant defect can be closed with Mersilene mesh supplemented if necessary by a myocutaneous flap. Postoperative radiotherapy is generally advised (unless the tumour is of low grade).

26.7.4 HEAD AND NECK

Sarcomas in the head and neck are often smaller at presentation than at other sites. Complete or wide excision may be impossible because of involvement or proximity of major neurovascular structures which would cause severe morbidity if resected. In the head and neck, unlike the extremities, local recurrence is a major cause of death (63% Eeles *et al.,* 1990). Wide excision and radiotherapy provide the best local control (Eeles *et al.,* 1990).

26.7.5 CHEMOTHERAPY

Some of the sarcomas common in the paediatric age group, such as rhabdomyosar-coma and Ewing's soft tissue sarcoma, are usually chemosensitive, and treatment with combination chemotherapy can dramatically reduce the incidence of distant metastases and increase survival (Chapter 30). Adult type soft tissue sarcomas are relatively chemoresistant. In advanced disease, doxorubicin as a single agent has overall response rates of about 25% (Elias, 1992). Ifosfamide (a cyclophosamide analogue) has a similar level of activity and is used at the Royal Marsden Hospital as a second line agent. Both have significant toxicity; doxorubicin on the myocardium and ifosfamide on the bone marrow. Combination chemotherapy such as doxorubicin plus ifosfamide or CYVADIC (cyclophosphamide/vincristine/doxorubicin/dacarbazine) has not shown any improvement in disease free or overall survival (Santoro *et al.,* 1990).

A number of trials of adjuvant chemotherapy in adults with high grade soft tissue sarcomas using doxorubicin singly or in combination have failed to demonstrate any survival advantage. Adjuvant chemotherapy should be considered investigational for soft tissue sarcomas at the present (Elias, 1992).

26.7.6 PULMONARY METASTASECTOMY

The lungs are the commonest and usually the only site of metastatic disease. Untreated most patients with pulmonary metastases die within 2 years, and chemotherapy has not been shown to prolong survival. Surgical resection of pulmonary metastases can lead to a 5 year survival of 10–35% (Barr *et al.,* 1992), but these are uncontrolled series and undoubtedly subject to case selection. The efficacy of pulmonary metastasectomy has not been tested in controlled trials against chemotherapy or localized radiotherapy.

In selecting patients for metastasectomy, several criteria should be fulfilled. The primary site should be controlled, there should be no extrapulmonary metastases, and the patient should be a good operative risk.

Favourable prognostic factors include a long disease free interval between treatment of the primary tumour and the appearance of pulmonary metastases (greater than 12 months); complete resectability of the pulmonary metastases and the persisting absence of local recurrence (Verazin *et al.*, 1992). As the number of metastases increases, the likelihood of complete resection is less. Verazin *et al.* (1992) report a longer disease free and overall survival in those with five metastases or less even when complete excision was possible in those with more lesions. Repeat operations for pulmonary metastases can be worthwhile. As a rule of thumb it should be remembered that if pulmonary metastases are visible on a chest X-ray then a CT of the thorax will identify approximately twice that number; also at thoracotomy twice the number of metastases will be found than were predicted from the CT of thorax (Swoboda *et al.*, 1992).

26.8   CURRENT RESEARCH

Improved reconstructive techniques have continued to reduce the amputation rate in extremity sarcomas. Isolated limb perfusion, using melphalan and tumour necrosis factor alpha (TNFα) can help salvage limbs with large bulky or unresectable tumours (Hill and Thomas, 1993). Hyperthermia is being used in conjunction with radiotherapy to increase sensitivity. Photodynamic therapy is being tried for retroperitoneal sarcomas. It is unlikely that the mortality figures will improve, however, until more effective chemotherapeutic agents are available.

REFERENCES

Alvarenga, J.C., Ball, A.B.S., Fisher, C. *et al.* (1991) Limitations of surgery in the treatment of retroperitoneal sarcoma. *British Journal of Surgery*, **78**, 912–6.

Ball, A.B.S., Fisher, C., Pittam, M. *et al.* (1990a) Diagnosis of soft tissue tumours by tru-cut biopsy. *British Journal of Surgery*, **77**, 756–8.

Ball, A.B.S., Cassoni, A., Watkins, R.M. and Thomas, J.M. (1990b) Silicone implant to prevent visceral damage during adjuvant radiotherapy for retroperitoneal sarcoma. *British Journal of Radiology*, **63**, 346–8.

Ball, A.B.S., Serpell, J.W., Fisher, C. and Thomas, J.M. (1991) Primary soft tissue tumours of the pelvis causing referred pain in the leg. *Journal of Surgical Oncology*, **47**, 17–20.

Barr, L.C., Skene, A.I. and Thomas, J.M. (1992) Metastasectomy. *British Journal of Surgery*, **79**, 1268–74.

Brennan, M.F., Casper, E.S., Harrison, L.B. *et al.* (1991) The role of multi modality therapy in soft tissue sarcoma. *Annals of Surgery*, **214**, 328–36.

Cohen, B.H. and Rothner, A.D. (1989) Incidence, types and management of cancer in patients with neurofibromatosis. *Oncology*, **3**, 23–30.

Collin, C., Godbold, J., Hadju, S. *et al.* (1987a) Localised extremity sarcoma; an analysis of factors affecting survival. *Journal of Clinical Oncology*, **5**, 601–12.

Collin, C., Hadju, S., Godbold, J. *et al.* (1987b) Localised operable soft tissue sarcoma of the upper extremity. *Annals of Surgery*, **205**, 331–9.

Cooper, C.S. and Stratton, M.R. (1991) Soft tissue tumours: the genetic basis of development. *Carcinogenesis*, **12**, 155–65.

Costa, J., Wenley, R.A., Glatskin, E. *et al.* (1984) The grading of soft tissue sarcomas: results of a clinico-histo-pathologic correlation in a series of 163 cases. *Cancer*, **53**, 530–41.

Davidson, T., Westbury, G. and Harmer, C.L. (1986) Radiation-induced soft tissue sarcoma. *British Journal of Surgery*, **73**, 308–9.

Davidson, T., Cooke, J., Parsons, C. and Westbury, G. (1987) Pre-operative assessment of soft tissue sarcomas by computed tomography. *British Journal of Surgery*, **74**, 474–8.

Eeles, R.A., Fisher, C., A'Hern, R.P. *et al.* (1990) Head and neck sarcomas: a review of 130 cases treated at the Royal Marsden Hospital 1944 to 1988. *British Journal of Cancer*, **62**, (suppl 11), 9.

Elias, A.D. (1992) The clinical management of soft tissue sarcomas. *Seminars in Oncology*, **19**, 19–25.

Enneking, W.F., Spanier, S.S. and Malawer, M.W. (1981) The effect of anatomic setting on the results of surgical procedures for soft parts sarcoma of the thigh. *Cancer*, **47**, 1005–22.

Fisher, C. (1992) Soft tissue sarcomas. *Clinical Oncology*, **4**, 322–6.

Fong, Y., Coit, B.G., Woodruff, J.M. and Brennan, M.F. (1993) Lymph node metastases from soft tissue sarcoma in adults. *Annals of Surgery,* **217,** 72–7.

Hadju, S.I. (1979) *Pathology of Soft Tissue Tumours,* Lea and Febinger, Philadelphia.

Hill, S., Fawcett, W.J., Sheldon, J. *et al.* (1993) Low dose tumour necrosis factor alpha and melphalan in hyperthermic isolated limb perfusion. *British Journal of Surgery,* **80** (8), 995–7.

Johnson, V.C., Feingold, M. and Tilley, B. (1990) A meta-analysis of exposure to phenoxyacid herbacides and chlorophenols in relation to risk of soft tissue sarcoma. *International Archives of Occupational and Environmental Health,* **62,** 513–20.

Karakousis, C.P., Emrich, L.J., Rao, U. and Krishnamsetty, R.M. (1986) Feasibility of limb salvage and survival in soft tissue sarcoma. *Cancer,* **57,** 484–91.

Kissin, M.W., Fisher, C., Carter, R.L. *et al.* (1986) Value of tru-cut biopsy in the diagnosis of soft tissue tumours. *British Journal of Surgery,* **73,** 742–4.

Kissin, M.W, Fisher, C,. Webb, A.J. and Westbury, G. (1987) The value of fine needle aspiration cytology in the diagnosis of soft tissue tumour: preliminary study on the excised specimen. *British Journal of Surgery,* **74,** 479–80.

Leibel, S.A., Tranbaugh, I.F., Wara, W.M. *et al.* (1982) Soft tissue sarcomas of the extremities. Survival and patterns of failure with conservative surgery and postoperative irradiation compared to surgery alone. *Cancer,* **50,** 1076–83.

Lindberg, R.L., Martin, R.G., Romsdahl, M.M. and Barkley, H.T. (1981) Conservative surgery with postoperative radiotherapy in 300 adults with soft tissue sarcoma. *Cancer,* **47,** 3291–7.

Markhede, G., Angervall, L. and Steiner, B. (1982) A multivariate analysis of the prognosis after surgical treatment of malignant soft tissue tumours. *Cancer,* **49,** 1721–33.

Menon, A.G., Anderson, K.M., Riccardi, V.M. *et al.* (1990) Chromosome 17p deletions and p53 gene mutations associated with the formation of malignant neurofibrosarcomas in von Recklinghausen's neurofibromatosis. *Proceedings of the National Academy of Sciences, USA,* **87,** 5435–9.

Robinson, M., Barr, L. Fisher, C. *et al.* (1990) Treatment of extremity sarcomas with surgery and radiotherapy. *Radiotherapy and Oncology,* **18,** 221–3.

Santoro, A., Rouesse, J. Steward, W. *et al.* (1990) A randomised EORTC study in advanced soft tissue sarcomas: ADM versus ADM plus IFX vs Cyvadic. *Proceedings of the American Society of Clinical Oncology,* **9,** 309.

Serpell, J.W., Ball, A.B.S., Robinson, M.H. *et al.* (1991) Factors influencing local recurrence and survival in patients with soft tissue sarcoma of the upper limb. *British Journal of Surgery,* **78,** 1368–72.

Sorensen, S.A., Mulvihill, J.J. and Nielsen, A. (1986) Long term follow up of von Recklinghausen's neurofibromatosis: survival and malignant neoplasms. *New England Journal of Medicine,* **314,** 1010–15.

Stewart, F.W. and Treves, N. (1948) Lymphangiosarcoma in postmastectomy lymphoedema. *Cancer,* **1,** 68–81.

Stotter, A.T., A'Hern, R.P., Fisher, C, *et al.* (1990) The influence of local recurrence of extremity soft tissue sarcoma on metastasis and survival. *Cancer,* **65,** 1119–29.

Suit, H.D. (1989) The George Edelsteyn Memorial Lecture: radiation in the management of malignant soft tissue tumours. *Clinical Oncology (Royal College of Radiologists),* **1,** 5–10.

Suit, H.D., Mankin, H.J., Wood, W.C. and Proppe, K.H. (1985) Preoperative, intraoperative and postoperative radiation in the treatment of primary soft tissue sarcoma. *Cancer,* **55,** 2659–67.

Suit, H.D., Mankin, H.J., Wood, W.C. *et al.* (1988) Treatment of the patient with stage MO soft tissue sarcoma. *Journal of Clinical Oncology,* **6,** 854–62.

Swoboda, L., Wertzel, H., Bonne, H. and Hasse, J. (1992) New developments in the surgery of pulmonary metastases. *Helvetica Chirurgica Acta,* **58,** 555–8.

Verazin, G.T., Warneke, J.A., Driscoll, D.L. *et al.* (1992) Resection of lung metastases from soft tissue sarcoma. *Archives of Surgery,* **127,** 1407–11.

Watkins, R.M. and Thomas, J.M. (1987) Role of computer tomography in selecting patients for hindquarter amputation. *British Journal of Surgery,* **74,** 711–14.

Westbury, G. (1987) Soft tissue sarcomas, in *Operative Surgery and Management,* 2nd edn, (Ed. G. Keen), Wright, Bristol, pp. 757–65.

Willett, C.G., Suit, H.D., Tepper, J.E., *et al.* (1991) *Cancer,* **68** (2), 278–83.

Wingreng, G., Fredrikson, M., Brage, H.N. *et al.* (1990) Soft tissue sarcomas and occupational exposures. *Cancer,* **66,** 806–11.

BONE TUMOURS

27

Gerald Westbury and Ross Pinkerton

27.1 INTRODUCTION

This chapter is concerned with primary malignant tumours of bone. While these account for 6% of cancers under the age of 14 years, they form only 0.2% of the total in the adult where by far the commonest form of skeletal cancer is metastatic disease from a primary lesion elsewhere, e.g. breast, bronchus, prostate, kidney, etc. Other lesions that can mimic primary skeletal cancer include certain chronic inflammations, fibrous dysplasia, exuberant callus following trauma, Paget's disease and hyperparathyroidism.

27.2 CLASSIFICATION (Dahlin, 1978)

This is based on the cytological characteristics of tumour cells together with the stroma they produce and is summarized in Table 27.1. Bone contains a wide range of cell types, some related specifically to bone formation, e.g. osteoblasts and chondroblasts, others which are common to most tissues, e.g. connective tissue cells and cells of the haemopoietic system which occupy the bone marrow. The commonest tumours within this overall uncommon group are osteosarcoma and chondrosarcoma, whose histological pattern can be related respectively to normal

Table 27.1 Malignant primary bone tumours

Tissue of origin or differentiation	Tumour
Bone	Osteosarcoma
	Parosteal sarcoma
Cartilage	Chondrosarcoma
	Primary
	Secondary
	Dedifferentiated
	Mesenchymal
	Clear cell
Haematopoietic tissue	Lymphoma
	Myeloma
Uncertain origin	Ewing's tumour
	Malignant giant cell tumour
	Adamantinoma
Soft tissues	Malignant fibrous histiocytoma
	Malignant vascular tumours, etc.
Notochord	Chordoma

bone and cartilage. Next in frequency is Ewing's tumour whose cells resemble no normal bone constituent. Chordoma is very rare; presumably it is derived from notochordal vestiges. Primary lymphomas of bone are histologically identical with the much commoner non-Hodgkin's lymphomas arising elsewhere. In contrast, myeloma, a tumour of plasma cells, is seldom seen outside the skeleton; it has been described in Chapter 22. Tumours identical with soft tissue sarcomas also occasionally arise primarily within bone; the majority of these are malignant fibrous histiocytomas. It should be noted that on rare occasions tumours identical with osteosarcoma, chondrosarcoma and Ewing's tumour arise primarily in the soft tissues.

27.3 DIAGNOSIS

Diagnosis is made by a combination of clinical, radiological and histological features. All factors must be taken into account. Age is an important feature. Osteosarcoma and Ewing's tumour occur mainly during the second decade of life, whereas metastatic bone disease is seldom seen before the third decade. Chondrosarcoma, on the other hand, is a disease mainly of the fourth to seventh decades. Metastases are usually multiple, although a solitary, or apparently solitary, secondary deposit can cause confusion. Site and age are important in the diagnosis of chordoma which affects older patients and arises either in the sacrum, the skull base or cervical spine. Fever and other systemic symptoms point to inflammatory pathology but Ewing's tumour can also be associated with these manifestations. The most useful radiological investigation for the purpose of diagnosis is a good quality plain radiograph (Stoker, 1987). Classical appearances are described for the various tumour groups but the appearances are not infrequently atypical and, for example, chronic osteomyelitis can show identical radiological appearances to osteosarcoma. The bone lesions of hyper-

parathyroidism may be radiologically and histologically indistinguishable from giant cell tumour. Tumours of bone can be associated with raised serum alkaline phosphatase levels but hyperparathyroidism will be distinguished by appropriate biochemical studies.

27.3.1 TISSUE DIAGNOSIS

An adequate biopsy will provide the definitive diagnosis in the majority of bone tumours, although in some instances the pathologist will be unable to report specifically without knowledge of the clinical picture and other investigations. Traditionally, biopsy has been undertaken by open operation but the use of X-ray guided fine needle aspiration cytology or core needle biopsy, where necessary with the high speed drill, is becoming increasingly popular. These techniques are especially useful for sites which are relatively difficult for surgical access, e.g. the vertebral column. Most bone tumours contain soft tissue elements and a rapid histological diagnosis is possible where the biopsy site has been carefully selected. Imprint preparations of fresh tissue can be helpful. In other cases it is necessary to await decalcification. When open biopsy is necessary it should be performed by a surgeon with special expertise in bone tumours and ideally by the surgeon who will undertake the definitive excisional surgery should this be contemplated as part of overall management.

27.4 OSTEOSARCOMA

27.4.1 AETIOLOGY

The peak incidence for osteosarcoma is in the second decade of life. Common sites are the metaphyses of the long bones, especially those around the knee joint; the lower end of the femur and the upper end of the tibia account for more than half the total followed by the upper end of the humerus. Males are more commonly affected than females in the proportion 3 : 2. Less commonly, osteosarcoma occurs in the jaws, the limb girdles, the vertebrae and rarely the bones of the feet and hands. The age incidence in these atypical sites tends to be higher.

Osteosarcoma usually arises without apparent cause. Trauma has been blamed but this is likely to be a coincidental event, since injuries are frequent at the sites and age of maximum occurrence. Known predisposing causes include Paget's disease of bone, multiple hereditary exostosis, polyostotic fibrous dysplasia and previous irradiation. Paget's osteosarcoma arises in later life reflecting the age distribution of the underlying disease. Osteosarcoma may also be a feature of retinoblastoma and the Li–Fraumeni syndrome, in which there may be germ line mutations of the RBI and p53 genes respectively.

27.4.2 PATHOLOGY

The histological hallmarks of osteosarcoma are malignant osteoblasts with the formation of tumour osteoid. Confusion can arise when there are substantial areas of chondroid or fibrous tissue in the stroma. The tumour usually arises in the central part of the metaphysis of a long bone. The cartilaginous epiphyseal plate acts as a barrier to longitudinal extension until late in the disease but there is free spread within the medulla away from the joint which extends beyond the level of the abnormality seen on the plain X-ray. Skip lesions can sometimes be found. Lateral spread involves the cortical bone which is often breached by the time of clinical presentation. There is usually a mixed pattern of bone destruction and new bone formation but some tumours are predominantly lytic and others sclerotic; pathological fracture may occur. Uncommonly the tumour appears to involve only the outer cortex and is termed periosteal sarcoma. A rare variant is the parosteal sarcoma which grows eventually to surround the shaft forming a collar of densely sclerotic tumour bone. Parosteal sarcoma must be clearly distinguished because it is a much less aggressive form of the disease with a long term survival in the order of 80% without systemic therapy.

Osteosarcoma metastasizes via the blood stream to the lungs and to other bones. Lymph node metastasis is rare and is associated with late stage, high grade tumours.

27.4.3 CLINICAL PRESENTATION AND INVESTIGATION

The typical patient is a teenage boy with a history of pain in the knee, followed by swelling and increasing local disability. These are common symptoms following sporting activity and the clinician must maintain a high index of suspicion if diagnosis is to be made at an early stage. Physical examination shows swelling, with or without joint effusion, local warmth, limitation of movement, tenderness and sometimes a palpable bony mass. The lesion may be highly vascular and even pulsatile (telangiectatic type). Uncommonly presentation is with a pathological fracture or metastases. Sarcoma arising in other sites produces relevant local symptoms and signs. Diagnosis of Paget's 'sarcoma' may be difficult initially because tumour symptoms are indistinguishable from those of the underlying disorder. Primary osteosarcoma does not cause systemic symptoms except in the late neglected case where there may be marked cachexia. The tumour may fungate through an incisional biopsy site where there is delay between the operation and definitive treatment.

Plain X-ray shows features which depend on the extent of tumour, the proportion of sclerotic to lytic change and the degree of cortical involvement. Invasion through the cortex may be followed by the laying down of new bone at right angles to the shaft, the classical sunburst appearance. Codman's triangles result from the formation of wedges of subperiosteal new bone at the gross proximal and distal edges of the cortical invasion. As has been stated, the plain film under-estimates the extent of tumour spread within the medullary cavity. A more accurate estimate is provided by isotope scanning, CT or most effectively MRI. CT or MRI also give useful information on the soft tissue extent of the tumour which may not be apparent on the plain film. Blood count and biochemistry are not helpful in diagnosis; there may be non-specific elevation of the serum alkaline phosphatase. The search for metastases includes lung CT and a skeletal radioisotope scan.

27.4.4 STAGING

Systems of tumour staging form a convenient shorthand method of documenting the extent of the disease and provide guidelines to prognosis and to the allocation of patients to various treatment regimens.

The TNM system (UICC TNM Classification of Malignant Tumours, 1978) and Enneking's surgical staging system (Enneking *et al.*, 1980) are similar in essence, differing mainly in that the TNM recognizes four histological grades (G) whereas Enneking uses a two grade scheme. Also in the TNM stage grouping, stage III is not defined and stage IV corresponds with Enneking's stage III. The TNM classification and stage grouping are shown in

Table 27.2. Each category is assessed both by physical examination and by imaging.

In clinical practice it is however sufficient to divide patients into those with localized or metastatic disease. With increasingly effective systemic chemotherapy the impact of tumour size or soft tissue infiltration has become less important. There remains, however, a major difference in outcome in those with metastases at presentation. Although a number with lung metastases may be curable, those with bone metastases or multifocal primary disease are virtually incurable.

Recent studies of biological factors such as tumour ploidy have suggested this may be a useful prognostic factor, and a near diploid karyotype carries a good prognosis (Look *et al.*, 1988).

27.4.5 TREATMENT

Prior to the introduction of cytotoxic therapy in the early 1970s surgery was the only reliably effective means of control at the primary site, and even after urgent amputation less that 20% of patients were alive at 5 years. This was usually a major amputation, e.g. through-hip disarticulation, mid-thigh amputation or forequarter amputation as dictated by the predominant sites of involvement. An alternative policy of initial radio-

Table 27.2 TNM classification and stage grouping

TNM classification				
T1	Tumour confined within cortex			
T2	Tumour invades beyond cortex			
N0	No regional node metastasis			
N1	Regional node metastasis			
G1–4	Well; moderately; poorly; undifferentiated			
Stage grouping				
IA	G1,2	T1	N0	M0
IB	G1,2	T2	N0	M0
IIA	G3,4	T1	N0	M0
IIB	G3,4	T2	N0	M0
III	Not defined			
IVA	Any G	Any T	N1	M0

therapy to the primary site was advocated by Cade (1955) in the hope of controlling the tumour for a sufficient length of time to allow the majority of patients who were doomed to metastases, mostly within a year of presentation, to avoid unnecessary mutilation. Amputation was to be reserved for those patients who passed a probationary period of 6–9 months without demonstrable secondary deposits. This scheme was often frustrated by the failure to achieve local control or to maintain it for the required length of time. These approaches were rendered obsolete and the strategy of management revolutionized by the advent of effective chemotherapy and the coincidental development of reconstructive orthopaedic techniques, which permitted resection and replacement of major segments of the long bones and adjacent joints. This dual advance has led to a significant reduction in mortality and in the requirement for major amputation.

27.4.6 CHEMOTHERAPY

Management of osteosarcoma requires close cooperation between the medical oncologist and the orthopaedic surgeon so that the timing and nature of surgery are optimal, both in terms of cancer control and functional outcome.

Initial studies using adjuvant chemotherapy given after amputation showed a reduction in metastatic relapse rates (Goorin *et al.*, 1987). The concept of preoperative chemotherapy was subsequently developed and has the advantage of achieving tumour reduction prior to surgery, thus facilitating conservative limb preserving procedures. It was suggested that the response to initial chemotherapy correlated with ultimate prognosis and in the case of a poor response, outcome could be improved by altering the chemotherapy regimen. This concept, however, remains unproven (Rosen *et al.*, 1982).

Randomized trials have now demonstrated clearly that both relapse free survival and overall survival are significantly improved by adjuvant chemotherapy using regimens including doxorubicin, cisplatin and high dose methotrexate (Link *et al.*, 1986; Eilber *et al.*, 1987). Intra-arterial chemotherapy has been used to try to increase effective drug concentration in tumour but is of unproven value (Jaffe *et al.*, 1985).

The gold standard chemotherapy programme at present appears to be a combination of doxorubicin/cisplatin as shown in Figure 27.1. In an EORTC trial this regimen has produced a 5 year disease free survival of 75% in patients presenting without metastases. In metastatic cases the 5 year survival is however less than 20%.

27.4.7 SURGERY

For sarcomas of the long bones the aim is limb conservation which, in selected patients and in the setting of multidisciplinary management, can be achieved without increasing the local recurrence rate and without detriment to survival (Marcove, 1984; Kemp, 1987). It is necessary to be able to clear the tumour with a wide surround of healthy muscle and to include the biopsy site *en bloc*. The provision of sound skin cover is essential. The resection should include the adjacent joint which is most often the knee joint. The line of bone section should be 6–7 cm beyond the level of disease as detected by scintiscan, CT or most accurately MRI. Replacement of bone or joint is usually undertaken with a custom built metallic endoprosthesis; one of the arguments for preoperative chemotherapy is the time required to manufacture this individually tailored item. The femoral component can be made adjustable to allow lengthening from time to keep pace with normal growth, provided the estimated deficit in limb length is not too great, i.e. in children aged around 7 years and over at the time of surgery. Stapling of the contralateral epiphyses may also be helpful. In the lower limb, amputation and the fitting of an artificial limb is functionally superior to

Primary chemotherapy
MRC regimen

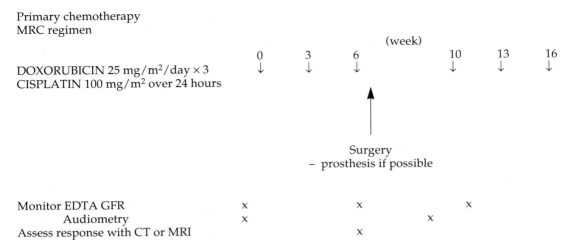

Figure 27.1   Treatment strategy in osteosarcoma.

severe disparity in limb length which follows loss of the major growth epiphyses about the knee joint. Amputation may also be the procedure of choice for extensive tibial tumours where most of the proximal bone must be resected and there may be difficulty in finding attachments for the muscles around the knee joint which results in poor function. Children in particular quickly adapt to amputation and acquire remarkable agility after a short time. Such arguments do not apply to the upper limb since no prosthesis can match the function of the hand. Alternative options to bone replacement with a metallic endoprosthesis include, for example, transposition of the patient's fibula to substitute for the resected humerus or grafting with autologous or cadaveric bone, although these latter procedures often require prolonged immobilization and there is a significant failure rate leading ultimately to amputation. These various considerations indicate the need to be selective about which patients are suitable for limb conservation procedures and early cosmetic results should not be the sole end point. An unusual but effective operation sometimes employed following resection of the lower femoral or upper tibial lesion is rotationplasty. The distal limb, with its nerves and vessels intact, is rotated so that the foot faces posteriorly and is fixed in this position to the proximal segment. This reconstructed, shortened member imparts far greater control to the artificial limb than does a conventional mid-thigh amputation stump.

Sarcomas of the jaws are best managed in a multidisciplinary head and neck unit where maxillectomy or mandibulectomy are accompanied by an expert programme of reconstruction and rehabilitation. Tumours of the vertebral column are not amenable to radical resection and at this and other sites where there is gross residual disease or narrow resection margins, adjuvant radiotherapy is helpful in reducing the likelihood of local failure.

27.4.8   SURGERY FOR PULMONARY METASTASES

Secondary deposits in the lungs may be detected at initial presentation or appear some time following treatment of the primary tumour. In either case this is an adverse prognostic occurrence but salvage is possible and an aggressive approach should be considered (Marina *et al.*, 1992). In general, a limited number of metastases would encourage a policy of resection, as would a satisfactory response to chemotherapy. The nature of second line chemotherapy will depend on the drugs given initially. Combinations of ifosfamide and etoposide are important second line agents.

27.4.9 THE ROLE OF RADIOTHERAPY

The introduction of chemotherapy has narrowed the indications for this method of treatment but radiotherapy is still of value in two situations. The first is adjuvant to surgery when resection is less than radical or frankly incomplete. The second is for palliation of painful bone metastases.

There have been trials of adjuvant pulmonary irradiation following treatment for the primary tumour, on the basis that micro metastases would be destroyed even by the necessarily limited dose that can be delivered to the whole lung. There was little benefit and this approach has in any event been outmoded by adjuvant chemotherapy which treats extrapulmonary sites in addition to the lungs.

27.5 EWING'S TUMOUR

27.5.1 AETIOLOGY

Prior to the introduction of cytotoxic therapy Ewing's tumour was the most lethal of all the primary neoplasms of bone. Less common than osteosarcoma, it shows a similar sex distribution with a male preponderance of approximately 3 : 2. The maximum age incidence is in the sec ond decade of life but compared with osteosarcoma a greater proportion affects patients in the first decade. The incidence rapidly declines thereafter and the disease is rare after middle age. Any bone may be affected but the commonest site is the femur followed by the pelvic girdle.

27.5.2 PATHOLOGY

This is a highly cellular tumour with little stroma. The cells are small, round and of uniform size. They may be morphologically indistinguishable from certain other small round cell tumours, including metastatic neuroblastoma, non-Hodgkin's lymphomas, histiocytosis, secondary undifferentiated carcinoma in older patients and, in the rare instance of primary soft tissue Ewing's tumour, embryonal rhabdomyosarcoma.

Differential diagnosis of these listed tumours has been greatly helped by modern immunohistochemistry and electron microscopy. Recent studies have also shown that many tumours within the Ewing's group of small round cell sarcomas exhibit neural differentiation and a specific chromosomal translocation, t11;22 (Rettig *et al.*, 1992). This translocation provides a useful diagnostic aid which is becoming widely available due to the increasing application of *in situ* hybridization techniques. It seems likely that Ewing's tumour of the soft tissues and the group of primitive neuroectodermal tumours (PNET) are part of the spectrum of the same disease process (Jurgens *et al.*, 1988a).

In the long bones the lesion characteristically, though not invariably, arises in the medulla of the central part of the shaft. It is a lytic process which spreads rapidly through the medullary cavity and also invades the cortex initially raising the periosteum before finally breaching it to invade the soft tissues. Some tumours produce reactive new bone with radiological changes which may resemble those of osteosarcoma. There may also be extensive areas of tumour necrosis which can liquify and grossly mimic pus.

Metastasis is to the lung and, more commonly than in osteosarcoma, to other bones. Spread to lymph nodes and the viscera is sometimes seen.

27.5.3 CLINICAL PRESENTATION AND INVESTIGATION

There is pain and swelling in relation to the affected bone associated with local heat and tenderness. This may be accompanied by fever and malaise so that osteomyelitis is suspected, a suspicion which is reinforced if the unwary surgeon opens the lesion and releases its sometimes pus-like necrotic contents.

Plain X-ray shows lytic changes which are usually extensive by the time the patient is first seen. There may be associated sclerosis due to the presence of areas of reactive new bones. Elevation of the periosteum following penetration of the cortex may produce characteristic parallel lines of new bone formation, the so-called onion skin appearance. Bone may, however, also be laid down in a sun-ray pattern, mimicking osteosarcoma. As for all bone tumours, the importance of jointly considering clinical, radiological and pathological evidence cannot be over-emphasized. Additional imaging procedures to determine the presence of metastases include chest X-ray, chest and abdominal CT, skeletal radioisotope scanning and bone marrow biopsy. Elevation of urine catecholamine levels indicates the diagnosis of metastatic neuroblastoma, but normal levels do not exclude this. The serum lactic dehydrogenase (LDH) level is a useful prognostic marker. Tissue diagnosis is obtained by needle or open surgical techniques. MRI scanning is very useful to determine the extent of intramedullary and soft tissue involvement and aids surgical planning (MacVicar *et al.*, 1992).

27.5.4   STAGING

Staging is based on known prognostic factors. Adverse features include large tumour volume, raised serum LDH and the presence of metastases. The association of poor prognosis with central location of the primary lesion relates to the usually greater mass of tumour, in for example the pelvis, than in the peripheral skeleton. As in the case of osteosarcoma, sophisticated staging systems are not required and in practice patients are generally grouped into localized or metastatic.

27.5.5   TREATMENT

The availability of effective cytotoxic drugs has transformed the outlook for patients with Ewing's tumour. The 3 year event free survival for non-metastatic cases is currently 65% though the results are less favourable in large volume lesions (see below) and in metastatic cases. Long term study is required for full evaluation of the results in each group. Chemotherapy forms the central pillar of multidisciplinary management and is the initial line of treatment both to eliminate micrometastases and for cytoreduction at the primary site. Ewing's tumour is very radiosensitive and prior to the advent of chemotherapy irradiation was used routinely for local control, which was maintained in the majority of patients until they died from metastatic disease usually within 2 years of presentation. Systemic treatment has significantly increased survival, which in some cases has allowed sufficient time for late relapse at the primary site especially for bulky disease. The combination of intensive chemotherapy, e.g. vincristine, actinomycin D, doxorubicin and cyclophosphamide or ifosfamide, with radiotherapy (Figure 27.2) results in prolonged local control in up to 80% of patients with small volume disease. However, there is an increasing trend to use surgery in certain circumstances, e.g. in dispensable bones such as the rib, fibula, etc. and at sites of bulky poor prognosis disease, e.g. the pelvis, where technically feasible. Amputation may be indicated as the initial surgical approach for tumours of the femur and tibia in infancy and early childhood because irradiation causes growth arrest of the epiphyses, importantly those about the knee joint. Resection and endoprosthetic replacement are not appropriate at this stage of skeletal immaturity as discussed for osteosarcoma, although these and other reconstructive techniques may be applicable in older patients. With large volume lesions, especially in the pelvis, where the radiation

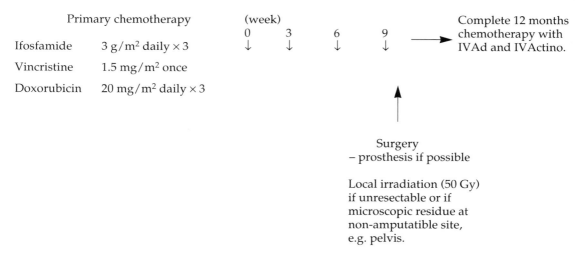

Figure 27.2 Treatment strategy for Ewing's sarcoma (UKCCSG regimen).

dose may be limited by intestinal toxicity and surgical resection is difficult, the outcome remains poorer (30–40% long term survival). An aggressive surgical policy for pelvic tumours with endoprosthetic reconstruction may well be responsible for recently improved results for this site (Jurgens *et al.*, 1988b; Burgert *et al.*, 1990).

New drug combination, alternative drug scheduling and the use of myeloblative chemo/radiotherapy with bone marrow rescue are currently under evaluation for bad risk patients and there is a trend towards more aggressive surgery to improve local control.

27.6 CHONDROSARCOMA

27.6.1 AETIOLOGY

Chondrosarcoma is principally a disease of middle and late life. It shows a slight preponderance for the male. The favoured sites are the limb girdles and the proximal ends of the femur and humerus. Other bones can be affected, e.g. the rib cage, and it also arises rarely in the laryngeal skeleton. The cause is unknown in most cases of so-called primary chondrosarcoma. Secondary chondrosarcoma arises in a pre-existing bony abnormality,

most often the cartilaginous cap of an osteochondroma, especially in patients with the multiple exostoses of diaphyseal aclasis. Malignant change in a previous benign enchondroma is believed to be very uncommon but it has been described in Ollier's disease, a rare condition where multiple enchondromas involve the hemiskeleton.

27.6.2 PATHOLOGY

Chondrosarcoma usually arises centrally within the bone of origin; less often it is situated peripherally originating either in an exostosis or at the surface of an otherwise apparently normal bone. Central lesions produce expansion and the formation of cortical new bone. They are often slow growing and not uncommonly have breached the periosteum by the time they present. There may be pathological fracture. Grossly the appearances are varied with discrete areas of cartilage, sometimes forming multiple nodules and sometimes areas of necrotic material especially in higher grade tumours. Histological grade correlates well with prognosis, varying from approximately 75% survival in grade I tumours to 15% in grade III. Well differentiated grade I chondrosarcoma can be difficult to distinguish from benign chondroma and the pathologist is helped by a formal surgical biopsy specimen with adjacent bone in which permeation of the marrow spaces by tumour indicates malignancy.

Secondary deposits are mainly to the lungs and occur far less commonly than in osteosarcoma. Metastasis can occur late, sometimes up to 10 years following initial management, as is also the case for local recurrence.

27.6.3   CLINICAL PRESENTATION AND DIAGNOSIS

The cardinal clinical features are pain and a bony mass. Because of the generally slow rate of growth the onset of symptoms may be insidious so that the lesion is locally advanced at initial presentation, particularly in the case of deeply situated parts of the pelvic skeleton. The diagnosis of chondrosarcoma should be suspected when a pre-existing exostosis becomes painful and increases in size, especially in diaphyseal aclasis where the family history provides a useful additional clue. It may not be easy to distinguish between benign chondroma and well differentiated chondrosarcoma; differential diagnosis calls for careful consideration of clinical and radiological features together with adequate surgical biopsy.

The X-ray appearance of central chondrosarcoma shows destructive changes sometimes with expansion of the shaft and scalloping of the cortex. There may be dense mottled calcification which is a characteristic feature. In secondary chondrosarcoma the radiological changes can lag behind the clinical signs but a soft tissue mass may be evident with irregular calcification or ossification and ultimately erosion of the parent exostosis.

27.6.4   TREATMENT

This is essentially surgical because chondrosarcoma is radio-resistant and unresponsive to cytotoxic agents. Every effort must be made to achieve complete surgical clearance with wide margins in view of the marked tendency to local recurrence which sometimes is not manifest until many years after operation.

In the limbs resection and endoprosthetic replacement play a major role. Tumours of the limb girdle may be amenable to the types of resection described above for osteosarcoma but complete surgical clearance is not always possible in these sometimes massive lesions. Attempts have been made to destroy the tumour residue by cryosurgery using liquid nitrogen (Marcove, 1984). Chondrosarcomas which are too extensive for consideration of standard surgical procedures can, in selected cases, be palliated by debulking via a limited incision (Ball *et al.*, 1991).

Although chondrosarcoma is generally unresponsive to irradiation even at the upper end of the therapeutic dose range, growth restraint is occasionally observed and this method of treatment can be considered as part of palliative management.

27.6.5   DEDIFFERENTIATED CHONDROSARCOMA

Dedifferentiation towards a more aggressive pattern is sometimes seen especially after repeated local recurrence. The dedifferentiated areas may be of spindle cell type or can show features of osteosarcoma. The clinical behaviour is that of the more malignant component and the patient is treated as appropriate for that tumour type.

27.6.6   MESENCHYMAL CHONDROSARCOMA

This is a rare entity with a predilection for the jaws and the ribs. It can also occur primarily in the soft tissues. It is an aggressive tumour with a high risk of metastases and, unlike the common forms of chondrosarcoma, is chemoresponsive. Multiagent regimens of the Rosen T 10 type (high dose methotrexate, vincristine, adriamycin, bleomycin, cyclophosphamide, actinomycin, cisplatin) have been found to be effective.

27.6.7 CLEAR CELL CHONDROSARCOMA

This is another rare variant which most commonly affects the upper ends of the femur and the humerus. The primary tumour is generally slow growing but it is capable of metastasis.

27.7 GIANT CELL TUMOUR

Giant cell tumour is a neoplasm found mainly in the epiphyses of long bones, most commonly at the lower end of the femur. The maximum age frequency is in the second and third decades of life and, unlike most bone tumours, it affects females somewhat more often than males. The cause is unknown, although a few cases have been described arising in Paget's disease of bone.

Giant cell tumours are locally destructive lesions which on rare occasions may exhibit malignant characteristics and metastasize.

27.7.1 PATHOLOGY

The multinucleated giant cell which gives this tumour its name and its lytic behaviour resembles the normal osteoclast and is believed to be simply reactive to the true tumour spindle cell which forms the stroma. Attempts to grade giant cell tumours according to the appearance of the stromal cells have failed to provide a reliable guide to prognosis; lesions with the blandest cellular features can metastasize. To the naked eye the lesion is soft, grey to red and haemorrhagic in appearance and produces thinning and expansion of the cortical bone. Although thinning may be extreme the periosteum is rarely breached. The tumour extends close up to the articular cartilage.

27.7.2 CLINICAL PRESENTATION AND INVESTIGATION

Patients present with pain and a bony mass; there is sometimes impairment of mobility in the adjacent joint. The radiograph typically shows a lytic lesion sited eccentrically within the epiphysis. The cortex is expanded and thinned sometimes to a degree which readily explains the classical, although uncommon, physical sign of egg shell cracking and the tendency to pathological fracture. The edge of the lesion on the metaphyseal side is not clearly defined and there is no reactive sclerosis.

Differential diagnosis is from other lesions with a prominent giant cell component, e.g. aneurysmal bone cyst, malignant fibrous histiocytoma and osteosarcoma showing a marked osteoclast reaction. Biochemical investigation should distinguish bone lesions due to hyperparathyroidism.

Neither the histological nor the radiographic appearances are predictive of malignancy, a rare event which usually follows previous treatment, especially when radiotherapy has been used.

27.7.3 TREATMENT

This is principally surgical because radiotherapy, while often successful in the past in arresting the disease and producing reossification, carries the risk of malignant change.

The ideal surgical treatment is total resection which is readily applicable to dispensable bones, e.g. the fibula, rib, etc. For lesions at major juxta-articular sites the choice rests between thorough curettage and filling of the cavity with bone chips or the more major procedure of resection and endoprosthetic replacement of the relevant bone and joint. Amputation is occasionally required when there is frank malignant change.

27.8 PRIMARY MALIGNANT LYMPHOMA OF BONE

27.8.1 AETIOLOGY

While the skeleton may be a site of metastasis in disseminated non-Hodgkin's lymphoma, this neoplasm can arise rarely as a primary lesion within bone. Previously described under the collective title of reticulum cell sarcoma, it is now recognized that primary bone lymphoma covers the same spectrum of histological subtypes as is found more commonly in the soft tissues (Chapter 26).

All age groups are affected; there is a moderate male preponderance. Any bone can be involved but the commonest site is the femur.

27.8.2   PATHOLOGY

The gross picture is one of diffuse bone destruction with a varying degree of reactive new bone formation. The cortex is commonly destroyed with soft tissue extension of disease. There may be pathological fracture. The most frequent histological type is diffuse histiocytic lymphoma.

27.8.3   CLINICAL PRESENTATION AND DIAGNOSIS

Presentation is with local pain and a bony mass. In lymphoma of the spine paraplegia may be an early symptom because of the associated soft tissue mass. There may be enlargement of the regional lymph nodes.

The radiological picture is non-specific: diffuse permeative bone destruction which is often extensive and associated with a variable degree of sclerosis. Cortical destruction with soft tissue extension is a typical feature. The definitive diagnosis is made by biopsy.

Full staging investigation of lymphoma is essential before the diagnosis can be accepted as a true primary bone lesion and also as a guide to prognosis and treatment (bone only, stage IE; bone and regional nodes, stage IIE).

27.8.4   TREATMENT

In adults the primary lesion is treated by radiotherapy to include the whole bone, any soft tissue extension and the regional lymph node fields if involved. The local control rate is excellent, in the order of 50%, and the role of surgery is usually restricted to the management of pathological fracture, e.g. by internal fixation of a long bone. The rarity of the condition has precluded randomized clinical trials of adjuvant cytotoxic therapy, but reports of small series suggest benefit and a cytotoxic regimen appropriate to the histological subtype is recommended (Rathmell *et al.*, 1992). Chemotherapy has been recommended as the sole treatment in children where late effects of irradiation are of concern (Haddy *et al.*, 1988; Coppes *et al.*, 1991).

27.9   MALIGNANT FIBROUS HISTIOCYTOMA

This entity, although rare, is the commonest of the soft tissue type sarcomas which arise within bone. As in the soft tissues, the diagnosis of true fibrosarcoma is now seldom made. Primary malignant vascular tumours and liposarcoma of bone are occasionally met.

Malignant fibrous histiocytoma (MFH) occurs across the age range, although mainly in the middle decades of life. It shows a slight preponderance for the male. It is distributed widely in the skeleton but occurs most often in the femur and tibia. Cases have been reported of MFH arising in Paget's disease of bone, postradiotherapy and at the site of previous bone infarcts.

27.9.1   PATHOLOGY

The histological appearances are those of MFH of the soft tissues. Grossly there is a mixture of destruction and reactive new bone formation. There may be pathological fracture.

27.9.2   CLINICAL PRESENTATION AND DIAGNOSIS

The clinical and radiological changes are non-specific and biopsy is required for definitive diagnosis.

27.9.3   TREATMENT

MFH of bone, unlike its soft tissue counterpart, regularly shows marked objective response to chemotherapy (den Heeten *et al.*, 1985). Therefore in this aggressive lesion it is reasonable to combine local management of the primary tumour, generally by resection and reconstruction, with an adjuvant cytotoxic regimen of osteosarcoma or soft tissue sarcoma type. Proof of survival benefit will require multicentre studies to accrue adequate numbers.

27.10 CHORDOMA

27.10.1 AETIOLOGY

This is a rare tumour which arises presumably from primitive notochordal rests. The sacrum is the commonest site followed by the spheno-occipital region and the cervical spine. It is a disease of the latter half of life and affects males more often than females.

Chordoma behaves as an indolent locally malignant lesion which grows slowly over many years but can occasionally metastasize.

27.10.2 PATHOLOGY

Grossly this is a lobulated, soft to firm greyish lesion which destroys bone and eventually erupts into the soft tissues. It may contain areas which to the naked eye resemble cartilage; there may be mucinous change and foci of calcification. Histology shows strands of the typical physaliphorous or bubble cells distended by the accumulation of intracytoplasmic mucus. In some tumours cells are scanty and the appearances may resemble chondrosarcoma. Chordoma invades the soft tissues and can grow to considerable size, particularly in the sacral area. Local recurrence is seen in the skin and soft tissues after operation but metastasis is uncommon.

27.10.3 CLINICAL PRESENTATION AND DIAGNOSIS

Longstanding pain is followed by pressure symptoms depending on the site. For sacral chordoma there is progressive impairment of nerve root function with disturbance of bladder and bowel control, root pain and weakness of the lower limbs. Spheno-occipital tumours may invade the air sinuses and orbits. Upward extension produces pressure effects on the adjacent structures at the base of the brain.

Imaging by CT or MRI will demonstrate the extent of bone destruction and soft tissue involvement. Biopsy is necessary to exclude chondrosarcoma and other tumours which occur respectively in the region of the sacrum and of the skull base.

Treatment is difficult because radical surgery provides the only hope of cure which, at the sites of origin of chordoma, is either impossible or involves the risk of major neurological damage. The possibility of surgical cure without major functional deficit is virtually restricted to sacral tumours below the level of the second segment (Bethke, 1991). This type of major surgery should be considered in younger fit patients. In the elderly and frail the slow growing nature of chordoma dictates a conservative policy. Radiotherapy can produce growth restraint and sometimes a small diminution in tumour volume which is a palliative benefit. Irradiation is also indicated to supplement incomplete or narrow surgical resection. Chemotherapy is without value.

27.11 ADAMANTINOMA OF LONG BONES

This rare and inappropriately named tumour is made up of epithelium-like cells whose origin is uncertain. It is possibly a sarcoma showing epithelial differentiation. By far the commonest site is the tibia.

It is a slowly growing lesion presenting with a long history of pain and showing mixture of lytic and sclerotic changes on radiological examination. Exceptionally it may metastasize.

Treatment is by surgical resection and bone replacement. Extensive tumours with soft tissue invasion may require amputation. Adamantinoma does not respond to irradiation or chemotherapy.

REFERENCES

Ball, A.B.S., Barr, L.C. and Westbury, G. (1991) Chondrosarcoma of the pelvis: the role of palliative debulking surgery. *European Journal of Surgical Oncology*, **17**, 135–7.

Bethke, K.P. (1991) Diagnosis and management of sacrococcygeal chordoma. *Journal of Surgical Oncology*, **48**, 232–8.

Burgert, E.O., Nesbit, M.E., Garnsey, L.A. *et al.* (1990) Multimodal therapy for the management of nonpelvic localized Ewing's sarcoma of bone: Intergroup Study IESS-II. *Journal of Clinical Oncology*, **8**, 1514–24.

Cade, S. (1955) Osteogenic sarcoma: a study based on 133 patients. *Journal of the Royal College of Surgeons of Edinburgh*, **1**, 79–116.

Coppes, M.J., Patte, C. Couanet, D. *et al.* (1991) Childhood malignant lymphoma of bone. *Medical and Pediatric Oncology*, **19**, 22–7.

Dahlin, D.C. (1978) *Bone Tumours*, 3rd edn, Charles C. Thomas, Springfield, Illinois.

den Heeten, G.J., Schraffordt-Koops, H., Kamps, W.A. *et al.* (1985) Treatment of malignant fibrous histiocytoma of bone. A plea for primary chemotherapy. *Cancer*, **56**, 37–40.

Eilber, F., Giuliano, A. Eckardt, J. *et al.* (1987) Adjuvant chemotherapy for osteosarcoma: a randomized prospective trial. *Journal of Clinical Oncology*, **5**, 21–6.

Enneking, W.F., Spanier, S.S. and Goodman, M.A. (1980) A system of staging of musculoskeletal sarcoma. *Clinical Orthopaedics and Related Research*, **153**, 106–20.

Goorin, A.M., Perez-Atayde, A., Gebhardt, M. *et al.* (1987) Weekly high-dose methotrexate and doxorubicin for osteosarcoma: the Dana-Farber Institute/The Children's Hospital – Study III. *Journal of Clinical Oncology*, **5**, 1178–84.

Haddy, T.B., Keenan, A.M., Jaffe, E.S. and Magrath, I.T. (1988) Bone involvement in young patients with non-Hodgkin's lymphoma: efficacy of chemotherapy without local radiotherapy. *Blood*, **72**, 1141–7.

Jaffe, N, Robertson, R., Ayala, A. *et al.* (1985) Comparison of intra-arterial cis-diamminedichloroplatinum II with high-dose methotrexate and citrovorum factor rescue in the treatment of primary osteosarcoma. *Journal of Clinical Oncology*, **3**, 1101–4.

Jurgens, H., Bier, V., Harms, D. *et al.* (1988a) Malignant peripheral neuroectodermal tumours. A retrospective analysis of 42 patients. *Cancer*, **61**, 349–57.

Jurgens, H., Exner, U., Gardner, H. *et al.* (1988b) Multidisciplinary treatment of primary Ewing's sarcoma of bone. A 6-year experience of a European Cooperative Trial. *Cancer*, **61**, 23–32.

Kemp, H. (1987) Limb conservation surgery for osteosarcoma and other primary bone tumours. *Ballière's Clinical Oncology*, **1**, 111–36.

Link, M.P., Goorin, A.M., Miser, A.W. *et al.* (1986) The effect of adjuvant chemotherapy on relapse-free survival in patients with osteosarcoma of the extremity. *New England Journal of Medicine*, **314**, 1600–6.

Look, A.T., Douglass, E.C. and Meyer, W.H. (1988) Clinical importance of near-diploid tumour stem lines in patients with osteosarcoma of an extremity. *New England Journal of Medicine*, 1988. **318**, 1567–72.

MacVicar, A.D., Olliff, J.F.C., Pringle, J. *et al.* (1992) Ewing sarcoma: MR imaging of chemotherapy-induced changes with histologic correlation. *Radiology*, **184**, 859–64.

Marcove, R.C. (1984) *Surgery of Tumours of Bone & Cartilage*, 2nd edn, Grune, Orlando, Florida, p. 240.

Marina, N.W., Pratt, C.B., Rao, B.N. *et al.* (1992) Improved prognosis of children with osteosarcoma metastasis to the lung(s) at the time of diagnosis. *Cancer*, **70**, 2722–7.

Rathmell, M.K., Gospodarowicz, S.B., Sutcliffe, R.M. *et al.* (1992) Localised lymphoma of bone: prognostic factors and treatment recommendations. *British Journal of Cancer*, **66**, 603–6.

Rettig, W.J., Garin-Chesa, P. and Huvos, A.G. (1992) Ewing's sarcoma: new approaches to histogenesis and molecular plasticity. *Laboratory Investigation*, **66**, 133–7.

Rosen, G., Caparros, B., Huvos, A.G. *et al.* (1982) Preoperative chemotherapy for osteogenic sarcoma: selection of postoperative adjuvant chemotherapy based on the response of the primary tumor to preoperative chemotherapy. *Cancer*, **49**, 1221–30.

Stoker, D.J. (1987) The place of radiology in diagnosis and management. *Baillière's Clinical Oncology*, **1**, 65–96.

UICC TNM Classification of Malignant Tumours (1987) Springer-Verlag, Berlin.

SKIN CANCER

Chris C. Harland and Peter S. Mortimer

28.1 INTRODUCTION

Skin cancer is the commonest human malignancy. Over 90% of cases comprise malignant melanoma, basal cell carcinoma (BCC) and squamous cell carcinoma (SCC). Skin cancer can be broadly classified as either **melanoma** (malignant melanoma) or **non-melanoma** (BCC, SCC, and others). Melanoma is derived from melanocytes, and BCC and SCC from keratinocytes. Thus, the majority of skin cancers are epidermal. In addition, the dermis and skin appendages (sweat glands, hair follicles, sebaceous glands) generate an array of other cutaneous malignancies. Malignant lymphomas, particularly the T-cell varieties, can begin in the skin.

The epidermis is vulnerable to the carcinogenic effects of ultraviolet irradiation, especially where the protective epidermal melanin content is low. Hence, skin cancer is prevalent in the white population of Australia, where 2.3% of the population over 40 years of age suffer from skin cancer at some stage during their lives (Giles *et al.*, 1988). Malignant melanoma is the most dangerous of skin cancers. Once it has been allowed to invade into the deeper dermis or fat, it has frequently metastasized to local regional lymph nodes or to other organs. There is currently no curative treatment for metastatic disease.

28.2 INCIDENCE AND EPIDEMIOLOGY

28.2.1 MELANOMA

There is an alarmingly high rate of increase of melanoma worldwide compared with other cancers. It is the most rapidly increasing cancer in Scotland, and in the USA reference has been made to the 'epidemic of melanoma'. It has been projected that from the year 2000, 1% of Americans will develop a melanoma within their lifetimes if the present rate of increase continues. Between 1960 and 1990 the incidence of cutaneous melanoma in the South West Thames region nearly doubled every decade for females and every two decades for males. The average annual rate for melanoma between 1987 and 1989 was 4.25 and 6.86 per 100 000 for men and women, respectively (Thames Cancer Registry, 1992). These figures are similar to those for the rest of the UK. Thus, UK females are at greater risk of developing melanoma than males. In females the commonest site of involvement is the lower leg, and in males it is the back. Prior to puberty melanoma is rare; its incidence increases steadily throughout adult life, reaching a plateau around the sixth decade. The mean age at which individuals develop melanoma is 45 years.

In England and Wales the death rate per million population attributable to melanoma in 1974 rose from 12 for men, and 15 for women, to 23 for each sex in 1991 (Office of Population Censuses and Surveys, England and Wales, 1993). The most important prognostic factor for patients with stage I, non-metastatic cutaneous melanoma is tumour thickness (Breslow, 1970). Melanomas less than 1.5 mm thick have a 5 year survival of over 90%, those with tumours 1.5–3.5 mm of 70%, and those with tumours over 3.5 mm of only 40%. Thus, early detection of melanoma in a population should improve survival statistics. There is evidence that this goal is being achieved in Scotland. Following an educational campaign, mortality for females has shown a downward trend (MacKie, 1992). Less important adverse prognostic indices include the presence of micro- or macroscopic ulceration, Clark level of microscopic invasion (level IV indicates that fat has been breached) and involvement of certain body sites (e.g. nail-bed). Male or elderly patients generally fare worse.

Episodic sunburn is more likely to induce melanoma than chronic sun exposure (Elwood, 1985). There has been a significant shift towards a sunbathing culture since 1930 with the result that the 'package holiday' industry has burgeoned. Thus, unacclimatized white skin is subject to sunburn at least once per year. This phenomenon is thought to explain why indoor professions are associated more strongly with melanoma than outdoor occupations.

28.2.2 NON-MELANOMA SKIN CANCER

The most prevalent of non-melanoma skin cancers is the basal cell carcinoma (BCC), also known as basal cell epithelioma and 'rodent ulcer'. Squamous cell carcinoma (SCC) is the second most common skin cancer. Their incidence rises progressively with age. Cumulative, chronic sun exposure and fair skin are important predisposing factors. Data from the South West Thames Cancer Registry indicate that the incidence of non-melanoma skin cancer is at least ten times greater than melanoma for males, and four times greater for females. Their true incidence has been underestimated owing to poor registration; many cases of BCC are diagnosed and treated without histological confirmation. An Australian study indicates that the true ratio of BCC to SCC is 4 : 1 and for BCC to melanoma is 34 : 1 (Giles *et al.*, 1988). BCC has an indolent growth pattern, so that it may not be noticed for many years. BCC very rarely metastasizes,

but neglected lesions can result in widespread tissue destruction. SCC have a propensity to metastasize once deeply invasive.

28.3 MANAGEMENT OF SKIN CANCER

Aspects of skin cancer management to be considered are prevention, clinical diagnosis, investigation, treatment, premalignant conditions and risk factors.

28.4 PREVENTION

Skin cancer is one of the four main malignancies which the Government has targeted for action in its White Paper, Health of the Nation (Department of Health, 1992), with the specific aim of curbing the rising incidence of skin cancer by the year 2005. This objective will be difficult to achieve due to the considerable lag period between excessive sun exposure and the development of skin cancer. The ultimate aim should be to reduce mortality. An intensified primary public awareness programme is of urgent national importance to alter attitudes in our sun-worshipping culture. Childhood sun exposure is a risk factor for melanoma in later life (McMichael and Giles, 1988), therefore the importance of protecting children's skin from strong sunlight should be emphasized. A secondary prevention education programme may promote early presentation of cutaneous melanoma (Doherty and MacKie, 1988). There is accumulating evidence that the ozone layer is being depleted by pollutants, permitting an increased amount of ultraviolet radiation (UVR) to penetrate the Earth's atmosphere. It is difficult to quantify the carcinogenic risk of additional UVR exposure. However, further UVR is like to add to the escalation of skin cancer. Only strict government policies worldwide will limit this effect.

28.5 CLINICAL DIAGNOSIS

Skin cancer is readily accessible for examination. It should therefore be possible to recognize it during its early stages. Early recognition is vital for the effective treatment of cutaneous melanoma.

28.5.1 MELANOMA

There are four major clinicopathological types of melanoma: superficial spreading, nodular, acral lentiginous and lentigo maligna melanoma. **Superficial spreading** lesions preferentially affect the female leg or male back. Between 50% and 70% of melanomas belong to this category. They are usually irregularly shaped plaques with variegate pigmentation (Figure 28.1). Tumour cells invade the dermis, but initially extend radially ('horizontal growth phase'). The tumour is presumed to enter a 'vertical growth phase' if untreated, at which stage lymphatic and vascular spread is more likely to occur. Therefore, early recognition is essential to effect a cure. **Nodular** lesions are commoner on the trunk. They are deemed to be in a vertical growth phase only, which may explain their high metastatic potential. **Acral lentiginous** melanomas occur on the palms and soles. They appear to have a protracted intra-epidermal phase before becoming invasive. **Lentigo maligna** melanoma presents on the chronically sun damaged facial skin of

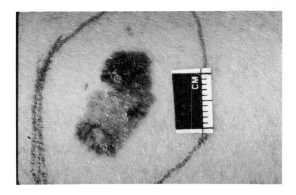

Figure 28.1 Superficial spreading malignant melanoma. Note the irregular border and variable pigmentation.

elderly persons. They are *in situ* melanomas, which invade the dermis after many years. Lesions have an irregular pattern of pigmentation, and may be extensive by the time of presentation (Figure 28.2). All categories of melanoma can undergo regression: that is ,an inflammatory response results in destruction of tumour cells with their eventual replacement by fibrosis. Regression is characterized clinically by areas of depigmentation which appear pink or inflamed. Curiously, this partially effective immune response is not associated with better prognosis.

Ideally, simple guidelines for the recognition of melanoma should improve early detection. Early detection implies that the melanoma is still thin, has not yet metastasized, and is therefore curable. In 1985, when an early detection campaign was established in the west of Scotland, a seven point checklist was devised for all family doctors. This included, in order: sensory change, often described as a greater awareness of the lesion but also mild itch; diameter of 1 cm or greater; growth of the lesion; an irregular edge; irregular pigment with different shades of brown and black in the lesion; inflammation; and crusting, oozing or bleeding. Melanomas were thought to be more likely to have three or more of these features. However, in 1985–89 the surface area of excised melanomas had decreased. Moreover, the inclusion of itch appeared to have precipitated the referral of an excessive number of benign lesions, such as moles and seborrhoeic warts. The seven point checklist was revised (Table 28.1). The current recommendation is that a patient with a pigmented lesion with any of the major signs – change in size, change in shape, change in colour – should be considered for referral, and that the presence of a minor feature – inflammation, crusting or bleeding, sensory change, diameter ≥ 7 mm – should be a further stimulus to referral (MacKie, 1990). The finding of satellite lesions and palpable lymph nodes indicates poor prognosis, and is irrelevant to

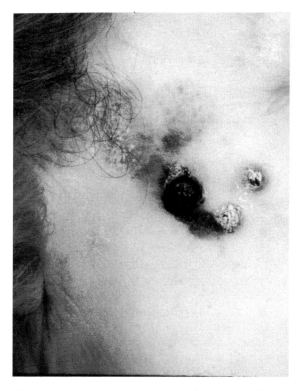

Figure 28.2 An extensive lentigo maligna melanoma on the face of an elderly patient. Invasive nodular melanoma has developed adjacent to an area of depigmentation (regression).

any checklist designed to promote early diagnosis.

A checklist is only a guideline. Unfortunately, recognition of melanomas is not simple. St George's Hospital Pigmented Lesion Clinic (PLC), which offers a rapid referral service to general practitioners in South London, reveals only 1 melanoma for

Table 28.1 Revised checklist for suspected malignant melanoma (MacKie, 1990)

Major signs	Minor signs
Change in size	Inflammation
Change in shape	Crusting or bleeding
Change in colour	Sensory change
	Diameter ⩾7 mm

every 40 referrals. In Scotland the pick-up rate is 1 in 20 referrals. Banal pigmented lesions, such as seborrhoeic keratoses and dermatofibroma, cause diagnostic confusion. At St George's Hospital PLC, 30% of lesions are subsequently diagnosed as seborrhoeic keratoses. There is even substantial disagreement between experienced dermatologists over the clinical diagnosis of pigmented naevi (Curley *et al.*, 1989). In addition, amelanotic melanoma can deceive patients and physicians owing to their absence of pigment. Subungual lesions mimic haematoma or fungal infection, and therefore escape early diagnosis.

Because of these difficulties, there has been recent interest in aids to clinical diagnosis. Skin surface microscopy is a relatively simple technique whereby a hand-held lens with fitted light source is applied directly on to the skin using an oil interface. The diagnostic accuracy is dependent on the observer's acumen, but readily discriminates between vascular, keratotic and melanocytic lesions. The development of computerized image analysis is expected to improve diagnostic accuracy (Steiner *et al.*, 1987). The authors are pursuing the use of high frequency, high resolution ultrasonography as a diagnostic aid; it can distinguish between seborrhoeic warts and melanoma. Ocular melanoma can be differentiated from haematoma and SCC metastasis by ultrasound (Coleman and Lizzi, 1983).

The diagnostic quagmire for melanoma contains seborrhoeic wart, dermatofibroma, subungual haematoma and solar lentigo, and haemangioma. In addition, pyogenic granuloma, a benign vascular proliferation, is similar in appearance to amelanotic melanoma.

28.5.2   BASAL CELL CARCINOMA

These slow growing tumours arise predominantly on sun exposed sites. Characteristically, they have the appearance of a pearl, with or without ulceration, over which dilated vessels course.

There are several clinicopathological types: cystic, morphoeic, pigmented, superficial, basisquamous and invasive. In clinical practice, it is important to distinguish between the well circumscribed lesions, which often resemble cysts ('cystic'), and those tumours with ill defined margins. The latter may be associated with either superficial scarring ('morphoeic') or, more worryingly, subcutaneous invasion. If the typical features of basal cell carcinoma (BCC) are indistinct, it is useful to pull the lateral skin borders taut, so that the pearly texture of the tumour margins become apparent. The authors have coined the term 'stretch test' for this poorly described but valuable technique (Figure 28.3). Following the detection of one BCC, further examination of the undressed patient is important, as multiple BCCs commonly occur.

It may be difficult to distinguish between BCC and SCC, trichoepithelioma, sweat gland tumours, radionecrotic ulcers and sebaceous hyperplasia. BCC on the lower limbs rarely exhibits the classical pearly appearance, but a protracted history is suggestive of the diagnosis.

28.5.3 SQUAMOUS CELL CARCINOMA

The evolution of squamous cell carcinoma (SCC) is more rapid that for BCC. Sun exposed sites are susceptible, especially the lower lip of smokers, helix of the ear and a bald scalp. Keratotic nodules eventually ulcerate to leave rolled tumour edges. Unlike BCC, SCC is often painful. Local lymph nodes should be palpated for evidence of metastatic spread.

Well differentiated SCC produces abundant keratin, which helps the clinician to

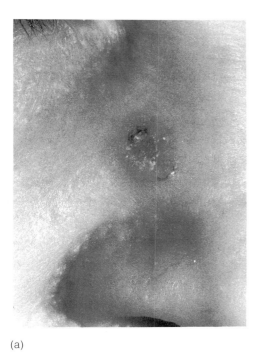

(a)

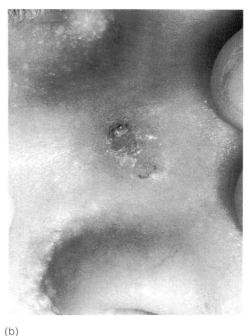

(b)

Figure 28.3(a) Ulcerated basal cell carcinoma with overlying telangiectasia. **(b)** The 'stretch test' has been helpful in demonstrating the pearly appearance as well as the tumour border.

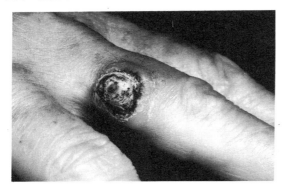

Figure 28.4 A well differentiated squamous cell carcinoma. A diagnostic feature is the abundant scaly, brown keratin produced by the tumour.

distinguish it from other tumours (Figure 28.4). Other conditions to be considered within the differential diagnosis are keratoacanthoma, BCC, viral warts, solar keratoses, Bowen's disease and chondrodermatitis helicis nodularis (CDHN). Keratoacanthoma manifests as a dome shaped nodule with a central keratin plug, which enlarges rapidly on sun exposed sites, but then involutes spontaneously to leave a scar. CDHN is an inflammatory condition affecting the cartilage of the ear; a pathognomic feature is local tenderness whilst sleeping on the affected side.

28.6   INVESTIGATION

Histopathological examination of suspected skin cancers is essential. **Excision biopsy** following local anaesthetic is a definitive treatment which furnishes a complete histological specimen. An **incision biopsy** for histological confirmation is sometimes appropriate in order to plan future management. Where there is diagnostic uncertainty over an atypical mole, a narrow excision margin is appropriate; a wider excision can be performed later. There is no convincing evidence that incisional biopsy of a melanoma promotes metastases.

A valuable incision biopsy technique involves the use of a **punch biopsy** needle.

This has a luminal diameter of 2–8 mm; a skewering action with the needle provides a core of tumour tissue, which can be retrieved by fine forceps. The tumour plug should be dissected carefully from its base to avoid crush-artefact to the specimen. Suturing is not always necessary, and a simple dressing may be all that is required. Therefore, the punch biopsy technique is quick and convenient. However, a scalpel biopsy usually provides a better orientated specimen for histological interpretation, and should be reserved for melanocytic lesions.

Cytological examination can be performed on a smear from the scraped surface of a BCC. Basal cells are characteristically dark blue, or basophilic, on haematoxylin and eosin stain. This technique is a less sensitive diagnostic technique than the incisional biopsy, but it is rapid and does not require a local anaesthetic. Similarly, a small fragment of BCC can be removed with a size 15 disposable blade without local anaesthetic, often painlessly, and is usually sufficient for histological confirmation prior to radiotherapy.

Histological examination of clinically obvious skin cancers is not always indicated. BCCs in the elderly do not necessarily require treatment, and multiple superficial BCCs are amenable to cryosurgery. Also, radiotherapists do not always insist on a histological diagnosis of a BCC with the classical clinical appearances.

Staging investigations for metastatic melanoma or SCC are indicated when the tumours are deeply invasive, and include liver function tests, chest X-ray and ultrasound examination of the liver. CT and NMR scans may be helpful, but are not employed routinely. The role of positron emission tomography and radioimmunoscintography in imaging melanoma metastases is being evaluated. Enlarged lymph nodes should be biopsied in order to determine further management. BCC rarely merits staging procedures, although inner canthus tumours can infiltrate the medial wall of the orbit. A skull

X-ray and CT or NMR scan would then be invaluable.

28.7 TREATMENT

The main treatment options for skin cancer are surgery (excision biopsy, Mohs micrographic surgery and cryosurgery), radiotherapy and drug therapy. Criteria which determine the choice of treatment include eradication of the tumour, cosmetic result (cosmesis) and costs in terms of time and money. The therapeutic approach is also dictated by the skin cancer *per se*.

28.7.1 SURGERY

The standard treatment for most skin cancers is **excision biopsy.** In general, the tumour is excised *in toto* with an elliptical margin, followed by the repair of the wound defect. The longitudinal axis of the ellipse should follow natural wrinkles or skin crease marks. This is best demonstrated by a preceding circular excision of the tumour, thereby allowing the defect to adopt an elliptical shape of least tension. Whenever possible, the wound should be closed directly along this axis with non-absorbable, monofilament nylon sutures, such as Ethilon or Prolene. Subcutaneous absorbable sutures, such as undyed Vicryl, may be required where the wound edges oppose with difficulty. Flaps and grafts are used for wounds which cannot be closed primarily.

(a) Melanoma

Primary invasive cutaneous melanoma is treated by excision biopsy. In the early 1960s, wide excision and skin grafting for even the thinnest lesions was a routine procedure, resulting in disfiguring, depressed, 'dinner plate' deformities. It was then shown that prognosis was directly related to the depth to which the melanoma cells had invaded the dermis (Breslow, 1970). Subsequently, excision margins for thinner melanomas shrank from the traditional 5 cm of uninvolved skin in all directions to 3 cm or less. An ongoing WHO trial suggests that survival is not adversely affected by 1 cm vs 3 cm excision margins for melanomas less than 2 mm thickness (Veronesi *et al.*, 1988). Many clinicians limit excision margins to 1 cm even for thicker lesions, but this practice has not been substantiated by randomized, prospective studies. *In situ* melanoma, which has no metastatic potential, merits narrower excision margins of 2–5 mm. Lentigo maligna melanoma may be too extensive to permit primary wound closure. Recurrence of disease may occur after extensive surgical removal, indicating that there is a 'field-defect' of premalignant melanocytes. As invasive melanoma may not eventuate during the patient's lifetime, a watch-and-see policy for lentigo maligna is frequently adopted with the aid of photographic documentation.

Prophylactic lymph node dissection for melanomas is practised in some centres, but 5 year survival figures have failed to demonstrate a convincing advantage compared with excision biopsy alone.

(b) Basal cell carcinoma

Surgery is often simpler for the patient, as fewer hospital visits are necessary. BCCs frequently extend beyond their visible borders, so that the optimum width of surgical margins is difficult to discern. Mohs micrographic surgery is the most accurate technique for ascertaining the actual extent of BCC. The tumour is first debulked, then a thin layer of tissue is excised with a 1–2 mm margin of normal appearing skin. Horizontal frozen sections of the excised tissue are prepared, stained and examined. Any residual tumour noted on microscopic examination is mapped and selectively excised, the process being repeated until the entire tumour is excised. Virtually 100% of tumours can be cured whilst sacrificing a minimum of unaffected skin.

Using the Mohs technique as the definitive guide of cure, it has been shown that a visually determined margin of 4 mm is required to totally eradicate 95% of tumours less than 2 cm in diameter (Wolf and Zitelli, 1987). This finding is supported by a retrospective study of 468 BCCs, in which excision of lesions plus a 3–5 mm margin of normal tissue resulted in a 5 year cumulative recurrence of 6.8% (Bart *et al.*, 1978). Therefore, 3 mm is the minimum recommended margin for excision of BCCs. Wider margins may be appropriate for large tumours or for those on locations with an associated high risk of recurrence, such as the eyelids, canthi, pinnae, nasolabial folds and alae nasi. Dermatological surgeons in North America reserve the use of Mohs micrographic surgery to these areas, or to morphoea-like BCC. In Britain there are fewer advocates of Mohs surgery. It is argued that it is not cost-effective because of its labour intensive nature. Nevertheless, it optimizes cure rates whilst minimizing unnecessary tissue destruction.

A simpler, quicker and cheaper surgical method for treatment of BCC is curettage and electrodissection (curettage and cautery). This method should be reserved for well defined BCCs. In crude terms, the tumour is scooped out following local anaesthetic. More technically, it is dissected away from its underlying stroma by virtue of a natural cleavage plane at this interface. The wound base is then cauterized. This procedure is repeated two or three times to ensure that residual tumour is destroyed whilst controlling haemorrhage. The wound heals by secondary intention. In experienced hands the cure rate for this technique is the same as for excision biopsy, and the cosmetic result is usually satisfactory. However, certain body sites, such as the nose, are prone to form depressed wounds. Unfortunately, removal margins cannot be evaluated histologically from the piecemeal specimen. Thus, purists never perform this technique.

Cryosurgery offers another rapid means of treating BCCs. Again, tumours must be care- fully selected. It is the treatment of choice for multiple, superficial BCCs on the trunk. Liquid nitrogen is applied or sprayed on to the tumour surface. An ice-ball of tissue develops beyond the tumour margins, which is then allowed to thaw slowly. Frozen tumour cells lyse following their expansion by ice. Frequently the treated area blisters and crusts, and the wound heals by secondary intention with good cosmesis. Usually the scar is flat and hypopigmented. Disadvantages of treatment include discomfort, blistering and absence of histological specimen. There is no reliable way of monitoring treatment reliably, so deeply invasive tumours should be avoided. In the future, high resolution real-time ultrasound might facilitate placement of a thermocouple needle at the tumour base to permit accurate measurement of the critical temperature required for tumour necrosis, $-20°C$ to $-35°C$.

(c) Squamous cell carcinoma

Surgical excision is the treatment of choice for SCC. As for BCC, recommended margins of excision have been arbitrary and variable. On the basis of Mohs micrographic surgery, minimum margins of 4 mm around the clinical borders have been proposed to achieve clearance rates of at least 95% (Brodland and Zitelli, 1992). Subclinical tumour extension and metastatic potential may be greater for SCCs which are poorly differentiated, greater than 2 cm in diameter, or located on the scalp, ears, eyelids, nose and lips. Wider margins have been suggested for these high risk tumours. The level of invasion is associated with increased mortality (Friedman *et al.*, 1983). Excision biopsies should include subcutaneous fat.

28.7.2 RADIOTHERAPY

(a) Melanoma

Melanoma is not particularly radiosensitive, but irradiation palliates metastatic bone pain and symptoms of raised intracranial pressure from cerebral secondaries. Superficial radiotherapy may be a viable option for treatment of lentigo maligna melanoma if excision biopsy is deemed to be too radical.

(b)   Non-melanoma skin cancer

Superficial radiotherapy is mainly used for the treatment of BCC. There is little to choose between surgery and radiotherapy. Both methods give at least a 95% cure over 5 years in experienced hands. Superficial radiotherapy is a painless treatment with very little risk to the patient. The treated area becomes crusted before healing. The choice between surgery and radiotherapy depends on the site of lesion, the patients' age, previous treatments and their preferred option.

Radiotherapy is indicated for certain body sites such as the nose, where the cosmetic results of surgery are frequently disappointing. The lower limbs and the dorsum of hands should be avoided; these areas heal better after surgery, particularly where there is photodamaged skin. Irradiation of the auricular cartilage can produce painful chondritis if it is breached by tumour. This adverse effect of radiotherapy is less common since the advent of electron beam therapy, which treats superficial cutaneous tumours effectively whilst minimizing irradiation of subcutaneous structures. Radiotherapy scars are atrophic, hypopigmented with telangiectasiae. These changes are mild initially, but become more marked over the years, even to the extent that radionecrotic ulcers occasionally develop, whereas surgical scars become less noticeable. In addition, there is a small risk of inducing skin cancer many years after treatment. For these reasons, radiotherapy is usually avoided for treatment of younger patients. If an irradiated BCC recurs, further radiotherapy is contraindicated because of the risk of radionecrosis. Nevertheless, the patient should be allowed to influence the choice between radiotherapy and surgery in

the first instance, having heard the pros and cons of both treatments.

Radiotherapy can be used for SCC. It is normally reserved for metastatic SCC with lymph node involvement.

28.7.3   DRUG THERAPY

As radiotherapy and surgery carry the risk of scarring, drug therapy appears to be an attractive alternative. 5% Fluorouracil (Efudix) is the most widely used topical cytotoxic for the treatment of non-invasive epidermal tumours. It is particularly effective for the treatment of Bowen's disease, extensive solar keratoses and multiple superficial BCC. However, the cream is highly irritant, and should only be prescribed to individuals who are likely to comply with treatment correctly. It is applied twice daily for up to 21 days, but should be stopped if severe inflammation or soreness develops.

The retinoids are synthetic oral vitamin A derivatives which have cytostatic properties. The rate of appearance of BCC is reduced in patients with xeroderma pigmentosa, but tumours rapidly recur on withdrawing therapy (Kraemer *et al.*, 1988). Their use is limited by numerous side-effects and expense. There is no clear-cut benefit from low dose retinoid therapy for any of the skin cancers (Tangrea *et al.*, 1992). Intralesional interferons are an alternative, non-surgical approach to the treatment of BCC. However, treatment is not 100% effective in the short term, multiple visits are necessary, and long term follow-up studies are not yet available.

Chemotherapy for melanoma has been disappointing. Adjuvant arterial limb perfusion for poor prognosis thick primary melanomas on the limbs is available in some centres, but its efficacy is unproven. Treatment of metastatic disease is essentially palliative. Short-lived responses are reported in 20–25% of treated patients. The most commonly employed regimen is DTIC. Newer immunotherapeutic approaches with interferons, interleukin 2 and tumour necrosis factor are being evaluated.

28.8   PATIENT FOLLOW-UP

Follow-up policies vary enormously according to the tumour, therapy and treatment centre. Many centres review patients frequently for 10 years or more. However, of those melanomas which recur, over 80% will have declared themselves within 3 years of treatment (Fusi *et al.*, 1993), and 72% of recurrences will have been noted by the patient (Ruark *et al.*, 1993). Even if metastatic disease is detected, further treatment is palliative. Nevertheless, valuable epidemiological data is gleaned from continued follow-up. Also, a second melanoma may be detected by scrupulous follow-up; patients who have one stage I cutaneous melanoma have an eight-fold relative risk of producing further melanomas. The risk is much higher if there is a family history of melanoma.

The approach to BCC follow-up can be more pragmatic. If an appropriate resection margin has been taken around the lesion, and histological margins are clear, the cost-benefit of continued follow-up is debatable. The authors discharge most patients having reviewed them once. Patients are at increased risk of further non-melanoma skin cancer, but clearly the prognostic implications are not the same as for melanoma. Patients with appropriately excised SCCs are reviewed for up to a year. Opinions vary; in the USA, it is standard practice to follow-up all patients with skin cancer for several years.

Excessive exposure to cutaneous carcinogens or predisposition to skin cancer may influence the decision to monitor for cutaneous malignancy. Risk factors and at-risk groups will now be considered.

28.9   RISK FACTORS

The risk of developing skin cancer is determined by a combination of environmental and genetic factors.

28.9.1   ULTRAVIOLET RADIATION

UVR is invisible light which can cause sunburn. Its carcinogenic effect on skin is influenced by the Earth's atmosphere, which absorbs many of the harmful short UVR wavelengths. Atmospheric absorption decreases as the angle of incidence of the solar rays increases. Thus skin cancer is more prevalent in decreasing latitudes. As much as 50% of UVR may reach the skin by reflection from the sand, water, snow and concrete surfaces.

The shortest wavelength in terrestrial sunlight is approximately 290 nm. By convention, UVR is subclassified as UVA (320–400 nm), UVB (290–320 nm) and UVC (<290 nm). UVB is a probably both an initiator and promoter of cutaneous carcinogenesis. Molecular alterations of DNA result in either cell death or malignant transformation. UVB also impairs immune surveillance of malignant cells (Streilein, 1991). UVA penetrates the atmosphere and skin more readily than UVB, but is less erythrogenic. UVA is associated with the ageing effects of chronic sunlight exposure. There is evidence that UVA may potentiate the carcinogenic effects of UVB (Chew *et al.*, 1988). Photochemotherapy for certain dermatoses incorporates UVA exposure with psoralen ingestion (PUVA), which enhances UVA erythema. PUVA is associated with a small risk of skin cancer (Lindelöf *et al.*, 1991). Commercial sunbeds emit UVA, UVB and even UVC, despite claims that they offer a safer UVA tan. It is presumed future studies will demonstrate a link between skin cancer and sunbed use.

An uncompromising message is of paramount importance in order for a public educational programme to be effective: no tan is healthy. The public should be encouraged to enjoy the sun, but to avoid the sun when it is hottest; to seek the shade or wear a broad-brimmed hat and cover up; to take extra care with children and babies; to wear a good quality pair of sunglasses; to use a sunscreen with an SPF greater than 10, probably with balanced UVB/UVA protection. These precautions are routinely enacted by many Australians.

28.9.2 IONIZING RADIATION

Carcinoma induced by radiotherapy is rarely seen since the development of sophisticated machinery and a greater understanding of radiobiology. BCCs occur following radiation of the face, scalp and trunk, whereas on the hands SCCs tend to arise. Radiation induced BCC of the scalp may be seen 20–50 years after X-ray treatment of the scalp for ringworm infection. BCCs and related tumours may also be a late complication of lumbar spine irradiation; polypoid lesions with the histological features of the premalignant fibroepithelioma of Pinkus have been reported. Postradiation sarcomas and atypical fibroxanthoma (pseudosarcoma of the skin) are even less common, and their clinical course is benign despite their highly anaplastic histological appearances. X-ray induced tumours should be excised.

28.9.3 CHEMICAL CARCINOGENS

A number of chemical carcinogens acting on the skin have been recognized. Coal tar, creosote oil, mineral oil, crude paraffin and cutting oil may be carcinogenic in unusual circumstances. Chimney sweeps were susceptible to scrotal cancer because of prolonged soiling of rugose skin with soot from coal fires. Cases of scrotal cancer due to lubricating and cutting oils have been described. Earlier this century arsenic was used as an ingredient of 'tonic' ('Fuller's Earth' or 'Parish's food'). It was also used as a treatment of syphilis. Elderly patients with keratotic intra-epithelial carcinomas on the palms and soles may have taken arsenical preparations. Arsenic ingestion is a cause of SCC and BCC.

28.9.4 WOUNDS

There are many anecdotal reports of carcinoma developing at sites of previous injury. Scarred areas undergoing cycles of healing and breakdown seem to be particularly susceptible. Malignant transformation may affect venous ulcers of the leg (Marjolin's ulcer).

28.9.5 HUMAN PAPILLOMA VIRUS

There is increasing evidence linking human papilloma viruses (HPVs) with skin cancer. HPV types 16 and 18 have been repeatedly detected in genital carcinomas and genital Bowen's disease. They are also implicated in some cases of non-genital skin cancers. Epidermodysplasia verruciformis is a rare, often hereditary disease, characterized by a generalized cutaneous infection with HPV, depressed cell-mediated immunity and a propensity for transformation of the warty lesions to SCC on predominantly sun exposed skin. HPV 5 and 8 are most closely associated with an oncogenic potential. HPV 16 has been identified in Bowen's disease (Kettler *et al.*, 1990) and SCC of the hands and feet (Eliezri *et al.*, 1990).

28.9.6 IMMUNOSUPPRESSION

Immunosuppression is associated with skin cancer. About a quarter of renal transplant patients in the UK have dysplastic skin lesions (Shuttleworth *et al.*, 1987). SCC usually occurs on sun exposed sites. Immunosuppressive drugs can result in an increased number of benign moles and a higher incidence of malignant melanoma (McLelland *et al.*, 1988). Kaposi's sarcoma, which frequently presents in the skin, is attributed to the immunosuppression of HIV infection.

28.9.7 GENETIC FACTORS

Genetic factors determining the risk of developing cutaneous melanoma include the presence of large number of banal moles, freckling, fair skin, blue eyes, red hair and clinically or pathologically dysplastic melanocytic naevi, and a history of severe blistering sunburn (MacKie *et al.*, 1989). About 50% of cutaneous melanomas originate within moles, or melanocytic naevi. Extensive congenital melanocytic naevi, some of which encompass a major proportion of the body surface, are more likely to undergo malignant transformation.

In general, it is accepted that dysplastic or atypical moles tend to be flatter and larger than most moles, with an ill defined blurred margin; there is colour variation and sometimes irregularity of edge. Individuals with dysplastic naevi are thought to have an increased risk of melanoma. The relative risk is about seven compared with a population without dysplastic naevi. This risk escalates to up to 400 if there is an additional family history of melanoma, and such individuals are said to have the familial dysplastic naevus syndrome. However, some authorities dispute the histological definition of dysplastic naevus (Clark and Ackerman, 1989). Consequently, others avoid this classification, and refer to the 'atypical mole syndrome' (AMS) as a **clinical** definition (Newton, 1993). Newton's definition also takes into account the unusual distribution of moles in AMS (Table 28.2).

Melanomas are a manifestation of the family cancer syndromes: Li–Fraumeni syndrome (LMS) and Lynch type II syndrome. LMS is a rare autosomal dominantly inherited syndrome, in which affected individuals develop multiple cancers in early adulthood. Recent evidence suggests that the human p53 tumour suppressor gene may be crucial, since germline p53 mutations have been discovered in affected families (Malkin *et al.*, 1990). The p53 suppressor protein is just one of the gene products which is thought to have an important role in the biology of human cutaneous melanoma.

A most striking example of genetic susceptibility to skin cancer is xeroderma pigmentosum, which is inherited as an autosomal recessive trait. It commonly results in death at an early age from multiple skin cancers. The extreme sensitivity of patients to UVR is attributed to a defective repair replication of DNA. Gorlin's syndrome (naevoid basal cell carcinoma syndrome) is transmitted by autosomal dominant inheritance, although there appears to be a high rate of spontaneous mutation accounting for sporadic cases. Multiple BCCs and palmar and plantar pits commonly appear during the second decade. Skeletal and central nervous system abnormalities are associated with the syndrome. Bony cysts of the mandible, frontal

Table 28.2 Scoring system for the atypical mole syndrome (AMS). Patients are said to be affected if they score 3 or more, but a score of 2 is suspicious of the AMS, especially in the presence of a melanoma (Newton, 1993).

Clinical features	Score
One or more iris melanocytic naevi	1
More than 100 moles (>2 mm in diameter) or more than 50 moles if aged < 20 or >50 years	1
2 or more clinically dysplastic moles	1
Moles on the anterior scalp	1
Moles abnormally distributed, e.g. buttocks and/or dorsum of the feet.	1
Total score	maximum of 5

bossing, bifid ribs, intracranial calcification and an increased risk of meduloblastoma and meningioma are associated features. Surgical excision is the preferred treatment of BCCs. Radiotherapy is said to be contraindicated because of the risk of inducing large numbers of BCCs within the irradiated area.

28.10 PREMALIGNANT CONDITIONS

28.10.1 SOLAR KERATOSES

Solar keratoses, or actinic keratoses, are ubiquitous in white, elderly populations. They represent areas of dysplastic epithelium on sun exposed skin. They present as erythematous, scaly patches which may be poorly defined. Their malignant potential is thought be extremely low; less than 1 in 1000 solar keratoses progress to SCC within 1 year (Marks *et al.*, 1988). Our aim is to treat symptomatic lesions only. Extensive solar keratoses can be regarded as a significant risk factor for non-melanoma skin cancer, and affected individuals should be carefully examined for evidence of BCC or SCC. Liquid nitrogen, applied for several seconds, is a well tolerated, effective treatment for solar keratoses, although recurrences frequently occur. Topical 5-fluorouracil is used for refractory areas. Topical retinoids (Retin A) reduce the size and number of solar keratoses if used regularly for 3–6 months, but cause erythema and irritation. 10–20% salicylic acid ointment can be used long term to reduce hyperkeratosis.

28.10.2 BOWEN'S DISEASE

Bowen's disease is an intra-epithelial SCC. Typically, erythematous, hyperkeratotic plaques have been present for many years. The risk of malignant transformation of Bowen's disease is much greater. Eventually 3–5% will develop into SCC, and therefore, treatment is advisable. Ideally lesions should be excised with a narrow margin. Cryotherapy and topical 5-fluorouracil are good alternatives for areas which would otherwise justify a skin graft. **Erythroplasia of Queyrat** is an uncommon intra-epidermal carcinoma, histologically similar to Bowen's disease, which affects the mucous membranes, particularly the penis. Well circumscribed, bright red, glistening plaques are situated on the glans penis. In this situation it can be considered as genital Bowen's disease. Erythroplasia responds to 5-fluorouracil. Untreated lesions may progress to SCC.

28.10.3 KERATOACANTHOMA

Keratoacanthoma is not truly premalignant, but has many of the features of malignancy during its evolution, when it can be difficult to distinguish from SCC both clinically and histologically. It is a rapidly growing squamous tumour which heals spontaneously within a few months to leave a residual scar. Treatment may reduce scarring. Since the tumour has a shallow, saucer shaped base, curettage and electrodissection is an excellent treatment. Radiotherapy is effective, but precludes histological analysis.

28.10.4 ORGANOID NAEVUS

The organoid naevus, or sebaceous naevus, is a hamartomatous malformation which comprises sebaceous glands, papillomatous hyperplasia of the epidermis, primordial hair follicles and apocrine sweat glands. It can be found in about 0.3% of all neonates. Solitary, circumscribed, pinkish, velvety, hairless plaques occur predominantly on the head and neck. At puberty the sebaceous glands mature, accounting for a more elevated, yellowish, waxy appearance; hence the synonym 'sebaceous naevus'. Malignant transformation occurs in over 5% of cases after adolescence, resulting in basal cell, sebaceous, apocrine and squamous carcinomas, most of which are of low grade malignancy. Excision of organoid naevi is advisable during early adulthood.

28.11 THE FUTURE

Future progress in skin cancer management will depend upon advances in prevention, early detection and treatment. Political intervention and public educational programmes will be of crucial importance. Molecular biology is expected to throw further light on the genetic aspects of melanoma, with the intriguing possibility that the relevant genes and oncogenes may be manipulated by drugs. There is concern that emphasis on these activities will lead to a hiatus in research development within the field of melanoma detection: without the necessary technology to reliably diagnose pigmented lesions, there is a risk that the advances on both a global and molecular scale will, in part, be wasted.

REFERENCES

Bart, R.S., Schrager, D., Kopf, A.W. *et al.* (1978) Scalpel excision of basal cell carcinomas. *Archives of Dermatology*, **114**, 739–42.

Breslow, A. (1970) Thickness, cross-sectional area and depth of invasion in the prognosis of cutaneous melanoma. *Annals of Surgery*, **172**, 902–8.

Brodland, D.G., Zitelli, J.A. (1992) Surgical margins for excision of primary cutaneous squamous cell carcinoma. *Journal of the American Academy of Dermatology*, **27**, 241–8.

Chew, S., Deleo, V. and Harber, L.C. (1988) Longwave ultraviolet radiation (UVA)-induced alteration of epidermal DNA synthesis. *Photochemistry and Photobiology*, **47**, 383–9.

Clark, W.H. and Ackerman, A.B. (1989) An exchange of views regarding the dysplastic nevus controversy. *Seminars in Dermatology*, **18**, 229–50.

Coleman, D.J. and Lizzi, F.L. (1983) Computerized ultrasonic tissue characterization of ocular tumours. *American Journal of Ophthalmology*, **96**, 165–75.

Curley, R.K., Cook, M.G., Fallowfield, M.E. and Marsden, R.A. (1989) Accuracy in clinically evaluating pigmented lesions. *British Medical Journal*, **299**, 16–18.

Department of Health (1992) *Health of the Nation – a strategy for health in England*, HMSO, London.

Doherty, V.R. and MacKie, R.N. (1988) Experience of a public educational programme on early detection of cutaneous malignant melanoma. *British Medical Journal*, **297**, 388–91.

Eliezri, Y.D., Silverstein, S.J. and Nuovo, G.J. (1990) Occurrence of human papillomavirus type 16 DNA in cutaneous squamous and basal cell neoplasms. *Archives of Dermatology*, **23**, 836–42.

Elwood, J.M., Gallagher, R.P., Hill, G.B. *et al.* (1985) Cutaneous melanoma in relation to intermittent and constant sun exposure. The Western Canada melanoma study. *International Journal of Cancer*, **35**, 427–33.

Friedman, H.I., Copper, P.H. and Wanebo, H.J. (1983) Prognostic and therapeutic use of microstaging of cutaneous squamous cell carcinoma of the trunk and extremities. *Cancer*, **56**, 1099–105.

Fusi, S. Ariyan, S. and Sternlicht, A. (1993) Data on first recurrence after treatment for malignant melanoma in a large patient population. *Plastic and Reconstructive Surgery*, **91**, 94–8.

Giles, G.G., Marks, R. and Foley, P. (1988) The incidence of non-melanocytic skin cancer in Australia. *British Medical Journal*, **296,** 13–17.

Kettler, A.H., Rutledge, M., Tschen, J.A. and Buffone, G. (1990) Detection of human papilloma virus in nongenital Bowen's disease by *in situ* DNA hybridization. *Archives of Dermatology*, **126**, 777–81.

Kraemer, K.H., DiGiovanna, J.J., Moshell, A.N. *et al.* (1988) Prevention of skin cancer in xeroderma pigmentosum with use of oral isotretinoin. *New England Journal of Medicine*, **318,** 1633–7.

Lindelöf, B., Sigurgeirsson, B., Tegner, E. *et al.* (1991) PUVA and cancer: a large-scale epidemiological study. *Lancet*, **338**, 91–3.

MacKie, R.M. (1990) Clinical recognition of early invasive malignant melanoma. *British Medical Journal*, **301**, 1005–6.

MacKie, R.M., Feudenberger, T. and Aitchison, T.C. (1989) Personal risk-factor chart for cutaneous melanoma. *Lancet*, **ii**, 487–90.

MacKie, R.M. and Hole, D. (1992) Audit of public education. Campaign to encourage earlier detection of malignant melanoma. *British Medical Journal*, **304**, 1012–5.

McLelland, J., Rees, A., Williams, G. and Chu, T. (1988) The incidence of immunosuppression-related skin disease in long-term transplant patients. *Transplantation*, **46**, 871–4.

McMichael, A.J. and Giles, G.G. (1988) Cancer in migrants to Australia extending the descriptive epidemiological data. *Cancer Research*, **48**, 751–6.

Malkin, D., Li, F.P., Strong, L.C. *et al.* (1990) Germline p53 mutations in a familial syndrome of breast cancer, sarcomas and other neoplasms. *Science*, **250**, 1233–8.

Marks, R., Jolley, D., Dorevitch, A.P. and Selwood, T.S. (1988) The incidence of non-melanocytic skin cancers in an Australian population: results of a five-year prospective study. *Medical Journal of Australasia*, **49**, 514–5.

Newton, J.A. (1993) Familial melanoma. *Clinical and Experimental Dermatology*, **18**, 5–11.

OPCS. (1993) *Cancer Statistics: registrations 1987*, HMSO, London.

Ruark, D.S., Shaw, H.M., Ingvar, C. *et al.* (1993) Who detects the first recurrence in stage I cutaneous malignant melanoma: patient or doctor? *Melanoma Research*, **3**, (Suppl 1), 44.

Shuttleworth, D., Marks, R., Griffin, P.G.A. and Salaman, J.R. (1987) Dysplastic epidermal change in immunosuppressed patients with renal transplants. *Quarterly Journal of Medicine*, **64**, 609–16.

Steiner, A., Pehamberger, H. and Wolff, K. (1987) *In vivo* epiluminescence microscopy of pigmented skin lesions. II Diagnosis of small pigmented skin lesions and early detection of malignant melanoma. *Journal of American Academy of Dermatology*, **17**, 584–91.

Streilein, J.W. (1991) Immunogenetic factors in skin cancer. *New England Journal of Medicine*, **325**, 884–7.

Tangrea, J.A., Edwards, B.K., Taylor, P.R. *et al.* (1992) Long-term therapy with low-dose isotretinoin for prevention of basal cell carcinoma: a multicentre clinical trial. *Journal of the National Cancer Institute*, **84**, 328–32.

Thames Cancer Registry. (1992) *Cancer in South West Thames 1987–1989*, Thames Cancer Registry, Sutton.

Veronesi, U., Cascinelli, N., Adamus, J. *et al.* (1988) Thin stage I primary cutaneous malignant melanoma. Comparison of excision with margins of 1 or 3 cms. *New England Journal of Medicine*, **318**, 1159–62.

Wolf, D.J. and Zitelli, J.A. (1987) Surgical margins for basal cell carcinoma. *Archives of Dermatology*, **123**, 340–4.

Michael Brada

29.1 EPIDEMIOLOGY

Primary tumours of the central nervous system (CNS) are uncommon, with an age adjusted incidence ranging from 6 to 12 per 100 000 population per year. Yet primary intracranial tumours are the second commonest neoplastic disease of childhood and the brain and spinal cord are a frequent site of metastatic disease.

Primary brain tumours have specific age predilection. Primitive neuroectodermal tumours (PNETs), pilocytic astrocytomas, craniopharyngiomas and optic nerve gliomas occur most frequently in childhood, intracranial germ cell tumours present in the teens and early twenties, while the incidence of most glial and meningeal tumours is highest in adults and increases with age. Gliomas constitute the largest histological group of primary brain tumours.

29.2 AETIOLOGY

29.2.1 INHERITED PREDISPOSITION

Type I neurofibromatosis (von Recklinghausen's disease, NF1) predisposes to the development of optic nerve/chiasma glioma as well as meningioma and other glial tumours. Type 2 neurofibromatosis (NF2; bilateral acoustic neuroma) is associated with increased incidence of meningiomas which are often multiple. Other genetic predispositions are shown in Table 29.1

29.2.2 ACQUIRED

Immune deficiency following organ transplantation and with HIV infection is associated with increased incidence of primary cerebral lymphoma. Cranial irradiation in childhood in the form of scalp irradiation for the treatment of tinea capitis (Ron *et al.*, 1988) and as prophylactic cranial irradiation in acute lymphatic leukaemia is associated with an increased risk of development of glioma and meningioma (Neglia *et al.*, 1991). Similar tumours have also been described following radiotherapy for benign tumours such as pituitary adenoma and craniopharyngioma.

29.3 MOLECULAR ASPECTS OF BRAIN TUMOUR BIOLOGY

Loss of heterozygosity with deletions on chromosome 22 has been identified in meningiomas in association with NF2 and in sporadic meningiomas, suggesting loss of suppressor gene as a predisposing factor in the aetiology of both types of meningioma (Seizinger *et al.*, 1987; Collins *et al.*, 1990). Haemangioblastomas in patients with von Hippel–Lindau syndrome are associated with an allele loss on chromosome 3. Specific gene locus has not been detected in glial tumours although a number of changes have been identified which are seen in glial tumours and some which accompany the progression of glioma from low to high grade. These include gains of chromosome 7, loss of part or whole

Table 29.1 Familiar disorders predisposing to a higher risk of primary CNS neoplasm

Familial predisposition	Associated brain neoplasms
Peripheral neurofibromatosis (von Recklinghausen's disease, NF1)	Optic nerve glioma Astrocytoma Ependymoma
Central neurofibromatosis (bilateral acoustic neurofibroma, NF2)	Meningioma
Gorlin's syndrome	Medulloblastoma
Tuberous sclerosis	Giant cell astrocytoma
Turcot's syndrome (familial adenomatous.polyposis and brain tumour)	Medulloblastoma Astrocytoma
von Hippel–Lindau syndrome	Haemangioblastoma

of chromosome 10, loss of material from chromosome 17 and amplification of epidermal growth factor receptor (EGF-R) gene in 30–40% of glial tumours (for review see Akbasak and Sunar-Akbasak, 1992). Gene amplification is often associated with mutation of the EGF-R gene and production of abnormal protein. Although the NF1 gene is present on chromosome 17 its direct association with glial tumours has not been demonstrated.

29.4 PATHOLOGY

Primary intracranial tumours may arise from any intracranial tissue including glia, neurones, meninges, vessels or endocrine apparatus. A modified WHO classification which defines tumour type on the basis of the putative cell of origin is shown in Table 29.2. The commonest brain tumours are of neuroepithelial origin and include low and high grade astrocytomas. Based on cellular and tissue features many of the brain tumours can be graded according to the degree of malignancy. However the distinction into benign and malignant neoplasms is not as clear as in systemic tumours. Apparently histologically benign tumours can be invasive and simply the presence of a space occupying lesion within the cranial cavity may be fatal. The majority of intracranial tumours do not metastasize but spread locally within the

CNS. Germ cell tumours can disseminate systemically via shunts while medulloblastomas and primary cerebral lymphomas may relapse outside the CNS without shunting.

29.5 CLINICAL MANIFESTATION AND DIAGNOSIS OF BRAIN TUMOURS

Patients with a brain tumour present with a combination of features of raised intracranial pressure, epilepsy and focal or global neurological deficit. Focal or generalized convulsions first appearing in adults indicate a structural brain lesion and may be the first or only presenting feature of a brain tumour.

The investigation of choice in patients with suspected brain tumour is CT scan or MRI. CT scan usually demonstrates distortion of normal brain architecture and the presence of a space occupying lesion of varying radiological density. The degree of enhancement following intravenous contrast is characteristic for each tumour type. Enhancing lesions have to be distinguished from abscess, multiple sclerosis, infection, sarcoid, vascular abnormalities and haemorrhage. Low density unenhancing lesions have to be differentiated from localized encephalitis, multiple sclerosis or infarction.

MRI provides similar information to CT scan with better contrast discrimination and more sophisticated display. It is superior in demonstrating lesions in the posterior and

Table 29.2 WHO classification of CNS tumours

I	Tumours of neuroepithelial tissue
A.	Astrocytic tumours including
	Astrocytoma
	Anaplastic (malignant) astrocytoma
	Glioblastoma
	Pilocytic astrocytoma
	Pleomorphic xanthoastrocytoma
	Subependymal giant cell astrocytoma
B.	Oligodendroglial tumours
C.	Ependymal tumours
D.	Mixed gliomas
E.	Choroid plexus tumours
F.	Neuroepithelial tumours of uncertain origin
G.	Neuronal and mixed neuronal-glial tumours
	including ganglioglioma, central neurocytoma, olfactory neuroblastoma
H.	Pineal tumours
	pineocytoma and pineoblastoma
I.	Embryonal tumours
	including neuroblastoma, ependymoblastoma, retinoblastoma and primitive neuroectodermal tumours (PNETs) especially medulloblastoma
II	Tumours of cranial and spinal nerves
	Schwannoma and neurofibroma
III	Tumours of the meninges
A.	Tumours of meningothelial cells
	Meningioma (bening, atypical and malignant)
B.	Mesenchymal, non-meningothelial tumours
	Benign or malignant (e.g. meningeal sarcoma)
C.	Primary melanocytic lesions
	Melanosis, melanocytoma and malignant melanoma
D.	Tumours of uncertain origin
	Haemangiopericytoma and haemangioblastoma
IV	Haemopoietic neoplasms
	including primary cerebral lymphoma and plasmacytoma
V	Germ cell tumours
	esp. germinoma and teratoma
VI	Cysts and tumour-like lesions
VII	Tumours of the anterior pituitary
	Pituitary adenoma
VIII	Malformations and local extensions of regional tumours
	craniopharyngioma
	chordoma, chondroma and chondrosarcoma
IX	Metastatic tumours

temporal fossi as it is free of bone artefacts although calcification and bone changes are more difficult to demonstrate. Cerebral angiography may help to distinguish vascular lesions (AVMs and aneurysms) from neoplasia and demonstrate the details of circulation prior to surgical intervention. MR angiography demonstrates larger vessels without the need for contrast angiography.

Positron emission tomography (PET) has currently little primary diagnostic role. The degree of glucose uptake and anaerobic glycolysis correlates with histological grade in glial tumours. FDG (fluorodeoxyglucose) uptake may help to distinguish tumour recurrence from necrosis following high dose focal irradiation. PET imaging is also used to study amino acid metabolism, nucleotide incorporation and the integrity of blood–brain barrier and blood–tumour barrier.

In the diagnosis of spinal tumours MRI with and without contrast (gadolinium EDTA) is the investigation of choice. If not available, plain X-ray and CT myelography are used although the enhancement characteristics of intrinsic cord lesions cannot be demonstrated.

29.6 TREATMENT OF BRAIN TUMOURS

29.6.1 MEDICAL MANAGEMENT

Prior to definitive diagnosis and before specific antitumour therapy patients with features of raised intracranial pressure are treated empirically with corticosteroids (initial oral dexamethasone 4 mg three to four times daily) and occasionally with osmotic diuresis (10–20% mannitol, 100–200 ml, given two or three times a day). This provides symptomatic relief and may also produce a transient improvement in focal neurological deficit. Corticosteroid dose should be gradually reduced and titrated against symptoms to the lowest effective level. In patients who derive little or no benefit they should be withdrawn. Once definitive antitumour therapy

has started it is important to monitor the dose closely and discontinue corticosteroids at the earliest opportunity to avoid potentially disabling long term side-effects. Epilepsy is treated with appropriate anticonvulsants.

29.6.2 SURGERY

Neurosurgical intervention as in other oncological surgery aims to obtain tissue for histological diagnosis and remove tumour with curative or palliative intent. However, the direct tumour involvement of eloquent regions in the brain increases the hazards of any surgical procedure, often with unacceptable consequences.

Neurosurgical techniques have seen great advances. Image directed stereotactic methods allow three dimensional (3D) localization and visualization of intracranial lesions. Stereotactically guided needle biopsy can obtain small tissue samples with high precision. It carries minimal morbidity and obviates the need for craniotomy. Surgical resection can also be aided by 3D image reconstructions from CT and MRI in the plane of resection and by intraoperative ultrasound and endoscopy. Awake craniotomy with electrophysiological mapping also allows for more controlled tumour resection with diminished morbidity. Traditional neurosurgical approaches involve access through a craniotomy, lifting a skull flap with biopsy or resection under direct vision. However, previously inaccessible sites to conventional craniotomy such as the region of the skull base can now be reached through novel transoral, facial or orbital approaches. Nevertheless, deep seated hemispheric or brain stem tumours cannot be removed without unacceptable neurological morbidity.

Benign tumours in accessible locations, such as meningiomas, small secretory pituitary adenomas, choroid plexus tumours and low grade (pilocytic) posterior fossa astrocytomas in childhood, can be cured by complete surgical excision. Malignant tumours are usually widely infiltrating and complete excision is rarely if ever possible. Tumour resection provides effective relief of symptoms but in most malignant tumours the influence of extent of resection on tumour control and survival is not clear. In patients with suspected malignant tumours surgery is frequently limited to a biopsy. Radical resection is important in some malignant tumours such as medulloblastoma.

Palliative surgical procedures such as shunting and cyst drainage are important components of treatment and palliative tumour resection may be useful in patients with symptomatic poorly chemo- and radio-responsive tumours.

29.6.3 RADIOTHERAPY

Radiotherapy is one of the most effective treatment modalities in the management of patients with intracranial tumours. In some rare malignant brain tumours such as germinoma, radiotherapy is curative. The excellent disease control following conservative surgery and radiotherapy in the more benign tumours, e.g. optic nerve glioma, pituitary adenoma and craniopharyngioma, has established radiotherapy as the essential component of treatment. Radical radiotherapy is also a potentially curative treatment in PNETs. In high grade gliomas radiotherapy achieves prolongation of disease free survival and survival. In low grade glioma and meningioma the role of radiotherapy is not proven beyond doubt and the suggestion of its effectiveness is based on selected series of patients receiving radiotherapy following incomplete tumour excision. Radiotherapy is also an effective palliative treatment in patients with brain metastases.

The amount of radiation which can be delivered to CNS tumours is limited by the radiation tolerance of the brain and spinal cord. Radiation damage can be classified according to time of appearance into early delayed and late delayed, although transient acute reactions also occur (Gutin *et al.*, 1991). Late radiation damage to the CNS is due to depletion of target population of oligodendrocytes and endothelial cells and leads to demyelination and necrosis and consequent neurological deficit specific to the damaged site. Late damage to the spine is expressed as progressive radiation myelopathy causing paraparesis. The risk of late injury is highly fractionation dependent with highest risk of damage following a large dose given in a few fractions. Neurological sequelae of radiation are also enhanced by chemotherapy given either within a short time of radiation or concurrently. Combination of methotrexate and brain irradiation causes severe leucoencephalopathy and combination of intrathecal cytosine arabinoside and radiation also produces severe damage.

Developing brain is particularly sensitive to injury and brain irradiation in young children results in severe neuropsychological impairment. Cranial irradiation is best avoided for children under 3–4 years of age. The likelihood of global damage diminishes with full myelination and beyond the age of 7 years the neurotoxicity is similar to that in adults. The pituitary gland is also sensitive to radiation with delayed pituitary failure which is dose dependent.

Conventional external beam radiotherapy is used either in the form of localized irradiation with two, three or four fields, or with extended field techniques treating the whole brain or the entire craniospinal axis. The precision of cranial irradiation has improved with the use of neurosurgically derived stereotactic technology. Highly localized radiation which achieves better sparing of normal tissue can be given by stereotactic external beam radiotherapy (SRT) (Brada and Graham, 1993) or by stereotactically guided interstitial radiotherapy. SRT, as fractionated or single fraction treatment (described as 'radiosurgery'), can be delivered either with a conventional linear accelerator with multiple non-coplanar fixed beams or multiple arcs of rotation or with a dedicated multi-headed cobalt unit (described as gamma knife). Linear accelerator based techniques can treat larger and irregular volumes and are more versatile while gamma knife produces a high precision treatment of smaller lesions. SRT is currently suitable only for volumes < 5 cm diameter. Stereotactic radiotherapy is used as single fraction treatment for eradication of small inoperable arteriovenous malformations and as single fraction or fractionated therapy it is being investigated in the treatment of small brain tumours, particularly solitary brain metastases.

29.6.4 CHEMOTHERAPY

Because of the presence of the blood–brain barrier (BBB) the effectiveness of chemotherapy has been considered to be limited on theoretical grounds. However the blood–tumour barrier (BTB) is usually permeable and the main determinant of the effectiveness of chemotherapy is most likely the primary chemosensitivity of the individual tumour types. Cranial germ cell tumours, PNETs and primary cerebral lymphomas are chemosensitive intracranial tumours and chemotherapy is being used with increasing frequency, although its precise role in the management of these tumours is not yet fully defined. Although the overall effectiveness of chemotherapy in gliomas is poor it occasionally achieves palliation in recurrent tumours and in an adjuvant setting produces marginal survival advantage (Stenning *et al.*, 1987).

29.6.5 NEW MODALITIES

Monoclonal and polyclonal antitumour antibodies have been tested in patients with intracranial tumours. Intrathecal administration of radiolabelled antibody has some effectiveness in metastatic lymphoid and some non-glial tumours with meningeal/CSF dissemination. Gene transfer techniques are being tested in the treatment of rodent brain tumour xenografts (Culver *et al.*, 1992).

Boron neutron capture therapy (BNCT), where the stable isotope boron-10 is irradiated with low energy thermal neutrons to produce α particles and lithium-7 nuclei is being exploited in the treatment of experimental gliomas (Barth *et al.*, 1992) and may have a potential clinical application.

29.6.6 REHABILITATION

Patients with CNS tumours frequently have major neurological deficit with physical disability as well as cognitive impairment, communication difficulties and personality change. All those with a reasonable life expectancy need active rehabilitation managed by a multidisciplinary rehabilitation team. Rehabilitation should not await the completion of specific therapy but should be started shortly after diagnosis as an integral part of management. The diagnosis of brain tumour and disability have a devastating psychological effect on the patient, the family and friends and all require sympathetic and practical support.

29.7 SPECIFIC BRAIN TUMOURS

29.7.1 GLIOMAS

Gliomas are neuroepithelial tumours arising from supporting glial tissue and are classified as astrocytomas, oligodendrogliomas and ependymomas. Astrocytomas constitute two-thirds of all gliomas and are graded on the basis of cytological and tissue features into Kernohan grades 1–4 or according to WHO classification into three grades of increasing malignancy as astrocytoma, anaplastic astrocytoma and glioblastoma. Pilocytic astrocytoma and giant cell astrocytoma are localized low grade gliomas and are classified separately.

(a) High grade astrocytomas

High grade astrocytomas are the most common primary malignant brain tumours and are classified into anaplastic astrocytoma and glioblastoma. The incidence increases with age and peaks between 65 and 75 years. Anaplastic astrocytoma and glioblastoma are distinguished by the degree of cellular anaplasia, pleomorphism, necrosis, and the presence of endothelial proliferation and haemorrhage. The grading of astrocytomas is difficult due to tumour heterogeneity and the potential sampling error when based on small tissue biopsy. In addition there is considerable interobserver variation. On CT scan high grade gliomas are usually inhomogeneous hyperdense masses enhancing after intravenous contrast and surrounded by peritumour oedema.

Treatment

Clinical suspicion of diagnosis requires histological confirmation usually by stereotactic biopsy. Surgical tumour debulking provides effective palliation of raised intracranial pressure and often improvement of neurological deficit. Although retrospective studies suggest that more extensive tumour resection is associated with prolonged survival (Wood *et al.*, 1988; Quigley and Maroon, 1991), there are no randomized studies addressing the issue and it is likely that it is the resectability of the tumour rather than the debulking itself which determines the outcome.

Radiotherapy is the mainstay of treatment and is effective in prolonging survival as demonstrated in randomized studies (Walker *et al.*, 1978; Kristiansen *et al.*, 1981). However, long term tumour control and survival remain poor. In patients with responding tumours radiotherapy together with rehabilitation also improve neurological deficit and quality of life. The current radiotherapy practice is to treat patients with daily fractions over a period of 6 weeks to a dose of 55–60 Gy

to the tumour and a margin of suspected infiltration 3–5 cm beyond the region of enhancement on CT scan. Radiotherapy can be delivered using 'accelerated fractionation' where the same dose is given two or three times a day over a shorter period of time. When compared to conventional fractionation survival is not significantly different but the overall duration of treatment is shortened.

Lower doses of radiation result in worse survival (Bleehen and Stenning, 1991), while increasing the dose of localized irradiation with stereotactic external beam radiotherapy or with brachytherapy may improve tumour control and is currently being tested in randomized trials. However additional high dose localized irradiation carries a risk of radiation necrosis within the high dose volume which is a cause of morbidity and may require surgical intervention.

Nitrosoureas (BCNU, CCNU, ACNU) are at present the most effective chemotherapeutic agents in the treatment of high grade gliomas. In randomized studies of adjuvant chemotherapy, the overall survival advantage is 9% at 1 year and 3% at 2 years with no increase in long term survival (Stenning *et al.*, 1987). Current debate centres on the value of adjuvant chemotherapy to an individual patient with high grade glioma. It is a reasonable practice not to offer routine adjuvant chemotherapy as the small potential benefit may be outweighed by treatment toxicity. However, the poor overall results should encourage clinicians to enter patients into randomized trials testing new treatment approaches.

New treatment approaches

Considerable research effort is directed to finding new ways of controlling malignant gliomas. As well as optimization of conventional treatment modalities, novel treatments are being tested in patients with recurrent high grade glioma and occasionally as adjuvant therapy.

Refinement of radiotherapy technology with stereotactically guided conformal radiotherapy allows for higher radiation doses without increasing toxicity. It achieves prolongation of disease control in patients with recurrent disease although there are no cures (Laing *et al.*, 1993a). We have to await the results of randomized studies to prove the effectiveness of stereotactic radiotherapy.

Conventional radiosensitizers have not prolonged survival and a new generation of selective radiosensitizers for proliferating tissues (BUDR and IUDR) are currently under test. New radiation modalities in the form of protons or neutrons have not so far demonstrated survival benefit (for review see Brada, 1989). Tumours can potentially be locally irradiated with BNCT (Barth *et al.*, 1992). The selectivity is based on the localization of uptake of boron containing compounds into the tumour and subsequent release of α particles and lithium nuclei on exposure to low energy thermal neutrons. BNCT is under intensive investigation in a number of centres but prior to introduction into clinical studies requires further technical development and preclinical testing.

Chemotherapy given in high dose together with autologous bone marrow transplantation has so far not been successful in the treatment of high grade gliomas (Mbidde *et al.*, 1988).

However, inhibition of DNA repair enzyme O^6 alkylguanine-DNA-alkyltranspherase may increase the activity of nitrosoureas and derivatives in selected patients. Targeted therapy has concentrated on antibodies to EGF-R which is overexpressed in some high grade gliomas. There are a number of other tumour targets for antibody therapy and these include tenascin and a mutated form of EGF-R which may be truly tumour specific.

Experimental brain tumours in rodents have been successfully treated by *in situ* retroviral-mediated transfer of Herpes thymidine kinase gene into proliferating brain tumour tissue and subsequent treatment with ganciclovir (Culver *et al.*, 1992).

Treatment recommendations and prognosis

The median survival of patients with high grade glioma treated with conservative surgery and radiotherapy is 40–50 weeks with only 10–20% of patients surviving 2 years. Old age, high histological grade and poor performance status are the most important adverse determinants of survival (Shapiro, 1986). Short history of symptoms, the absence of convulsions and limited resection are additional poor prognostic features of lesser significance. The current treatment recommendation is biopsy or tumour debulking fol-

Table 29.3   The Royal Marsden Hospital treatment policy in patients with high grade glioma

Prognostic category	Age (years)	Performance status (KPS)	Policy	RT regimen
Favourable	<65	KPS >40	Radical RT	Daily: 55–60 Gy in 30 fractions once a day accelerated: 55 Gy in 34 fractions twice daily
Unfavourable	≥65	KPS >40	Palliative RT or no treatment	30 Gy in 6 fractions in 2 weeks
	<65	KPS <40		

Chemotherapy: no routine chemotherapy but patients are asked to enter into multicentre randomized studies of adjuvant therapy.
Radiotherapy target volume: tumour plus 3–5 cm margin.
RT, radiotherapy; KPS, Karnofsky performance score.

lowed by radiotherapy (Table 29.3). The treatment has to be tailored to the patient's age and general condition. In severely disabled and elderly patients with a short life expectancy it may be appropriate not to offer active treatment. In addition to palliative care, and specific antitumour treatment, patients and families require sympathetic care and intensive support from many professionals within a neuro-oncology team

(b)   Low grade gliomas

Low grade gliomas include low grade astrocytomas (defined as grades I and II astrocytomas on Kernohan grading and as astrocytoma on WHO classification), oligodendrogliomas, mixed oligo-astrocytomas and low grade ependymomas as well as a subgroup of localized gliomas (see above). They present with slow onset and a long history of features of intracranial tumour and presentation with convulsions is particularly common. On CT scanning low grade gliomas tend to be of low density without enhancement and are occasionally associated with calcification. The MR features are equivalent with low signal intensity lesion on T1 and high intensity on T2 images without gadolinium enhancement.

Astrocytomas are usually infiltrating tumours occurring in all age groups while pilocytic astrocytomas are well localized and present predominantly in childhood in the posterior fossa although there are hemispheric histological counterparts in adults. Oligodendrogliomas and mixed oligoastrocytomas which consist of both astrocytic and oligodendroglial components occur in all age groups with a peak incidence between 40 and 60 years.

Ependymomas project from ependymal surfaces, most commonly the floor of the fourth ventricle, and less frequently from the canal of the spinal cord, or the lateral and third ventricles and may also arise in the brain parenchyma. Ependymomas are graded

into low and high grade variants. The term ependymoblastoma is reserved for PNET with ependymal differentiation.

Treatment

Posterior fossa pilocytic astrocytomas, particularly of the cystic type, and low grade ependymomas of the fourth ventricle are best treated with radical resection. Other low grade gliomas, in particular astrocytomas and oligodendrogliomas, often diffusely involve cerebral parenchyma and are not fully excisable. They are usually biopsied with debulking as a palliative procedure in selected patients.

The role of radiotherapy in the treatment of low grade gliomas is controversial and is currently being tested in prospective randomized studies, although retrospective studies of incompletely excised tumours suggest a survival advantage (Shaw *et al.*, 1989). Radiotherapy is an effective symptomatic treatment. It stabilizes or improves the neurological deficit caused by the tumour. The practice in the Royal Marsden Hospital is conventional radiotherapy technique to a localized volume including the abnormal region seen on CT/MRI and a 2–4 cm margin to a dose of 55–60 Gy over a period of 6 weeks.

Patients with ependymoma are at 8–10% risk of developing spinal seeding via the CSF pathway and the incidence relates to tumour grade, tumour localization and tumour control at the primary site (Vanuytsel and Brada, 1991; Vanuytsel *et al.*, 1992). As there is no evidence that prophylactic spinal irradiation prevents spinal seeding, neuraxis irradiation in ependymoma is no longer recommended.

The prognosis in low grade gliomas relates to histology, age, performance status and the extent of resection (Shaw *et al.*, 1989; Vanuytsel *et al.*, 1992). The 5 year survival rate for patients with pilocytic astrocytoma is approximately 85% and for patients with astrocytoma, oligodendroglioma and mixed oligo-astrocytoma 50%. The 5 year survival of patients with low grade cranial ependymomas is also 50–60%.

(c)   Brain stem gliomas

Glial tumours may involve any region of the brain including the thalamus, hypothalamus and the brain stem from mid brain to pons and medulla. Patients with brain stem tumours present with a variety of cranial nerve palsies and other posterior fossa signs often causing severe disability. Excision of brain stem tumours is not possible and frequently even surgical biopsy is considered hazardous. The prognosis of verified and unverified brain stem gliomas is poor and relates to histological grade and resectability. Radiotherapy is the mainstay of treatment and frequently results in neurological improvement. The dose fractionation schedules are similar to those of low grade gliomas.

29.7.2   MENINGIOMAS

Meningiomas comprise 10–20% of intracranial tumours and their frequency increases with age. They arise in the arachnoid villi of the meninges in the cerebral convexity, the falx and less frequently sphenoid and suprasellar region, posterior fossa and the tentorium. Most meningiomas are encapsulated solitary tumours attached to the dura. In patients with NF2 they may be multiple. Invasion of the brain parenchyma in benign meningiomas is rare but tumours may invade adjacent skull eliciting an osteoblastic reaction which can be seen on skull X-ray.

Meningiomas present in an indolent fashion with gradual development of focal deficit and occasionally deterioration in intellectual function and personality, which may pass unnoticed. The characteristic CT appearance of a meningioma is a well defined extra-axial mass with attachment to the meningeal surface. It is usually uniformly hyperdense, showing homogeneous enhancement with contrast.

There are a number of histological variants of benign meningioma describing the predominant cell pattern. The histological subgroups have no prognostic significance except haemangiopericytic and angioblastic forms which are considered to have a worse prognosis. More aggressive behaviour of meningioma is also associated with higher mitotic rate, necrosis and cellular atypia. Malignant meningeal sarcoma has the appearance of a spindle cell sarcoma and is an invasive malignant tumour.

Treatment

The primary treatment of benign meningioma is complete surgical resection. Tumours which are poorly accessible through conventional craniotomy (e.g. sphenoid) can be approached through skull base techniques, which improve access and may allow for complete tumour excision. Radiotherapy is reserved for patients with incomplete excision of benign meningioma. Retrospective studies suggest that an extended course of high dose treatment (55–60 Gy in 6 weeks) localized to the residual tumour site halves the risk of recurrence (Barbaro *et al.*, 1987; Glaholm *et al.*, 1990). Radiotherapy has also been recommended as adjuvant treatment following incomplete excision of malignant meningioma, although the effectiveness is not proven. Patients with recurrent meningioma after previous surgery and radiotherapy may be considered for stereotactic radiotherapy/radiosurgery providing surgery is not feasible and the tumour is of appropriate size.

Meningiomas and meningioma cultures contain progesterone and androgen receptors and their inhibition leads to tumour responses in tumour models *in vitro* and *in vivo*. The antiprogesterone agent mifepristone has shown some clinical activity and is currently under test.

Prognosis

The prognosis in patients with meningioma is determined by extent of surgery, tumour histology and neurological performance status. The recurrence rate following complete excision of benign meningioma is less than 3%. Incompletely excised benign tumours following radiotherapy have a 5 year progression free survival of 80–85% (15–20% recurrence rate) (Glaholm *et al.*, 1990). Prognosis in patients with completely excised malignant meningioma/sarcoma is poor, with a median survival of less than 1 year.

29.7.3 PRIMITIVE NEUROECTODERMAL TUMOURS

PNETs have a common histological appearance of densely cellular masses of uniform small oval or round cells. They include medulloblastoma, ependymoblastoma and pineoblastoma. Medulloblastomas are the commonest PNETs as well as the commonest brain tumour in childhood, although in adults they represent only 1–2% of intracranial tumours. They arise from the cerebellum and may invade the fourth ventricle, brain stem and extend inferiorly as far as the foramen magnum. Medulloblastomas and PNETs have a tendency to seed through the subarachnoid space to the spinal cord and distant intracranial sites.

Patients with medulloblastoma present with cerebellar signs and occasionally brain stem cranial nerve palsies and hydrocephalus. MRI is the investigation of choice and demonstrates a homogeneously enhancing posterior fossa mass with distortion of the fourth ventricle. Histological confirmation is necessary to distinguish medulloblastoma from other posterior fossa tumours such as ependymoma, glioma and solitary cerebellar metastasis and usually awaits definitive surgery.

Treatment and prognosis

Patients with suspected medulloblastoma require radical surgery and craniospinal irradiation. Following surgery full staging investigations include CSF cytology for the presence of malignant cells and a myelogram or spinal MRI to detect occult spinal seeding. Postoperative radiotherapy is indicated in all patients regardless of the extent of tumour resection. The whole craniospinal axis is irradiated to a dose of 30–35 Gy and this is followed by a boost to the posterior fossa to a total dose of 55 Gy. Isolated spinal seeding is treated with a local boost.

Adjuvant chemotherapy has been tested in large randomized trials. Although there is no overall survival advantage for the whole group of patients with medulloblastoma, those with poor prognostic factors which include evidence of metastatic disease, brain stem involvement and incomplete tumour excision, show a survival benefit with chemotherapy (Evans *et al.*, 1990; Tait *et al.*, 1990). The adjuvant chemotherapy regimens tested were usually given after radiotherapy and include CCNU and vincristine. Newer treatment regimens include a combination of cisplatin or carboplatin, cyclophosphamide and occasionally anthracyclines and are given prior to definitive radiotherapy. Such treatment approaches are currently tested in randomized trials.

With present treatment strategies the 5 year survival of children with medulloblastoma is 50–60%. The chance of recurrence beyond the first 5 years is less than 10%. The most frequent site of relapse is the primary site in the cerebellum, although the disease may recur elsewhere in the brain and in the spine and occasionally in the bone marrow. Reported survival rates in adults are comparable to those obtained in children and treatment strategies are identical (Bloom and Bessell, 1990) although current randomized studies do not include adults.

29.7.4 PINEAL TUMOURS

Germ cell tumours including germinoma and teratoma represent more than 60% of the tumours in the pineal region, and germinomas which are histologically equivalent to testicular seminomas are the commonest type. Pineal tumours may also be of pineal parenchymal origin (pineocytoma or pineo-blastoma) or gliomas (Bloom, 1983) (Table 29.4).

Table 29.4   Lesions around the third ventricle

Region	Lesion
Sellar and parasellar	Pituitary adenoma
	Craniopharyngioma
	Germ cell tumour
	Langerhan's cell
	histiocytosis
	Sarcoid granuloma
	Optic chiasmal glioma
	Benign cyst
	Other gliomas
Pineal	Germinoma
	Teratoma
	Pineocytoma
	Pineoblastoma
	Glioma

Pineal region tumours usually present with hydrocephalus and features of compression of the quadrigeminal plate with paresis of upward gaze and pupils unresponsive to light or accommodation (Parinaud's syndrome). Most pineal tumours are hyperdense on CT scanning and show contrast enhancement with equivalent MR characteristics. It is not possible to differentiate individual tumour types on imaging alone.

Cranial germ cell tumours as their testicular and ovarian counterparts may secrete alphafetoprotein (AFP) or human chorionic gonadotrophin (HCG). The detection of AFP in plasma or CSF is specific for non-seminomatous germ cell tumour (teratoma) while HCG may be elevated in teratoma or germinoma.

All patients with pineal tumours should have assessment of serum tumour markers prior to biopsy. In the absence of elevated tumour markers, diagnosis should be confirmed by a biopsy which is either stereotactically guided or performed under endoscopic vision. Occasionally such a procedure is considered hazardous and response to a small dose of local irradiation in the initial phase of treatment has been used as a diagnostic test. A reduction in the size or complete disappearance of pineal tumour following 20 Gy of localized radiation is compatible with the diagnosis of germinoma.

Management

Serum/CSF AFP and HCG should be measured prior to histological verification. Biopsy is recommended in most cases of unverified pineal tumour with normal markers. In the presence of hydrocephalus patients are considered for shunting. However, if germ cell tumour is suspected, shunting may increase the risk of systemic seeding and should be delayed to enable spontaneous drainage which may occur following successful primary therapy. Postsurgical staging in germ cell tumours should include CSF markers and CSF cytology as well as myelogram or high resolution spinal MRI.

The role of surgical excision in the management of pineal tumours is controversial. It is a potentially hazardous procedure with no obvious benefit in germinoma, pineoblastoma or glioma. However, the excision of a residual teratoma following chemotherapy and radiotherapy and primary excision of localized pineocytoma may be curative.

Radiotherapy is the treatment of choice in localized pineal germinoma and is curative in most patients. Local radiotherapy to the pineal region is given to a dose of 40–50 Gy. The addition of craniospinal irradiation depends on staging of disease and therefore the perceived risk of CNS seeding (Brada and Rajan, 1990). Spinal irradiation reduces the risk of spinal relapse but this should be balanced against the potential toxicity of wide field irradiation, particularly in children with incomplete skeletal growth and in girls whose ovaries may be included in the radiation field. Localized germinoma is therefore treated with craniospinal irradiation to 25–30 Gy except in prepubertal children and women where this can be given on an individual basis. This is followed by a boost to the primary site to a dose of 40–45 Gy.

Cranial germ cell tumours are chemosensitive and potentially curable with chemotherapy (Allen *et al.*, 1987). Chemotherapy is being exploited as part of primary treatment in disseminated or locally extensive germinoma and as the treatment of choice in verified teratomas. Disseminated germinoma should be treated either with craniospinal irradiation and a boost or with a short course of cisplatin/carboplatin containing chemotherapy followed by craniospinal irradiation to a dose of 25–30 Gy and a boost to 40–45 Gy. Teratomas are best treated with primary chemotherapy with platinum/carboplatin containing regimens used in systemic testicular tumours. This is followed by craniospinal axis irradiation and a boost to the primary site. Residual masses in the pineal region may be excised or treated with stereotactic external beam radiotherapy.

In patients with pineoblastoma, craniospinal axis irradiation is mandatory and is followed by a boost. The technique and doses are identical to those used in medulloblastoma. The role of radiotherapy in pineocytoma is not clear.

29.7.5 PRIMARY CEREBRAL LYMPHOMA

Primary cerebral lymphoma (PCL) is a non-Hodgkin's lymphoma (NHL) localized to the CNS and is usually a B-cell diffuse large cell type. PCL is associated with immune deficiency (part of AIDS or following organ transplantation) or arises sporadically and the frequency increases with age.

Clinical presentation of PCL is indistinguishable from other brain tumours. On CT scan-

ning there are single or multiple masses which are iso or hyperdense with frequent evidence of subependymal spread. An additional feature suggestive of lymphoma is an apparent CT response to corticosteroids. However, the imaging features are not sufficiently diagnostic and lesions may be indistinguishable from glioma. Histological confirmation is therefore mandatory. Following the histological diagnosis of PCL further staging is restricted to CSF cytology. In the absence of a known preceding history of NHL there is no need for further systemic staging with chest and abdominal CT scan or bone marrow.

(a) Treatment of sporadic PCL

Surgery should be confined to a diagnostic biopsy and debulking surgical excision has no therapeutic role. Historically radiotherapy had been the mainstay of treatment (Nelson *et al.*, 1992). The recommended dose is 40 Gy to the whole brain followed by a boost of 15–20 Gy to the primary site, with craniospinal axis irradiation reserved for patients with positive CSF cytology. Radiotherapy produces dramatic radiological and clinical responses but the median survival is only 12–18 months with the majority of patients relapsing in the CNS and no long term cures (Brada *et al.*, 1990; Nelson *et al.*, 1992).

Patients with PCL respond to a variety of chemotherapy regimens which include conventional NHL protocols (such as CHOP or MACOP-B) or regimens designed to cross the BBB such as high dose methotrexate (Hochberg *et al.*, 1991). They have been given prior to radiotherapy, after radiation and at the time of relapse. There are no randomized studies comparing the different treatment approaches although the current results of treatment with combined modality regimens (primary chemotherapy followed by radiotherapy) and primary chemotherapy with BBB disruption suggest a prolongation of

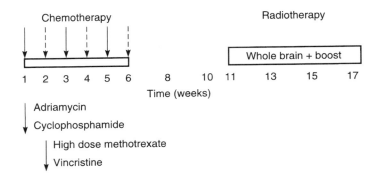

Figure 29.1 Treatment regimen for patients with primary cerebral lymphoma currently under investigation at the Royal Marsden Hospital.

median survival with a possible increase in the number of long term survivors (Neuwelt *et al.*, 1991; De Angelis *et al.*, 1992). The excellent initial responses to chemotherapy and the effectiveness of chemotherapy in systemic NHL would therefore argue in favour of a combined modality approach with chemotherapy first. The protocol currently tested at the Royal Marsden Hospital is shown in Figure 29.1. Intrathecal chemotherapy with methotrexate is recommended only in patients with positive CSF cytology. Patients unable to tolerate intensive treatment, either because of age or poor general condition, should receive radiotherapy alone.

(b) Treatment of PCL in AIDS

The management of malignant disease in patients with AIDS depends on the severity of the AIDS complex. In patients with frequent opportunistic infections the presence of PCL has a further adverse effect on prognosis and treatment is aimed at palliation. The usual regimen is whole brain irradiation to a dose of 30 Gy in 10 fractions. More aggressive radiotherapy or combined treatment are reserved for patients with normal bone marrow reserve where PCL is the only presentation in an HIV-positive patient.

29.7.6 CRANIOPHARYNGIOMAS

Craniopharyngiomas are benign neoplasms arising from epithelial rests in the suprasellar region associated with Rathke's pouch. They mostly present in childhood, although may occur at all ages with an apparent second peak at 50–60 years. Craniopharyngiomas are partly solid and partly cystic tumours lined by stratified squamous epithelium. Small islands of epithelium may breach the capsule surrounding the tumour.

The enlarging suprasellar mass may compress and adhere to adjacent structures which include the optic nerves and chiasma, the pituitary, hypothalamus and the third ventricle. Presenting features depend on the structures affected and include endocrine, visual and mental disturbances and hydrocephalus.

CT or MRI scan are frequently diagnostic and show a partly cystic and solid suprasellar mass with calcification in the cyst wall. Rarely a pituitary adenoma with cystic change and calcification may mimic this appearance. The differential diagnosis also includes aneurysm of the circle of Willis, suprasellar germinoma, optic chiasmal glioma, Langerhans cell histiocytosis and benign cyst (Table 29.4, above).

Therapy

Hydrocephalus requires urgent shunting, tumour decompression or both. Total excision is curative treatment in selected patients, particularly young children, although it carries a high morbidity and mortality (10–20%). The wall of the craniopharyngioma is firmly adherent to surrounding structures and attempts at complete removal may lead to damage which includes severe endocrine deficiency and hypothalamic damage with altered temperature control, fluctuating level of consciousness and uncontrolled obesity. Following incomplete surgery alone, the risk of recurrence is high (65–75%). Radiotherapy is highly effective in controlling the growth of craniopharyngioma. The recommended dose is 50 Gy in 30–33 daily fractions using a localized three field technique. Following conservative surgery and radiotherapy, the recurrence rate is 10–20% with 80–100% 5 year and 70–90% 10 year survival (Brada and Thomas, 1993; Rajan *et al.*, 1993).

The recommended treatment policy is therefore conservative surgery (aspiration or partial resection of craniopharyngioma) followed by radical local radiotherapy (Brada and Thomas, 1993). Radiation may result in unacceptable damage in young children who should be treated with radical or limited excision with radiotherapy reserved for the time of recurrence (Jose *et al.*, 1992), allowing the child to reach an age when radiation can be given more safely. In the initial phases of treatment the cystic component of craniopharyngioma may enlarge with further fluid accumulation causing local damage with visual deficit and hydrocephalus. Patients therefore require intensive ophthalmological and clinical monitoring and urgent aspiration and shunting. Reaccumulation of cystic fluid following conventional surgery and radiotherapy can be treated with further aspiration and instillation of radioactive colloidal chromic phosphate, gold or yttrium.

29.7.7   PITUITARY ADENOMAS

Pituitary adenomas are slowly proliferating benign tumours arising from the cells of the anterior pituitary. They present either with endocrine syndromes of hypersecretion (galactorrhoea/prolactinoma, acromegaly, Cushing's syndrome, and rarely gonadotrophin or thyroxin hypersecretion) or due to an enlarging mass arising out of the pituitary fossa, causing compression of the visual apparatus, particularly the optic chiasm. Initial investigations in patients with suspected pituitary adenoma include plain skull X-ray (which may reveal enlargement of the sella) and endocrine assessment particularly of prolactin level. CT or MRI scans reveal an iso- or hyperdense mass arising from the pituitary fossa which enhances with contrast.

(a)   Treatment of hormone secreting tumours

Prolactinomas

Initial treatment of prolactinoma is with bromocriptine. This can be followed by local radiotherapy which provides lasting tumour and hormonal control. In the absence of satisfactory response to medical treatment tumours can be resected.

Acromegaly

Hypersecretion of growth hormone is best treated with attempted complete tumour removal, usually by transphenoidal resection. Patients with persistently elevated growth hormone following surgery can be temporarily treated with bromocriptine or somatostatin analogues. Further persistent elevation is successfully treated with local radiotherapy, although there is a considerable delay in the normalization of growth hormone levels. New, long acting somatostatin analogues may become the initial treatment of choice in patients with raised growth hormone without a significant tumour mass.

Cushing's syndrome

Following failure of medical therapy patients should be treated along the lines of acromegaly, with initial resection and radiotherapy reserved for patients failing conventional treatment. Patients with ACTH secreting pituitary adenoma treated by bilateral adrenalectomy are at risk of developing Nelson's syndrome and should receive prophylactic pituitary irradiation.

(b)   Treatment of non-secreting adenomas

Initial treatment of non-secreting pituitary adenoma is surgical resection, usually by the transphenoidal route. This provides decompression of the visual apparatus. Pituitary adenomas particularly with suprasellar extension are rarely controlled by surgery alone and most incompletely excised tumours should also receive radiotherapy. The recommended radiotherapy dose is 45–50 Gy in 25–30 fractions using a localized technique to include the tumour and a margin. The morbidity of this treatment is minimal with 1–2% risk of optic neuropathy and 1% risk of second tumour at 10 years (Brada *et al.*, 1992). Following conservative surgery and radiotherapy, the 10 year control rate of non-secreting pituitary adenomas is 95% (Brada *et al.*, 1993).

29.7.8   OPTIC NERVE GLIOMA

Optic glioma is an indolent low grade astrocytoma of the optic pathways which occurs predominantly in childhood and is frequently associated with NF1. Visual disturbance with restriction of visual field and acuity is the commonest presenting feature with occasional headache. The tumour mass may also compress surrounding structures and cause hydrocephalus. Imaging with MRI or CT shows enhancing tumour of the optic chiasm or optic nerves. A biopsy is rarely required, particularly in patients with neurofibromatosis. However, in cases of doubt, histological confirmation can be sought with stereotactic biopsy.

The overall management has to take into account age, visual impairment and other disabilities as well as the apparent natural history of the tumour. The majority of optic nerve gliomas are indolent and providing they are not causing immediate or impending damage can be followed with interval scans and clinical and ophthalmological examination. A proportion of tumours stabilize and do not require further treatment. Progressing tumours in young children can be treated initially with carboplatin containing chemotherapy to allow for postponement of definitive treatment or occasionally tumours anterior to chiasma can be resected. Localized radiotherapy is effective at arresting further tumour growth with excellent long term survival (Bataini *et al.*, 1991; Jenkin *et al.*, 1993); it also improves the visual deficit in 20–30% of patients, and stabilizes vision in the majority (Horwich and Bloom, 1985) The risk of radiation induced damaged to normal brain is reduced providing the treatment is delayed beyond 4 years or older.

In summary the majority of patients with indolent slowly progressive or stable tumours do not require immediate therapy. They should be carefully followed with ophthalmological examination and scanning. Intervention in the form of radiotherapy, surgery or chemotherapy should be reserved for patients with progressive disease.

29.7.9   ACOUSTIC NEUROMA

VIIIth cranial nerve neurilemomas are benign encapsulated tumours which occur either as unilateral sporadic tumours or bilateral tumours as part of NF2. Rarely nerve sheath tumours may arise from the Vth and IXth cranial nerves. Patients present with progressive neural deafness and vestibular dysfunction and involvement of adjacent VIIth and Vth nerves or the brain stem. MRI scan shows a cerebello-pontine angle mass which enhances with gadolinium.

Tumours are frequently indolent and intervention depends on the size and rate of progression (Bederson *et al.*, 1991). Small unilateral tumours are best excised, although conventional surgery carries a high risk of deafness and risk of VIIth nerve damage. New microsurgical techniques reduce these risks. Stereotactic radiotherapy/radiosurgery is a non-invasive alternative which carries little immediate morbidity, although deafness is frequent particularly following treatment of larger tumours (Flickinger *et al.*, 1991).

29.7.10 GANGLIOGLIOMA

Gangliogliomas and gangliocytomas are neuronal tumours composed of mature gangliocytes supported by glial cells. They are indolent tumours and their behaviour does not correlate with the degree of histological differentiation of the glial elements. They present as primary intracranial tumours with some predilection for temporal lobe usually in children and young adults. The definitive treatment is by limited surgery. The role of radiotherapy is not clear. Five and 10 year survival ranges from 80% to 90%.

29.7.11 SKULL TUMOURS

The skull bones may be the site of primary bone and cartilage tumours particularly chondrosarcoma and chondroma and occasionally osteosarcoma. The skull may also be the site of an eosinophilic granuloma or benign cystic tumours. Tumours are particularly frequent in the clivus/skull base and they are most frequently chordomas which arise from the remnants of primitive notochord. In addition to clivus, chordomas, typically involve the sacrococcygeal region.

Most skull base tumours have infiltrative properties with destruction and invasion of surrounding structures. Surgery is the treatment of choice in chordoma, chondroma and chondrosarcoma. Skull base surgical approaches enable more radical tumour removal although complete excision of invasive tumours is frequently not possible. Local radiotherapy is not usually curative and is reserved for palliation (Fuller and Bloom, 1988). Localized conformal irradiation with protons to high doses may achieve better tumour control than conventional external beam radiotherapy (Austin-Seymour *et al.*, 1989).

29.7.12 BRAIN METASTASES

Tumours with particularly high risk of brain and meningeal metastases include small cell lung cancer, lymphoblastic and Burkitt's type lymphoma and acute lymphatic leukaemia. Because of the high incidence of other solid tumours, metastatic disease in the brain is seen most frequently in patients with breast and non-small cell lung cancer. Brain metastases present usually as multiple intracranial lesions or less frequently as solitary masses or as meningeal disease.

Clinical presentation is typical of features of brain tumour with focal or global neurological impairment frequently with confusional state and multiple deficits. One or more enhancing masses seen on CT or MRI should be distinguished from other multiple lesions such as abscesses, rare opportunistic infections or primary cerebral lymphoma. In the absence of known systemic malignancy patients should undergo limited investigations to exclude tumours treatable systematically such as breast, prostate or small cell lung cancer and rarely lymphoma or thyroid cancer. In the presence of known systemic malignancy biopsy is only indicated if there are unusual features such as a solitary lesion in a patient otherwise free of disease. Patients presenting with lesions suggestive of metastases without a known primary site must undergo a careful systemic examination, including rectal and pelvic examination and chest X-ray, prior to biopsy to exclude any easier site for obtaining tissue.

The treatment of brain metastases is aimed at palliation. Multiple metastases of chemosensitive tumours such as testicular teratoma, lymphoma or small cell lung cancer can be treated with chemotherapy providing the disease is considered chemosensitive. The majority of patients with multiple metastases should receive short palliative course of whole brain irradiation such as 20 Gy in 5 fractions which achieves neurological improvement in 60–70% of patients. Higher doses of conventional radiotherapy with more protracted treatment have no further palliative or survival benefit (Borgelt *et al.*, 1980; Coia, 1992). However, the overall prognosis of patients with multiple metastases is poor with a median survival of 4 months.

Solitary metastases are best treated radically either by surgical excision (Patchell *et al.*, 1990) or by stereotactic radiotherapy/radiosurgery (Laing *et al.*, 1993b). Additional whole brain radiotherapy is also recommended although it is not of proven benefit.

29.8 SPINAL CORD TUMOURS

The incidence of primary spinal cord tumours is low and ranges from 0.8 to 2.5 per 100 000 population per year. The most frequent tumours affecting the spinal cord are secondary deposits which are usually extradural arising from the vertebral bodies or paravertebral masses and occasionally intradural either extra- or intramedullary. Primary spinal cord tumours, spinal ependymoma and astrocytoma are usually intramedullary (Table 29.5).

29.8.1 CLINICAL PRESENTATION AND INVESTIGATIONS

Patients with extradural spinal cord compression present with back pain at the level of the lesion and impairment of neurological function at the affected spinal level and below. Below the affected level there is impairment of long tract function with paraparesis or

Table 29.5 Spinal cord tumours

Site	Tumour
Intradural	
Intramedullary	Ependymoma
	Astrocytoma
	Metastasis
Extramedullary	Meningioma
	Neurofibroma
	Cauda equina ependymoma
	Metastasis
Extradural	Metastasis
	Lymphoma
	Extension of paraspinal mass

paraplegia and loss of sensation of pain and temperature. This is frequently associated with bladder and bowel sphincter dysfunction causing urinary retention and constipation or incontinence. Intramedullary tumours produce loss of local function over several spinal segments particularly involving spinothalamic tract fibres and loss of neurological function below the level of the tumour. In patients with intrinsic spinal cord tumour the sphincter function is usually spared. Tumours involving the cauda equina typically present with local pain, loss of sphincter control and lower limb weakness with saddle anaesthesia.

Plain X-ray may reveal bony destruction suggestive of metastatic disease with erosion of lamina or pedicle, fracture or collapse of the vertebral body and paraspinal soft tissue mass. The current investigation of choice is spinal MRI with gadolinium enhancement. It demonstrates a mass, delineates the longitudinal extent of spinal tumour and determines the enhancement characteristics. If MRI is not available myelography may show block to the flow of contrast or expanded spinal cord. CT scan through the spinal levels with contrast (CT myelography) considerably improves the diagnostic potential of myelography.

29.8.2 PRIMARY SPINAL CORD TUMOURS

(a) Spinal ependymomas

Spinal cord ependymomas are histologically identical to their cranial counterparts and can be differentiated into low and high grade tumours. Low grade myxopapillary ependymomas have a predilection for cauda equina and conus medullaris arising from the conus or the filum terminale as intradural extramedullary masses. Low or high grade ependymomas also involve cervical, thoracic or lumbar cord as intramedullary tumours (Table 29.5).

Low grade cauda equina and conus medullaris tumours can usually be completely excised with no need for further therapy. Complete resection of intramedullary tumours elsewhere is frequently difficult and may lead to severe neurological deficit. Following incomplete excision local radiotherapy confined to the region of the tumour and a margin is recommended. The prognosis in ependymomas relates largely to the tumour grade and in low grade tumours to the extent of excision. Following partial excision and radiotherapy the 5 and 10 year progression free survival is 50–60% (Whitaker *et al.*, 1991).

(b) Spinal astrocytoma

Spinal astrocytomas are rare intramedullary tumours that histologically resemble cranial astrocytomas. The treatment includes surgery and radiotherapy although complete excision is usually not possible because of the infiltrative nature of the tumours. The rationale for localized postoperative radiotherapy is equivalent to that advocated for intracranial gliomas. Patients with high grade tumours have poor prognosis with frequent intracranial recurrence of disease which is usually not prevented by prophylactic cranial irradiation.

29.8.3 METASTATIC SPINAL CORD TUMOURS

Metastatic spinal cord tumours usually arise from bone or surrounding soft tissue masses and cause spinal cord compression. Rarely tumour metastases may be intramedullary. The aim of therapy is functional improvement and pain control. The most important determinant of functional outcome is pretreatment functional status. Early diagnosis of spinal cord compression before complete loss of neurological function may forestall paraplegia and allow for recovery of useful function.

Patients with suspected spinal cord compression from metastatic disease should have initial plain spinal X-ray followed by spinal MRI or myelography if MRI is not available. In the absence of known primary disease, tissue should be obtained for histological examination. Initial treatment in patients with suspected spinal cord compression includes corticosteroids (usually dexamethasone 4 mg orally 6 hourly). Further treatment decision depends on the patient's general condition, functional status, tumour type and the extent of primary and metastatic disease.

Spinal cord compression by tumours of unknown histology and primary site and the progression of neurological deficit despite radiotherapy are an indication for surgery. However longstanding paraplegia rarely recovers and surgery may be withheld. Patients with tumours of known poor radioresponsiveness should also be considered for surgery first. Posterior cord compression is best relieved by posterior approach through a decompressive laminectomy. Disease arising from a vertebral body may be approached through a lateral or anterior approach. Removal of a vertebral body requires grafting and the spine may need subsequent stabilization. Such an intensive procedure is only suitable for patients with a good long term prognosis and limited metastatic disease. Patients with radioresponsive tumours and with common solid tumours such as breast, lung and prostatic carcinoma should be treated with initial radiotherapy. A short 1 week course of radiotherapy with direct treatment to the spine carries no morbidity and is usually sufficient. Chemotherapy can be used as initial treatment in tumours such as teratoma or lymphoma. The prognosis in patients with metastatic spinal cord compression is determined by the overall disease status and the degree of functional impairment.

REFERENCES

Akbasak, A. and Sunar-Akbasak, B. (1992) Oncogenes: cause or consequence in the development of glial tumors. *Journal of the Neurological Sciences*, **111**, 119–33.

Allen, J.C., Kim, J.H. and Packer, R.J. (1987) Neoadjuvant chemotherapy for newly diagnosed germ-cell tumours of the central nervous system. *Journal of Neurosurgery*, **67**, 65–70.

Austin-Seymour, M., Munzenrider, J., Goitein, M. *et al.* (1989) Fractionated proton radiation therapy of chordoma and low-grade chondrosarcoma of the base of the skull. *Journal of Neurosurgery*, **70**, 13–17.

Barbaro, N.M., Gutin, P.H., Wilson, C.B. *et al.* (1987) Radiation therapy in the treatment of partially resected meningiomas. *Neurosurgery*, **20**, 525–8.

Barth, R.F., Soloway, A.H., Fairchild, R.G. and Brugger, R.M. (1992) Boron neutron capture therapy for cancer. *Cancer*, **70**, 2995–3007.

Bataini, J.P., Delanian, S. and Ponvert, D. (1991) Chiasmal gliomas: results of irradiation management in 57 patients and review of literature. *International Journal of Radiation Oncology, Biology, Physics*, **21**, 615–23.

Bederson, J.B., von Ammon, K., Wichmann, W.W. and Yasargil, M.G. (1991) Conservative treatment of patients with acoustic tumours. *Neurosurgery*, **28**, 646–51.

Bleehen, N.M. and Stenning, S.P. (1991) A Medical Research Council trial of two radiotherapy doses in the treatment of grades 3 and 4 astrocytoma. *British Journal of Cancer*, **64**, 769–74.

Bloom, H.J.G. (1983) Primary intracranial germ cell tumours. *Clinics in Oncology*, **2**, 233–57.

Bloom, H.J.G. and Bessell, E.M. (1990) Medulloblastoma in adults: a review of 47 patients treated between 1952 and 1981. *International Journal of Radiation Oncology, Biology, Physics*, **18**, 763–72.

Borgelt, B., Gelber, R., Kramer, S. *et al.* (1980) The palliation of brain metastases: final results of the first two studies by the radiation therapy oncology group. *International Journal of Radiation Oncology, Biology, Physics*, **6**, 1–19.

Brada, M. (1989) Back to the future – radiotherapy in high grade gliomas. *British Journal of Cancer*, **60**, 1–4.

Brada, M., Dearnaley, D., Horwich, A. and Bloom, H.J.G. (1990) Management of primary cerebral lymphoma with initial chemotherapy: preliminary results and comparison with patients treated with radiotherapy alone. *International Journal of Radiation Oncology, Biology, Physics*, **18**, 787–92.

Brada, M., Ford, D., Mason, M. *et al.* (1992) Risk of second brain tumour following conservative surgery and radiotherapy of pituitary adenoma. *British Medical Journal*, **304**, 1343–6.

Brada, M. and Graham, J.D. (1993) Stereotactic external beam radiotherapy, in *Image Directed Surgery of Brain Tumours*, (ed. D.G.T. Thomas), Churchill Livingstone, London, pp. 149–67.

Brada, M. and Rajan, B. (1990) Spinal seeding in cranial germinoma. *British Journal of Cancer*, **61**, 339–40.

Brada, M., Rajan, B., Traish, D. *et al.* (1993) The long-term efficacy of conservative surgery and radiotherapy in the control of pituitary adenomas. *Clinical Endocrinology*, **38**, 571–8.

Brada, M. and Thomas, D.G.T. (1993) Craniopharyngioma revisited. *International Journal of Radiation Oncology, Biology, Physics*, **27**, 471–5.

Coia, L.R. (1992) The role of radiation therapy in the treatment of brain metastases. *International Journal of Radiation Oncology, Biology, Physics*, **23**, 229–38.

Collins, V.P., Nordensköld, M. and Dumanski, J.P. (1990) The molecular genetics of meningiomas. *Brain Pathology*, **1**, 19–24.

Culver, K.W., Ram, Z., Wallbridge, S. *et al.* (1992) *In vivo* gene transfer with retroviral vector-producer cells for treatment of experimental brain tumours. *Science*, **256**, 1550–2.

De Angelis, L.M., Yahalom, J., Thaler, H.T. and Kher, U. (1992) Combined modality therapy for primary CNS lymphoma. *Journal of Clinical Oncology*, 10, 635–43.

Evans, A.E., Jenkin, D.T., Sposto, R. *et al.* (1990) Results of a prospective randomised trial of radiation therapy with and without CCNU, Vincristine and Prednisone. *Journal of Neurosurgery*, **72**, 572–82.

Flickinger, J.C., Lunsford, L.D., Coffey, R.J. *et al.* (1991) Radiosurgery of acoustic neurinomas. *Cancer*, 67, 345–53.

Fuller, D.B. and Bloom, J.G. (1988) Radiotherapy for chordoma. *International Journal of Radiation Oncology, Biology, Physics*, **15**, 331–9.

Glaholm, J., Bloom, H.J.G. and Crow, J.H. (1990) The role of radiotherapy in the management of intracranial meningiomas: The Royal Marsden Hospital experience with 186 patients. *International Journal of Radiation Oncology, Biology, Physics*, **18**, 755–61.

Gutin, P.H., Leibel, S.A. and Sheline, G.A. (1991) *Radiation Injury to the Nervous System*, Raven Press, New York.

Hochberg, F.H., Loeffler, J.S. and Prados, M. (1991) The therapy of primary brain lymphoma (Review). *Journal of Neuro-Oncology*, **10**, 191–201.

Horwich, A. and Bloom, H.J.G. (1985) Optic gliomas: radiation therapy and prognosis. *International Journal of Radiation Oncology, Biology, Physics*, **11**, 1067–79.

Jenkin, D., Angyalfi, S., Becker, L. *et al.* (1993) Optic glioma in children: surveillance, resection, or irradiation? *International Journal of Radiation Oncology, Biology, Physics*, **25**, 215–25.

Jose, C.C., Rajan, B., Ashley, S. *et al.* (1992) Radiotherapy for the treatment of recurrent craniopharyngioma. *Clinical Oncology*, **4**, 287–9.

Kristiansen, K., Hagen, S., Kollevold, T. *et al.* (1981) Combined modality therapy of operated astrocytomas grade III and IV. Confirmation of the value of postoperative irradiation and lack of potentiation of bleomycin on survival time: a prospective multicenter trial of the Scandinavian Glioblastoma Study Group, *Cancer*, **47**, 649–52.

Laing, R.W., Warrington, A.P., Graham, J. *et al.* (1993a) Efficacy and toxicity of fractionated stereotactic radiotherapy in the treatment of recurrent gliomas (phase I/II study). *Radiotherapy and Oncology*, **27**, 22–39.

Laing, R.W., Warrington, A.P., Hines, F. *et al.* (1993b) Fractionated stereotactic external beam radiotherapy in the management of brain metastases. *European Journal of Cancer*, **29A**, 1387–91.

Mbidde, E.K., Selby, P.J., Perren, T.J. *et al.* (1988) High dose BCNU chemotherapy with autologous bone marrow transplantation and full dose radiotherapy for grade IV astrocytoma. *British Journal of Cancer*, **58**, 779–82.

Neglia, J.P., Meadows, A.T., Robinson, L.L. *et al.* (1991) Second neoplasms after acute lymphatic leukemia in childhood. *New England Journal of Medicine*, **325**, 1330–6.

Nelson, D.F., Martz, K.L., Bonner, H. *et al.* (1992) Non-Hodgkin's lymphoma of the brain: can high dose, large volume radiation therapy improve survival? Report on a prospective trial by the Radiation Therapy Oncology Group (RTOG): RTOG 8315. *International Journal of Radiation Oncology, Biology, Physics*, **23**, 9–17.

Neuwelt, E.A., Goldman, D.L., Dahlborg, S.A. *et al.* (1991) Primary CNS lymphoma treated with osmotic blood–brain barrier disruption: prolonged survival and preservation of cognitive function. *Journal of Clinical Oncology*, **9**, 1580–90.

Patchell, R., Tibbs, P., Walsh, J. *et al.* (1990) A randomised trial of surgery in the treatment of single metastases to the brain. New England Journal of Medicine, **322**, 494–500.

Quigley, M.R. and Maroon, J.C. (1991) The relationship between survival and the extent of the resection in patients with supratentorial malignant gliomas. *Neurosurgery*, **29**, 385–9.

Rajan, B., Ashley, S., Gorman C. *et al.* (1993) Craniopharyngioma – long term results following limited surgery and radiotherapy. *Radiotherapy and Oncology*, **26**, 1–10.

Ron, E., Modan, B., Boice, J.D. *et al.* (1988) Tumours of the brain and nervous system after radiotherapy in childhood. *New England Journal of Medicine*, **319**, 1033–9.

Seizinger, B.R., De La Monte, S., Atkins, L. *et al.* (1987) Molecular genetic approach to human meningioma: loss of genes on chromosome 22, *Proceedings of the National Academy of Sciences*, **84**, 5419–23.

Shapiro, W.R. (1986) Therapy of adult malignant brain tumours: what have the clinical trials taught us? *Seminars in Oncology*, **13**, 38–45.

Shaw, E., Daumas-Duport, C. and Scheithauer, B. (1989) Radiation therapy in the management of low-grade supratentorial astrocytomas. *Journal of Neurosurgery*, **70**, 853–61.

Stenning, S., Freedman, L. and Bleehen, N. (1987) An overview of published results from randomized studies of nitrosoureas in primary high grade malignant glioma. *British Journal of Cancer*, **56**, 89.

Tait, D., Thornton-Jones, H., Bloom, H. *et al.* (1990) Adjuvant chemotherapy for medulloblastoma: the first multi-centre controlled trial of the International Society of Paediatric Oncology (SIOP I). *European Journal of Cancer*, **26**, 464–9.

Vanuytsel, L., Bessell, E.M., Ashley, S.E. *et al.* (1992) Intracranial ependymoma: long-term results of a policy of surgery and radiotherapy. *International Journal of Radiation Oncology, Biology, Physics*, **23**, 313–19.

Vanuytsel, L. and Brada, M. (1991) The role of pro-phylatic spinal irradiation in localised intra-cranial ependymoma. *International Journal of Radiation Oncology, Biology, Physics*, **21**, 825–30.

Walker, M.D., Alexander, E., Hunt, W.E. *et al.* (1978) Evaluation of BCNU and/or radiotherapy in the treatment of anaplastic gliomas. *Journal of Neurosurgery*, **49**, 333–43.

Whitaker, S., Bessell, E., Ashley, S. *et al.* (1991) Post operative radiotherapy in the management of spinal cord ependymoma. *Journal of Neuro-surgery*, **74**, 720–8.

Wood, J.R., Green, S.B. and Shapiro, W.R. (1988) The prognostic importance of tumor size in malignant gliomas: a computed tomographic scan study by the Brain Tumor Cooperative Group. *Journal of Clinical Oncology*, **6**, 338–43.

Ross Pinkerton

30.1 INTRODUCTION

Cancer in childhood is very rare in comparison with adult malignancies, but remains the commonest cause of non-accidental death in childhood. Conventionally, children of 15 years of age or less are classified as 'paediatric' patients. Because a number of cancers affect the older child and young adolescent, e.g. Ewing's sarcoma, osteosarcoma and Hodgkin's disease, most paediatric oncology units will treat patients up to 16 or 17 years. The needs of the child and young adolescent are very different from the adult and it is no longer acceptable for any child with cancer to be managed in an adult cancer unit, no matter how skilled the physicians or radiotherapists are in their particular field. The majority of children with cancer are treated in general hospital paediatric units, although a specialist children's unit sited within a comprehensive cancer centre, adequately staffed with paediatric trained nurses and medical personnel is an alternative.

The incidence of the commoner tumours in children under 15 years is listed in Table 30.1. The management of childhood leukaemia differs little from that in the adult, although the outcome is better (Chapter 20).

30.2 AETIOLOGY AND MOLECULAR ASPECTS

Because childhood cancer is rare it is very difficult to draw firm conclusions regarding aetiological factors, particularly any contribution from the environment. Childhood leukaemia has been the focus of intense speculation and case control studies to try and determine whether factors such as environmental radiation, either from nuclear generating or reprocessing plants or natural radon exposure, contribute. Clustering of cases has been described and an increased incidence of leukaemia in the children of fathers involved in the nuclear industry was suggested, then refuted (Gardner *et al.* 1990; Henshaw *et al.*, 1990; Kinlen, L.J. 1993). The impact of viral infection possibly related to lack of herd immunity in isolated areas has been postulated. It is hoped that the recently commenced national case control study on childhood cancers within the UK will throw light on these factors. In this study all children with cancer will be compared with age matched controls and most of the factors which have been put forward as having a contributory role will be evaluated.

The primary role of Epstein–Barr virus (EBV) in Burkitt's lymphoma has been extensively studied and an indirect association between infection and common acute lymphoblastic leukaemia has been postulated. It is possible that the rapid proliferation of lymphocyte precursors during early infancy, at which time the child is exposed to a variety of infectious agents, leads to a mutational event resulting in leukaemia (Greaves, 1988).

Epidemiological data on Hodgkin's disease suggests that where rates of infection during infancy are high the disease occurs at a

Table 30.1 Annual incidence of malignant disease per million children 15 years of age or less

Diagnostic group	Annual rates per million
Total	106.7
Leukaemias	
Acute lymphoblastic	29.7
Acute non-lymphoblastic	6.0
Chronic myeloid	0.8
Lymphomas	
Hodgkin's disease	4.1
Non-Hodgkin	6.1
Brain and spinal	
Ependymoma	3.1
Astrocytoma	8.9
Medulloblastoma	5.0
Sympathetic nervous system	
Neuroblastoma	7.0
Retinoblastoma	3.5
Kidney	
Wilms' tumour	7.2
Renal carcinoma	0.1
Liver	
Hepatoblastoma	0.8
Hepatic carcinoma	0.2
Bone	
Osteosarcoma	2.4
Ewing's sarcoma	1.7
Soft tissue sarcomas	
Rhabdomyosarcoma	4.2
Fibrosarcoma	0.8
Gonadal and germ cell	
Non-gonadal germ cell	0.9
Gonadal germ cell	1.5
Epithelial	
Adrenocortical carcinoma	0.3
Thyroid carcinoma	0.3
Nasopharyngeal carcinoma	0.3

Data from United Kingdom Cancer Childrens Study Group and Children's Cancer Registry.

younger age and tends to be of mixed cellularity.

A variety of chromosomal abnormalities are associated with specific malignancies and in some cases may be a primary event (Table 30.2). Three major molecular mechanisms have been proposed for the development of childhood cancer; the loss of a tumour suppressor gene, leading to uncontrolled cell division, the translocation of an oncogene to a site which influences its function, and thirdly mutation in a growth regulatory gene, such as p53.

In retinoblastoma (chromosome 13q 14) and Wilms' tumour (chromosome 11p 13) the tumour suppressor gene on each allele must be lost for tumour to occur. The Knudson 'Two-hit' hypothesis suggests that these mutational events occur sequentially. The first may be an inherited mutation arising in the

Table 30.2 Abnormalities of chromosomes which have been reported in paediatric malignancies

Chromosomal abnormalities	Malignancy
t(8:21), (15:17)	Acute myeloid leukaemia
t(8:22), (8:14), (2:8)	B-cell leukaemia and lymphoma
t(4:11)	High count ALL, especially infants
t(1:19)	Pre-B ALL
t(11:14)	T-cell ALL
t(9:22)	Chronic myeloblastic leukaemia
Monosomy 7	Myelodysplastic syndrome
Deletion 11p	Wilms' tumour
Deletion 13q	Retinoblastoma, osteosarcoma
t(11:22)	Ewing's sarcoma and primitive neuroectodermal tumour
t(2:13)	Alveolar rhabdomyosarcoma
Deletion 1p	Neuroblastoma
t(2:5)	Large cell anaplastic lymphoma
Inversion 17q	Astrocytoma
Inversion 12p	Germ cell tumour
Deletion 22q	Meningioma
t(x;18)	Synovial sarcoma
Isochrome 12p	Malignant germ cell tumour

germ line with the second event occurring later specifically in retinal or renal cells. In non-familial retinoblastoma both mutational events occur in the retinal cell population and this explains the later onset of sporadic, compared to familial, disease (Knudson, 1971).

Juxtaposition of an oncogene occurs in Burkitt's lymphoma, in which the c-*myc* gene on chromosome 8 is translocated adjacent to the immunoglobulin heavy chain locus on chromosome 14 or the kappa or lambda light chain gene loci on chromosomes 2 and 22 respectively. As in chronic myeloid leukaemia where the c-*abl* oncogene is juxtaposed with the *bcr* gene on chromosome 22, this chromosomal configuration leads to growth disregulation.

Much interest has been attached to the role of the *p53* gene. This gene may play a role in temporarily arresting cell division when there has been DNA damage, allowing time for repair. Mutations of the *p53* gene protein can be detected immunohistochemically and are very common in many adult and childhood tumours. In the Li–Fraumeni syndrome a somatic mutation of the *p53* gene has been reported, which may be the primary predisposing factor to a variety of cancers, including rhabdomyosarcoma (Li and Fraumeni, 1969).

30.3 BRAIN TUMOURS

Central nervous system neoplasms are the commonest solid tumours in childhood and may be divided into six pathological subgroups (Table 30.3). Astrocytoma (particularly low grade) and medulloblastoma or primitive neuroectodermal tumour (PNET) are the commonest in this age group. To some extent the tumour type can be predicted by the location of the tumour. Supratentorial tumours include cerebral astrocytoma, lateral ventricular ependymoma and, rarely, craniopharyngioma. In the small infant cerebral PNET, choroid plexus papilloma, meningioma and teratoma occur.

Infratentorial tumours are commonly medulloblastoma or PNET, astrocytoma, brain stem glioma and third ventricular ependymoma (Table 30.4).

Table 30.3   Pathological subgroups of the commoner tumours involving the central nervous system in children

Gliomas
    Astrocytoma
    Ependymoma
    Oligodendroglioma
    Glioblastoma
    Mixed glioma

Neuroectodermal tumours
    Medulloblastoma
    PNET (primitive neuroectodermal tumour)

Neurinoma
    Optic nerve glioma

Pineal
    Pineoblastoma
    Pineocytoma

Germ cell
    Germinoma
    Teratoma
        Differentiated
        Undifferentiated

Craniopharyngioma

The symptoms at presentation will reflect the site of the tumour. For example, medulloblastoma will often produce nystagmus and ataxia, whereas parietal tumours will lead to focal weakness and visual disturbance may be the result of a suprachiasmal lesion. With brain stem tumours multiple cranial nerve palsies may be seen. Non-specific symptoms such as severe, recurrent or persisting headaches are rare in children and should be regarded as highly suspicious. In small infants macrocephaly with bulging anterior fontanelle may be apparent early in the disease course.

30.3.1   STAGING

As metastatic disease beyond the neuraxis is extremely rare, clinical staging in brain tumours reflects the degree of tumour remaining after an attempted primary resection. For most tumours this is the single most important prognostic factor. MRI and CT scan play a vital role in both pre- and post-

Table 30.4   Anatomical site of central nervous system tumours in childhood

Supratentorial		Cerebral astrocytoma
		Frontal
		Temporal
		Parietal
		Lateral ventricle ependymoma
		Craniopharyngioma
	Especially < 1 year	Primitive neuroectodermal tumour
		Choroid plexus papilloma
		Meningioma
		Teratoma
Infratentorial		Astrocytoma
		Medulloblastoma
		Brain stem glioma
		3rd ventricle ependymoma
Intraspinal	Extradural	Neuroblastoma
		Sarcoma
		Lymphoma
	Intradural	Neurofibromatosis
		Dermoid
		Lipomata
	Intramedullary	Astrocytoma

operative assessment. It is important to be aware, however, of the limitations of imaging following surgery due to postoperative artefact caused by localized oedema or haemorrhage. In tumours such as medulloblastoma and PNET careful spinal imaging with contrast myelography and CSF cytology remain mandatory. Even high resolution MRI has not yet replaced these procedures.

30.3.2 TREATMENT STRATEGY

Specific aspects of the commoner tumour types are dealt with individually but in general surgery and radiotherapy provide the mainstay of treatment. Insertion of a ventricular peritoneal or ventriculo-atrial shunt may produce a dramatic improvement in symptoms where definitive resection is not possible. If at all possible, however, initial resection should be attempted and even where the initial imaging suggests unresectability a biopsy should be obtained. This is of particular importance with the advent of increasingly effective chemotherapy and the necessity to confirm the histological subtype prior to planning treatment. Despite this there remains some deep tumours of the brain stem where the diagnosis will be a clinical one based on imaging. The use of stereotactic techniques has improved the diagnostic yield in such tumours.

Where appropriate following surgery doses of 40–50 Gy are given to the primary site with 24–30 Gy to the whole brain. In tumours such as medulloblastoma and ependymoma where there is a risk of spinal seeding whole neuraxis radiation is performed.

30.3.3 TUMOUR SUBTYPES

(a)   Astrocytoma

Low grade tumours have an overall cure rate of around 60% at 5 years using surgery and radiotherapy. In the case of high grade tumours the cure rate is around 25%.

Combination chemotherapy comprising agents such as vincristine, actinomycin, CCNU (Comustine) and cisplatin have to date had little impact on survival of either high grade or low grade glioma, although responses are seen and one randomized study has demonstrated significant benefit using vincristine, prednisolone and CCNU (Pendergrass *et al.*, 1987; Sposto *et al.*, 1989).

(b)   Ependymomas

These tumours arising from the lining of the ventricle occur both above and below the tentorium. Although often well differentiated they may behave in a locally aggressive manner and also seed into the spinal fluid. Treatment is essentially surgical with radiotherapy of the whole neuraxis (Wallner *et al.*, 1986).

(c)   Medulloblastoma

This is the commonest infratentorial tumour and occurs in the cerebellum. Tumours contain variable degrees of neural differentiation often with rosette formation. The desmoplastic variety is usually more superficial and thus more readily resectable. With primary surgery followed by whole brain and spinal irradiation a 5 year survival around 40–50% is achieved. With extensive spinal metastases at presentation this is approximately 20%. Because of the high chemosensitivity of this tumour in phase II studies of patients relapsing following radiotherapy, extensive studies have been carried out using either primary chemotherapy or as an adjuvant following surgery and radiotherapy. For example, regimens including vincristine, CCNU, steroids, cisplatin, etoposide and ifosfamide have been used. At present either the 8 in 1 regimen (Pendergrass *et al.*, 1987) or combinations of carboplatin, etoposide and vincristine are most commonly used (Castello *et al.*, 1990, Lefkowitz *et al.*, 1990). Despite the routine use of adjuvant chemotherapy in many centres,

Vincristine 1.5 mg/m^2	weekly $\times$ 10
Carboplatin 500 mg/m^2 daily $\times$ 2	6 weekly $\times$ 2
Etoposide 100 mg/m^2 daily $\times$ 3	(alternately)
Cyclophosphamide 1500 mg/m^2 with mesna	6 weekly $\times$ 2

Figure 30.1 Outline of the European SIOP PNET III protocol for medulloblastoma and primitive neuroectodermal tumours.

its role is still an area of some controversy (Tait *et al.*, 1990). The current SIOP group is evaluating in a prospective randomized study the value of intensive adjuvant treatment, combining carboplatin, vincristine, etoposide alternating with cyclophosphamide, etoposide and vincristine (Figure 30.1).

The term 'primitive neuroectodermal tumour' is now increasingly replacing the term 'medulloblastoma'. In the past this term was confined to what were in effect medulloblastoma occurring in the supratentorial region. These are histologically and biologically identical and treatment is therefore the same. Tumours at this site are more commonly seen in the infant and because of the significant neurological sequelae associated with whole brain irradiation in infants under 3 years there is an increased tendency to rely on chemotherapy alone in this age group. In some cases chemotherapy is given to produce a response which is sufficiently durable to delay the need for radiotherapy until maximum brain growth has occurred.

(d) Brain stem gliomas

These are the most feared of all paediatric brain tumours. They commonly arise in the pons and although are of low grade histology are particularly difficult to treat. Complete resection is usually impossible and radiotherapy remains the mainstay of treatment.

Cure rates are generally less than 20% despite attempts to improve this with modifications in radiotherapy and scheduling. Moreover, aggressive chemotherapy has to date had little impact (Wolff *et al.*, 1987).

(e) Optic gliomas

These low grade astrocytomas may be associated with Von Recklinghausen syndrome. Symptom progression may be very slow with gradual onset of visual defect or obstructive hydrocephalus. In the older child radiation will generally produce a survival of over 70% but in the small infant where radiation is to be avoided a wait and watch policy may be appropriate. Adjuvant chemotherapy with low dose vincristine and actinomycin may be of use (Horwich and Bloom, 1985; Packer *et al.*, 1988).

The management of other rare brain tumours such as craniopharyngioma or meningioma is similar to that in adults (Chapter 29).

30.4 LYMPHOMAS

The clinical features of Hodgkin's disease in the child are little different from those in the adult and initial staging investigations are similar. Lymphangiography is not done in children and because of the increasing use of systemic chemotherapy there is no indication for a diagnostic laparotomy and splenectomy. Abdominal nodes should be evaluated with a high resolution CT scan.

The emphasis of different treatment modalities differs, however, in childhood. Because of the very high cure rate (overall > 90% of children will survive) there is considerable concern about late effects, both of radiotherapy and chemotherapy.

In the current UKCCSG protocol patients with high cervical stage IA Hodgkin's disease are treated with involved field radiotherapy (30 Gy). Bilateral fields are used to reduce neck asymmetry. With this approach about 20% of patients will relapse due to undetected disease at other sites but the majority, if not all, of these are curable with subsequent chemotherapy. All other stages receive ChlVPP (Chlorambucil, Vinblastine, Procarbazine, Prednisolone) chemotherapy. Usually six to eight courses are given (Figure 30.2). It is unlikely that this regimen causes sterilization in girls but all boys will be sterilized. The risk of second malignancies exists, although to date this is less than 1% in several hundred thus treated. Irradiation is not given even to patients with bulky mediastinal disease, provided a complete remission is achieved with chemotherapy. The difficulty of interpreting a small residual mediastinal mass on CT scan is being addressed in a prospective study of high dose gallium scanning versus biopsy. It is likely that such residual imageable abnormalities are fibrosis in the majority of cases and will resolve with time (Ekert *et al.*, 1988; Radford *et al.*, 1988).

The VEEP (Vincristine, Etoposide, Epirubicin, Prednisolone) regimen is being evaluated in a limited number of centres, but concern about its efficacy compared to ChlVPP limits its use to boys, in order to avoid sterilization (O'Brien *et al.*, 1992). ABVD (Adriamycin, Bleomycin, Vinblastine, DTIC) alone or alternating with MOPP (Mustine, Vincristine, Procarbazine, Prednisolone) is a widely used regimen in children (Ekert *et al.*, 1988; Fryer *et al.*, 1990; Leverger *et al.*, 1990).

30.4.1 NON-HODGKIN'S LYMPHOMA

In childhood virtually all non-Hodgkin's lymphomas (NHLs) are high grade and the complex classifications for adult lymphomas are not now used. There are four main categories: diffuse lymphoblastic T cell, diffuse lymphoblastic B cell, lymphoblastic non-B non-T and 'others'. The latter category includes large cell anaplastic Ki-1 positive lymphoma, peripheral T-cell lymphoma and true malignant histiocytosis.

It has been clearly demonstrated that most paediatric lymphoblastic lymphomas should be treated on the basis of immunophenotype. T lymphoblastic lymphoma receive an identical protocol to that used for acute lymphoblastic leukaemia (Figure 30.3). B-cell disease is treated with a pulsed cyclophosphamide based regimen, as shown in Figure

Days 1–14	CHLORAMBUCIL	6 mg/m^2 orally daily (maximum 10 mg)
Days 1–14	PROCARBAZINE	100 mg/m^2 orally daily (maximum 150 mg/day)
Days 1–14	PREDNISOLONE	30 mg/m^2 orally daily (not to exceed 40 mg/day)
Days 1 *and* 8 only	VINBLASTINE	6 mg/m^2 i.v. stat (maximum 10 mg)

Figure 30.2 The Ch1VPP regimen for Hodgkin's disease used by the UK Childrens Cancer Study Group.

Induction	Consolidation	CNS directed therapy	Continuing chemotherapy
Vincristine	Daunorubicin	High dose methotrexate	6-Mercaptopurine
Asparaginase	Cytarabine	with folinic acid	Methotrexate
Prednisolone	6 Thioguanine	rescue	Vincristine
I.T. methotrexate	Etoposide		Prednisolone
Weeks 1–4	Weeks 4 and 23	Weeks 6, 8, 10	for 2 years

Figure 30.3 Regimen used by the UK Childrens Cancer Study Group for T-cell non-Hodgkin's lymphoma based on the UKALL XD ALL regimen.

30.4. In stages I and II disease either cyclophosphamide or doxorubicin may be omitted to avoid late sequelae. Traditionally patients with > 25% infiltration of bone marrow are classified as 'leukaemia' and while this may be of prognostic significance with some protocols, does not influence the general treatment strategy. With B-cell acute lymphoblastic leukaemia (ALL) there is a particularly high incidence of CNS disease and therefore a more intensive CNS directed chemotherapy programme is used.

Because of the exquisite chemosensitivity of both B-cell and T-cell lymphoma, an initial phase of non-intensive chemotherapy using vincristine and prednisolone may be indicated. This avoids the additional complications of chemotherapy if severe tumour lysis and renal failure occur. Intensive hyperhydration with up to 4 litres/m^2 per day of intravenous fluid plus allopurinol is mandatory prior to commencing chemotherapy, and very close monitoring during induction is required. Early dialysis or haemofiltration should be instituted in the event of persisting severe hyperkalaemia or hyperphosphataemia.

Occasionally in a very sick child with massive thoracic disease, often presenting with superior vena caval obstruction, sedation or anaesthesia for diagnostic procedures may be dangerous and lead to respiratory obstruction. In this situation treatment with vincristine and prednisolone is appropriate, making a presumptive diagnosis on clinical grounds and within 24–48 hours pathological material may be obtained.

In T-cell NHL 5 year survival is around 70% for stages III and IV disease (Wheeler *et al.*, 1990). The outcome in B-cell NHL has improved markedly with increased intensity of chemotherapy and currently is around 75% for both stages III and IV disease (Murphy *et al.*, 1986; Patte *et al.*, 1986; Philip *et al.*, 1987).

30.5 SOFT TISSUE SARCOMA

30.5.1 RHABDOMYOSARCOMA

This tumour arises from embryonal striated muscle precursor cells. The commonest histological subgroups of childhood rhabdomyosarcoma are the embryonal and alveolar types. This division is based upon appearances on conventional staining. The embryonal rhabdomyosarcoma consists mainly of spindle shaped cells or a more undifferentiated small round cell tumour, in which the diagnosis may depend on immunohistochemical staining with desmin and myoglobin. The alveolar subgroup has micro-architecture resembling pulmonary alveoli lined with loosely arranged tumour cells. This division is of prognostic importance, the alveolar subgroup having a significantly poorer outcome with standard treatment (Heyn *et al.*, 1989). Within the embryonal subgroup the botryoid form is of particularly good prognosis and often presents as a mucosa lined, grape like

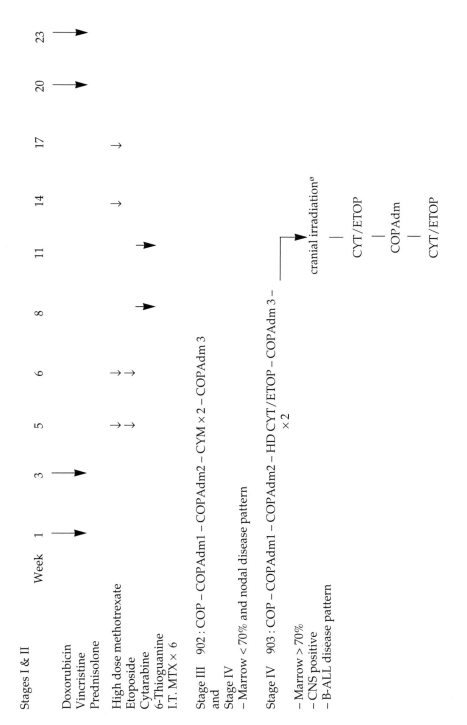

Figure 30.4 Regimen used for localized and advanced non-Hodgkin's lymphoma by the UK Childrens Cancer Study Group. ø, only given to those CNS positive. COP = cyclophosphamide, vincristine, prednisolone; COPAdm = cyclophosphamide, vincristine, prednisolone, doxorubicin, high dose methotrexate; CYM = cytarabine, high dose methotrexate; HD CYT-ETOP=high dose cytarabine, etoposide.

Table 30.5   Sites and degree of invasiveness of rhabdomyosarcoma in relation to outcome

Primary site	% of patients	4 year survival rate (%) T_1	T_2
Orbit	10	90	85
Head and neck	12	80	50
Parameningeal	17	60	50
Bladder, prostate	13	80	50
Other genitourinary sites	15	95	60
Limbs	13	60	40
Other	20	50	45

mass at sites such as the vagina, bladder or auditory canal (Newton *et al.*, 1988).

The molecular basis of rhabdomyosarcoma remains unclear, although the demonstration of a consistent t(2;13) translocation in the alveolar histological subtype may give a clue to the site of the causal gene. Loss of heterozygosity on chromosome 11 occurs frequently in embryonal rhabdomyosarcoma.

The commonest sites of this tumour are shown in Table 30.5. The parameningeal subgroup including tumours in nasopharynx, paranasal sinuses, middle ear and base of skull still have a relatively poor outcome.

Tumour presentation will depend on the site of the primary tumour. There may be superficial swelling, bleeding from nasopharynx, bladder, vagina or middle ear. Orbital tumours can cause ptosis and strabismus. The disseminated alveolar sarcoma may present with evidence of myelosuppression and in some cases hypercalcaemia.

The commonly used staging systems are either the IRS (Intergroup Rhabdomyosarcoma Study Group) or the SIOP (International Society for Paediatric Oncology) systems (Tables 30.6, 30.7). Mandatory initial investigations include chest X-ray and CT scan of chest, CT scan or ultrasound of abdomen, technetium bone scan and bone marrow aspirate and biopsy. The primary tumour should be measured using either CT or MRI scans. In the SIOP staging system particular emphasis is put on the extent of the primary disease, whether this remains limited to the organ of origin or whether there is regional extension. This division is of clear prognostic importance (Rodary *et al.*, 1991).

Table 30.6   American IRS Grouping System for rhabdomyosarcoma

Group I	Localized disease, completely resected
	Confined to organ or muscle of origin
	Infiltration outside organ or muscle of origin; regional nodes not involved
Group II	Regional disease, grossly resected
	A: Grossly resected tumours with microscopic residue
	B: Regional disease, completely resected, in which nodes may be involved and/or extension of tumour into an adjacent organ present
	C: Regional disease with involved nodes, grossly resected, but with evidence of microscopic residue
Group III	Incomplete resection or biopsy with gross residual disease
Group IV	Distant metastases present at onset

Table 30.7 European SIOP Staging System for rhabdomyosarcoma

Clinic stage	Invasiveness	Size	Nodal status	Metastasis status
I	T_1	a or b	N0	M0
II	T_2	a or b	N0	M0
III	T_1 or T_2	a or b	N1	M0
IV	T_1 or T_2	a or b	N0 or N1	M1

T_1, confined to organ of origin; T_2, involving adjacent organ(s) or tissues(s) ± effusion or multiple tumours in single organ. a, ≤ 5 cm diameter; b, > 5 cm diameter;

The traditional approach of initial aggressive surgery and early wide field irradiation has now been replaced by primary chemotherapy with delayed resection and conservative radiotherapy. Only in the case of small localized primaries with no distant disease is primary excision recommended. Primary chemotherapy is designed to reduce the mutilating effects of surgery or radiotherapy and increase the likelihood of complete excision once maximal tumour shrinkage is achieved. Where complete remission is obtained radiation is generally omitted (Table 30.8).

Chemotherapy comprises cyclophosphamide or ifosfamide combined with actinomycin D and vincristine. The addition of anthracyclines has not been shown to be of benefit. The replacement of cyclophosphamide by ifosfamide remains controversial, although improved response rates have been claimed (Treuner *et al.*, 1989; Crist *et al.*, 1990). (Figure 30.5).

Treatment in rhabdomyosarcoma is tailored to the primary site and the age of the child.

30.5.2 OTHER SOFT TISSUE SARCOMAS

Although tumours of the orbit can be cured by radiotherapy and non-intensive chemotherapy such as vincristine and actinomycin D, the cosmetic effects on facial bone growth have encouraged the use of primary chemotherapy with either VAC or IVA, followed by limited surgical resection of residual tumour if complete remission (CR) is not achieved (Heyn *et al.*, 1986).

With a parameningeal primary CR following chemotherapy is less common and cannot

Table 30.8 Outline treatment strategy for rhabdomyosarcoma depending on initial extent of tumour

Localized, resectable tumour
Surgery – if complete   VA × 10/52
            – incomplete   IVA × 4 courses
Regional, unresectable tumour
Primary chemotherapy   IVA or VACA
                                                                       × 4–6 courses depending on site

Delayed surgery
Irradiate if no CR achieved or parameningeal with bone erosion
Metastatic
More intensive multidrug regimen, e.g. add platinum-etoposide
? Megatherapy with marrow rescue

VA – vincristine, actinomycin; IVA – ifosfamide, vincristine, actinomycin; VACA – vincristine, actinomycin, cyclophosphamide, adriamycin.

	Day 1	Day 2	Day 3	
IFOSFAMIDE 3 g/m2	↓	↓	↓	+ MESNA and HYDRATION
VCR 1.5 mg/m2	↓			
ACT.D 1.5 mg/m2	↓			

Figure 30.5 Details of the IVA regimen used by the SIOP and UK Childrens Cancer Study Group for rhabdomyosarcoma.

be achieved with surgery. Radiotherapy localized to the primary site is given following chemotherapy (Raney *et al.*, 1987).

Paratesticular tumours have a good prognosis. Initial staging lymphadenectomy is unnecessary and if there is no evidence of lymph nodes on CT scan chemotherapy alone is usually curative (Hamilton *et al.*, 1989).

With tumours of the bladder, prostate, vagina and uterus radical surgery is not indicated, as in many cases CR is achieved with chemotherapy alone, enabling conservation of normal anatomy and function (Raney *et al.*, 1990). Residual tumour can be resected or locally irradiated. In some cases small volume residual disease can be treated by interstitial radiotherapy using iridium wires, either directly implanted or placed in moulds (Gerbaulet *et al.*, 1985).

Fibrosarcoma, synovial sarcoma, liposarcoma and neurofibrosarcoma occur rarely in childhood, and although these are less chemosensitive than rhabdomyosarcoma it is usually appropriate to attempt primary chemotherapy if non-mutilating surgery is not feasible at presentation.

Soft tissue sarcomas in the infant under 1 year of age are particularly difficult as despite apparently aggressive histological features these tumours may behave in a comparatively indolent manner. Low dose chemotherapy with vincristine and actinomycin D may be sufficient (Weiss and Lackman, 1989).

30.6 NEUROBLASTOMA

Neuroblastoma is the commonest abdominal tumour in children and usually presents under 3 years of age. The tumour arises from fetal neural cells (neuroblasts) which migrate from the neural crest to the sympathetic ganglia and adrenal glands. The tumour may thus arise at any site of sympathetic nerve tissue. Approximately 40% arise in the adrenal, 40% at other abdominal sites and 15% in the thorax.

It appears that there are at least two distinct biological entities, ranging from stage 4S which regresses spontaneously, to the highly aggressive metastatic form presenting in children over 1 year of age. Up to 2% of neonatal autopsies reveal the presence of primitive neuroblastic tissue indistinguishable from tumour, suggesting a high rate of spontaneous regression in normal children. In stage 4S disease, which almost invariably occurs in children under 1 year of age, there is often extensive infiltration of liver, with marrow or skin disease. Conservative management may be appropriate with the spontaneous resolution of the tumour over a period of weeks or months. Occasionally low dose chemotherapy or radiotherapy to hepatic tumour may be necessary because of respiratory difficulty (Suarez *et al.*, 1991).

The International Neuroblastoma Staging System is shown in Table 30.9 (Brodeur *et al.*,

Table 30.9 International Neuroblastoma Staging system

Stage 1	Localized tumour confined to the area of origin; complete gross excision, with or without microscopic residual disease; identifiable ipsilateral and contralateral lymph nodes negative macroscopically
Stage 2a	Unilateral tumour with incomplete gross excision; identifiable ipsilateral and contralateral lymph nodes negative microscopically
Stage 2b	Unilateral tumour with complete or incomplete gross excision; with positive ipsilateral regional lymph nodes; contralateral lymph nodes negative microscopically
Stage 3	Tumour infiltrating across the midline with or without regional lymph node involvement; or, unilateral tumour with contralateral regional lymph node involvement; or, midline tumour with bilateral regional lymph node involvement
Stage 4	Dissemination of tumour to distant lymph nodes, bone, bone marrow, liver and/or other organs (except as defined in stage 4S)
Stage 4S	Localized primary tumour as defined for stage 1 or 2 with dissemination limited to liver, skin and/or bone marrow

1988) Recently a number of biological prognostic factors have been demonstrated and are summarized in Table 30.10 (Look *et al.*, 1991).

Commonly, neuroblastoma presents as an abdominal mass with associated systemic symptoms due to metastatic disease. These include general malaise, bone pain, anaemia, fever and weight loss. With primary intraspinal disease there may be signs of cord compression. Hypertension at presentation may occur either due to renal vascular compression or tumour release of catecholamines. Diarrhoea has been described in association with mature ganglioneuroblastoma due to the release of vasoactive intestinal peptides.The so called 'dancing eyes syndrome' is a rare presentation often associated with well differentiated thoracic tumours. The reason for the cerebellar ataxia in this syndrome is unclear. With extensive disease exophthalmos and peri-orbital discoloration may occur and there may be evidence of bruising and petechiae due to the tumour infiltration of bone marrow.

The diagnostic criteria defined by the International Neuroblastoma Study Group comprises either an unequivocal pathological diagnosis based on tumour biopsy using appropriate immunohistochemistry or unequivocal bone marrow infiltrate with raised urinary catecholamines (Brodeur *et al.*, 1988).

The initial staging should include technetium bone scan, bilateral bone marrow aspirate and trephines and CT scan of primary site to determine nodal involvement and degree of infiltration across the midline. Metaiodobenzylguanidine (mIBG) scanning is used increasingly. This radio-iodinated compound is taken up by sympathetic neural tissue and scans are positive in neuroblastoma or phaeochromocytoma. It provides a highly

Table 30.10 Biological prognostic factors in neuroblastoma

Factors	Good	Intermediate	Poor
Ferritin levels	Normal	–	Abnormal (raised)
NSE levels (ng/ml)	< 20	20–100	> 100
No. of n-*myc* copies	2	3–10	> 10
Ploidy	Hyperdiploid		Diploid
Chromosome 1	Normal		Abnormal

sensitive and specific method of determining disease extent, both at presentation and following treatment (Hoefnagel *et al.*, 1987).

Pathological classifications in neuroblastoma are essentially based on the degree of tumour differentiation, ranging from the mature ganglioneuroblastoma, where there is a predominance of differentiated ganglionic cells, to the completely undifferentiated small round cell tumour, where the pathological diagnosis relies on the demonstration of immunohistochemistry consistent with a tumour of neural origin. These markers include PGP 9.5 and neurone specific enolase.

Stages I and II tumours are usually well differentiated and have few adverse biological factors. These are curable by surgery alone and no adjuvant chemotherapy or radiotherapy is necessary. In stage IIB where there is nodal involvement a short course of chemotherapy is generally given and this should carry as few late effects as possible. High doses of cyclophosphamide are avoided and carboplatin generally has replaced cisplatin (Matthay *et al.*, 1989) (Table 30.11).

In stage III disease preoperative chemotherapy with a platinum/etoposide based regimen will usually shrink the mass sufficiently to permit complete resection. Local radiotherapy is given if resection is incomplete. The survival in such cases now exceeds 60% at 5 years, largely due to the increased rate of complete resection following effective primary chemotherapy (Haase *et al.*, 1991).

Stage IV disease with metastases to bone, bone marrow, liver, nodes or skin now carries a cure rate of between 10% and 20% following very intensive chemotherapy, and in some cases megatherapy with autologous bone marrow rescue. In stage IV patients' age is a strong prognostic value and patients under 18 months do significantly better than older children. In the former group the cure rate is around 50%. The OPEC/OJEC regimen is shown in Figure 30.6, as is the more intensive rapid COJEC. The value of increased dose intensity is currently under study by the European Neuroblastoma Study Group.

mIBG targeted irradiation may have a role in treating residual disease following initial chemotherapy and is also being investigated as primary treatment (Lewis *et al.*, 1991).

The possibility of screening for neuroblastoma is currently under evaluation. Japanese studies have suggested that the incidence of metastatic disease is reduced by checking for urinary catecholamine in young infants. The disadvantage of this, however, is that a number of patients with tumours that will spontaneously resolve may receive unnecessary surgery or even chemotherapy (Murphy *et al.*, 1991).

30.7 WILMS' TUMOUR

Wilms' tumour or nephroblastoma arises due to an aberration in the normal metanephric blastema cell population. As discussed earlier deletion of the short arm of chromosome 11 is

Table 30.11 Outline treatment strategy in neuroblastoma

Stages 1 and 2A	Surgery alone.
Stage 2B	OPEC/OJEC × 6 courses then surgery
Stage 3	OPEC/OJEC × 6–8 courses then surgery; irradiation if incomplete resection
Stage 4	OPEC/OJEC or more intensive high dose intensity variant then surgery; *high dose melphalan with autologous marrow rescue
Stage 4S	Observe; low dose irradiation or chemotherapy if required

OPEC/OJEC – vincristine, cisplatin or carboplatin (JM8) alternately, etoposide, cyclophosphamide.
* Not given to infants < 1 year at diagnosis.

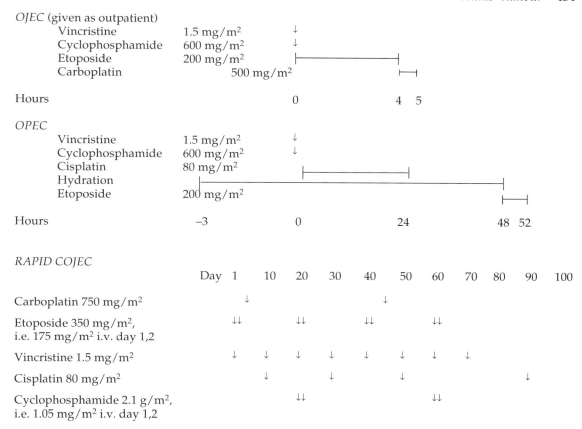

Figure 30.6 Outline of the chemotherapy regimens used by the UK Childrens Cancer Study Group and the European Neuroblastoma Study Group (ENSG) for advanced neuroblastoma.

occasionally found in tumour tissue, suggesting that loss of a tumour suppressor gene may be of primary aetiological importance.

In some patients Wilms' tumour is associated with aniridia and hemihypertrophy of trunk and limbs. In the Drash syndrome the tumour occurs in conjunction with nephritis and in some cases pseudohermaphroditism. In Beckwith's syndrome there is a high incidence of Wilms' tumour.

The pathological subclassification of Wilms' tumour is of considerable prognostic value. The majority of tumours fall within the so called 'favourable' group. In these tumours there is evidence of three subtypes (triphasic):

blastema, epithelial and stromal elements. The unfavourable subgroup which covers less than 10% of patients is usually anaplastic or sarcomatous. These differ in terms of clinical behaviour and chemotherapy responsiveness. The clear cell sarcoma tends to metastasize to bone and the rhabdoid to brain. Increasingly these tumour subgroups are regarded as separate entities from the classic Wilms' tumour.

The common presentation is as an asymptomatic abdominal mass, which may reach considerable size before being picked up. In only 10% of cases does haematuria or hypertension occur. Occasionally patients have a low grade intermittent fever.

Initial staging investigations include ultra-sound and, ideally, CT scan of the abdomen to clarify the intactness of the tumour capsule and the presence of nodal involvement. These are of importance if primary surgery is to be attempted. Doppler ultrasound and CT scan have a role in determining whether the vena cava is involved. This is one of the firm contraindications to attempting primary surgery. Chest X-ray is mandatory to exclude lung deposits but the role of a CT scan remains controversial. It is possible that this sensitive technique may upstage patients inappropriately and this is the subject of prospective study in the UK.

There is a tendency to use preoperative chemotherapy routinely. The European SIOP group recommend primary treatment with vincristine and actinomycin D, whereas the American National Wilms' Tumour Study Group still recommends primary surgery to be attempted if possible (Lemerle *et al.*, 1983; D'Angio *et al.*, 1989).

Although in some centres the diagnosis is made on clinical grounds relying on imaging and normal urinary catecholamines, it is preferable to perform either an open or tru-cut biopsy of the tumour prior to commencing therapy. The American National Wilms' Tumour Study Group staging system is shown in Table 30.12.

Treatment strategy is summarized in Table 30.13. The cure rates by stage are: stages I and II, 90%; III, 80%; IV, 60%. Cyclophosphamide has been omitted because it does not increase efficacy and may cause sterilization in males. Irradiation to the tumour bed is limited to those with initially unresectable disease who have incomplete resection after primary chemotherapy. It is also used in some patients with unfavourable histology. The need for lung irradiation in patients with initial pulmonary metastases is also a subject of debate. If there is a rapid disappearance of lung metastases on the CT scan after two to three courses of chemotherapy, radiotherapy is probably unnecessary (DeKraker *et al.*, 1990). In about 5% of cases disease is bilateral at presentation. Primary chemotherapy is designed to shrink the tumour on both sides thus enabling conservative partial nephrectomy

Table 30.12   Staging system for Wilms' tumour devised by the American National Wilms' tumour study group

Stage I	Tumour is limited to the kidney and is completely excised. The surface of the renal capsule is intact. Tumour not ruptured before or during removal. No residual tumour at or beyond the margins of resection. The tumour may have been biopsied.
Stage II	Tumour extends beyond the kidney, but is completely excised. There is regional extension of the tumour, i.e. penetration through the outer surface of the renal capsule into perirenal soft tissues. Vessels outside the kidney substance are infiltrated or contain tumour thrombus. There has been local spillage of tumour confined to the flank. There is no residual tumour at or beyond the margins of excision.
Stage III	Residual non-haematogenous tumour confined to the abdomen. Any one or more of the following may be present: a. Lymph nodes on biopsy are found to be involved in the renal hilum para-aortic chain or beyond b. Diffuse peritoneal contamination by tumour such as spillage beyond the flank before or during surgery or by tumour growth which has penetrated through the peritoneal surface c. Implants on peritoneal surfaces d. The tumour extends to the surgical margins either micro- or macroscopically
Stage IV	Deposits beyond stage III
Stage V	Bilateral tumours at diagnosis

Table 30.13   Outline treatment strategy for Wilms' tumour in relation to stage at presentation

Stage I	Vincristine (1.5 mg/m^2) weekly × 10
Stage II	Vincristine, actinomycin (1.5 mg/m^2) 3 weekly × 6/12
Stage III	Vincristine + alternating actinomycin + doxorubicin (40 mg/m^2) 3 weekly × 12/12
Stage IV	Vincristine + simultaneous actinomycin + doxorubicin (30 mg/m^2) × 12/12
Stages III and IV	Primary tumour is resected after 2–3 months' chemotherapy
	Irradiation to the primary site is only used if surgery is incomplete or lymph nodes are involved
	Lung irradiation is given in stage IV if CR on CT is not achieved by 12 weeks

to be carried out once maximum response has been achieved (Coppes *et al.*, 1989).

30.8   LIVER TUMOURS

Malignant primary liver tumours in childhood are usually hepatoblastoma or hepatocellular carcinoma. Rhabdomyosarcoma, angiosarcoma and teratoma are also occasionally seen.

The histological pattern in hepatoblastoma may resemble perinatal hepatocytes (fetal type) or more primitive cells (embryonal type). A third anaplastic highly undifferentiated form also occurs. The cytology of hepatocarcinoma resembles that in adult disease (Kasai and Watanabe, 1970).

Because the management of these two tumours is identical in childhood, they will be considered together.

These tumours usually present as an abdominal mass, which may be associated with marked abdominal distention and discomfort. On initial investigation plain X-ray may show some calcification within the tumour and ultrasound localizes the mass to the liver. CT scan is mandatory to assess initial operability. Alphafetoprotein levels in serum are raised in about 80% of hepatoblastomas and about half of hepatocarcinomas. This marker is useful both in assisting in diagnosis and assessment of response to primary chemotherapy or surgery. Technetium bone scan and CT scan of chest complete staging investigations.

In a small percentage of patients where the tumour is small and very localized primary surgery is the treatment of choice. This is followed by a short course of chemotherapy such as single agent doxorubicin. In the majority of cases, however, combination chemotherapy is used to shrink the tumour and facilitate ultimate complete resection (Weinblatt *et al.*, 1982). Only if the tumour can ultimately be resected is cure possible and preoperative MRI scan or angiography play an important role. The PLADO (Platinum–Doxorubicin) regimen is shown in Figure 30.7 and in general six to eight courses are given prior to surgery. With this strategy approximately 60% of children are cured, including those with initial metastatic disease In the event of incomplete resection radiotherapy is usually given, although the efficacy of this is questionable. (Habrand, 1991).

30.9   GERM CELL TUMOURS

Although the same range of histological subtypes of malignant germ cell tumours may occur in children as in adults, the majority are yolk sac tumours. Thus alphafetoprotein levels are almost invariably raised and provide a useful guide to both diagnosis and response to treatment. There may also be a mixed histological pattern with trophoblastic elements producing beta human chorionic gonadotrophin (βHCG).

Testicular teratomas (orchioblastoma) usually present as a painless swelling,

```
                                                                    Surgery
(week)
                        0       3       6       9      12      15
Cisplatin               ↓       ↓       ↓       ↓       ↓       ↓
100 mg/m²
over 24 hours

Doxorubicin             ↓       ↓       ↓       ↓       ↓       ↓         irradiate if
25 mg/m² daily × 2                                                        incompletely
                                                                         resected
```

Figure 30.7   The SIOP chemotherapy regimen and treatment strategy for management of malignant liver tumours in childhood.

although occasionally there may be extensive nodal involvement. Initial surgery should never be through the scrotal skin as this carries a risk of tumour contamination and will not achieve adequate excision of the potentially involved spermatic cord. Following removal through an inguinal excision, if microscopically complete, the patient is followed with no adjuvant chemotherapy. Provided the serum alphafetoprotein levels fall to normal this is curative. Routine staging examinations include chest X-ray/CT scan of chest and abdomen and technetium bone scan. Dysgerminomas and yolk sac tumours are the commonest histological type of ovarian tumour in childhood, and with localized disease unilateral salpingo-oophorectomy without postoperative radiation or chemotherapy should be curative (Flamant *et al.*, 1978; Weinblatt and Ortega, 1982). Even in the absence of a serum marker this conservative approach may be followed using regular CT scan or ultrasound follow-up. In the event of a local recurrence the salvage rate should be high with effective chemotherapy.

The sacrococcygeal teratoma in the neonate is usually of benign well differentiated subtype. Complete resection including excision of the coccyx is usually curative (Whalen *et al.*, 1985). Occasionally there may be yolk sac or undifferentiated teratomatous elements, in which case if excision is incomplete adjuvant chemotherapy is required. Again

the overall cure rate is high (Mann *et al.*, 1989).

Mediastinal germ cell tumours, often of mixed histological type, may be very bulky at presentation and have a less good prognosis than the other tumours mentioned above. With effective chemotherapy and resection of any residual imageable abnormality the cure rate should exceed 50%.

For metastatic disease, bulky unresectable tumours or if tumour markers fail to decline after resection, chemotherapy is given, using effective non-sterilizing regimens such as carboplatin, etoposide, bleomycin (Figure 30.8). Cure rate should exceed 80%. Cisplatin, in particular at high dose, cyclophosphamide or anthracyclines are not indicated for first line treatment in children (Pinkerton *et al.*, 1990).

30.10   RETINOBLASTOMA

This embryonal tumour arises in the neuroectodermal tissue of the retina. In about 60% of cases it is unilateral, the remainder are bilateral, although there is a very rare trilateral form in which a lesion is found in the pineal or anterior third ventricular region. This tumour is of particular interest because it provides a model for the molecular basis of carcinogenesis (Benedict *et al.*, 1988; Dryja *et al.*, 1989) and has contributed to the understanding of the *p53* gene (Stratton *et al.*, 1990).

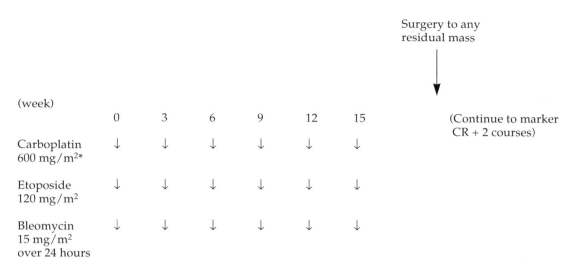

Preferably dose based on EDTA GFR formula; mg = [EDTA ml/min + (15 × SA)] × 6

Figure 30.8 The UK Childrens Cancer Study Group chemotherapy regimen for unresectable malignant germ cell tumours.

Invariably this tumour occurs below 3 years of age, and may present with visual loss or loss of the normal red reflex when light is shone directly into the eye. Strabismus can occur or there may be secondary glaucoma due to multiple lesions. Clinical staging is based on the extent of tumour infiltration along the optic nerve and an initial assessment under anaesthesia is mandatory. MRI or CT scan will provide information on which the initial treatment decision is based.

A conservative eye-sparing procedure is inadvisable if there is involvement of the optic disc or where there is a high risk of heavy choroidal invasion, accompanying either glaucoma or retinal detachment. In these situations primary surgery may be required. Conservative treatment is with sophisticated radiotherapy technique delivered either by surface applicator or external beam (Harnett *et al.*, 1987). Over 80% of children are cured. Chemotherapy is generally reserved for the small number of patients who recur, either locally or at distant sites. Similar drugs to those used in the treatment of neuroblastoma have been shown to be effective.

Close follow-up with examination under anaesthesia should be done every 3–4 months for 2 years and then 6 monthly for up to 5 years. In the UK the majority of children are followed in one of two national centres. Where there is no previous family history and one affected child, other children have about a 5% chance of being affected. By contrast, the offspring of a parent with bilateral disease has a 50% chance of being affected. If a parent has unilateral retinoblastoma and a previous child has been affected, then any subsequent child has a 50% chance of being involved.

The use of molecular techniques to detect loss of heterozygosity on chromosome 13 has enabled screening of children, avoiding the necessity for close follow-up if shown to be normal. It has also enabled antenatal screening to be done, although the issue of whether elective termination is justified in a highly curable tumour remains controversial (Lee *et al.*, 1987).

30.11   LANGERHANS' CELL HISTIOCYTOSIS

Although this is not a malignant disorder, because in some cases it may require treatment with chemotherapy it is usually managed by paediatric oncologists.

Langerhans' cell histiocytosis (LCH), which was previously known as histiocytosis X, covers a range of clinical disorders. These used to be divided on the basis of clinical extent into eosinophilic granuloma of bone, Letterer–Siwe disease of skin and lung and Hand–Schüller–Christian disease with multisystem involvement. In fact, these all involve the same cellular disorder and are now included under the single diagnosis of LCH.

Demonstration of the Langerhans' cell, a mononuclear cell with a lobulated nucleus is pathognomonic of LCH. There is often a reactive proliferation of phagocytic histiocytes, polymorphs and lymphocytes. The Langerhans' cell on electron microscopy contains a racquet shaped organelle known as the Burbeck granule. Special stains which are positive in LCH include S100, alpha D mannosidase and the monoclonal marker CD1 (Chu *et al.*, 1987).

From a management point of view LCH is considered either as a single system or multisystem disorder. Single system disease is readily curable, irrespective of site. This may be bone, skin, ear or lymph nodes. No treatment may be required as spontaneous remission can occur. In the case of an isolated bone lesion, diagnostic curettage may produce spontaneous healing. Topical mustine has been used with good effect for refractory aural discharge.

Multisystem disease in addition to the above may involve lung, liver, spleen and bone marrow. The infant with multisystem disease has the worst prognosis with up to 40% dying of disease and may require multiagent chemotherapy. In general, treatment is commenced with vincristine and prednisolone and etoposide is introduced for resistant cases (McLelland *et al.*, 1990).

30.12   LATE EFFECTS

As more than half of all children with cancer can now expect to be cured of their disease, it is of increasing importance that they are cured 'at least cost'. Late sequelae may be the consequence of any of the three main treatment modalities, surgery, radiation or chemotherapy. With improved primary chemotherapy multilating surgical procedures can now be avoided in most patients. It is therefore the late consequences of chemotherapy and radiotherapy which have received most attention. (Meadows and Hobbie, 1986; Pinkerton, 1992).

The major late complication of radiotherapy in the young child is bony undergrowth. This may be of considerable cosmetic importance in the case of the child with an orbital rhabdomyosarcoma, where facial asymmetry may be marked. Hemi-abdominal irradiation for Wilms' tumour will produce underdevelopment of soft tissue and musculature. With mantle irradiation for Hodgkin's disease undergrowth of the clavicles leads to posture deformity and hypoplastic thorax. Irradiation fields which include the hip may result in aseptic necrosis or slipped femoral epiphyses. Where possible long bone epiphyses should be avoided in the younger child but this must not be allowed to compromise the effectiveness of radiotherapy.

Growth can also be affected by an indirect influence of radiotherapy on endocrine function. Subtle abnormalities in hypothalamic, pituitary and thyroid function will influence linear growth. Overt growth hormone deficiency is uncommon, except in patients receiving total body irradiation prior to bone marrow transplant procedures, but is also seen in children irradiated for brain tumours. Close follow-up of such patients and early institution of growth hormone therapy is of importance if growth deficiency is to be optimally corrected (Brown *et al.*, 1983; Sanders *et al.*, 1986; Clayton *et al.*, 1988).

Neurological sequelae from whole brain irradiation have been extensively studied and in children with leukaemia subtle deficits in specific areas of learning, such as numeracy, have been reported. These effects are clearly age related and for this reason cranial irradiation is avoided in children under 3 years if possible (Jannoun, 1983).

There is still a considerable amount to be learned about the dose–effect relationship for many drug related toxicities and long term follow-up of patients at clinics specifically designed to consider these sequelae is essential. Treatment related infertility is one of the most important, both to parents and the children. Sperm banking may be feasible in some adolescent males, although the topic of sperm collection is clearly a sensitive one and needs to be handled with delicacy. In many cases the adolescent is unable to produce an adequate sample. Alkylating agents, such as cyclophosphamide, chlorambucil and procarbazine will almost invariably cause sterility in boys but the ovary is considerably more resistant and most girls probably retain fertility (Aubier *et al.*, 1989).

Attempts to reduce the toxicity of anthracyclines with prolonged infusion schedules are being evaluated, as are alternative analogues such as epirubicin. Cardiac protection using iron chelaters, such as cardioxane, are also under assessment (Lipshultz *et al.*, 1991; Yeung *et al.*, 1991). Bleomycin should be avoided if possible, particularly a weekly schedule. It is likely that a 3 weekly infused schedule will have minimal pulmonary toxicity. Similarly, BCNU, particularly at high dose, has unacceptable late lung toxicity and should be avoided.

Around 5% of cancer patients will develop a second tumour as a result of their treatment. The precise contributory factors still require some clarification, but at present a high dose of alkylating agent, particularly when combined with radiation, is the major factor. The epipodophyllotoxins, particularly teniposide, given in a frequent dose (weekly or more often) have recently been implicated (Pui *et al.*, 1991).

The primary goal of therapy in any children's cancer is to cure the patient and it is important that some late effects, while causing understandable concern, should not be overemphasized and result in a compromise on cure rates. Cosmetic abnormalities may have to be accepted, as may infertility and a low risk of second tumours.

REFERENCES

Aubier, F., Flamant, F., Brauner, R. *et al.* (1989) Male gonadal function after chemotherapy for solid tumors in childhood. *Journal of Clinical Oncology*, **7**, 304–9.

Benedict, W.F., Fung, Y-K.T. and Murphree, A.L. (1988) The gene responsible for the development of retinoblastoma and osteosarcoma. *Cancer*, **62**, 1691–4.

Brodeur, G.M., Seeger, R.C., Barrett, A. *et al.* (1988) International criteria for diagnosis, staging and response to treatment in patients with neuroblastoma. *Journal of Clinical Oncology*, **6**, 1874–81.

Brown, I.H., Lee, T.J., Eden, O.B. *et al.* (1983) Growth and endocrine function after treatment for medulloblastoma. *Archives of Disease in Childhood*, **58**, 722–7.

Castello, M.A., Clerico, A., Deb, G. *et al.* (1990) High dose carboplatin in combination with etoposide (JET Regimen) for childhood brain tumours. *American Journal of Pediatric Hematology Oncology*, **12**, 297–300.

Chu, A., D'Angio, D.J., Favara, B. *et al.* (1987) Histiocytosis syndromes in children. *Lancet*, **i**, 208–9.

Clayton, P.E., Morris-Jones, P.H., Shalet, S.M. and Price, D.A. (1988) Growth in children treated for acute lymphoblastic leukaemia. *Lancet*, **i**, 483–5.

Coppes, M.J., DeKraker, J., van Dijken, P.J. *et al.* (1989) Bilateral Wilms' tumor: long-term survival and some epidemiological features. *Journal of Clinical Oncology*, **7**, 310–15.

Crist, W.M., Garnsey, L., Beltangady, M. *et al.* (1990) Prognosis in children with rhabdomyosarcoma: A report of the Intergroup Rhabdomyosarcoma Studies I and II. *Journal of Clinical Oncology*, **8**, 443–52.

D'Angio, G.J., Breslow, N., Beckwith, B. *et al.* (1989) Treatment of Wilms' tumor. Results of the third

National Wilms' Tumor Study. *Cancer*, **64**, 349–60.

DeKraker, J., Lemerle, J., Voute, P.A. *et al.* (1990) Wilms' tumor with pulmonary metastases at diagnosis: the significance of primary chemotherapy. *Journal of Clinical Oncology*, **7**, 1187–90.

Dryja, T.P., Mukai, S., Petersen, R. *et al.* (1989) Parental origin of mutations of the retinoblastoma gene. *Nature*, **339**, 556–8.

Ekert, H., Waters, K.D., Smith, P.J. *et al.* (1988) Treatment with MOPP or ChlVPP chemotherapy only for all stages of childhood Hodgkin's disease. *Journal of Clinical Oncology*, **6**, 1845–50.

Flamant, F., Caillou, B., Pejovic, M-H. *et al.* (1978) Prognostic factors in malignant germ cell tumors of the ovary in children excluding pure dysgerminoma. *European Journal of Cancer*, **14**, 901–6.

Fryer, C.J., Hutchinson, R.J., Krailo, M. *et al.* (1990) Efficacy and toxicity of 12 courses of ABVD chemotherapy followed by low dose regional radiation in advanced Hodgkin's disease in children: a report from the Children's Cancer Study Group. *Journal of Clinical Oncology*, **8**, 1971–80.

Gardner, M.J., Snee, M.P., Hall, A.J. *et al.* (1990) Results of case-control study of leukaemia and lymphoma among young people near Sellafield nuclear plant in West Cumbria. *British Medical Journal*, **300**, 423–9.

Gerbaulet, A., Panis, X., Flamant, F. *et al.* (1985) Iridium after loading curietherapy in the treatment of pediatric malignancies. The Institute Gustave Roussy Experience. *Cancer*, **56**, 1274–9.

Greaves, M.F. (1988) Speculations on the cause of childhood acute lymphoblastic leukemia. *Leukemia*, **2**, 120–5.

Habrand, J.L. (1991) Role of radiotherapy in hepatoblastoma and hepatocellular carcinoma in children and adolescents: results of survey conducted by the SIOP Liver Tumour Group. *Medical and Pediatric Oncology*, **19**, 208.

Hamilton, C.R., Pinkerton, C.R. and Horwich, A. (1989) The management of paratesticular rhabdomyosarcoma. *Clinical Radiology*, **40**, 314–17.

Harnett, A.N., Hungerford, J.L., Lambert, G. *et al.* (1987) Modern lateral external beam (lens sparing) radiotherapy for retinoblastoma. *Ophthalmic Paediatrics and Genetics*, **8**, 53–61.

Haase, G.M., O'Leary, M.C., Ramsay, N.K.C. *et al.* (1991) Aggressive surgery combined with intensive chemotherapy improves survival in poor-risk neuroblastoma. *Journal of Pediatric Surgery*, **26**, 1119–24.

Henshaw, D.L., Eatough, J.P. and Richardson, R.B. (1990) Radon as a causative factor in induction of myeloid leukaemia and other cancers. *Lancet*, **335**, 1008–1–12.

Heyn, R., Beltangady, M., Hays, D. *et al.* (1989) Results of intensive therapy in children with localized alveolar extremity rhabdomyosarcoma: report from the Intergroup Rhabdomyosarcoma Study. *Journal of Clinical Oncology*, **7**, 200–7.

Heyn, R., Ragab, A., Romey, B. *et al.* (1986) Late effects of therapy in orbital rhabdomyosarcoma in children. A report from the Intergroup Rhabdomyosarcoma Study. *Cancer*, **57**, 1738–43.

Hoefnagel, C.A., Voute, P.A., DeKraker, J. and Marcuse, H.R. (1987) Radionuclide diagnosis and treatment of neural crest tumours using iodine-131-meta-iodobenzylguanidine. *Journal of Nuclear Medicine*, **28**, 308–14.

Horwich, A. and Bloom, H.J.G. (1985) Optic gliomas; radiation therapy and prognosis. *International Journal of Radiation Oncology, Biology, Physics*, **11**, 1067–79.

Jannoun, L. (1983) Are cognitive and educational development affected by age at which prophylactic therapy is given in acute lymphoblastic leukemia? *Archives of Disease in Childhood*, **58**, 953–8.

Kasai, M. and Watanabe, I. (1970) Histological classification of liver cell carcinoma in infancy and childhood and its clinical evaluation. *Cancer*, **24**, 551–63.

Kinlen, L.J. (1993) Can paternal preconceptional radiation account for the increase of leukaemia and non-Hodgkin's lymphoma in Seascale? *British Medical Journal*, **306**, 1718–21.

Knudson, A.G. (1971) Mutation and cancer: statistical study of retinoblastoma. *Proceedings of the National Academy of Sciences USA*, **68**, 820–3.

Lee, W-H., Bookstein, R., Hong, F.D. *et al.* (1987) Human retinoblastoma susceptibility gene: cloning identification and sequence. *Science*, **235**, 1394–9.

Lefkowitz, I.B., Packer, R.J., Siegel, K.R. *et al.* (1990) Results of treatment of children with recurrent medulloblastoma/primitive neuroectodermal tumors with lomustine, cisplatin, and vincristine. *Cancer*, **65**, 412–17.

Lemerle, J., Voute, P.A., Tournade, M.F. *et al.* (1983) Effectiveness of pre-operative chemotherapy in Wilms' tumor: results of an International Society of Paediatric Oncology (SIOP) clinical trial. *Journal of Clinical Oncology*, **1**, 604.

Leverger, G., Oberlin, O., Quintana, E. *et al.* (1990) ABVD vs MOPP/ABVD before low-dose radiotherapy in CS IA-IIA childhood Hodgkin's disease: a prospective randomized trial from the French Society of Pediatric Oncology. *Proceedings of the American Society of Clinical Oncology,* **9,** 1060.

Lewis, I., Lashford, L.S., Fielding, S. *et al.* (1991) A phase I/II study of [131]I mIBG in chemo-resistant neuroblastoma. *Advances in Neuroblastoma Research,* **3,** 463–9.

Li, F.P. and Fraumeni, J.F. (1969) Rhabdomyosarcoma in children: epidemiologic study and identification of a familial cancer syndrome. *Journal of the National Cancer Institute,* **43,** 1365–73.

Lipshultz, S.E., Colan, S.D., Gelber, R.D. *et al.* (1991) Late cardiac effects of doxorubicin therapy for acute lymphoblastic leukemia in childhood. *New England Journal of Medicine,* **324,** 808–15.

Look, A.T., Hayes, F.A., Shuster, J. *et al.* (1991) Clinical relevance of tumor cell ploidy and N-myc gene amplification in childhood neuroblastoma: pediatric oncology group study. *Journal of Clinical Oncology,* **9,** 581–91.

McLelland, J., Broadbent, V., Yeoman, E. *et al.* (1990) Langerhans cell histiocytosis; a conservative approach to treatment. *Archives of Disease in Childhood,* **65,** 301–3.

Mann, J.R., Pearson, D., Barrett, A. *et al.* (1989) Results of the United Kingdom Children's Cancer Study Group's malignant germ cell tumour studies. *Cancer,* **63,** 1657–67.

Matthay, K.K., Sather, H.N., Seeger, R.C. *et al.* (1989) Excellent outcome of stage II neuroblastoma is independent of residual disease and radiation therapy. *Journal of Clinical Oncology,* **7,** 236–44.

Meadows, A. and Hobbie, W. (1986) The medical consequences of cure. *Cancer,* **58,** 524–8.

Murphy, S.B., Bowman, W.P., Abromowitch, M. *et al.* (1986) Results of treatment of advanced-stage Burkitt's lymphoma and B cell (SIg+) fractionated cyclophosphamide and coordinated high-dose methotrexate and cytarabine. *Journal of Clinical Oncology,* **4,** 1732–9.

Murphy, S.B., Cohn, S.L., Craft, A.W. *et al.* (1991) Do children benefit from mass screening for neuroblastoma? *Lancet,* **337,** 344–46.

Newton, W.A. Jr, Soule, E.H., Hamoudi, A.B. *et al.* (1988) Histopathology of childhood sarcomas, Intergroup rhabdomyosarcoma studies I and II:

Clinicopathologic correlation. *Journal of Clinical Oncology,* **6,** 67–75.

O'Brien, M.E.R., Pinkerton, C.R., Kingston, J. *et al.* (1992) 'VEEP' in children with Hodgkin's disease – a regimen to decrease late sequelae. *British Journal of Cancer,* **65,** 756–60.

Packer, R.J., Sutton, L.N., Bilaniuk, L.T. *et al.* (1988) Treatment of chiasmatic/hypothalamic gliomas of childhood with chemotherapy: an update. *Annals of Neurology,* **23,** 79–85.

Patte, C., Philip, T., Rodary, C. *et al.* (1986) Improved survival rate in children with stage III and IV B-cell non Hodgkin's lymphoma and leukemia using a multiagent chemotherapy: results of a study of 114 children from the French Pediatric Oncology Society. *Journal of Clinical Oncology,* **4,** 1219–29.

Pendergrass, T.W., Milstein, J.M., Geyer, J.R. *et al.* (1987) Eight drugs in one day chemotherapy for brain tumours: experience in 107 children and rationale for preradiotherapy chemotherapy. *Journal of Clinical Oncology,* **5,** 1221–31.

Philip, T., Pinkerton, R., Biron, P. *et al.* (1987) Effective multiagent chemotherapy in children with advanced B-cell lymphoma: Who remains the high risk patient? *British Journal of Haematology,* **65,** 159–64.

Pinkerton, C.R. (1992) Avoiding chemotherapy related late effects in children with curable tumours. *Archives of Disease in Childhood,* **67,** 1116–1119.

Pinkerton, C.R., Broadbent, V., Horwich, A. *et al.* (1990) JEB – a carboplatin based regimen for malignant germ cell tumours in children. *British Journal of Cancer,* **62,** 257 -62.

Pui, C-H., Ribeiro, R.C., Hancock, M.L. *et al.* (1991) Acute myeloid leukemia in children treated with epipodophyllotoxins for acute lymphoblastic leukemia. *New England Journal of Medicine,* **325,** 1682–7.

Radford, J.A., Cowan, R.A., Flanagan, M. *et al.* (1988) The significance of residual mediastinal abnormality on the chest radiograph following treatment for Hodgkin's disease. *Journal of Clinical Oncology,* **6,** 940–6.

Raney, R.B. Jr, Gehan, E.A., Hays, D.M. *et al.* (1990) Primary chemotherapy with or without radiation therapy and/or surgery for children with localized sarcoma of the bladder, prostate, vagina, uterus, and cervix. A comparison of the results in Intergroup Rhabdomyosarcoma Studies I and II. *Cancer,* **66,** 2072–81.

Raney, B., Tefft, M., Newton, W.A. *et al.* (1987) Improved prognosis with intensive treatment of children with cranial soft tissue sarcomas arising in nonorbital parameningeal sites. *Cancer*, **59**, 147–55.

Rodary, C., Gehan, E., Flamant, F. *et al.* (1991) Prognostic factors in 951 nonmetastatic rhabdomyosarcoma in children: report from the International Rhabdomyosarcoma Workshop. *Medical and Pediatric Oncology*, **19**, 89–95.

Sanders, J.E., Pritchard, S., Mahoney, P. *et al.* (1986) Growth and development following marrow transplantation for leukaemia. *Blood*, **68**, 1129–35.

Sposto, R., Ertel, I.J., Jenkin, R.D.T. *et al.* (1988) The effectiveness of chemotherapy for treatment of high-grade astrocytoma in children; results of a randomized trial. A report from the Children's Cancer Study Group. *Journal of Neuro-oncology*, **7**, 165–77.

Stratton, M.R., Moss, S., Warren, W. *et al.* (1990) Mutation of the p53 gene in soft tissue sarcomas: association with abnormalities of the RB1 gene. *Oncogene*, **5**, 1297–301.

Suarez, A., Hartmann, O., Vassal, G. *et al.* (1991) Treatment of stage IV-S neuroblastoma: A study of 34 cases treated between 1982 and 1987. *Medical and Pediatric Oncology*, **19**, 473–7.

Tait, D.M., Thornton-Jones, H., Bloom, H.J.G. *et al.* (1990) Adjuvant chemotherapy for medulloblastoma: the first multi-centre control trial of the International Society of Paediatric Oncology (SIOP I). *European Journal of Cancer*, **26**, 461–9.

Treuner, J., Koscielniak, E. and Keim, M. (1989) Comparison of the rates of response to ifosfamide and cyclophosphamide in primary unresectable rhabdomyosarcoma. *Cancer Chemotherapy and Pharmacology*, **24** (suppl 1), 5, 48–50.

Wallner, K.E., Wara, W.M., Sheline, G.E. and Davis, R.L. (1986) Intracranial ependymomas: results of treatment with partial or whole brain irradiation without spinal irradiation. *International Journal of Radiation Oncology, Biology, Physics*, **12**, 1937–41.

Weinblatt, M.E. and Ortega, J.A. (1982) Treatment of children with dysgerminoma of the ovary. *Cancer*, **49**, 2608–11.

Weinblatt, M.E., Siegel, S.E., Siegel, M.M. *et al.* (1982) Preoperative chemotherapy for unresectable primary hepatic malignancies in children. *Cancer*, **50**, 1061–4.

Weiss, A.J. and Lackman, R.D. (1989) Low-dose chemotherapy of desmoid tumours. *Cancer*, **64**, 1192–4.

Whalen, T., Mahour, G., Landing, B. and Wooleyt, M.M. (1985) Sacrococcygeal teratomas in infants and children. *American Journal of Surgery*, **150**, 373.

Wheeler, K. and Chessells, J.M. (1990). UKALL X– an effective treatment for stage III mediastinal non-Hodgkin's lymphoma. *Archives of Disease in Childhood*, **65**, 252–4.

Wolff, S.N., Phillips, G.L. and Herzig, G.P. (1987) High-dose carmustine with autologous bone marrow transplantation for the adjuvant treatment of high-grade gliomas of the central nervous system. *Cancer Treatment Reports*, **71**, 183–5.

Yeung, S.T., Yoong, C., Spink, J. *et al.* (1991) Functional myocardial impairment in children treated with anthracyclines for cancer. *Lancet*, **337**, 816–18.

NEUROENDOCRINE TUMOURS

Diana Tait

The definition of the term 'neuroendocrine tumour' is a matter of dispute and for the purpose of this chapter will be taken to mean those tumours arising from the 'diffuse neuroendocrine system'.

31.1 NEUROENDOCRINE NETWORK

Living organisms require an internal communication system and chemical signals, in the form of regulatory peptides, often provide this service. During the 1970s, immunological methods demonstrated that neurones and endocrine cells could produce immunologically identical signals with the synthesis of peptides such as somatostatin, substance P, gastrin, vasoactive intestinal polypeptide (VIP) and adrenocorticotrophic hormone (ACTH). This discovery challenged the traditional concept of distinct neural and endocrine transmission, and suggested that these signals, shared by nerve cells and peripheral endocrine glands, could provide a communication network between body and brain. Thus evolved the concept of the neuroendocrine system which structurally is composed of endocrine/paracrine cells disseminated in epithelial tissues and intrinsic neurones forming continuous ganglionic chains in the submucosa and muscle layers. Outside the brain, the gastro-entero-pancreatic system is the richest source of regulatory peptides, but production is widespread and particularly marked throughout the bronchial tree, bladder and skin.

31.2 INCIDENCE

Individually, these are all rare tumours and precise figures on incidence are not available. However, as many of the tumours in this group are benign in histological appearance and nature, it is likely that many are undetected and unreported. For example, in pathological review of appendix specimens the overall incidence of carcinoid is reported to be from 1 in 150 to 1 in 1000.

31.3 AETIOLOGY

For the most part, nothing is known about the aetiology of this group of tumours. The exception to this is their occurrence as part of two well characterized hereditary syndromes. Multiple endocrine neoplasia Type I (MEN I) is an inherited disorder of autosomal dominant type encompassing tumours of the parathyroid gland, anterior pituitary and endocrine pancreas. The genetic defect has now been identified and maps to the long arm of chromosome II (11q13) (Larsson *et al.*, 1988). It appears that the MEN I gene belongs to the group of oncogenes known as tumour suppresser genes. Multiple endocrine neoplasia Type II (MEN II) occurs as two types, IIa and IIb, each of which encompasses medullary thyroid carcinoma, phaeochromocytoma and parathyroid adenoma. In addition, MEN IIb is associated with a marfanoid habitus and mucosal neuromas. The gene responsible for these two syndromes is probably the same and is on the long arm of chromosome 10. Like MEN I, inheritance is of autosomal dominant type.

31.4   PATHOLOGY

Virtually all eukaryotic cells contain some secretory organelles but, in addition, neuroendocrine cells (neuronal and endocrine) contain two characteristic secretory organelles. According to their electron microscopic appearance, these are referred to as small neuroendocrine vesicles and neuroendocrine granules. The identification of tumour as being of neuroendocrine origin relies on the demonstration of these neurosecretory organelles either by silver (argyrophil) staining, electron microscopy or immunocytochemistry.

Immunophenotypically, these tumours are distinctive and typically show a mixed epithelial and endocrine pattern. Of the epithelial markers, cytokeratins, carcinoembryonic antigen (CEA) and epithelial membrane antigen (EMA) are most commonly encountered. The endocrine markers can be considered one of two types, general and specific. The former consist of peptides such as chromogranin, neurone specific enolase (NSE), protein gene product 9.5 (PGP9.5), synaptophysin and serotonin. The latter group includes individual peptides such as gastrin, somatostatin, insulin, glucagon and calcitonin.

Neuroendocrine tumours typically have the features of low grade malignant neoplasms, although aggressive variants can occur. The usual features are therefore a distinctive regular microscopic architecture with only infrequent mitotic figures and minimal nuclear polymorphism. The typical appearance of a carcinoid tumour is shown in Figure 31.1.

31.4.1   CLASSIFICATION

There is no recognized classification of these tumours and indeed the subject is sur-

rounded by confusion and debate. For simplicity's sake, categories can be defined according to the site of origin of the tumour. Thus, for those arising in the gastrointestinal tract or bronchial tree, the term carcinoid is usually applied; in the pancreas these are referred to as islet cell tumours and further subdivided according to peptide production; in the skin the term Merkel cell tumour is used; in the thyroid they are known as medullary carcinomas. This latter type is covered in Chapter 39 and will not be dealt with here.

Carcinoids are the most commonly occurring tumours and can be further subdivided by microscope appearance into typical carcinoids, atypical carcinoids (sometimes considered the equivalent of carcinomas with neuroendocrine features), and small cell tumours. Anatomical site has some bearing on this histological spectrum, with tumours of gastrointestinal origin mainly being typical carcinoids whereas the bronchial tree displays all three types with small cell lung cancer being the commonest. Small cell lung cancer is fully discussed in Chapter 40 on lung tumours.

Phaeochromocytoma is a tumour of the organized rather than the diffuse neuroendocrine system. In other words, it arises in a discrete neuroendocrine organ, the adrenal medullary. However, as the commonest type of tumour arising from the organized system it deserves mention, particularly as it shares much of the features of presentation, investigation and treatment with the tumour described in this chapter.

31.5   PRESENTATION

Presenting features are determined by peptide production and tumour encroachment on adjacent normal structures. Because of the diversity of this group of tumours, a vast range of symptoms can be encountered and the present account will be confined to the commonest groups.

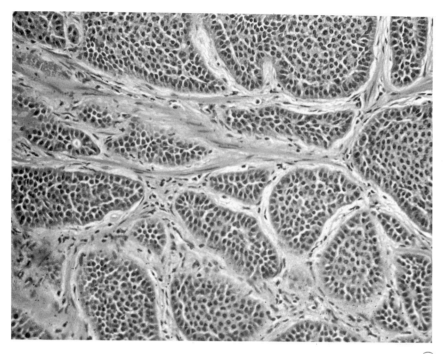

(b)

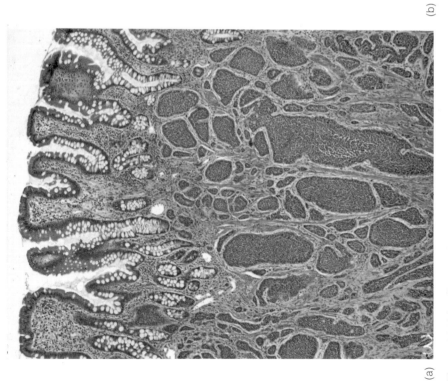

(a)

Figure 31.1(a) Carcinoid tumour of the ileum. Intact ileal mucosa overlies the tumour which is infiltrating the submucosal connective tissues. (Haematoxylin and eosin, × 60.) **(b)** A higher power view of the same tumour. The characteristic packeted or insular growth pattern is apparent. Cellular and nuclear pleomorphism is minimal. No mitoses are seen here. (Haematoxylin and eosin, × 240.)

31.5.1 PEPTIDE RELATED SYMPTOMS

The 'carcinoid syndrome' is a clinical entity resulting from the secretion of vasoactive amines, particularly 5-hydroxytryptamine (5HT), prostaglandins and tachykinins, from carcinoid tumour cells. The presence of the syndrome usually implies liver metastases and is generally accompanied by high levels of the 5HT catabolite, 5-hydroxy indole acetic acid (5-HIAA), in the urine. The most prominent clinical manifestation of this syndrome is flushing, a feature often precipitated by alcohol or stress. The next most common symptom, diarrhoea, is often accompanied by intestinal colic. Less common, but typical, features include bronchial asthma and right-sided heart failure as a result of tricuspid or pulmonary valve stenosis.

The commonest pancreatic islet cell tumour, the insulinoma, usually presents with hypoglycaemic episodes related to excessive insulin secretion, often induced by fasting or exercise. The gastrinoma, along with other neuroendocrine tumours, is responsible for secretion of excessive gastrin and consequently for the peptic ulceration seen in the Zollinger–Ellison syndrome. The clinical features of the glucagonoma syndrome include a necrolytic migratory erythematous rash, stomatitis, glossitis, cheilitis, vaginitis and nail changes. The other discrete pancreatic islet cell tumour, the VIPoma, is exceedingly rare and is characterized by excessive watery diarrhoea, hypokalaemia and hypochlorhydria caused by secretion of VIP.

31.5.2 TUMOUR MASS RELATED SYMPTOMS

Gastrointestinal carcinoids may be detected as a result of bowel obstruction although a range of minor and more chronic gastrointestinal symptoms have been attributed to them. Bronchial carcinoids arise endobronchially, frequently in the major bronchi, and usually present with bronchial obstruction and/or haemophysis.

Merkel cell tumours have no particular distinguishing features and may resemble other primary skin neoplasms such as squamous carcinoma, basal cell carcinoma, amelanotic melanoma and adnexal carcinomas. They usually occur in sun exposed skin areas.

31.6   INVESTIGATION

The appropriate line of investigation will vary with tumour type and cannot be covered comprehensively in this chapter. In general however there are two diagnostic scenarios. First, in those tumours producing symptoms as a result of a tumour mass encroaching on adjacent structures, the approximate site of the tumour will be known and the diagnostic work-up will be similar to that pursued for others tumours at that site. Having identified the tumour mass, diagnostic confirmation can only be obtained by biopsy and pathological examination. Second, and more commonly, symptoms arise from hormone production. In this situation, excessive levels of the suspected responsible hormone may be identified first and localization of the tumour will be attempted secondarily.

31.6.1   PEPTIDE DETECTION

Peptide products are detected by radioimmunoassay on serum samples.

31.6.2   TUMOUR LOCALIZATION

Intrathoracic and intra-abdominal neuroendocrine tumours may be localized by standard imaging techniques such as ultrasound, CT and MRI. However, gastrointestinal tumours, particularly those in the small bowel, are difficult to visualize with these techniques. The same is true for some pancreatic tumours, particularly where the sort of precision required for planning a surgical procedure is necessary (Figure 31.2).

An alternative approach is to utilize the functional capacity of these tumours which,

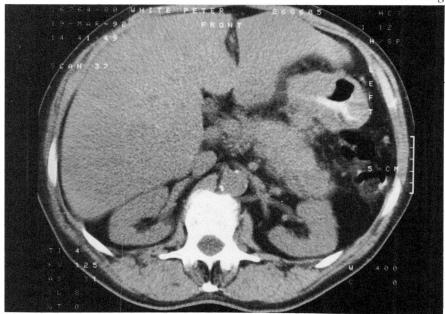

Figure 31.2 CT scan of the upper abdomen showing a diffusely swollen pancreas but no clear delineation of tumour margins.

with the aid of radiopharmaceuticals and scintigraphy, may be capable of demonstrating small volume disease and unsuspected metastases. Methods under investigation, include the two described below.

Somatostatin is a neuropeptide widely distributed in neural and endocrine cells in brain, peripheral neurones, endocrine pancreas, the gastrointestinal tract, thyroid and, to a lesser extent, a number of other tissues.

Efforts to synthesize a somatostatin analogue with properties suitable for scintigraphy resulted in the production of octreotide. Initial studies suggest that indium labelled octreotide may be a useful approach in localizing carcinoids, pancreatic tumours and Merkel cell tumours (Lamberts *et al.*, 1990a, b).

Meta-iodobenzylguanidine (mIBG) has structural similarities to both guanethidine and the endogenous catecholamines, and can be radiolabelled with iodine isotopes. The radiolabelled form has the ability to image functional abnormalities, and abnormalities, of the catecholamine pool. Tissues rich in sympathetic nerves, such as the adrenal glands and sympathetic chains, can be clearly visualized after intravenous injection. Tumours which arise from these structures, such as neuroblastoma and phaeochromocytoma, are mostly positive for mIBG and this has become a useful diagnostic tool and also has value in terms of therapy and of monitoring response to treatment. Greater sensitivity can be achieved by the use [124]I-labelled mIBG in combination with positron emission tomography (Ott *et al.*, 1992). Because many carcinoid tumours, and some other neuroendocrine tumours, produce and secrete catecholamines, mIBG has been used in their localization. Figure 31.3 shows uptake of [123]ImIBG in a patient with metastatic carcinoid who later went on to therapy with [131]ImIBG. The CT appearance of the abdominal mass demonstrated by mIBG is shown in Figure 31.4. However, because of the rarity of these tumours there are as yet no substantial

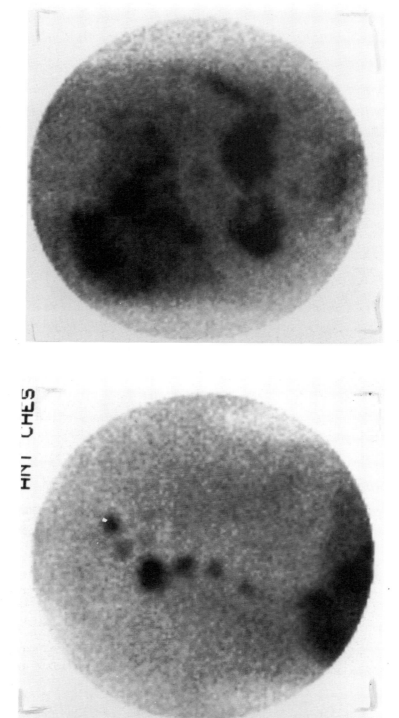

Figure 31.3 [^{123}I]IBG scan in a patient with metastatic carcinoid showing uptake in: **(a)** mediastinal nodes; **(b)** liver metastases and an abdominal mass.

series and therefore it is not possible to quote the percentage of tumours in which uptake can be demonstrated.

31.7 MANAGEMENT

In broad terms, the appropriate management policy will depend on the degree of malignancy and metastatic status of an individual tumour.

31.7.1 SURGERY

Where technically feasible, benign localized lesions are best treated by surgical excision which is potentially curative. Tumours in which this is most likely to be the appropriate manoeuvre are gastrointestinal carcinoids, bronchial carcinoids and insulinomas. In carcinoids, total excision will result in a cure rate of 90%. Surgery may be appropriate in other pancreatic tumour types, although the tendency for malignant behaviour is much greater. However, even in patients with metastatic disease there may be a case for debulking surgery in order to alleviate symptoms as even tumours with a malignant appearance may have a relatively slow growth rate and patients have a life expectancy of several years.

Where curative surgery is being attempted, tumour margins should be localized as precisely as possible prior to surgery. Apart from standard imaging procedures, there are a number of different ways to acquire this

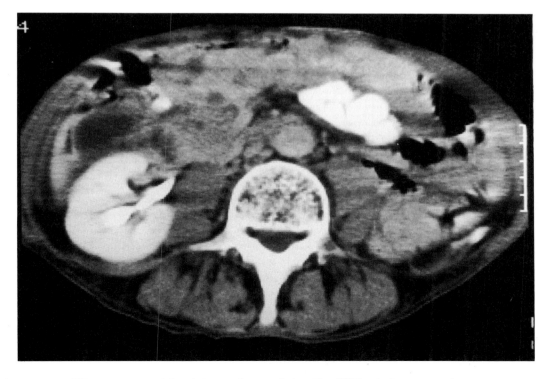

Figure 31.4 CT appearance of the abdominal mass defined by [123I] mIBG scanning (Figure 31.3). A 4 cm tumour lies anterior to the right renal vessels and this extends across the anterior abdomen in the line of the greater omentum.

information. For insulinomas, percutaneous transhepatic venous catheterization with sampling for insulin and C-peptide levels has been reported to be effective. By demonstrating the most distal extent of tumour, piecemeal removal of the pancreas at operation is avoided. In those carcinoids and pancreatic tumours which are somatastatin receptor positive, radiolabelled octreotide can aid in the definition of tumour site and extent.

31.7.2 RADIOTHERAPY

The rarity of neuroendocrine tumours and their long and varied natural history makes it difficult to assess response to any treatment modality. Despite this, it has been well documented that at least some carcinoid tumours are responsive to radiotherapy and that this may provide a useful means of palliation and a possibility of cure in patients with localized disease.

The limited data available on the radiosensitivity of carcinoids suggests that nonfunctional tumours are more sensitive than those with peptide production and associated syndromes (Keane *et al.*, 1981). In 14 syndromic patients, there was no incidence of regression equal to, or greater than, 50% and only five patients showed minimal detectable response. By contrast, two of seven nonfunctional tumours achieved a complete response and one a partial response with more than 50% reduction in tumour volume. It is interesting to note that the complete responses were achieved with relatively low doses, 20–25Gy in 20–25 fractions, and that in using this dose to the whole abdomen useful palliation was achieved in 25% of patients with gastrointestinal tumours. Recently, the Memorial Sloan–Kettering experience in the palliation of patients with metastatic carcinoma has been reported (Schupak and Wallner, 1991). Radiation response of metastatic carcinoid in brain, bone and spinal cord was found to be similar to that of other metastatic cancers, with overall response

rates of 63%, 88% and 92% respectively. However, liver metastases were not successfully treated and the median survival of patients in this group was only 11 weeks. In the Sloan–Kettering series, radiotherapy doses were also low, although higher than in the Keane series, ranging from 27 to 40 Gy. Although no dose–response relationship could be demonstrated, probably because of marked heterogeneity in terms of site of disease and extent, carcinoids do appear to be relatively radiosensitive tumours. These reports encourage the use of radiotherapy in unresectable primary disease, although in the curative setting higher doses are likely to be required and the radiosensitivity of adjacent normal tissue structures is obviously a limiting factor, particularly for tumours arising in the pancreas and gastrointestinal tract.

31.7.3 MEDICAL TREATMENT

Cytotoxic drug therapy has been investigated in carcinoid tumours but only four conventional drugs have single agent activity of 20% or more: adriamycin, 5-fluorouracil (5-FU), streptozotocin and dacarbazine (DTIC). In combination, 5-FU and streptozotocin appear to be the most effective agents with a response rate of 63% (Moertel and Hanley, 1979). However, activity of this level is not a universal finding and chemotherapy is generally not justified as a first line approach in view of limited responses and significant toxicity (Öberg and Eriksson, 1989).

There are other medical approaches to the management of neuroendocrine tumours but the aims are the same; to relieve symptoms by decreasing hormone levels and to reduce tumour growth. In carcinoids, serotonin antagonists are effective in modifying the diarrhoea and colic, and occasionally also the flushing. Long acting somatostatin analogues can reduce 5-HT levels and also influence the symptoms of carcinoid syndrome (Engelman, *et al.*, 1967). In gastrinomas, selective H_2-receptor blocking agents are effective in controlling the hypersecretory disorder, but obviously have no inhibitory affect on tumour growth.

Somatostatin appears to exert an inhibitory effect on peptide hormone secretion from nearly all endocrine tissues and has been demonstrated in nerves and epithelial cells of many organs of the gastro-entero-pancreatic system. In addition, a growth inhibiting affect on several organs has been demonstrated in animals (Vinik *et al.*, 1981). Natural somatostatin is however not a suitable therapeutic agent because of its short half-life which limits its use to intravenous infusion. The long acting somatostatin analogue, octreotide, can however can be given subcutaneously and used for long term treatment (Bauer *et al.*, 1982), and a number of studies have reported the use of this agent in neuroendocrine tumours (Kvols *et al.*, 1986; Ahlman and Tisell, 1987). A recent series reported on 23 patients with malignant mid-gut carcinoid tumours who were treated with octreotide twice a day for 6 months. An objective response was seen in 28%, which lasted 6–30 months, stable disease was observed in 35% and disease progressed in the remaining 36% (Öberg *et al.*, 1991). The natural history of these tumours makes it difficult to be optimistic about such a result.

Interferon is the biological response modifier which has been most investigated in neuroendocrine tumours. A report of a clinical trial of human leucocyte interferon in malignant carcinoid tumours gave an objective response rate of 49% with a median duration of 34 months (Öberg *et al.*, 1986). The same group has recently published more extensive results on 111 patients treated with interferon and compared them with 19 patients given streptozotocin and 5-FU. With interferon, 42% demonstrated a significant biochemical response and 15% of these also had a greater than 15% reduction in tumour size. Median duration of response was 34 months. In the chemotherapy group, two patients had a biochemical response which

lasted 3–5 months and overall the median survival for this group was 8 months. In the interferon treated patients, the median survival was reported to be 80+ months (Öberg and Eriksson, 1991).

31.8 CURRENT RESEARCH

31.8.1 DIAGNOSIS, PROGNOSIS AND MONITORING OF RESPONSE TO THERAPY

Advances in molecular biology have permitted the detection of specific nucleic acid sequences using techniques such as *in-situ* hybridization (ISH). The unique advantage of ISH is that the localization of nucleic acid is superimposed on cellular structure, thus allowing this cellular localization of DNA and RNA sequences in a heterogeneous population. This approach is currently being used to investigate hormone and peptide mRNA synthesis in a range of neuroendocrine tumours (Funa, 1991). Though currently experimental, this approach may be complimentary to immunohistocytochemistry in diagnosing neuroendocrine tumours and, in addition, may provide useful prognostic information. Furthermore, as the natural history of these tumours makes monitoring and evaluation of response to therapy extremely difficult, ISH may provide a more sensitive measure of tumour activity. On a more general level, understanding of peptide synthesis and activity in neuroendocrine tumours may provide a means of harnessing neuroendocrine activity in a wider range of tumours (Larsson, 1990).

Developments in molecular biology have been extensively applied in the multiple endocrine neoplasia syndromes. Genetic screening by linkage analysis allows selections of gene carriers with a high degree of accuracy, making it possible to concentrate laborious biochemical screening efforts on family members at risk of developing the syndromes. Biochemical screening, and detection, of MEN I lesions in young asymptomatic individuals decreases the age of diagnosis by many years and allows the possibility of early therapeutic intervention. It has not yet been established, and it will be extremely difficult to do so, whether early intervention will have any impact on mortality (Larsson and Öberg, 1991).

31.8.2 THERAPY

Identification of neuroendocrine peptides, and their receptors, provide an attractive therapeutic avenue. As previously discussed, this has already been explored but is likely to be extended to further peptides in the future. In addition, developments in radiopharmacy broaden the potential application of isotope therapy.

The results achieved with biological response modifiers are encouraging further investigation in this area. Also, as it has been suggested that the mechanism of action of these substances may be quite distinct from that employed by endocrine receptor based therapies, the two might be used in combination to advantage (Creutzfeldt *et al.*, 1991).

REFERENCES

Ahlman, H. and Tisell, L.-E. (1987). The use of a long-acting somatostatin analogue in the treatment of advanced endocrine malignancies with gastrointestinal symptoms. *Scandinavian Journal of Gastroenterology*, **22**, 938–42.

Bauer, W., Griner, U. and Doepfner, W. (1982) SMS 201–995: A very potent and selective octapeptide analogue of somatostatin with prolonged action. *Life Science*, **31**, 1133–40.

Creutzfeldt, W., Bartsch, H.H., Jacubaschke, U. and Stöckmann, F. (1991). Treatment of gastrointestinal endocrine tumours with interferon-α and octreotide. *Acta Oncologica*, **30**, 529–35.

Engelman, K., Lovenberg, W. and Sjoerdsma, A. (1967) Inhibition of serotonin synthesis by parachlorophenylalanine in patients with the carcinoid syndrome. *New England Journal of Medicine*, **277**, 1103–8.

Funa, K. (1991). *In situ* hybridization for detection of hormone and peptide mRNA in carcinoid tumors. *Acta Oncologica*, 30, 457–61.

Keane, T.J., Rider, W.D., Hardwood, A.R. *et al.* (1981) Whole abdominal radiation in the management of metastatic gastrointestinal carcinoid tumor. *International Journal of Radiation Oncology, Biology, Physics*, **7**, 1519–21.

Kvols, L.K., Moertel, C.G., O'Connell, M.J. *et al.* (1986) Treatment of the malignant carcinoid syndrome: evaluation of a long-acting somatostatin analogue. *New England Journal of Medicine*, **315**, 663–6.

Lamberts, S., Hofland, L.I., Van Koetsveld, P.M. *et al.* (1990a) Parallel *in-vivo* and *in-vitro* detection of functional somatostatin receptors in human endocrine pancreatic tumours. Consequences with regard to diagnosis, localisation and therapy. *Journal of Clinical Endocrinology and Metabolism*, **71**, 566–74.

Lamberts, S.W.J., Bakker, W.H., Reubi, J.C. and Krenning, E.P. (1990b) Somatostatin-receptor imaging in the localisation of endocrine tumours. *New England Journal of Medicine*, **323**, 1246–9.

Larsson, B.S. and Öberg, K. 1991, Genetic and clinical characteristics of multiple endocrine neoplasia type I. *Acta Oncologica*, **30**, 485–8.

Larsson, C.S., Öberg, K., Nakamura, Y. and Nordenskiöld, M. (1988) Multiple endocrine neoplasia type I gene maps to chromosome 11 and is lost in insulinoma. *Nature*, **332**, 85–7.

Larsson, L.I. (1990) Tracing of neuroendocrine peptides and their corresponding mRNA's unravelling the neuroendocrine network. *Acta Haematologica*, **38**, 9–14.

Moertel, C.G. and Hanley, J.A. (1979) Combination chemotherapy trials in metastatic carcinoid tumour and the malignant carcinoid syndrome. *Cancer Clinical Trials*, **2**, 327–34.

Öberg, K. and Eriksson, B. (1989) Medical treatment of neuroendocrine gut and pancreatic tumors. *Acta Oncologica*, **28**, 425–31.

Öberg, K. and Eriksson, B. (1991) The role of interferons in the management of carcinoid tumors. *Acta Oncologica*, **30**, 519–22.

Öberg, K., Norheim, I. and Lind, E. (1986) Treatment of malignant carcinoid tumors with human leukocyte interferon. Long-term results. *Cancer Treatment Review*, **70**, 1297–304.

Öberg, K., Norheim, I. and Theodorsson, E. (1991) Treatment of malignant midgut carcinoid

tumours with a long-acting somatostatin analogue octreotide. *Acta Oncologica*, **30**, 503–7.

Ott, R.J., Tait, D., Flower, M. *et al.* (1992) Treatment
planning for I[311]-mIBG radiotherapy and neural
crest tumours using I[241]-mIGB positron emission
tomography. *British Journal of Radiology*, **65**,
787–91.

Schupak, K.D. and Wallner, K.E. (1991) The role of
radiation therapy in the treatment of locally
unresectable or metastatic carcinoid tumors.
*International Journal of Radiation Oncology,
Biology, Physics*, **20**, 489–95.

Vinik, A.I., Gaginella, T.S. and O'Dorisio, T.M.
(1981) The distribution and characterisation of
somatostatin-like immunoreactivity in epithelial
cells, submucosa, and muscle of the rat stomach
and intestine. *Endocrinology*, **109**, 1921–6.

PROSTATE CANCER

32

David P. Dearnaley

32.1 INTRODUCTION

Prostate cancer presents an increasing health problem in all developed countries and is now the most frequently diagnosed male malignancy in the USA with 106 000 cases per annum. Although affecting predominantly the ageing male population, prostate cancer ranks second to lung cancer in mortality from malignant disease in men in western countries and in the USA it has been calculated that men dying from carcinoma of the prostate lose on average 9 years of life (National Cancer Institute, 1989). Although in many countries 50% or more of men present with metastatic disease, 'prostate awareness' and programmes of early detection mean that there is an increasing incidence of early localized disease, particularly in North America and Western Europe. Early detection of disease is aided by use of the serum marker prostatic specific antigen (PSA), but it is as yet unclear whether early detection or 'screening' for prostate cancer will make any impact on mortality from the disease.

The natural history of prostate cancer varies widely with a high prevalence of localized (incidental) cancer at one end of the spectrum and rapid progression to metastases and death at the other. The optimal management for most men remains uncertain. The likelihood of disease progression and death must be considered in relation to the probability of death from intercurrent illnesses, and also the relative effectiveness and morbidities of available treatment options. For men with apparently localized disease 'curative' options include radical radiotherapy or nerve sparing radical prostatectomy. Alternatively a 'watchful waiting' policy may be adopted, introducing treatment at the time of clinically relevant disease progression. For reasons that are not clearly understood, prostate cancer disseminates most frequently to bone producing the characteristic pattern of osteoblastic skeletal metastases. Androgen deprivation remains the mainstay of management, using either orchidectomy or the modern pharmacological equivalents with LHRH agonists or anti-androgen drugs which may be more acceptable to the patient. The median duration of response is between 12 and 18 months and new avenues of drug development are required. After metastatic prostate cancer has escaped from initial hormone manipulation the palliation of bone pain and other symptoms with appropriate supportive measures, including radiotherapy, remains a major clinical challenge.

32.2 EPIDEMIOLOGY AND AETIOLOGY

Prostate cancer incidence rises with increasing age. Only 1–2% of cases are diagnosed at less than 55 years and 85% are 65 years old or more. Autopsy studies have demonstrated microscopic foci of well differentiated prostatic adenocarcinoma in 30–40% of men 75 years or over (Breslow *et al.*, 1977). There are very large variations in clinical incidence and mortality from prostate cancer throughout the world. The USA and Scandinavia have

Table 32.1   Age standardized prostate cancer mortality and incidence rates per 100 000 men aged 30–74 in various countries in 1985

Country	Mortality rate 1985	Recent 5 year trends	Incidence rate 1985 (from selected regional Cancer Registries)	Recent 5 year trends*
US blacks	{17.5	1.5	151.6	3.1
US whites			88.5	12.6
Norway	22.2	7.8	63.6+	5.7
UK (England and Wales)	15.2	7.2	32.9	14.1
Japan	3.3	8.4	10.1	30.2

Data from Coleman, *et al.*, 1993.
* Recent trends: estimated mean percentage change per 5 year period in the age specific rates (30–74 years) over a 15 year interval centred around 1980. Parentheses denote recent trends not significant at 5% level.
+ National Cancer Registry.

the highest incidence rates, the lowest being found in Asia, but the frequency of prostate cancer has increased in many countries in the past two decades (Table 32.1). Part of the increase in incidence may be apparent rather than real and due to the increased reporting of incidental foci of adenocarcinoma in transurethral resection specimens taken for the treatment of benign prostate hypertrophy (BPH). However, improving longevity in western societies can be expected to produce an overall increase in mortality from prostate cancer over the coming decades.

The wide international variation suggests that environmental factors are implicated in the aetiology and that a western lifestyle leads to an increased risk of disease. The age adjusted prevalence of 'incidental' prostate cancer is similar in Japan and the USA (Yatani *et al.*, 1982) despite a ten fold difference in clinical incidence, indicating that a promoting rather than an initiating carcinogen may be responsible for international differences. Similarly, migrant studies reveal that the clinical incidence of prostate cancer rises in succeeding generations when populations move from low to high incidence areas, e.g. from Japan to Hawaii. It has been suggested that there is a correlation with a high fat diet (pos-

itive) and diet rich in yellow and green vegetable (inverse) which may act on the prostate through modification of circulating sex hormones (Hill and Wynder, 1979). This might give a lead to possible methods of primary prevention, although currently it is not known which hormones are implicated and their mode of action. Other risk factors which have been investigated, usually with equivocal results, include physical activity, occupational exposure to cadmium, sexual activity and BPH (Meikle and Smith, 1990). Recently it has been suggested that vasectomy may correlate with an increased incidence of prostate cancer, although this finding remains controversial (Guess, 1993) A study performed on Atomic Energy Authority employees suggested that exposure to radiation correlated with mortality from prostate cancer (Beral *et al.*, 1985).

It is also likely that genetic factors are important as there is evidence for the familial aggregation of prostate cancer. A number of studies have shown that the relative risk to first degree relatives of prostate cancer cases is approximately 2 (Dearnaley *et al.*, 1993). This risk is markedly increased if first and second degree relatives are affected or if the age of the proband is less than 65 years (Cannon *et al.*, 1982). Although it is believed that prostate cancer can be associated with some familial types of breast cancer and with the Li–Fraumeni syndrome, the responsible gene has not been identified and there is no evidence to implicate the p53 or breast cancer I (BrCa1) genes.

32.3   PATHOLOGY

The considerable majority of prostate cancers are adenocarcinomas and arise from the glandular epithelium of the peripheral zone of the prostate. Other types of primary carcinoma are very uncommon. Primary transitional and squamous cell cancers are described but may also be secondary to primary tumours in the bladder. Carcinoid and small cell carcinomas may arise *de novo* or develop from prostate adenocarcinomas. These tumours may be chemosensitive but are highly malignant with a very poor prognosis. Sarcomas represent approximately 0.1% of prostatic malignancy. Rhabdomyosarcomas are described in younger patients. Leiomyosarcomas occur

usually after the age of 50. Non-Hodgkin's lymphoma may arise within the prostate and both chronic lymphocytic and acute leukaemias may cause prostatic infiltration. Secondary tumours of the prostate will most commonly arise from direct infiltration from bladder cancers, but secondary deposits from primary tumours such as malignant melanoma and bronchial carcinoma are described.

Histological recognition of prostatic adenocarcinoma can be difficult, particularly if only small fragments of tissue from fine needle biopsies are presented to the histopathologist. The recognition of well differentiated tumours depends on the overall assessment of architecture and a variety of grading systems have been proposed which correlate with clinical outcome (Gallee *et al.*, 1990). The systems in most common usage are those of Gleason (Gleason *et al.*, 1974) and Mostofi (Mostofi, 1976). The Gleason system analyses the histological structure of prostate cancer using low power magnification, dividing appearances into five grades (Table 32.2). The

Table 32.2   Histological grading of prostate cancer

Gleason System

Grade 1	Very well differentiated carcinoma with uniform gland pattern
Grade 2	Well differentiated carcinoma with some variation in size and shape of glands
Grade 3	Moderately differentiated adenocarcinoma either: a. polymorphic differentiated glands separated by abundant stroma arranged in poorly defined clumps, or b. well defined cribriform or papillary masses which generally correspond to intraduct spread
Grade 4	Poorly differentiated adenocarcinoma. Tumour clumps are poorly defined and differentiated with fixed glands widely infiltrating prostatic stroma
Grade 5	Undifferentiated carcinoma. Carcinoma with no or minimal very poorly differentiated gland formation, and marked stromal infiltration. Central necrosis may be present in tumour cell masses

Histological grade (2–10) is sum of scores of primary and secondary morphological patterns

Mostofi System

Grade 1	Well differentiated glands with slight nuclear anaplasia
Grade 2	Moderately well differentiated with gland formation and moderate nuclear anaplasia
Grade 3	Poorly or undifferentiated tumour with slight or no glandular formation and marked nuclear anaplasia

majority of tumours do not have a uniform appearance and this system takes account of such variability by scoring both a primary and secondary pattern. The overall grade is the sum of the two histological patterns and is scored from 2 to 10. The Mostofi system divides prostate cancer into three grades and considers both histological structure and cytological features of the tumour (Table 32.2). Grading systems have been shown to correlate with tumour stage, incidence of seminal vesicle and lymph node involvement, occurrence of distant metastases and survival. However, the reproducibility of such systems is not high and there is considerable intra- and inter-pathologist variability (Gallee *et al.*, 1990).

32.3.1 TUMOUR MARKERS

There are three biochemical markers for the assessment and monitoring of prostate cancer:

1. Prostatic acid phosphatase (PAP)
2. Prostate specific antigen (PSA)
3. Alkaline phosphatase (Alk P).

PAP is elevated in less than 20% of apparently localized prostatic cancers and high levels carry an adverse prognosis. Approximately 60–70% of patients with metastatic disease will have elevated levels and in these men it is a useful marker of disease response.

PSA is an organ specific serine protease specific for prostatic tissue but not for prostatic cancer. It was first identified in 1979 and has replaced PAP in most clinical situations (Stamey *et al.*, 1987; Hetherington *et al.*, 1988). It has an established role in the monitoring of treatment of metastatic disease. More than 95% of patients with disseminated disease will have elevated levels (> 4 ng/ml). Failure of levels to normalize following androgen deprivation indicates a poor prognosis. Following the development of hormone resistant disease, PSA levels are elevated in

approximately 80% of patients and changes in PSA can be used to monitor response to second line treatments. In patients with localized disease PSA levels give a guide to the extent of disease spread. PSA levels < 20 ng/ml are unlikely to be associated with extracapsular disease or metastases, although considerably higher levels can be seen in patients with apparently localized but bulky disease. Following treatment with radical prostatectomy, PSA levels should fall to undetectable levels and continuing elevation of PSA levels indicates the presence of residual disease. Following radical radiotherapy PSA levels fall slowly but would be expected to return to normal after a period of 6–12 months (Stamey *et al.*, 1989). It has been suggested that PSA can be incorporated in strategies for screening for early prostate cancer. However patients with benign prostatic hypertrophy may also have elevated levels and further work is needed to establish the sensitivity, specificity and predictive value of different values of PSA used in conjunction with digital rectal examination (DRE) and transrectal ultrasound (TRUS) (Dearnaley *et al.*, 1993).

Alkaline phosphatase is a non-specific marker for advanced bone disease, elevated levels correlating with osteoblastic activity. Raised levels may also occur in Paget's disease of bone and liver disease.

32.4   PRESENTATION, ASSESSMENT AND STAGING

Early prostate cancer is usually asymptomatic. As tumours most commonly arise in the peripheral zone of the prostate, symptoms of prostatism are relatively late events unless accompanied by additional benign prostatic hyperplasia. Haematuria, haematospermia and perineal discomfort are sometimes associated with localized disease. Metastases most commonly present with painful bone metastases and may be associated with weight loss, cachexia and anaemia. In the UK prostate cancer is usually diagnosed following the evaluation of obstructive symptoms or because of the development of painful bone metastases. In North America diagnosis is more commonly made when the disease is localized because rectal examination is performed as part of routine medical checks and PSA estimations are increasingly being performed on asymptomatic men.

The extent of evaluation of a man with apparently localized disease depends in part upon the treatment options considered appropriate. Rectal examination may be as accurate as currently available radiological tests for determining the extent of local disease. TRUS evaluation can be used to accurately guide transrectal or transperineal biopsies, giving a higher yield of positive results than finger guided biopsies. TRUS can also define small (approximately 5 mm) clinically undetectable lesions which may for example be found in men having PSA evaluations as part of early detection programmes. CT or MRI examination of the pelvis is valuable in defining macroscopic lymph node involvement which makes patients unsuitable for radical treatment, but will miss microscopic or minimal lymph node involvement. Increasing levels of PSA correlate with increasing bulk and stage of disease but absolute levels do not clearly differentiate between different stages. Elevated levels of acid phosphatase are very commonly associated with the development of metastases. Bone scan is the most sensitive test for detection of skeletal metastases and should be performed on all patients considered for radical local treatment. For patients presenting with metastases clinical examination, blood count, biochemical assessment of renal and liver function, PSA estimation and relevant skeletal X-rays and bone scan provide adequate information in most cases.

Histological confirmation of the diagnosis should be obtained before treatment. Previously this has frequently been made on the chippings from transurethral resection. This is not an ideal method of diagnosis as most tumours arise in the periphery of the gland and unless needed for the relief of obstructive symptoms, guided transrectal or perineal biopsies are to be preferred. Fine needle aspiration biopsy of the prostate can also be used but needs an experienced cytopathologist for adequate interpretation of results.

There are two commonly used clinical staging systems (Table 32.3). Local disease extent classified according to the TNM system approximates to the subclassification A–C of the Whitmore–Jewett system, but the former UICC system has the advantage of separating the assessment of primary tumour, lymph nodes and metastases.

32.5 MANAGEMENT

32.5.1 TREATMENT OF LOCALIZED PROSTATE CANCER

Localized prostate cancer usually progresses slowly with an estimated doubling time of 2 years based on PSA estimations (Stamey *et al.*, 1987). Controversy will continue to surround the optimal management for an individual patient until we have more accurate tools to predict local behaviour and metastatic potential of prostatic carcinomas. Treatment options need to balance the probability of progression, clinical deterioration and death from prostate cancer with competing causes of death. Clearly this balance varies between different patients and population groups with different life expectancies. At present it seems reasonable to offer curative therapy to men judged to have a life expectancy of 10 years or more, although there is no compelling evidence that a close 'watch policy' with deferred treatment until the time of clinical progression would produce inferior results. The relative merits of radical radiotherapy and surgery depend both on local tumour control probability and treatment morbidity. No adequate study has compared these treatments alternatives (Paulson *et al.*, 1982;

Table 32.3   Clinical staging systems of prostate cancer

TNM Classification of Prostate Cancer (Modified from Schröder *et al.*, 1992)

T0		**No evidence of primary tumour**
T1		**Clinically unapparent tumour, impalpable and not visible by imaging**
	T1a	Tumour an incidental finding in ≤ 5% of resected tissue
	T1b	Tumour an incidental finding in > 5% of resected tissue
	T1c	Tumour identified by needle biopsy (e.g. because of raised PSA)
T2		**Tumour confined within prostate**
	T2a	Tumour involves ≤ half a lobe
	T2b	Tumour involves > half a lobe but not both lobes
	T2c	Tumour involves both lobes
T3		**Tumour extends through the prostate capsule**
	T3a	Unilateral extracapsular extension
	T3b	Bilateral extracapsular extension
	T3c	Tumour invades seminal vesicles
T4		**Tumour is fixed or invades adjacent structures**
	T4a	Tumour invasion of bladder neck, external sphincter or rectum
	T4b	Tumour invasion of levator muscles or fixed to pelvic side wall

Regional lymph nodes

N0	No regional lymph nodes metastasis
N1	Metastasis in a single regional lymph node, ≤ 2 cm in greatest dimension
N2	Metastasis in a single regional lymph node, 2 cm–≤ 5 cm in greatest dimension, or multiple regional lymph nodes, ≤ 5 cm in greatest dimension
N3	Metastasis in a single regional lymph node, > 5 cm in greatest dimension

Distant metastases

M0	No distant metastasis
M1	Distant metastasis
M1a	Non-regional lymph node(s)
M1b	Bone(s)
M1c	Other site(s)

Whitmore–Jewett Staging System

A1	Microscopic focus of well differentiated adenocarcinoma in up to three foci of transuretheral specimens or enucleation; clinically not apparent on rectal examination
A2	Tumour not well differentiated or present in more than three areas
B1	Asymptomatic palpable nodule < 1.5 cm; normal surrounding prostate; no capsular extension; normal acid phosphatase
B2	Diffuse involvement of gland; no capsular extension; normal acid phosphatase
C	Extensive local tumour with penetration through the capsule; contiguous spread may involve seminal vesicles, bladder neck, lateral side wall of pelvis; acid phosphatase may be elevated; normal bone scan
D1	Metastases to pelvic lymph nodes below aortic bifurcation; acid phosphatase may be elevated
D2	Bone or lymph node metastases above aortic bifurcation or other soft tissue metastases

Hanks, 1988) and both are considered as standard management options for patients with disease confined to the prostate.

Radical radiotherapy is used in all stages of localized disease. Radical prostatectomy is generally restricted to younger fit patients and there is general agreement that positive lymph nodes or clinical evidence of extra-prostatic extension contraindicates surgery. The development of nerve sparing radical prostatectomy techniques may allow up to 50% of men (depending on case selection) to retain potency and urinary continence rates are in excess of 95%. The alternative policy of 'watchful waiting' has been advocated for all stages of localized disease because of the uncertainty of disease progression and treatment effectiveness. Hormone therapy alone may be used for advanced localized (T3 and T4) disease as many of these men will develop metastases as their first site of failure.

(a) Treatment of T1 disease

The probability of disease progression in untreated T1 tumours is determined by the histological grade and extent of glandular involvement (Epstein *et al.*, 1986; McNeal *et al.*, 1986; Lowe and Listrom, 1988; Johansson *et al.*, 1989; Chodak *et al.*, 1994). For well differentiated focal disease the probability of progression at 5 and 10 years is between

2% and 9%, and 18% respectively; cancer deaths at 5 and 10 years have been reported at 4% and 12% respectively. Radical local treatment is therefore not usually indicated, with a possible exception of the young patient with life expectancy of 15 years or more. Patients treated with radical prostatectomy can be expected to enjoy a survival similar to that of an age matched population (Gibbons *et al.*, 1989). There have been relatively few patients in this category treated with radical radiotherapy, but in a small series of 20 patients the 15 year overall survival was 90% (Bagshaw *et al.*, 1988). For patients with poorly differentiated or more diffuse (T1B) prostate cancer progression rates are considerably higher and have been estimated at between 36% and 39%, and 68% at 5 and 10 years respectively and cancer deaths at 5 and 10 years at about 8% and 20% respectively. In patients treated by radical prostatectomy, approximately 10% of patients with organ confined disease will develop progression and if the specimen had positive margins this figure will rise to 25% (Paulson *et al.*, 1988). The results following radical radiotherapy are shown in Table 32.4. Between 93% and 98% of patients can be expected to remain free of local recurrence at 10 years with a relapse free survival of 76% and overall survival of 62–76%. The variability in results reflects differences in tumour extent and histology. Twenty-four per cent

Table 32.4 Results of external beam radiotherapy for prostate cancer: outcome at 5, 10 and 15 years

Stage	Local Recurrence (%)			Relapse free survival (%)			Overall survival (%)		
	5 yr	10 yr	15 yr	5 yr	10 yr	15 yr	5 yr	10 yr	15 yr
T1 (No. 145)	3–6	3–8	8	84–85	76–77	72	83–95	62–76	46
T2 (No. 1023)	12–14	17–26	32	66–78	40–60	42	75–78	46–57	36
T3/4 (No. 1595)	12–26	19–31	25–56	43–60	27–46	22–40	58–72	35–42	27

Summary of results from largest reported series: Hanks *et al.*, 1987; Zagars *et al.*, 1987; Perez *et al.*, 1989; Goffinet and Bagshaw, 1990.

of patients with T1B disease may have positive pelvic lymph nodes if subjected to staging lymphadenectomy (Smith *et al.,* 1983) and in a small surgically staged series of patients treated with radiotherapy all 16 men remained recurrence free following a median follow-up of 7 years (Hanks, 1991).

(b)   Results in T2 prostate cancer

The estimated rate of progression for stage T2 disease followed expectantly are 54%, 66% and 100% at 5, 10 and 15 years respectively with associated cancer deaths of 0, 17% and 50% (Whitmore, 1988). Patients treated by radical prostatectomy have been reported as having a survival identical to that of an age matched population (Gibbons *et al.,* 1989). The classical series reported by Belt and Schröder in 1972 showed survival rates of 78%, 55%, 31% and 20% at 5, 10, 15 and 20 years respectively, but further review of this series demonstrated that only 16% of the patients died of prostate cancer. The results of treatment with radical radiotherapy are shown in Table 32.4. Local disease control is achieve in over 85% of patients at 5 years, and 75% at 10 years. Relapse free survival is between 66% and 78% at 5 years and 40% and 60% at 10 years with overall survival of approximately 75% at 5 years and 46–58% at 10 years. As expected, patients with stage T2 disease who have had a negative staging lymphadenectomy have a more favourable outcome, and in a subgroup of surgically staged patients treated in RTOG study 7706, the 10 year local control rate was 84% with cause specific survival of 86% and overall survival of 63% which exceeded that of an age matched population (Hanks *et al.,* 1991). Similarly, 51 surgically staged patients treated at Stanford had a 10 year actuarial disease free survival of 96% and overall survival of 85% (Bagshaw *et al.,* 1987). These results are comparable to the best reported after radical prostatectomy.

(c)   Stages T3 and T4 prostate cancer

The outcome for the majority of patients with advanced localized disease is determined by the development of metastases. In the Stanford series disease recurrence occurred in 52% of patients at 5 years, 66% at 10 years and 72% at 15 years (Goffinet and Bagshaw, 1990). Local control, however, can be obtained in most patients (Table 32.4), but failures increase with length of follow-up rising to between 25% and 56% at 15 years. Although radiotherapy achieves long term clinical local control of disease, it is likely that most patients have subclinical metastases at the time of treatment and local therapy is unlikely to have a major impact on survival. This hypothesis is supported by the results of the recent MRC study which has compared radiotherapy alone, radiotherapy plus orchidectomy and orchidectomy (Fellows *et al.,* 1992). This prospective randomized study showed that radiotherapy gave no survival advantage over orchidectomy and that the orchidectimized patients had a longer disease free interval, there being a delay in the appearance of metastases.

(d)   Lymph node positive disease

Prostate cancer frequently spreads to the pelvic lymph nodes, most commonly involving the internal and external iliac and presacral lymph node groups. The likelihood of lymph node involvement is related to both tumour stage and histological grade. Involvement is most unusual for T1A well differentiated disease but rises to approximately 24% for T1B and T2 tumours and 58% for T3 disease (Smith Jr *et al.,* 1983). The median time to disease progression whether or not local treatment is given is of the order of 1–2 years. In a group of pathological staged patients treated with radical radiation the 5 year relapse free survival for 61 lymph node positive patients was only 2% and survival less than 20% compared to 48% and 70%

respectively in 85 lymph node negative cases (Goffinet and Bagshaw, 1990). The optimal management for this group of patients is uncertain. Most commonly in the UK management will be with a policy of immediate or deferred hormone treatment for asymptomatic patients, or hormone therapy alone if significant symptoms are present. Radiotherapy, however, is usually successful in maintaining long-term clinical control within the pelvis and can be considered for patients who do not wish to have hormone therapy or if the hormone response is inadequate.

(e) Radiotherapy

Radical prostate irradiation should be given using a linear accelerator using at least 6 MeV for optimal dose distributions. Treatment should be carefully planned to minimize the dose to particularly the posterior rectal wall and bladder to avoid chronic radiation complications. Prostate cancers are slow growing and maximal tumour responses are achieved over periods of many months.

Presently CT gives the most accurate method of localization of the prostate and seminal vesicles for radiotherapy planning. Ideally 5 mm slice intervals should be used to accurately locate the superior and inferior aspects of the gland. CT planning and treatment should be carried out with the bladder comfortably full in order to reduce the volume of bladder wall in the treatment volume and this manoeuvre also has the advantage of displacing small and large bowel away from the high dose area. Rectal contrast should be avoided during planning procedures as rectal distension displaces the prostate. Although the lateral and anteroposterior margins of the prostate are clearly defined on CT, tumour extension in the bladder base (superiorly) and the prostatic apex (inferiorly) are less easy to define on axial slices. The urethral bulb is a useful landmark to define the inferior extent of the target volume.

For patients with T1 and T2 disease treatment should be given to prostate and base of seminal vesicles alone as an RTOG study has shown no advantage from additional treatment of the pelvic lymph nodes (Asbell *et al.*, 1988). A second RTOG study in patients with T3 tumours or enlarged pelvic lymph nodes randomized patients between prostate and pelvic radiotherapy or prostate, pelvic and para-aortic irradiation (Pilepich *et al.*, 1986) and again no difference was detected in recurrence or survival between the different treatment arms. However, the appropriate radiation treatment volume for T3 or poorly differentiated prostate cancers remains controversial and it is uncertain whether prostate and pelvic treatment is of additional benefit to prostate radiation alone. Most centres in the UK adopt the latter option and a retrospective review of Royal Marsden Hospital patients showed no difference in outcome whether or not additional pelvic irradiation was given (Dearnaley *et al.*, 1992). However, similar retrospective reviews from North American Centres have come to the opposite conclusion (Bagshaw, 1980; McGowan, 1981). If the pelvic lymph nodes are included the radiation target volume should include the internal and external iliac, common iliac and presacral lymph nodes groups. Such pelvic treatments are usually given using three or four field 'box' techniques but the dose must be limited to no more than 45–50 Gy or significant small bowel damage may result. The radiation field arrangements for the prostate will either be with a four field arrangement of opposing anterior and posterior and lateral fields or using anterior and posterior oblique fields when greater sparing of the posterior rectal wall is achieved (Figures 9.6 and 9.9). The optimal dose using conventional 2 Gy fractions is 60 Gy for T1 lesions, 64–66 Gy for T2 tumours, but local control may be improved by escalating the dose to 70 Gy for T3 cancers (Table 32.5) (Hanks *et al.*, 1988), although this higher dose is undoubtedly associated with an

Table 32.5   Radiation dose and local recurrence

| Dose | *Actuarial risk (%) of developing infield recurrence* | | | | | |
| | *Stage A (No. 168)* | | *Stage B (No. 724)* | | *Stage C (No. 624)* | |
(Gy)	*3 yr*	*5 yr*	*3 yr*	*5 yr*	*3 yr*	*5 yr*
< 60	0	–	15	29	28	37
60–64	5	–	6	18	24	36
65–70	2	4	9	12	17	28
> 70	0	0	7	16	14	19

Data from US Patterns of Care Studies (Hanks *et al.*, 1988).
– Too few patients for reliable estimate.

increased incidence of late complications. Satisfactory results have been reported with a variety of hypofractionated treatment schedules varying from 50 Gy in 20 fractions over 4 weeks (Duncan *et al.*, 1993), 50 Gy in 16 fractions over 21 days (Read and Pointon, 1989), and 36 Gy in 6 treatments in over 5 weeks (Collins *et al.*, 1991), but these schedules have not been prospectively compared with 'conventional' treatment.

The acute side-effects of radical irradiation include symptoms resulting from inflammation of both rectum – causing mucus discharge and rectal bleeding – and bladder – causing dysuria and frequency. Bladder infections are relatively common during radiotherapy and should be promptly treated with antibiotics. Diarrhoea may be helped by codeine or loperamide and proctitis by administration of steroid enemas. Late complications most commonly effect the rectum and rectal bleeding is the most frequent complaint followed by persistent tenesmus and mucus discharge. Haematuria and increased frequency of micturition may occur; urinary incontinence is most usually related to the need for repeated transurethral resections. Major complications requiring surgical correction are very uncommon and have occurred in less than 1% of patients treated at the Royal Marsden Hospital, although more minor effects such as transient bleeding may affect 30% of patients (Dearnaley *et al.*, 1992). The incidence of complications is clearly related to

radiotherapy technique and dose (Hanks *et al.*, 1987). The incidence of impotence following radical radiotherapy has been rather poorly documented and is probably of the order of 30%, but much depends on the vigour of the patient before treatment (Banker, 1988).

Although the incidence of clinically significant local recurrence is low after radiotherapy, post-treatment biopsies (12–24 months after radiotherapy) remain positive in approximately 15% of men treated for small T2 tumours rising to 79% for large T3/T4 cancers (Scardino and Bretas, 1987). Positive biopsies are associated with a marked increase in risk of disease recurrence. Strategies for improving control rates include the 'neoadjuvant' use of LHRH treatment (Shearer, *et al.*, 1992) currently undergoing extensive prospective randomized study by the RTOG group in the USA and 'conformal' radiotherapy techniques using 'state of art' imaging and beam shaping devices to deliver radiation more precisely, which may permit a safe increase in radiation dose (Lichter, 1992).

Interstitial irradiation has been extensively used in a number of centres during the 1970s and 1980s. However, long term follow-up of patients treated with permanent implants using ^{125}I-labelled seeds have shown generally inferior results to external beam therapy (Kuban *et al.*, 1989). These poor clinical results are probably explicable because of the very low dose rate of irradiation delivered and dose inhomogeneity due to poor geometric distribution of seeds in such implants. An alternative approach is to use temporary interstitial implants using iridium wires held in place by a rigid peritoneal template. (Porter *et al.*, 1988). Although impressive local control rates have been reported, considerable expertise is essential and significant bladder or rectal toxicity may be seen in up to 10% of patients.

32.5.2.   TREATMENT OF METASTATIC DISEASE

(a)   Hormone therapy

Prostatic epithelial cells depend on the presence of androgens for normal growth and development. Androgen deprivation reduces cell proliferation and causes cell death by the mechanism of apoptosis or programmed cell death. The majority of prostate cancers retain at least a partial dependence on androgens, and androgen withdrawal from men with symptomatic metastatic prostate cancer produces some of the most dramatic responses that can be seen in cancer treatment. Approximately 80% of patients derive subjective benefit and the median duration of response is from 12 to 24 months. However, prostate cancers eventually become androgen independent and the median duration of survival of patients with widespread disease is about 2.5 years, although some 20% may survive 5 years. If hormonal therapy is used for patients with advanced localized disease the median survival is 4.5 years (Veterans Administration Cooperative Urological Research Group, 1967).

Orchidectomy has been used for the treatment of prostatic disease for 100 years, but the effects of androgen deprivation using either orchidectomy or oestrogens were first comprehensively described by Huggins and Hodges in 1941. Despite the long history of hormonal treatment there is still considerable

uncertainty as to what comprises optimal therapy and there remains considerable debate both about the type and timing of treatment and it is also uncertain whether adjuvant hormonal therapy is of value as it is in breast cancer.

The currently used hormonal treatments have their principal action on androgen biosynthesis (Figure 32.1). Although the testes are the major site of androgen production, approximately 5% of circulating testosterone may come from the adrenals. Testosterone is metabolized within prostate cells by the enzyme 5 alpha reductase to the active metabolite dihydrotesterone which interacts with the androgen receptor. Following orchidectomy there is a rise of luteinizing hormone-releasing hormone (LHRH) and luteinizing hormone (LH) together with follicle stimulating hormone (FSH). Side-effects are those of loss of libido and impotence and hot flushing may also be troublesome. Oestrogens act mainly by a central mechanism blocking LHRH secretion by the hypothalamus and inhibiting LH secretion by the pituitary, and hence testosterone secretion by testis. Oestrogens may have some additional peripheral actions of uncertain significance which include a direct cytocidal effect on prostate cancer cells and also a decrease in free testosterone levels by increasing sex-hormone binding globulin (SHBG) levels. As well as causing impotence the major complication from oestrogens is the increase in cardiovascular complications mediated by the reduction of anti-thrombin 3 levels and increased platelet aggregation. Cardiovascular morbidity from oestrogens is usually manifest within a year of starting treatment and is sufficiently common to negate any beneficial effects of treatment on survival (Blackard *et al.*, 1973). Additionally gynaecomastia occurs in the majority of men, although this side-effect can be substantially reduced by giving low doses of radiotherapy before (but not after) starting oestrogen therapy. Although the cardiovascular side-

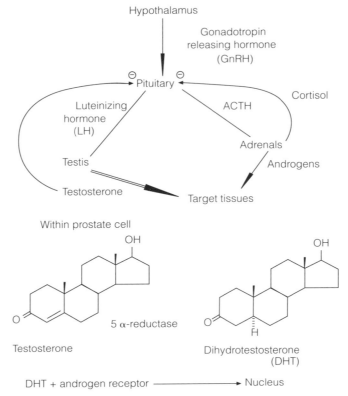

Figure 32.1   Androgen biosynthesis. (Reproduced by permission of Professor M. Jarman.)

effects of stilboestrol can be reduced by lowering the dose from 5 mg to 1 mg per day, 3 mg stilboestrol are required for adequate androgen suppression and oestrogen treatment has fallen into disrepute as first line management. The 1980s saw the development of the LHRH agonists which are given by convenient once monthly subcutaneous depot injection. Usually the pituitary responds to the pulsatile release of LHRH from the hypothalamus. Continuous stimulation by LHRH agonists results in inhibition of LH secretion and a reduction in LHRH receptors. Androgen levels are suppressed to castrate levels and the side-effects of these agents are essentially similar to those of orchidectomy. The initial LHRH treatment, however, causes a temporary elevation of LH secretion and

therefore testosterone levels for approximately 2 weeks. This action may stimulate prostate cancer growth and 'flare' reactions may occur including increases of bone pain, spinal cord compression or urinary obstruction. It is advisable to block this effect by giving an antiandrogen for several days before and after the first depot LHRH injection. There are two classes of antiandrogens. The non-steroidal group (flutamide, nilutamide and more recently casodex) are pure antiandrogens and compete with androgens for binding sites at the androgen receptor in the nucleus of prostate cancer cells. Their use is associated with a rise in LH and testosterone levels as the negative feedback of androgens on the pituitary is blocked. The secondary rise in testosterone level may partially negate the efficacy of non-steroidal antiandrogen therapy and these agents are not routinely used as first line monotherapy. The side-effects associated with treatment include gynaecomastia (resulting from increased peripheral aromatization of testosterone) and gastrointestinal upset (particularly flutamide), but libido may be maintained. Cyproterone acetate is a steroidal antiandrogen which has additional progestational effects which inhibit gonadotrophin secretion and so lower testosterone levels to castrate levels. This dual action makes cyproterone acetate suitable as a first line hormone therapy. Side-effects are those of androgen deprivation; thromboembolic risks are markedly less than with oestrogens but liver dysfunction and fatigue have been reported. Compliance with regular three times daily medication may be less satisfactory than for once monthly LHRH depot injections.

There is currently great controversy over the significance of the small amounts of androgen produced from the adrenals and its role in response to hormone therapy. Initial reports (Labrie *et al.*, 1987) claimed significant advantages for 'maximal androgen blockade' using orchidectomy in combination with an antiandrogen over standard mono therapy and a total of 21 prospective randomized studies have subsequently been performed (Van Tinteren and Dalesio, 1993). The first of these studies was reported by the National Cancer Institute and showed a small survival advantage, particularly for patients with good performance status and small volumes of disease (Crawford *et al.*, 1990). These findings have been correlated by a second study again adding flutamide LHRH therapy which compared to orchidectomy alone gave significant improvements in time to first progression and a 7-month improvement in median survival (Keuppens *et al.*, 1993). However, these results are currently in contrast with other studies and although maximal androgen blockade can reasonably be recommended for patients with good performance

status and small volumes of disease standard first line management for other patients should be considered as orchidectomy, treatment with LHRH agonists or cyproterone acetate. The conclusions from some of the major randomized studies of hormone therapy in prostate cancer are summarized in Table 32.6. The VACURG studies apparently showed no advantage for active hormone therapy as compared to placebo, but patients assigned to placebo in these studies subsequently received a variety of hormone treatments and a more realistic conclusion from this study was that there could be no difference detected between immediate or deferred hormone treatment. Currently the MRC are completing a large study to examine this aspect of timing of hormone treatment in patients with asymptomatic advanced localized or metastatic disease. We also need to learn whether there is a similar benefit to adjuvant hormone therapy in prostate cancer as in breast cancer. Data from patients with positive lymph node desections at the time of radical prostatectomy (Zincke *et al.*, 1987) suggest that the time to progression can be lengthened from some 10–22 months to between 60 and 100 months with immediate endocrine therapy. It is not certain whether such findings will translate into a survival advantage, but currently RTOG and European Organization for Research and Treatment of Cancer (EORTC) studies of adjuvant therapy with radical radiotherapy are addressing this question.

(b) Treatment of hormone relapsed prostate cancer

Progressive prostate cancer is characterized by general debility, anorexia, malaise and most particularly bone pain. In contrast to the dramatic responses of initial hormone therapy, second line manoeuvres produce responses in at most 30% of patients and these are usually of slight degree and short duration. Our practice is to recommend

Table 32.6 Prospective randomized studies of hormone treatment in advanced prostate cancer

Study	Treatments compared	Findings
VACURG I (Blackard *et al.*, 1973)	P vs S vs O + P vs O + S	Increased cardiovascular toxicity of S. Immediate and deferred treatment equivalent
VACURG II (Veterans Administration Cooperative Urological Research Group, 1967)	P vs S (0.2 mg) vs S (1 mg) vs S (5 mg)	1 mg S equivalent to 5 mg S but with reduced cardiovascular toxicity. 0.2 mg S ineffective
EORTC (Pavone-Macaluso *et al.*, 1986)	CPA vs S vs MPA	CPA equivalent to S with less cardiovascular toxicity. MPA inferior progression free and overall survival
EORTC (Smith *et al.*, 1986)	S vs EMP	Equivalent progression free and overall survival. S increased cardiovascular toxicity, EMP increased gastrointestinal toxicity
The Leuprolide Study Group, 1988	LHRH vs S	Equivalent response and survival. LHRH less toxicity
Waymont *et al.*, 1992	LHRH vs S	
Kaisary *et al.*, 1991	LHRH vs O	Equivalent response and survival
National Cancer Institute (Crawford *et al.*, 1989)	LHRH + F vs LHRH + P	MAB increased progression free and overall survival by 2.5 months and 7 months
Medical Research Council	Immediate versus deferred androgen ablation	Awaited

P, placebo; S, stilboestrol; O, orchidectomy; CPA, cyproterone acetate; MPA, medroxprogesterone; EMP, estramustine phosphate; F, flutamide; CAB, complete androgen blockade.

continuation of androgen suppression as rising testosterone levels may further stimulate prostate cancer growth. The addition of cortisone acetate (Plowman *et al.*, 1987) acts by suppressing ACTH levels and adrenal production of androgen and is arguably as effective as more expensive alternatives. Second line responses are most likely to be seen in patients who have derived substantial benefit from their initial hormone manoeuvres and alternative strategies include the addition of antiandrogens or oestrogens. In these patients response can be monitored using PSA levels and if no response is seen within a few weeks such measures should be abandoned. High dose ketoconazole has been shown to have some clinical activity and interferes with synthesis of testosterone precursors both in the adrenal glands and testis. The antihelminthic suramin represents a potentially exciting new class of drug inhibiting a variety of growth factors, but the 'therapeutic window' is very narrow and the potential for neurotoxicity high. Cytotoxic chemotherapy has a very limited role. Elderly patients with extensive bone marrow involvement tolerate treatment poorly and toxicity is high unless patients are carefully selected. Reported response rates of a variety of agents are between 10% and 20%, but responses are short lived. Estramustine phosphate (a combination of oestradiol and nitrogen mustard) has been reported to produce response rates up to 30%, but when formally tested in prospective studies has failed to show additional benefit over standard treatments.

Radiotherapy remains the most valuable single option for palliating bone pain. Eighty per cent of patients have significant pain relief using a single treatment of 8 Gy and in general this is to be preferred to longer fractionated courses (Price *et al.*, 1986). Frequently, however, there is very widespread bony disease and multiple sites of discomfort which can be effectively managed by wide field or hemibody irradiation. This technique treats half of the body at a time to a dose of 8 Gy (6 Gy for upper half to avoid lung toxicity). Again some 80% of patients can be expected to benefit and the duration of relief is frequently for the remaining life span of the patient. Hemibody irradiation is, however, inappropriate for patients who are in poor general condition and can produce marked malaise in addition to organ specific toxicities. Recently, the value of the bone metastasis seeking isotope strontium-89 has been studied (Dearnaley *et al.*, 1992; Porter *et al.*, 1993). Although expensive this isotope has been shown to give effective palliation in 70–80% of patients and, compared to external beam techniques, it slows the onset of development of new sites of bony discomfort. Spinal cord compression from extradural metastases is a particularly devastating and common complication in prostate cancer. Careful neurological examination should always be made if the patient presents with new sites of back pain. MRI is now the investigation of choice and prompt radiotherapy should be given. Outcome depends on the ambulatory status of the patient at the time of treatment and the natural history of their disease – in particular patients presenting for the first time with prostate cancer and spinal cord compression may have extended periods of survival with additional hormone treatment and carefully fractioned courses of treatment are indicated for these patients (Kuban *et al.*, 1986). The biphosphonate group of drugs is currently being evaluated in prostate cancer and may have a useful additional role to play in pain control, particularly for patients with widespread pain who are unsuitable for radiotherapy because of extensive bone marrow infiltration.

32.6 CONCLUSIONS

Real progress in the treatment and understanding of prostate cancer has been slow, although this already common disease can only become a greater health problem with increasing longevity of the population. Strategies for prevention and early detection need to be developed and rigorously tested. Local treatment options need to be compared in prospective studies and the value of adjuvant hormone therapy determined. Hormone refractory disease remains a major challenge. As for other common solid tumours, progress in developing more effective systemic treatment has stalled. New approaches are required and prostate cancer is a good model for the development of these new approaches being common and having an excellent marker of response in PSA. Advances in molecular biology will give new insights into the mechanisms controlling cancer growth and cell death which may lead to the identification of new targets for therapeutic intervention.

REFERENCES

Asbell, S.O., Krall, J.M., Pilepich, M.V. *et al.* (1988) Elective pelvic irradiation in stage A2, B carcinoma of the prostate: Analysis of RTOG 77-06. *International Journal of Radiation Oncology, Biology, Physics*, **15**, 1307–16.

Bagshaw, M.A. (1980) External radiation therapy of carcinoma of the prostate. *Cancer*, **45**, 1912–21.

Bagshaw, M.A., Cox, R.S. and Ray, G.R. (1988) Status of radiation treatment of prostate cancer at Stanford University. *National Cancer Institute Monographs*, **7**, 47.

Bagshaw, M.A., Ray, G.R. and Cox, R.S. (1987) Selecting initial therapy for prostate cancer. Radiation therapy perspective. *Cancer*, **60**, 521–5.

Banker, F.L. (1988) The preservation of potency after external beam irradiation for prostate cancer. *International Journal of Radiation Oncology, Biology, Physics*, **15**, 219–20.

Belt, E. and Schröder, F.H. (1972) Total perineal prostatectomy for carcinoma of the prostate. *Journal of Urology*, **107**, 91–6.

Beral, V., Inskip, H. and Fraser, P. (1985) Mortality of employees of the United Kingdom Atomic Energy Authority. *British Medical Journal*, **291**, 440–7.

Blackard, C.E., Byar, D.P. and Jordan, W.P. Jr (1973) Orchiectomy for advanced prostatic carcinoma: a re-evaluation. *Urology*, **1**, 553–60.

Breslow, N., Chan, C.W. and Dhom, G. (1977) Latent carcinoma of prostate at autopsy in seven areas. *International Journal of Cancer*, **20**, 680–8.

Cannon, L., Bishop, D.T., Skolnick, M. *et al.* (1982) Genetic epidemiology of prostate cance in the Utah Mormon geneology. *Cancer Surveys*, **1**, 47–69.

Chodak, G.W., Thisted, R.A., Gerber, G.S. *et al.* (1994) Results of conservative management of clinically localised prostate cancer. *New England Journal of Medicine*, **330**, 142–8.

Coleman, M.P., Esteve, J., Damiecki, P. *et al.* (1993) Trends in cancer incidence and mortality. *IARC Scientific Publications*, **121**.

Collins, C.D., Lloyd-Davies, R.W. and Swan, A.V. (1991) Radical external beam radiotherapy for localised carcinoma of the prostate using a hypofractionation technique. *Clinical Oncology*, **3**, 127–32.

Crawford, E.D., Eisenberger, M.A. and McLeod, D.G. (1989) A controlled trial of leuprolide with and without flutamide in prostatic carcinoma. *New England Journal of Medicine*, **321**, 419–24.

Dalesio, O. (1992) Complete androgen blockade in prostate cancer: an overview of randomized trials. *Prostate*, **(Suppl. 4)**, 111–14.

Dearnaley, D.P., Bayly, R.J., A'Hern, R.P. *et al.* (1992) Palliation of bone metastases in prostate cancer, hemibody irradiation or stontium-89? *Clinical Oncology*, **4**, 101–7.

Dearnaley, D.P., Eeles, R., Syndikus, I. *et al.* (1992) External beam radiotherapy for localised prostate cancer: long term follow-up in 443 patients – 11th Annual Meeting ESTRO Malmö, Sweden – 1–4 September. *European Society for Therapeutic Radiology and Oncology*, **24**, (Suppl), S80 (Abstr. 315).

Dearnaley, D.P., Price, A., Chamberlain, J. *et al.* (1993) Grand Round – Prostate Cancer. Report of a meeting of physicians and scientists, Institute of Cancer Research and the Royal Marsden Hospital. *Lancet*, **342**, 901–5.

Duncan, W., Warde, P., Catton, C.N. *et al.* (1993) Carcinoma of the prostate: results of radiotherapy (1970–1985). *International Journal of Radiation Oncology, Biology, Physics*, **26**, 203–10.

Epstein, J.I., Paull, G., Eggleston, J.C. and Walsh, P.C. (1986) Prognosis of untreated stage A1 prostatic carcinoma: a study of 94 cases with extended follow-up. *Journal of Urology*, **136**, 837–9.

Fellows, G.J., Clark, P.B., Beynon, L.L. *et al.* (1992) Treatment of advanced localised prostatic cancer by orchiectomy, radiotherapy, or combined treatment. A Medical Research Council Study. *British Journal of Urology*, **70**, 304–9.

Gallee, M.P.W., Ten Kate, F.J.W., Mulder, P.G.H. *et al.* (1990) Histological grading of prostatic carcinoma in prostatectomy specimens: comparison of prognostic accuracy of five grading systems. *British Journal of Urology*, **65**, 368–75.

Gibbons, R.P., Correa, R.J., Jr, Bannen, G.E. and Weissman, R.M. (1989) Total prostatectomy for clinically localised prostatic cancer: long-term results. *Journal of Urology*, **141**, 564–6.

Gleason, D.F., Mellinger, G.T. and The Veterans Administration Cooperative (1974) Prediction of prognosis for prostatic adenocarcinoma by combined histological grading and clinical staging. *Journal of Urology*, **111**, 58.

Goffinet, D.R. and Bagshaw, M.A. (1990) *Radiation Therapy of Prostate Carcinoma: thirty year experience at Stanford University. Treatment of Prostatic Cancer – facts and controversies*, Wiley-Liss, New York.

Guess, H.A. (1993) Is vasectomy a risk factor for prostate cancer? *European Journal of Cancer*, **29A**, 1055–9.

Hanks, G.E. 1988, More on the uro-oncology research group report of radical surgery vs radiotherapy for adenocarcinoma of the prostate. *International Journal of Radiation Oncology, Biology, Physics*, **14**, 1053–7.

Hanks, G.E. (1991) Radiotherapy or surgery for prostate cancer? Ten and fifteen year results of external beam therapy. *Acta Oncologica*, **30**, 231–7.

Hanks, G.E., Asbell, S., Krall, J.M. et al. (1991) Outcome for lymph node dissection negative T-1b, T-2 (A-2, B) prostate cancer treated with external beam radiation therapy in RTOG 77-06. *International Journal of Radiation Oncology, Biology, Physics*, **21**, 1099–103.

Hanks, G.E., Diamond, J.J., Krall, J.M. et al. (1987) A ten year follow-up of 682 patients treated for prostate cancer with radiation therapy in the United States. *International Journal of Radiation Oncology, Biology, Physics*, **13**, 499–505.

Hanks, G.E., Krail, J.M., Martz, K.L. et al. (1988) The outcome of treatment of 313 patients with T-1 (UICC) prostate cancer treated with external beam irradiation. *International Journal of Radiation Oncology, Biology, Physics*, **14**, 243–8.

Hetherington, J.W., Siddall, J.K. and Cooper, E.H. (1988) Contribution of bone scintigrapy, prostatic acid phosphatase and prostate-specific antigen to the monitoring of prostatic cancer. *European Urology*, **14**, 1–5.

Hill, P.B. and Wynder, E.L. (1979) Effect of vegetarian diet and dexamethasone on plasma prolactin, testosterone and dehyroepiandrosterone in men and women. *Cancer Letters*, **7**, 273–82.

Huggins, C. and Hodges, C.V. (1941) The effect of castration, of estrogen and of androgen injection on serum phosphatases in metastatic carcinoma of the prostate. *Cancer Research*, **1**, 292.

Johansson, J.E., Adami, H.O., Andersson, S.O. et al. (1989) Natural history of localised prostatic cancer. *Lancet*, **i**, 799–803.

Kaisary, A.V., Tyrrell, C.J., Peeling, W.B. and Griffiths, K. (1991) Comparison of LHRH analogue ('Zoladex') with orchiectomy in patients with metastatic prostatic carcinoma. *British Journal of Urology*, **67**, 502–8.

Keuppens, F., Whelan, P., Carneirode Moura, J.L. et al. for the members of the European Organisation for Research and Treatment of Cancer – Genitourinary Group (1993) Orchidectomy versus goserelin plus flutamide in patients with metastatic cancer (EORTC 30853). *Cancer*, **72**, 3863–69.

Kuban, D.A., el-Mahdi, Sigfred, S.V. et al. (1986) Characteristics of spinal cord compression in adenocarcinoma of prostate. *Urology*, **28**, 364.

Kuban, D.A., El-Mahdi, A.M. and Schellhammer, P.F. (1989) Prognosis in patients with local recurrence after definitive irradiation of prostatic carcinoma. *Cancer*, **63**, 2421–5.

Labrie, F., Dupont, A. and Giguere, M. (1987) Combination therapy with flutamide and castration (orchiectomy or LHRH agonist): the minimal endocrine therapy in both untreated and previously treated patients. *Journal of Steroid Biochemistry*, **27**, 525–32.

The Leuprolide Study Group (1998) Leuprolide versus diethylstilbestrol for metastatic prostate cancer. *New England Journal of Medicine*, **311**, 1281–6.

Lichter (1992) *Seminars in Radiation Oncology*. W.B. Saunders, New York.

Lowe, B.A. and Listrom, M.B. (1988) Incidental carcinoma of the prostate: an analysis of the predictors of progression. *Journal of Urology*, **140**, 1340–4.

McGowan, D.G. (1981) The value of extended field radiation therapy in carcinoma of the prostate. *International Journal of Radiation Oncology, Biology, Physics*, **7**, 1333.

McNeal, J.E., Bostwick, D.G., Kindrachuk, R.A. et al. (1986) Patterns of progression in prostate cancer. *Lancet*, **i**, 60–3.

Meikle, A.W. and Smith, J.A. (1990) Epidemiology of prostate cancer. *Urological Clinics of North America*, **17**, 709–18.

Mostofi, F.K. (1976) Problems of grading carcinoma of the prostate. *Seminars in Oncology*, **3**, 161–9.

National Cancer Institute (1989) NCI cancer statistics review 1973–1986 including a report on status of cancer control. NIH publication. *United States Department of Health and Human Services*, **89**, 2789.

Paulson, D.F., Lin, G., Hinshaw, W. and Stephani, S. (1982) Radical surgery versus radiotherapy for adenocarcinoma of the prostate. *Journal of Urology*, **128**, 502–4.

Paulson, D.F., Robertson, J.F., Daubert, L.M. and Walther, P.J. (1988) Radical prostatectomy in stage A prostatic adenocarcinoma. *Journal of Urology*, **140**, 535–9.

Pavone-Macaluso, M., De Voogt, H.J. and Viggiano, G. (1986) Comparison of diethylstilboestrol, cyproterone acetate and medroxyprogesterone acetate in the treatment of advanced prostatic cancer: final analysis of a randomized phase III trial of the European Organization for Research on Treatment of Cancer Urological Group. *Journal of Urology*, **136**, 624–31.

Perez, C.A., Garcia, D., Simpson, J.R. et al. (1989) Factors influencing outcome of definitive radiotherapy for localized carcinoma of the prostate. *Radiotherapy and Oncology*, **16**, 1–21.

Pilepich, M.V., Krall, J.M., Johnson, R.J. *et al.* (1986) Extended field (periaortic) irradiation in carcinoma of the prostate analysis of RTOG 75-06. *International Journal of Radiation Oncology, Biology, Physics*, **12**, 345–51.

Plowman, P.N., Perry, L.A. and Chard, T. (1987) Androgen suppression by hydrocortisone without aminoglutethimide in orchiectomised men with prostatic cancer. *British Journal of Urology*, **59**, 225–31.

Porter, A.T., Chir, M.B.B., Scrimger, J.W. and Pocha, J.S. (1988) Remote interstitial afterloading in cancer of the prostate preliminary experience with the microselectron. *International Journal of Radiation Oncology, Biology, Physics*, **14**, 571–5.

Porter, A.T., McEwan, A.J.B., Powe, J.E. *et al.* (1993) Results of a randomized phase III trial to evaluate the efficacy of strontium-89 adjuvant to local field external beam irradiation in the management of endocrine resistant metastatic prostate cancer. *International Journal of Radiation Oncology, Biology, Physics*, **25**, 805–13.

Price, P., Hoskin, P.J., Easton, D. *et al.* (1986) Prospective randomised trial of single and multi-fraction schedules in the treatment of painful bone metastases. *Radiotherapy and Oncology*, **6**, 247–55.

Read, G. and Pointon, R.C.S. (1989) Retrospective study of radiotherapy in early carcinoma of the prostate. *British Journal of Urology*, **63**, 191–5.

Scardino, P.T. and Bretas, F. (1987) Interstitial radiotherapy, in *Adenocarcinoma of the Prostate*, (eds A.W. Bruce and J. Trachtenberg), Springer-Verlag, London, pp. 145–58.

Schröder, F.H., Hermanek, P., Dennis, L. *et al.* (1992) TNM classification of prostate cancer. *Prostate*, **4**, (Suppl), 129–38.

Shearer, R.J., Davies, J.H., Gelister, J.S.K. and Dearnaley, D.P. (1992) Hormonal cytoreduction and radiotherapy for carcinoma of the prostate. *British Journal of Urology*, **69**, 521–4.

Smith, J.A. Jr, Seaman, J.P., Gleidman, J.B. and Middleton, R.G. (1983) Pelvic lymph node metastasis from prostatic cancer: influence of tumor grade and stage in 452 consecutive patients. *Journal of Urology*, **130**, 290–2.

Smith, P.H., Suciu, S., Robinson, M.R.G. *et al.* (1986) Comparison of effect of diethylstilbestrol with low dose estramustine phosphate in treatment of advanced prostatic cancer: final analysis of phase III trial of European Organisation for Research on Treatment of Cancer. *Journal of Urology*, **136**, 619–23.

Stamey, T.A., Kabalin, J.N. and Ferrari, M. (1989) Prostate specific antigen in the diagnosis and treatment of adenocarcinoma of the prostate. III. Radiation treated patients. *Journal of Urology*, **141**, 1084–90.

Stamey, T.A., Yang, N., Hay, A.R. *et al.* (1987) Prostate specific antigen as a serum marker for adenocarcinoma of the prostate. *New England Journal of Medicine*, **317**, 909–16.

Van Tinteren, H. and Dalesio, O. (1993) Systematic overview (meta-analysis) of all randomized trials of treatment of prostate cancer. *Cancer*, **72**, 3847–50.

Veterans Administration Cooperative Urological Research Group (1967) Treatment and survival of patients with cancer of the prostate. *Surgery, Gynecology and Obstetrics*, **124**, 1011.

Waymont, B., Lynch, T.H., Dunn, J.A. *et al.* (1992) Phase III randomised study of 'Zoladex' versus stilboestrol in the treatment of advanced prostate cancer. *British Journal of Urology*, **69**, 614–20.

Whitmore, W.F., Jr (1988) Panel discussion: management of stage B1 and B2 disease, in *Multidisciplinary Analysis of Controversies in the Management of Prostate Cancer*, (eds D.S. Coffey, M.I. Resnick, F.A. Door and J.P. Karr), Plenum Press, New York, pp. 143–4.

Yatani, R., Chigusa, I., Akazaki, K. *et al.* (1982) Geographic pathology of latent prostatic carcinoma. *International Journal of Cancer*, **29**, 611–16.

Zagars, G.K., von Eschenback, A.C., Johnson, D.E. and Oswald, M.J. (1987) Stage C adenocarcinoma of the prostate: an analysis of 551 patients treated with external beam radiation. *Cancer*, **60**, 1489–99.

Zincke, H., Utz, D.C., Thule, P.M. and Taylor, W.F. (1987) Treatment options for patients with stage D1 (TO-3 N1-2 MO) adenocarcinoma of prostate. *Urology*, **30**, 307–15.

BLADDER CANCER

33

Alan Horwich

33.1 INTRODUCTION

Bladder cancer encompasses a wide spectrum of disease ranging from the superficial papilloma adequately treated by transurethral resection alone to locally advanced and metastatic bladder cancer which can be one of the most rapidly progressive and debilitating of neoplasms. The molecular basis for this diversity is now being established and will provide a considerable impetus to the development of more successful treatment programmes. At present there is considerable controversy over the management of localized invasive disease where important contributions can come from surgeons, radiation oncologists and chemotherapists and there is no doubt that optimal management is multidisciplinary.

33.2 INCIDENCE

The incidence of bladder cancer rises steeply after the fifth decade of life. The incidence rates for the white population of the USA for individuals aged 60–69 years are 91.2 per 10^5 for males and 25.9 per 10^5 for females and these incidences are almost doubled in the 70–79 old age group. The male to female ratio in western countries is 3 to 1.

33.3 AETIOLOGY

33.3.1 CARCINOGENS

At the end of the nineteenth century an association between bladder cancer and employment in a chemical dye works was established (Rehn, 1904). This association was supported when 2-naphthylamine was shown to cause bladder cancer in experimental animals; the techniques also revealed related carcinogens which were employed in the aniline dye and in the rubber industries. In man the aromatic amines are detoxified by N-acetyl transferase. However the rate of acetylation does not appear to correlate with the development of cancer (Cartwright *et al.*, 1982).

33.3.2 CIGARETTE SMOKING

A smoker has a two to six times greater risk of developing bladder cancer than a non-smoker. Analysis of cigarette smoke has shown the presence of aromatic amines. There is some suggestion that the prognosis is better in patients who have stopped smoking at the time of diagnosis of bladder cancer (Anthony and Thomas, 1970).

33.3.3 SCHISTOSOMIASIS

This infection is common in many parts of Africa especially in Egypt. Chronic infection is associated with epithelial dysplasia, squamous metaplasia and squamous cell cancer.

33.3.4 EXSTROPHY OF THE BLADDER

This is known to be associated with the development of adenocarcinomas of the bladder.

33.3.5   DRUGS

There have been a number of reports of bladder cancers developing in patients who were previously treated with cyclophosphamide (Pearson and Soloway, 1978). A much slower time course of cancer induction is associated with the use of phenacetin.

33.3.6   MOLECULAR GENETICS

A mutated *ras* oncogene was first identified in the EJ human bladder cancer cell line and subsequently activated *ras* oncogenes have been found in a range of human tumours. This abnormality is found in approximately 10% of bladder cancers (Fujita *et al.*, 1984; Malone *et al.*, 1985). Bladder cancer has been associated with a number of chromosome abnormalities, suggesting loss of tumour suppressive genes (Table 33.1) (Presti *et al.*, 1991).

33.4   PATHOLOGY

The very great majority of urothelial tumours presenting in the UK are transitional cell carcinomas which can be graded histologically based on the number of cell layers in the urothelium, the range of cell sizes, the nuclear polarization and pleomorphism and the number of mitoses. Pure squamous carcinomas and adenocarcinomas of the bladder do

occur but are exceedingly rare. Even more rare are lymphomas and sarcomas of the bladder.

Adenocarcinomas are typically associated with the congenital malformation exstrophy. Squamous cancers are the commonest type found in a background of bladder schistosomiasis and indeed this is the commonest cancer found in countries where schistosomiasis is endemic such as Egypt.

Pathological staging of bladder cancer is based on the depth of invasion as listed in Table 33.2. The primary tumours are divided into two groups. Superficial cancers do not extend beyond the mucosa and submucosa and constitute approximately 80% of transitional cell carcinomas at presentation. The natural history of these tumours is to recur after superficial resection though whether these recurrences are true recurrence of the original tumour or whether they are new tumours forming within a diseased urothelium has not been determined unequivocally. Multiple synchronous tumours are clonally related and are unlikely therefore to represent a series of new tumours (Sidransky *et al.*, 1992).

Invasive tumours are staged as T2 and T3 if they invade bladder muscle and T4 if they invade adjacent organs. Pelvic lymph node involvement is found in approximately 20% of patients with T2/T3 tumours and 40–50% of patients with T4 tumours. Pelvic lymph

Table 33.1   Bladder cancer: molecular genetics

| | P *values* | | | | |
	Loss *3p*	*Loss* *11p*	*Loss* *17p*	*Loss* *18q*	*Altered* *Rb*
Grades 1/2,3	0.004	0.32	0.06	0.30	0.09
Stage					
superficial/invasive	0.01	0.09	0.01	0.42	0.05
Vascular invasion	0.13	0.07	0.04	0.48	0.30
Involved nodes	0.23	0.47	0.36	0.57	0.34

From Presti *et al.*, 1991.

Table 33.2   TNM staging of bladder cancer (1987)

Grade	Urinary bladder
Tis	*In situ*: 'flat tumour'
Ta	Papillary non-invasive
T1	Subepithelial connective tissue
T2	Superficial muscle (inner half)
T3	Deep muscle or perivesical fat
T3a	Deep muscle (outer half)
T3b	Perivesical fat
T4	Prostate, uterus, vagina, pelvic wall, abdominal wall
N1	Single ≤ 2 cm
N2	2 cm < single ≤ 5 cm; multiple ≤ 5 cm
N3	> 5 cm
M0	No distant metastasis
M1	Distant metastastasis

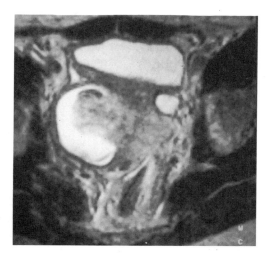

Figure 33.1 CT scan showing tumour within a diverticulum posterior to the bladder.

node involvement confers a poor prognosis and is a harbinger of more widespread disease in 80% of cases (Smith and Whitmore, 1981). Common sites of metastasis include other lymph node areas, especially the para-aortic region, liver, lungs and bone.

33.5   PRESENTATION

Most cases of bladder cancer present with macroscopic haematuria (Hendry *et al.*, 1981). Thus any patient with the symptom of red coloured urine requires investigations designed to diagnose or exclude a urological malignancy. Patients may also have dysurea and frequency of micturition associated either with infection of urine or sometimes extensive carcinoma-*in-situ* of bladder urothelium.

Haematuria is confirmed by urine analysis and in many cases the diagnosis of transitional carcinoma of the bladder can be made by cytological analysis of the voided urine or bladder washings.

Useful radiological investigations include intravenous urography, which has the advantage of revealing disease in the upper urinary tracts as well as providing functional information and evidence of obstruction. CT scanning of bladder cancer can reveal multiple tumours and also can indicate when the tumour has extended through the bladder wall. In addition it can reveal tumour within a diverticulum (Figure 33.1). However it is poor at discriminating the level of invasion of bladder wall. CT scan can also reveal pelvic lymph node enlargement. This technique has now largely superseded lymphography. MRI can also discern pelvic lymphadenopathy and extent of tumour within the bladder, and may offer some advantages in non-axial views (Figure 33.2).

Clinical staging is based on an examination under anaesthetic and cystourethroscopy. In this setting the finding of induration within the bladder wall following complete resection of a bladder tumour has been taken to indicate a T3 lesion. Clinical T stage is based on bimanual examination and pathological examination of the resected specimen; however, it should be emphasized that the pathologist is rarely able to distinguish a T2 from a T3 tumour except following cystectomy. There is often considerable disparity between clinical T staging and the pathological T stage of the excised bladder (Kenney *et al.*, 1970).

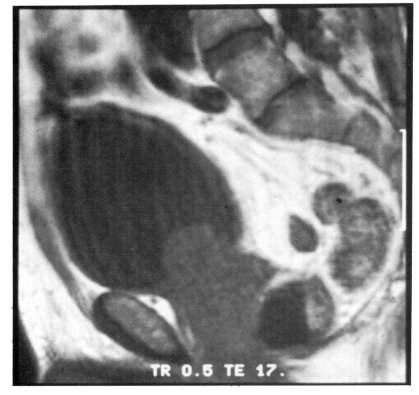

Figure 33.2   Sagittal MRI showing tumour extension through the postero-inferior bladder wall.

33.6   PROGNOSIS

Clinical T staging does provide information of considerable importance, as shown in Table 33.3. Within individual stages there are other factors which contribute important information.

Superficial tumours treated by resection will recur in approximately 60–70% of cases and this is more likely with multiple tumours, larger tumours, tumours of higher grade, and where there is carcinoma-*in-situ* in the bladder mucosa. A recent multivariate analysis co-ordinated by the Medical Research Council found that the most significant prognostic factors in superficial bladder cancer were whether presentation was with single or multiple tumours and whether the bladder was free from evidence of recurrence

3 months after the original resection (Table 33.4) (Parmar *et al.*, 1989). This form of study can be used to decide which patients should have more intensive treatment such as intravesical chemotherapy.

Of considerable concern are those patients with superficial bladder tumours who recur with more advanced disease and this appears to be most common in patients with grade 3 lesions. Radiotherapy has been advocated for these tumours but it is uncertain whether this approach will improve on the results of superficial resection with or without chemotherapy and currently a trial under the auspices of the Medical Research Council Urological Cancer Working Party is comparing these approaches.

For more advanced tumours the significant prognostic factors include histological grade,

Table 33.3 Bladder cancer prognostic factors: the Royal Marsden Hospital 1972–90

Variable	No.	% 5 yr S*
Male	1289	25.7
Female	494	23.1
T1	227	60.9
T2	274	38.8
T3	627	16.8
T4	424	5.9
N0	596	28.4
N+	342	11.1
G1	152	60.2
G2	500	30.1
G3	792	13.5
TCC	1361	26.5
SCC	87	12.6
≤ 4 cm	322	35.2
> 4 cm	217	14.2
M0	1135	28.0
M1	130	1.5

* S – survival

age of the patient, the presence of hydronephrosis, pathological evidence of lymphatic or vascular invasion in the primary tumour, and aneuploidy and the absence of ABO antigen expression (Raghavan *et al.*, 1990). Overexpression of the epidermal growth factor receptor has been associated with a poorer prognosis (Neal *et al.*, 1985; Wood *et al.*, 1992). It has been suggested that squamous metaplasia of a transitional carcinoma may indicate a poorer prognosis, but this has not been supported in all studies. Multivariate analysis of just under 400 patients with T3 cancer suggested that the major factors for invasive disease were the size of the primary tumour and the presence of lymphatic invasion or lymph node metastases (Babiker *et al.*, 1989).

Patients presenting with metastatic disease may benefit from therapy but the median survival is less than 1 year.

33.7 MANAGEMENT

33.7.1 SUPERFICIAL BLADDER CANCER

The standard initial management is transurethral resection which should achieve complete removal of tumour. Since tumours may be multiple the procedure should begin by carefully noting the location of all tumours and then the resection should be systematic. Diathermy coagulation should not be employed in initial treatment of what is thought to be a superficial tumour, since it will prevent detailed histological examinations. Tumours in a diverticulum may be difficult to resect partly because of access and partly because the muscle thickness may be extremely limited, and in many cases these tumours are better approached by partial cystectomy.

The main complications of transurethral resection include haemorrhage, infection, perforation and vesico-ureteric reflux (Dick *et al.*, 1980). The procedure carries a mortality of approximately 0.6%.

Regular follow-up check cystoscopies of the bladder are mandatory in patients with superficial bladder cancer and the usual practice is to perform a first check cystoscopy after approximately 3 months and thereafter at 6 monthly intervals for the next few years. In the patients who have remained free of recurrence for 5 years it is probably safe to continue assessments by urine cytology alone.

(a) Intravesical chemotherapy

This technique is appropriate for patients with superficial tumours with a high risk of recurrence, e.g. such as those who have previously suffered recurrence or those who present with multiple synchronous tumours. A range of agents have been used includ-

Table 33.4   Superficial bladder cancer: Medical Research Council (Parmar *et al.*, 1989). (417 Patients, 1981–84, thiotepa; 502 patients, 1984–86, mitomycin)

Parameter	2 years recurrence free (%)
3 month cystoscopy*+	30
–	66
Solitary*	69
Multiple	42
Diameter (max.)	
≤ 2.5 cm	71
2.6–4.9 cm	51
≥ 5 cm	38
Grade 1	64
Grade 2	62
Grade 3	38
Posterior Wall	
Yes	56
No	69

Stage Ta or T1 not significant.
* Significant on multivariate analysis.

ing thiotepa (triethylenethiophosphoramide), Epodyl (triethylene glycol diglycerol ether), mitomycin C and Bacillus Calmette-Guérin (BCG). The usual practice is to treat frequently in the early weeks after the initial transurethral resection and then to follow this by monthly maintenance instillations for 6 months or 1 year. The agents most widely used in the UK at present are mitomycin C and BCG. In the MRC study of adjuvant intravesical chemotherapy the recurrence rate by 2 years was reduced from 60% to 40% by the use of mitomycin C (Tolley *et al.*, 1988). BCG is also effective at reducing the recurrence of superficial bladder cancers, albeit at the risk of severe cystitis. It is unclear whether intravesical therapies reduce the risk of progression to more advanced disease. This only occurs in some 15–20% of patients presenting with superficial cancers.

Cystoprostatectomy is considered in patients with multiple tumours resistant to intravesical chemotherapy, but also for early recurrence of high grade tumours and for widespread carcinoma-*in-situ*.

33.7.2   LOCALIZED MUSCLE INVASIVE BLADDER CANCER

The treatment of these stages of transitional carcinoma of the bladder is controversial. Major modalities currently employed include radiotherapy alone, preoperative radiotherapy and cystectomy, partial cystectomy, radical cystectomy with urinary diversion, radical cystectomy with bladder reconstruction, or neoadjuvant chemotherapy with either radiotherapy or cystectomy. The treatment decision has been discussed by Soloway (1990), who suggests that partial cystectomy is rarely appropriate but could be considered for patients with small localized tumours especially at the dome of the bladder where removal of the tumour with a margin of normal tissue will allow function of the remaining bladder.

Radical radiotherapy allows bladder conservation, but it is important that regular check cystoscopies are performed following this treatment. Results equivalent to those produced by cystectomy have been claimed (Blandy *et al.*, 1980) and this has been supported by prospective randomized trial (Bloom *et al.*, 1982).

The more standard approach in the USA would be to perform a bilateral pelvic lymph node dissection followed by cystoprostatectomy. The choice of urinary diversion following removal of the bladder includes the traditional ileal conduit bladder and various forms of continent urinary diversion.

More recently, neoadjuvant chemotherapy has been advocated for locally advanced bladder cancers since responses of primary tumour to chemotherapy are seen quite frequently. However, to date this approach has not been extensively supported by results of randomized trial.

The final choice of treatment should depend upon full discussion with the patient of the advantages and disadvantages of the various approaches. At the Royal Marsden Hospital the major initial approaches include radical radiotherapy for patients with T2 or T3 disease, or alternatively cystectomy with continent urinary diversion. For patients who have relapsed after radiotherapy salvage cystectomy with ileal conduit is considered safer than to attempt a reconstruction. Patients with large T3 tumours, T4 tumours or suspicion of lymph node involvement are considered for neoadjuvant chemotherapy prior to local treatment.

(a) Radical radiotherapy for bladder cancer

In selected patients radical radiotherapy results in a 60–70% complete response rate and where no recurrence occurs patients may have persisting good bladder function and quality of life (Lynch *et al.*, 1992). However, radiotherapy is associated with a significant local failure rate and thus requires a monitoring policy in order to detect local recurrence at a time when salvage cystectomy may be curative. Initial cystectomy achieves the higher local control rate but the curative potential is mitigated by metastatic recurrence and it is considered that the majority of patients treated with radiotherapy who fail locally would also be those who would suffer metastatic failure.

For a treatment approach based on bladder conservation it is important to select patients whose pretreatment bladder function is satisfactory, i.e. to exclude those either with incontinence or with a severely contracted bladder. Also, to avoid a high recurrence rate, radical radiotherapy should be reserved for patients with tumours less than about 7 cm in maximum diameter and ideally less than 5 cm. Patients with associated pelvic inflammatory disease or inflammatory bowel disease may suffer increased side-effects.

Radiotherapy technique

Issues which have not yet been resolved include whether the initial treatment volume should include pelvic lymph nodes and, secondly, the need to irradiate to full dose the entire bladder rather than merely the tumour with a margin. The practice at the Royal Marsden Hospital is to plan the patient using a CT scan and to confine the target volume to the bladder with a 1 cm margin in most cases. The policy is to treat with the bladder empty in order to limit the size of the target volume. Occasionally small bladder tumours are treated in two phases, with the first phase confined to the tumour with a minimum 2 cm margin and treating with the bladder full. After 20% of the dose has been given the target volume is changed to encompass the whole bladder with the bladder empty.

The usual policy has been to use a three field plan with an anterior and two wedged lateral fields or anterior and two posterior oblique fields. The standard fractionation

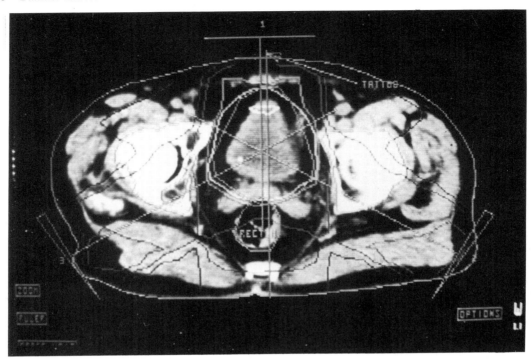

Figure 33.3   Radiation isodose distribution planned on axial CT image for radiotherapy of bladder cancer.

regimen has been 64 Gy in 32 fractions over 6.5 weeks, although more recently we have investigated a technique of accelerated fractionation treating with a 1.8 Gy fraction in the morning and 2 Gy fraction in the afternoon on each of 16 treatment days and allowing a short gap after the first week of treatment such that the final prescription is to a dose of 60.8 Gy in 32 fractions over 26 days. This approach is currently being evaluated in a randomized trial. Finally in patients in poor general medical health or those who are being treated with palliative intent we have employed a fractionation regimen consisting of 6 Gy fractions delivered once per week to a total dose of between 24 Gy and 36 Gy depending upon the indication. This approach seeks to avoid both frequent hospital visits and acute radiation reactions. A typical field arrangement is shown in Figure 33.3

Using standard fractionation most patients suffer some side-effects during radiotherapy. These consist of an increase in frequency of micturition associated with nocturia and in severe cases there may be dysuria and strangury requiring analgesic. Similarly, some patients suffer increase in frequency of bowel movements. All patients are warned of the risk that radiation may be associated with late side-effects including persisting frequency of micturition or diarrhoea or episodic haematuria or rectal bleeding. An appropriate planning technique and treatment prescription should limit the risk of severe late side-effects to less than 3% or 4% of patients.

(b)   Primary surgery

The initial procedure is usually lymphadenectomy from the bifurcation of the aorta down to include external and internal iliac nodes bilaterally. This then proceeds to cysto-prostatectomy in male patients or anterior exenteration in female patients. Methods of urinary diversion have included the uretero-sigmoidostomy or the non-refluxing ileal conduit (Skinner, 1982).

For optimal surgical results patient selection is important. Patients must be well motiv-ated and appreciate the need for self-care of the diversion. Possible complications include the loss of sexual potency in the male and loss of vagina in the female, and ideally the patient should be seen preoperatively by the stoma therapist. The stoma site should be selected to avoid a skin crease and should be well away from iliac crest. Preoperatively both physiotherapy to prevent lung com-plications and also bowel preparation are important. In recent series operative mortality is less than 4% (Skinner *et al.*, 1980; Brannan *et al.*, 1981; Mathur *et al.*, 1981).

In specialist centres excellent results can be achieved in selected patients treated by radical cystectomy with immediate lower urinary tract reconstruction by ileocystoplasty (Skinner *et al.*, 1991). In 126 consecutive patients 94% maintained good continence and the early complication rate was only 11% with an operative mortality of 1.6%. The rela-tively low incidence of local recurrence has argued against the need for preoperative radiation therapy (Montie *et al.*, 1984; Skinner and Lieskovsky, 1984) (7% and 9% local recurrence respectively). A prospective ran-domized trial comparing preoperative radi-ation with cystectomy alone did not show any survival difference (Anderström *et al.*, 1983).

(c) Neoadjuvant or adjuvant chemotherapy

The theoretical basis for this approach is that the majority of patients with locally invasive bladder cancer develop metastases within 3 years of their original treatment; the second major platform for this approach has been the demonstration of long term disease free sur-vival in some patients treated with chemo-therapy for metastatic disease, as discussed later in this chapter. Theoretically chemo-therapy may be more effective in treating the presumed subclinical micrometastases at the time of definitive initial local treatment. Set against this is the fact that not all patients need systemic therapy, and single agent neoadjuvant chemotherapy based either on methotrexate (Figure 33.4) or on cisplatin has been shown to be ineffective in prospective randomized trials (Shearer *et al.*, 1988; Wallace *et al.*, 1991).

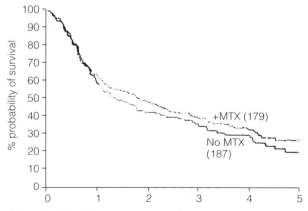

Figure 33.4 Results of the CUCG (Co-operative Urological Cancer Group) trial of neoadjuvant and adjuvant methotrexate in T3 bladder cancer (Shearer *et al.*, 1988).

The perceived advantages of neoadjuvant compared with adjuvant therapy are that the response of primary tumour can be assessed, the extent of local surgery may be reduced, and systemic micrometastases are treated earlier.

The response of the primary tumour following combination chemotherapy has been encouraging. Of four trials of a combination of cyclophosphamide, adriamycin and cisplatin involving 83 patients there was a 22% complete response at cystectomy, and of seven trials based on the combination MVAC (methotrexate, vinblastine, adriamycin and cisplatin) of 138 evaluable patients there was a 30% complete response at cystectomy (Scher and Splinter, 1990). Though the response to chemotherapy has been shown to have prognostic significance (Scher *et al.*, 1989), this does not necessarily indicate a cause/effect relationship since response may occur in a better prognosis group of patients who were destined to do well with local therapy alone. Therefore, the results of neoadjuvant treatment require evaluation in prospective randomized trials. The Medical Research Council is currently co-ordinating an international trial comparing neoadjuvant CMV (cisplatin, methotrexate and vinblastine) with local treatment alone. The planned accrual of 1000 patients is almost complete, but as yet the approach of neoadjuvant chemotherapy has not been proven.

There has been more limited evaluation of adjuvant combination chemotherapy **following,** surgery though this has some advantages since the need for adjuvant chemotherapy can be based on the pathological findings and reserved for those either with extension of tumour though the bladder wall or with pelvic node involvement. A randomized trial reported to show the benefit of adjuvant chemotherapy (Skinner *et al.*, 1990) has been strongly criticized because of the method of treatment allocation and analysis. More recently a small trial adjuvant chemotherapy in patients with either advanced primaries or node involvement has also been reported to show benefit for those receiving adjuvant chemotherapy (Stockle *et al.*, 1992). At present the role of adjuvant chemotherapy remains unresolved. A small randomized trial comparing neoadjuvant and adjuvant chemotherapy revealed no significant difference (Logothetis *et al.*, 1992).

33.7.3   METASTATIC BLADDER CANCER

Metastatic bladder cancer is a rapidly progressing neoplasm associated with significant symptoms, especially where nodal disease causes vascular obstruction or bone disease causes pain. Patients with small volume lung or liver disease may be relatively asymptomatic, in which case the timing of palliative treatments should be considered carefully in

Table 33.5   Chemotherapy regimens for bladder cancer

MVAC	Methotrexate 30 mg/m^2	Days 1, 15, 22
	Vinblastine 3 mg/m^2	Days 2, 15, 22
	Doxorubicin 30 mg/m^2	Day 2
	Cisplatinum 70 mg/m^2	Day 2
	Cycle 28 days	
CMV	Cisplatinum 100 mg/m^2	Day 2
	Methotrexate 30 mg/m^2	Day 1
	Vinblastine 4 mg/m^2	Day 1
	Cycle 21 days	

order not to reduce the quality of the limited remaining life of the patient.

Options of palliation include the use of combination chemotherapy, single agent chemotherapy or symptomatic measures such as local palliative radiotherapy and/or analgesics.

Standard combination chemotherapy regimens are illustrated in Table 33.5. The MVAC regimen was developed at the Memorial Sloan–Kettering Cancer Center in the 1980s. It achieved complete remission rates in the range of 15–30% with approximately twice these proportions achieving partial remissions. However the median survival of patients is only approximately 1 year and less than 20% of patients survive 2 years with exact numbers depending on patient selection. Prospective randomized trials of this particular regimen compared either with single agent cisplatin (Loehrer *et al.*, 1992) or with the combination of cisplatin, adriamycin and cyclophosphamide (Logothetis *et al.*, 1990) have both shown the superiority of MVAC. The regime has not been formally compared with CMV; however, the pilot studies would not suggest a major difference in efficacy between the two regimens (Harker *et al.*, 1985).

Both regimens are associated with severe side-effects including nausea, vomiting, alopecia, lethargy, neuropathy and mucositis. Additionally patients may be very difficult to treat since both cisplatin and methotrexate can be associated with renal toxicity and many patients with bladder cancer, either due to age, general medical problems or the specific consequences of their tumours, may have poor renal function prior to consideration for any chemotherapy.

Thus the use of combination chemotherapy requires skilled and experienced judgement and a full discussion with the patient. Those destined to benefit usually reveal this within a month of beginning chemotherapy and it is rarely useful to persist with chemotherapy unless objective early response can be documented.

Recent reports indicate that moderate increases in dose intensity have not been associated with improved response rates (Scher *et al.*, 1993; Seidman *et al.*, 1993).

In the medically fit patient MVAC is a reasonable choice of combination chemotherapy regimen; however, serious consideration should be given to deferring treatment in the asymptomatic patient and to stopping chemotherapy in the patient who does not demonstrate rapid response. In less fit patients a low toxicity outpatient regimen would be desirable and a current Medical Research Council trial is comparing the combination of methotrexate and vinblastine with the more standard cisplatin, methotrexate and vinblastine.

33.8 NEW APPROACHES AND CONCLUSION

Bladder cancer presents considerable therapeutic challenges because of the range of treatment techniques available, the complexity of these techniques and the distressing symptoms associated with progression of the disease and in some cases with the treatments themselves. Superficial bladder cancer carries a good prognosis, but because of the propensity for local recurrence this is a tumour requiring considerable resources from urological surgeons and additionally there is concern that some 15–20% of patients progress to a more advanced form of the tumour.

Localized muscle invasive bladder cancer is curable in 20–50% of patients. The choice of whether to base treatment on radiotherapy or on surgery will depend on a full discussion of the alternative treatment morbidities and on the resources available. As neither modality leads to entirely satisfactory results, it is appropriate to explore the use of adjuvant combination chemotherapy; the role of this modality is not yet established.

For patients with metastatic disease combination chemotherapy offers a 15–30% chance of complete remission; however, for the majority of patients there will be little or only transient response and the benefit would be outweighed by the side-effects of chemotherapy. A small proportion of patients have responses lasting more than 2 years and it would be of great benefit to predict which patients would benefit in order to protect the remainder from unnecessary toxicity.

There is considerable investigation of the basic biology of bladder cancer documenting a range of common chromosome abnormalities (Presti *et al.*, 1991). The identification of the underlying oncogene and tumour suppressor gene aberration associated with progression of this neoplasm should provide targets for design of more effective drugs.

REFERENCES

Anderström, C., Johansson, S., Nilsson, S. *et al.* (1983) A prospective randomised study of pre-operative irradiation with cystectomy or cystectomy alone for invasive bladder carcinoma. *European Urology*, **9**, 142–7.

Anthony, H.M. and Thomas, G.M. (1970) Bladder tumours and smoking. *International Journal of Cancer*, **5**, 266–72.

Babiker, A., Shearer, R.J. and Chilvers, C.E. (1989) Prognostic factors in a T3 bladder cancer trial. Co-operative Urological Cancer Group. *British Journal of Cancer*, **59**, 414–44.

Blandy, J.P., England, H.R., Evans, J.W. *et al.* (1980) T3 bladder cancer — the case for salvage cystectomy. *British Journal of Urology*, **52**, 506–10.

Bloom, H.J., Hendry, W.F., Wallace, D.M. and Skeet, R.G. (1982) Treatment of T3 bladder cancer: controlled trial of preoperative radiotherapy, and radical cystectomy versus radical radiotherapy, second report review. *British Journal of Urology*, **54**, 136–51.

Brannan, W., Ruselier, H.A., Ochsner, M. and Randrup, E.R. (1981) Critical evaluation of I-stage cystectomy – reducing morbidity and mortality. *Journal of Urology*, **125**, 640–2.

Cartwright, R.A., Glashan, R.W., Rogers, H.J. *et al.* (1982) Role of N-acetyltransferase phenotypes in bladder carcinogenesis: a pharmacogenetic epidemiological approach to bladder cancer. *Lancet*, **ii**, 842–6.

Dick, A., Barnes, R., Hadley, H. *et al.* (1980) Complications of transurethral resection of bladder tumours: prevention, recognition and treatment. *Journal of Urology*, **124**, 810 –11.

Fujita, J., Yoshida, O., Yashohito, Y. *et al.* (1984) Ha-*ras* oncogenes are activated by somatic alterations in human urinary tract tumours. *Nature*, **309**, 464–6.

Harker, W.G., Meyers, F.J., Freiha, F.S. *et al.* (1985) Cisplatin, methotrexate, and vinblastine (CMV): an effective chemotherapy regimen for metastatic transitional cell carcinoma of the urinary tract. A Northern California Oncology Group Study. *Journal of Clinical Oncology*, **3**, 1463–70.

Hendry, W.F., Manning, N., Perry, N.M. *et al.* (1981) The effects of a haematuria service in the early diagnosis of bladder cancer, in *Bladder Cancer: principles of combination therapy*, (eds R.T.D. Oliver, W.F. Hendry and H.J.G. Bloom), Butterworths, London, pp. 223–4.

Kenney, G.M., Hardner, G.J. and Murphy, G.P. (1970) Clinical staging of bladder tumours. *Journal of Urology*, **104,** 720–23.

Loehrer, P.J., Einhorn, L.H.S., Elson, P.J. *et al.* (1992) A randomised comparison of cisplatin alone or in combination with methotrexate, vinblastine, and doxorubicin in patients with metastatic urothelial carcinoma: a Cooperative Group Study. *Journal of Clinical Oncology*, **10,** 1066–73.

Logothetis, C.J., Dexeus, F.H., Finn, L. *et al.* (1990) A prospective randomised trial comparing MVAC and CISCA chemotherapy for patients with metastatic urothelial tumours. *Journal of Clinical Oncology*, **8,** 1050–5.

Logothetis, C.J., Finn, L. and Amato, R. (1992) Escalated (ESC) MVAC +/– rhGm–CSF (Schering–Plough) in metastatic transitional cell carcinoma (TCC): preliminary results of a randomised trial. *Proceeding of the American Society of Clinical Oncology*, **11**, 202 (Abstr).

Lynch, W.J., Jenkins, C., Flower, C.G. *et al.* (1992) The quality of life after radical radiotherapy for bladder cancer. *British Journal of Urology*, **70**, 519–21.

Malone, P.R., Visvanathan, K.V., Ponder, B.A.J. and Summerhayes, I.C. (1985) Oncogenes and bladder cancer. *British Journal of Urology*, **57,** 664–7.

Mathur, V.K., Krahn, H.P. and Ramsey, E.W.S. (1981) Total cystectomy for bladder cancer. *Journal of Urology*, **125**, 784–6.

Montie, J.E., Straffon, R.A. and Stewart, B.H. (1984) Radical cystectomy without radiation therapy for carcinoma of the bladder. *Journal of Urology*, **131**, 477–82.

Neal, D.E., Bennett, M.K., Hall, R.R. *et al.* (1985) Epidermal growth factor receptors in human bladder cancer: comparison of invasive and superficial tumours. *Lancet*, **ii**, 366–8.

Parmar, M.K.B., Freedman, L.S., Hargreave, T.B. and Tolley, D.A. (1989) Prognostic factors for recurrence and follow-up policies in the treatment of superficial bladder cancer: report from The British Medical Research Council Subgroup on Superficial Bladder Cancer (Urological Cancer Working Party). *Journal of Urology*, **142**, 284–8.

Pearson, R.M. and Soloway, M.S. (1978) Does cyclosphosphamide induce bladder cancer? *Urology*, **4**, 437–47.

Presti, J.C.J., Reuter, V.E., Galan, T. *et al.* (1991) Molecular genetic alterations in superficial and locally advanced human bladder cancer. *Cancer Research*, **51**, 5405–9.

Raghavan, D., Shipley, W.U., Garnick, M.B. *et al.* (1990) Biology and management of bladder cancer. *New England Journal of Medicine*, **322**, 1129–38.

Rehn, L. (1904) Weitere Erfahrungen über Blasengeschwülste bei Farbarbeitern. *Verhandlungen der Deutschen Gastroenterologie Chirurgie*, **33**, 231–40.

Scher, H.I., Geller, N.L., Curley, T. and Tao, Y. (1993) Effect of relative cumulative dose-intensity on survival of patients with urothelial cancer treated with M-VAC. *Journal of Clinical Oncology*, **11**, 400–7.

Scher, H., Herr, H., Sternberg, C. *et al.* (1989) Neo–adjuvant chemotherapy for invasive bladder cancer. Experience with the M–VAC regimen. *British Journal of Urology*, **64**, 250–6.

Scher, H.I. and Splinter, T.A. (1990) Chemotherapy for invasive bladder cancer: neo-adjuvant versus adjuvant. *Seminars in Oncology*, **17**, 555–65.

Seidman, A.D., Scher, H.I., Gabrilove, J.L. *et al.* (1993) Dose-intensification of MVAC with recombinant granulocyte colony-stimulating factor as initial therapy in advanced urothelial cancer. *Journal of Clinical Oncology*, **11**, 408–14.

Shearer, R.J., Chilvers, C.F., Bloom, H.J. *et al.* (1988) Adjuvant chemotherapy in T3 carcinoma of the bladder. A prospective trial: preliminary report. *British Journal of Urology*, **62**, 558–64.

Sidransky, D., Frost, P., Von Eschenbach, A. *et al.* (1992) Colonal origin of bladder cancer. *New England Journal of Medicine*, **326**, 737–40.

Skinner, D.G. (1982) Management of invasive bladder cancer. A meticulous pelvic node dissection can make a difference. *Journal of Urology*, **128**, 34–6.

Skinner, D.G., Crawford, E.D. and Kaufman, J.J. (1980) Complications of radical cystectomy for carcinoma of the bladder. *Journal of Urology*, **123**, 640–3.

Skinner, D.G., Daniels, J.R., Russell, C.A. *et al.* (1991) The role of adjuvant chemotherapy following cystectomy for invasive bladder cancer: prospective comparative trial. *Journal of Urology*, **145**, 459–67.

Skinner, D.G. and Lieskovsky, G. (1984) Temporary cystectomy with pelvic node dissection compared to preoperative radiation therapy plus cystectomy in management of invasive bladder cancer. *Journal of Urology*, **131**, 1069–72.

Skinner, E.C., Lieskovsky, G. and Skinner, D.G. (1990) The technique of radical cystectomy. *AUA Update Series Lesson 7*, **IX**, 50–5.

Smith, J.A. and Whitmore, W.F.J. (1981) Salvage cystectomy for bladder cancer after failure of definitive irradiation. *Journal of Urology*, **125**, 643–5.

Soloway, M.S. (1990) Follow up of patients receiving treatment for superficial bladder cancer with mitomycin C and BCG. *Progress in Clinical and Biological Research*, **350**, 71–0.

Stockle, M., Meyenburg, W., Wellek, S. *et al.* (1992) Advanced bladder cancer (stages pT3b, pT4a, pN1 and pN2): improved survival after radical cystectomy and 3 adjuvant cycles of chemotherapy. Results of a controlled prospective study. *Journal of Urology*, **148**, 302–7.

Tolley, D.A., Hargreave, T.B., Smith, P.H. *et al.* (1988) Effect of intravesical mitomycin C on recurrence of newly diagnosed superficial bladder cancer: interim report from the Medical Research Council Subgroup of Superficial Bladder Cancer (Urological Cancer Working Party). *British Medical Journal*, **296**, 1759–61.

Wallace, D.M.A., Raghavan, D., Kelly, K.A. *et al.* (1991) Neo-adjuvant (pre-emptive) cisplatin therapy in invasive transitional cell carcinoma of the bladder. *British Journal of Urology*, **67**, 608–15.

Wood, D.P., Fair, W.R. and Chaganti, R.S.K. (1992) Evaluation of epidermal growth factor receptor DNA amplification and mRNA expression in bladder cancer. *Journal of Urology*, **147**, 274–7.

TESTICULAR CANCER

Alan Horwich

34.1 INTRODUCTION

Most types of testicular cancer are curable in all stages. The majority are germ cell tumours with a peak incidence in the third decade of life, and the very success of treatment increases the importance of the risks of long term toxicity. Germ cell tumours also present an interesting model for tumour response partly because they are extremely sensitive to both chemotherapy and radiotherapy, but also because they elaborate specific tumour markers which provide a sensitive index of residual tumour burden within the individual patient.

34.2 INCIDENCE

As shown in Figure 34.1 the incidence of testicular cancer has been rising especially in the young age peak between 20 and 40 years of age, where the incidence has almost doubled over the last 25 years, to reach 9 per 100 000. This rise in incidence has been apparent for the last 60 years and is, therefore, unlikely to be associated with the social and sexual revolutions of 1960s and 1970s, and it has been noted in most western societies including the USA, Australasia and Western Europe. In the USA it is striking that the rise in incidence is apparent only in white males (Schottenfeld *et al.*, 1980). There are approximately 900 new registrations of testicular cancer per year in England and Wales where a white male has a 1 in 500 lifetime risk of developing the disease (Davies, 1981).

The peak incidence of seminoma is some 10 years later than that of malignant teratoma as shown as Figure 34.2. Germ cell cancers are uncommon over the age of 50 years though spermatocytic seminomas are commoner in older men. In the older age group testicular lymphoma becomes more common than germ cell tumours.

34.3 AETIOLOGY

Germ cell tumours are commoner in patients giving a history of testicular maldescent, especially when bilateral. Since maldescent of the testis is also increasing in incidence at the present time it seems likely that the rise in testicular cancer incidence will continue over the next 20 years. It has been estimated that there is a 5–10-fold increase in relative risk of germ cell tumour in patients with unilateral maldescent and also approximately the same level of increased risk applies to brothers of patients with testicular germ cell cancers (Senturia *et al.*, 1985; Forman *et al.*, 1992).

There has been considerable investigation of the role of oestrogens during the mother's pregnancy, either endogenous or in the form of diethylstilboestrol medication; however, the evidence is not strong as yet (Schottenfeld *et al.*, 1980). Further information on the aetiology of testicular cancer will come from a prospective study of 6000 consecutive male births at the Radcliffe Infirmary in Oxford, where details of pregnancy, cryptorchidism and subsequent medical history are being collected.

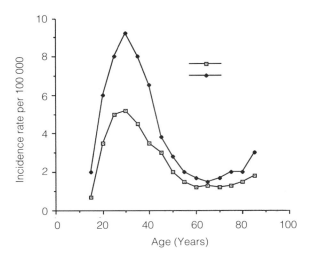

Figure 34.1 The incidence of testicular cancer by age, comparing 1964–68 (—□—) with 1979–82 (—◆—).

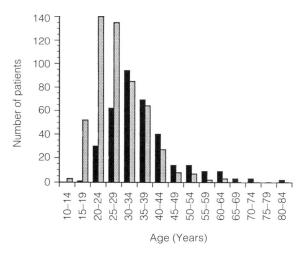

Figure 34.2 Age incidence of seminoma (■) compared to all non-seminomas (▨).

The great majority of germ cell tumours arise in association with carcinoma-*in-situ* of the testis, a lesion apparent on testicular biopsy of a small proportion of patients investigated for infertility. The very great majority of patients with carcinoma-*in-situ* of the testis will go on to develop a germ cell tumour, and this has been assessed particularly in the context of the contralateral testis of men with testicular cancer. It is known that 2–5% of men with testicular cancer develop a contralateral tumour. Studies from Denmark have found carcinoma-*in-situ* in the contralateral testis of approximately 5% of men with unilateral testicular cancer and careful follow-up has shown that the risk of progression to invasive tumour of the contralateral testis was 50% within 5 years (Von der Maase *et al.,* 1986). If this lesion was not present it was exquisitely rare to develop a testicular germ cell tumour. The rarity of germ cell tumours and invasive method of making the diagnosis of testicular carcinoma-*in-situ* have argued against its use in screening.

34.4 PATHOLOGY

The main histological classifications of testicular germ cell tumours are shown in Table 34.1. The major difference is that the WHO classification is based on listing all the morphologies discerned within a particular tumour, whereas the British Testicular Tumour Panel Classification groups the relatively heterogeneous tumour into a much more limited list. The distribution of primary tumours seen at the Royal Marsden Hospital between 1980 and 1988 was analysed, and of 876 patients 40% were pure seminomas, 15% were combined teratomas with seminoma and the remainder were varieties of nonseminomas, often called teratomas in the UK. Of malignant teratomas the great majority are either malignant teratoma intermediate (MTI) or malignant teratoma undifferentiated (MTU).

The two major subtypes of seminoma are classical seminoma and the much more rare spermatocytic seminoma. Classical seminomas may be associated with syncytial giant cells and with elevated serum concentrations of human chorionic gonadotrophin (HCG), placental alkaline phosphatase (PLAP) and lactate dehydrogenase, especially its isoenzyme LDH-1.

Microscopically, classical seminoma is identical to dysgerminoma of the ovary and is composed of large uniform polygonal cells with prominent nuclei. Cells have abundant cytoplasm which may be eosinophilic and contain glycogen and lipid. The connective tissue often shows a prominent lymphocytic infiltration and there may be a granulomatous reaction associated with the tumour. In some cases the tumour shows a high mitotic rate associated with cellular and nuclear pleomorphism and areas of necrosis and there may be difficulty in distinguishing the tumour from malignant teratoma undifferentiated.

Testicular teratoma occasionally presents with tissue which is apparently fully differentiated. In infants and young children these are associated with a benign course. However, in the young adult age group they should be regarded as the most indolent end

Table 34.1 Histological classifications

British Testicular Tumours Panel (Pugh and Cameron, 1976)	World Health Organization (Mostofi and Sobin, 1977)
Seminoma	Seminoma
Teratoma differentiated (TD)	Teratoma Mature Immature
Malignant teratoma intermediate (MTI)	Teratoma with malignant transformation, embryonal carcinoma and teratoma
Malignant teratoma undifferentiated (MTU)	Embryonal carcinoma Polyembryoma
Malignant teratoma trophoblastic (MTT)	Choriocarcinoma with or without embryonal carcinoma and/or teratoma
Yolk sac tumour	Yolk sac tumour

of the spectrum of MTI and this is a pattern consistent with metastases. More than 50% of malignant teratomas are of the MTI subtype, often described as teratocarcinoma in the American literature. These are composed of a combination of embryonal carcinoma cells admixed with other elements of teratoma with patterns of differentiation of the somatic tissues being heterogeneous often resembling cartilage, lung, brain or gastrointestinal epithelium. The histology of metastases may be different from the primary (Ray *et al.*, 1974).

MTU or embryonal carcinoma is composed of large polygonal cells with large irregular nuclei. Cell boundaries may be indistinct and cells often form a solid or syncytial arrangement. Mitoses are frequent. Papillary or pseudoglandular patterns occur and epithelial-like cells may form cystic spaces. Areas of necrosis are common.

Other less common patterns of malignant non-seminomatous germ cell tumour include yolk sac tumours associated with a production of alphafetoprotein (AFP) and trophoblastic tumours associated with production of human chorionic gonadotrophin (HCG), but either of these types can occur together with the more common MTU and MTI variety or together with seminoma, in which case the combined tumour is regarded for clinical purposes as a non-seminoma.

Pathological analysis can help with clinical decisions. In particular it appears that tumours invading testicular lymphatics or blood vessels are more likely to metastasize. In the context of chemotherapy for metastatic non-seminomas it has been suggested that a prominent fibrous reaction in the testis indicates a good prognosis (Freedman *et al.*, 1987; Mead *et al.*, 1992).

34.5 TUMOUR MARKERS

AFP is an embryonal protein produced by yolk sac and by fetal liver. It is thought to serve a function similar to albumin in the fetus and usually serum levels fall dramatically at the time of birth. In germ cell tumours AFP production is associated with yolk sac differentiation and this is taken to indicate the presence of a non-seminomatous component of the tumour. False positive serum assay of AFP may occur in the context of liver damage secondary to drugs, alcohol, infection or metastases and AFP is also a tumour marker for hepatocellular carcinoma.

HCG is usually produced from trophoblastic tissue in the placenta and in germ cell tumours production is mainly from syncytiotrophoblastic cells. It is a polypeptide consisting of alpha and beta subunits, however the alpha unit is found in other hormones such as luteinizing hormone whereas the beta subunit is specific and thus forms the basis of immunoassay. HCG is produced as a tumour marker in a range of tumours, especially those deriving from the upper gastrointestinal tract, the bladder and bronchus, but occasionally other malignancies.

Tumour markers can be helpful in diagnosis, though usually the presence of a tumour within the testis is clinically apparent. The marker is more useful in occult or extra-gonadal presentation, especially those arising in the anterior mediastinum (Childs *et al.*, 1993). Tumour markers can also be very useful in monitoring response to therapy and can be used as a monitor to detect relapse. Their use as a target for immunolocalization or targeted therapy is experimental.

Other markers in germ cell tumours include placental alkaline phosphatase, found mainly in serum of patients with seminoma, lactate dehydrogenase and neurone specific enolase (Mason, 1991).

34.6 PRESENTATION

The majority of testicular germ cell tumours present with a mass in the testis and the early stage of this is a small hard nodal which is usually painless. Subsequently the testis becomes hard and heavy and there may be intermittent pain especially following mild trauma. Approximately 10% of germ cell tumours present in a non-gonadal site; this is either because they are true extragonadal primaries or because the primary tumour in the testis has remained occult and occasionally has regressed.

Despite the relative ease of detecting a testicular primary tumour, a number of reports have indicated significant delay following detection of an abnormality by the patient. For example, in a review of 257 patients from the Royal Marsden Hospital diagnosed between 1980 and 1986 the median delay was 2.5 months, but the range went up to 3 years (Chilvers *et al.* 1989). Approximately equal numbers of patients fell into the three delay categories 0–49 days, 50–99 days and 100 days or more. Longer delay was associated with more advanced presentation, though in our analysis this did not have an impact on survival. Differential diagnosis of a testicular mass includes inflammatory disease and ultrasound scanning of the testis and may help in the differential diagnosis. The diagnosis is usually confirmed by inguinal orchidectomy, since this technique reduces the possibility of scrotal contamination and also allows high ligation of the spermatic cord. Testicular prostheses are available. In a patient with an increased risk of contralateral germ cell tumour, such as those with either a history of maldescent or with an atrophic contralateral testis (Berthelsen *et al.*, 1982), a contralateral testicular biopsy may reveal carcinoma-*in-situ*, in which case progression to germ cell tumour can be prevented by low dose radiotherapy. Alternatively, the absence of carcinoma-*in-situ* allows reassurance. In this patient population the impact of treatment on fertility should be considered as discussed in Chapter 16.

34.7 INVESTIGATION AND STAGING

Following definition of the histology the usually staging procedures are sequential assay of serum HCG and AFP levels together with a CT scan of thorax, abdomen and pelvis. The pattern of malignant dissemination of germ cell tumours is relatively predictable and for pure testicular seminoma it would be very rare for the patient to present with more widespread metastases without involvement of abdominal lymph nodes, and it has therefore been argued that the patient who has a normal abdominal CT scan does not need a thoracic scan. Non-seminomas metastasize more widely, though there is a particular predilection for spread to retroperitoneal nodes and the lung fields with somewhat less common sites including supradiaphragmatic lymph nodes, liver, bone and brain. Table 34.2 shows the Royal Marsden Hospital staging classification which is widely employed throughout Europe, and Table 34.3 indicates both the distribution of patients in relationship to this stage and also the 3 year survival probability determined for patients treated with chemotherapy for metastatic non-seminoma between 1982 and 1986. The survival figures for metastatic seminoma are somewhat similar or if anything 5–10% higher than for most non-seminomas. For patients presenting without any evidence of metastases the 3 year survival rate should be more than 95% and the patterns of recurrence of testicular germ cell tumours would indicate that the 3 year survival approximates to cure (Peckham *et al.*, 1988).

34.8 MANAGEMENT

34.8.1 STAGE I TESTICULAR NON-SEMINOMA

In the past, patients in the UK were treated with adjuvant radiotherapy to the draining lymph nodes in the para-aortic region and the ipsilateral pelvis. However, with the development of effective combination chemotherapy this approach has largely been abandoned, and the standard management in the UK is called surveillance and comprises an active policy of close monitoring at least the

Table 34.2   The Royal Marsden Hospital Staging Classification

Stage	Definition
I M	Rising postorchidectomy markers only
II	Abdominal lymphadenopathy
A	< 2 cm
B	2–5 cm
C	> 5 cm
III	Supradiaphragmatic lymphadenopathy
O	No abdominal disease
ABC	Abdominal node size as in stage II
IV	Extralymphatic metastases
L1	≤ 3 lung metastases
L2	> 3 lung metastases all < 2 cm diameter
L3	> 3 lung metastases 1 or more > 2 cm
H+	Liver involvement

Table 34.3   Medical Research Council prognostic factors analysis

Category	Stage	Treatment period 1976–82		Treatment period 1982–86	
		No. of patients	3 year survival (%)	No. of patients	3 year survival (%)
Small volume	I M	18	83	78	95
	II III AB	106	87	253	92
	IV L1 L2 AB	70	75	200	90
Large volume	IIC IIIC	104	85	82	82
	IV L1 L2 C	43	77	37	89
Very large volume	IV L3 H+	117	54	145	90

first 3–4 years following orchidectomy. This approach was introduced by Peckham and colleagues in 1979 (Peckham *et al.*, 1982), when it was found that approximately a third of clinical stage I patients would recur with the predominant pattern of recurrence within the first 18 months after orchidectomy. With this policy of surveillance recurrence is detected when the disease volume is small, and salvage chemotherapy is highly effective such that even in a multicentre study the overall cure rate of these patients is 98% (Freedman *et al.*, 1987). Subsequently the Medical Research Council co-ordinated a prospective study of surveillance based on 12 collaborating institutions; 458 patients were registered between 1984 and 1987; approximately 40% of

relapses were with small volume abdominal nodes and a further 20% with small volume lung metastases. Approximately 15% do not have any radiological evidence of relapse, but the recurrence is diagnosed by sequential marker assay. In an analysis of primary tumour histology the MRC study demonstrated four independent prognostic factors for relapse:

1. Vascular invasion
2. Lymphatic invasion
3. The presence of undifferentiated cells
4. The absence of the yolk sac elements.

If each of these factors scored zero if absent and 1 if present, a prognostic index could be constructed, such that patients with 3 or 4 risk factors would be predicted to have a risk of recurrence of approximately 50%. This has given rise to a new approach to management of patients with high risk stage I non-seminoma, namely the use of adjuvant chemo-therapy. The pilot study of only 2 cycles of adjuvant chemotherapy using bleomycin, etoposide and cisplatin (see below) has demonstrated that this modest amount of treatment is sufficient to prevent relapse in the vast majority of cases, and for some patients the side-effects of this limited chemotherapy are preferable to the anxiety of a prolonged surveillance policy. Patients with a lower risk of recurrence continue to be managed by surveillance and the current sur-veillance policy at the Royal Marsden Hospital is illustrated in Table 34.4.

In the USA and some European countries, there is an alternative approach to the man-agement of the patient with stage I testicular non-seminoma, and that is to perform a staging retroperitoneal lymph node dissec-tion (RPLND). It is argued that this provides an early measure of the likelihood of recur-rence since patients whose lymph nodes do not contain metastatic tumour, have a risk of relapse of only 10%, whereas those with metastases in retroperitoneal nodes may be cured by the surgical procedure especially when the number of metastases are limited and their size is small. Alternatively the pro-cedure may provide an early and reliable in-dication of the need for chemotherapy (Williams *et al.*, 1987). In the past this approach was strongly criticized because of the frequency with which RPLND was fol-lowed by ejaculatory failure. However, fol-lowing the demonstration of the relevant autonomic nerve pathways subserving ejacu-lation a nerve sparing technique has been devised following which this side-effect is rare (Donohue *et al.*, 1990). Nevertheless, the approach of RPLND in clinical stage I non-seminoma has not found favour in the UK, partly because the operation is unnecessary in the majority of patients who do not have metastatic disease, and partly because of the resource and experience required for the 3–5 hour nerve sparing technique. Overall, survival in stage I non-seminoma of testis is extremely high whichever management policy is adopted and treatment choices are determined by patterns of side-effects (Horwich, 1993).

34.8.2 METASTATIC NON-SEMINOMA

The standard treatment is with 4 cycles of combination chemotherapy based on bleo-mycin, etoposide and cisplatin (BEP) (Table 34.5). Chemotherapy is generally well toler-ated in the relatively young age group of patients who suffer testicular non-seminoma,

Table 34.4 *Testicular tumours*: teratoma stage I surveillance

	Month												
	0	*1*	*2*	*3*	*4*	*5*	*6*	*7*	*8*	*9*	*10*	*11*	*12*
OPD		+		+		+		+		+		+	
MARKERS	+	+	+	+	+	+	+	+	+	+	+	+	
CXR	+	+	+	+	+	+	+	+	+	+	+	+	
CT chest and abdomen			+				+			+			+

Year 2: OPD q 3/12 CT abdo. at 24 months.
Year 3: OPD q 4/12 CT abdo. at 36 months.
Year 4: OPD q 6/12.
Then annually.
OPD, Outpatient visit; CXR, chest X-ray; CT, computer tomographic scan.

Table 34.5 BEP chemotherapy for germ cell tumours

Bleomycin	30U	Days 2, 9, 16
Etoposide	120 mg/m^2	Days 1, 2, 3
Cisplatinum	20 mg/m^2	Days 1, 2, 3, 4, 5
	21 day cycle	

and is also highly effective with an overall cure rate of approximately 85% (Dearnaley *et al.*, 1991; Mead *et al.*, 1992).

Combination chemotherapy based on platinum greatly improved the prognosis of patients with metastatic non-seminoma and in the UK represents standard treatment for all patients with evidence of metastatic disease. The prognosis is influenced adversely by increasing the bulk of disease and by increasing concentration of tumour markers, and a multivariate analysis (Mead *et al.*, 1992) showed that significant independent factors included:

1. More than 20 lung metastases
2. Mediastinal mass more than 5 cm diameter
3. The presence of bone, liver or CNS metastasis
4. Presence of AFP over 1000 U/l or HCG over 10 000 U/l.

This form of prognostic factor analysis has lead to the concept of risk related chemotherapy for metastatic germ cell tumours (Horwich, 1991). Patients with good prognosis are candidates for low toxicity treatment approaches and those with an adverse prognosis are candidates for increased intensity of chemotherapy and frequently clinical trials are stratified in this way.

Chemotherapy toxicity depends on the specific choice of drugs, drug doses and the number of cycles administered, which influence the cumulative drug dose. As discussed above the standard BEP schedule is administered for 4 cycles, a new cycle beginning every 3 weeks. The main acute side-effects are nausea and vomiting especially in the few days following cisplatin administration, but these can usually be counteracted by the combination of dexamethasone and metoclopramide or in more resistant cases ondansetron. Alopecia secondary to etoposide is complete, but recovers following treatment. There is moderate myelosuppression with a nadir in white blood count at 10–14 days following the start of chemotherapy. However, infective complications and haemorrhage are rare. Cisplatin causes renal tubular damage, and treatment based on this drug implies a 20–25% permanent reduction in glomerular filtration rate. Cisplatin can also cause a dose dependent high tone hearing loss and a sensory peripheral neuropathy. Bleomycin is usually well tolerated but may cause a flu-like reaction unless concomitant steroids are given and additionally may cause skin rashes. Skin pigmentation occurs at the sites of inflammation and Raynaud's phenomenon may occur following completion of therapy. The most serious complication of bleomycin is pneumonitis which may progress to an irreversible fibrosis. This complication occurs in 1–2% of patients treated to the total standard cumulative dose of 360 units. Testicular germ cell chemotherapy causes a lowering of sperm count but in the majority of patients presenting with a normal sperm count there is full recovery (Chapter 16).

There have been a number of approaches to reducing the toxicity of chemotherapy. The use of BEP rather than the combination of platinum vinblastine and bleomycin is less toxic both in terms of bone marrow suppression and in terms of abdominal cramps, and furthermore BEP was more effective in patients with advanced stages of disease (Williams *et al.*, 1987). It is unclear that any of the components of the BEP regimen can be deleted, although a number of trials have addressed the need for bleomycin because of its lung toxicity. For the best prognostic group of patients it would appear that 4 cycles of EP are as effective as BEP (Stoter *et al.*, 1986). However, if only 3 cycles of chemotherapy are used EP was markedly inferior to BEP (Loehrer *et al.*, 1991). Our standard practice is to use 4 cycles of BEP chemotherapy deleting bleomycin from the last cycle.

It is at present unclear whether cisplatin can safely be replaced by carboplatin and indeed the evidence against this is increasing (Bajorin *et al.*, 1993). There is also strong retrospective evidence that the dose levels of both etoposide and cisplatin should be maintained at least at the levels indicated in Table 34.5.

In patients with adverse presentations there have been a range of attempts at increasing the aggressiveness of chemotherapy, including the use of alternating non-cross-resistant regimens such as the alternation of platinum vincristine methotrexate bleomycin with actinomycin D, cyclophosphamide and etoposide (Newlands *et al.*, 1986), or the use of short intercycle intervals (Horwich *et al.*, 1989; Lewis *et al.*, 1991). Simple doubling of the cisplatin dose has not proved to be more effective, but was very toxic.

At present no modification has been proved to be definitely more effective than the standard BEP chemotherapy in patients with adverse presentations. Our policy in these patients is to intensify chemotherapy using the C-BOP/BEP regimen (Figure 34.3) which includes the strategies of intensive induction and infusional bleomycin; a pilot study of 21 patients presenting with adverse prognostic factors has been extremely encouraging since 19 of these patients have remained continuously alive and disease free since completion of treatment (Horwich 1993).

34.8.3 POSTCHEMOTHERAPY LYMPHADENECTOMY

Residual masses are found following completion of chemotherapy in approximately 25% of patients. Analysis of 231 patients treated by postchemotherapy lymphadenectomy at the Royal Marsden Hospital between 1976 and 1990 revealed residual undifferentiated cancer in approximately 20%, though this was much less common if surgery had been undertaken following initial chemotherapy rather than following salvage chemotherapy. Lymphadenectomy in this setting provides both therapeutic benefit and information of prognostic value in planning future treatments (Hendry *et al.*, 1993). Approximately half of all patients reveal differentiated teratoma in the excised mass. In these patients the benefits of excision are:

1. To prevent the side-effects of slow cystic enlargement.
2. To prevent the possibility of late malignant change.

Thus for most patients excisional surgery is recommended if assessment following chemotherapy reveals a residual mass. This may be impossible in patients with multiple sites of metastases and anaesthetic caution is warranted in patients early after completion of high doses of bleomycin therapy. We do not routinely recommend excision of retroperitoneal lymph nodes which have returned to within normal size limits following chemotherapy, though occasionally late cystic enlargement of one of these nodes indicates that residual differentiated teratoma was present.

34.8.4 STAGE I SEMINOMA

Since seminoma is exquisitely radiosensitive and rarely spreads beyond retroperitoneal nodes the rationale for low dose adjuvant radiotherapy to these sites has influenced practice for more than 30 years. The usual field is indicated in Figure 34.4 and the treatment prescription is usually to treat the nodes to a mid plane dose of 25–30 Gy in 15–20 fractions over 3–4 weeks, using parallel-opposed equally weighted anterior and posterior portals shaped by lead blocks into a configuration known as a 'dog-leg' or sometimes

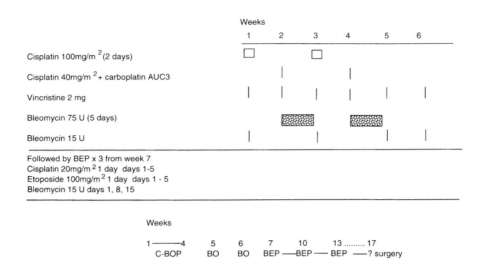

C-BOP

Weeks

	1	2	3	4	5	6

Cisplatin 100mg/m^2(2 days)

Cisplatin 40mg/m^2+ carboplatin AUC3

Vincristine 2 mg

Bleomycin 75 U (5 days)

Bleomycin 15 U

Followed by BEP x 3 from week 7
Cisplatin 20mg/m^2 1 day days 1-5
Etoposide 100mg/m^2 1 day days 1 - 5
Bleomycin 15 U days 1, 8, 15

Weeks

1————4   5   6   7   10   13 17
     C-BOP   BO   BO   BEP ——BEP—— BEP ——? surgery

Figure 34.3 The current Royal Marsden Hospital schedule of intensive chemotherapy for adverse presentations of non-seminoma.

a 'hockey stick' field. The upper border of the field is at the lower edge of the tenth dorsal vertebral body and the width of the field in the para-aortic region is limited by the radiosensitivity of the kidneys such that treatment planning is aided by an intravenous urogram to enable treatment of the ipsilateral renal lymph node. This treatment policy is highly effective and review of 232 patients treated at the Royal Marsden Hospital indicated a relapse rate of 2% and cause-specific survival of 100% (Hamilton *et al.*, 1986).

The concern over this treatment policy is based partly on the possibility of late side-effects from radiation including induction of second cancers. However, the evidence for this is somewhat scanty. Surveillance for seminomas has been investigated as a research protocol and the Royal Marsden Hospital series of just over 100 patients revealed that approximately 15% of patients with stage I seminomas have occult metastases, predominately in the para-aortic region. Since the pattern of recurrence is slow and

since the absence of a sensitive serum marker makes detection of recurrence difficult, we have now abandoned surveillance as a standard treatment policy.

34.8.5 STAGES IIA AND IIB SEMINOMA

Again the standard treatment for this extent of seminoma is radiotherapy to the para-aortic and ipsilateral pelvic lymph nodes. Radiation dose is usually slightly higher, with involved nodes taken to a total of 35 Gy using the same fractionation regimen as previously described for stage I seminoma. The prognosis is excellent with approximately 85–90% of patients remaining relapse free. Most of the remainder can be effectively treated with combination chemotherapy as described below.

In the past the recurrence rate after radiotherapy for stage II seminoma was reduced by adding mediastinal and cervical irradiation fields, but with the demonstrated efficacy of chemotherapy to treat more wide-

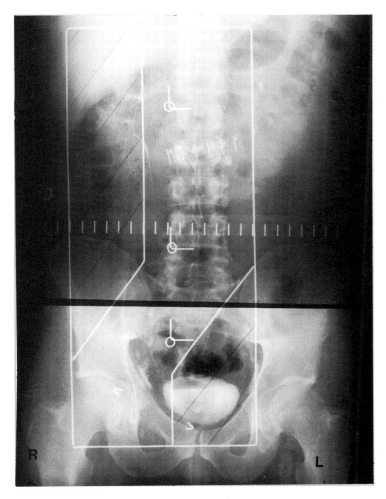

Figure 34.4 Simulator radiograph of field designed for radiotherapy postorchidectomy for stage I seminoma.

spread disease and with the problem of mylo-suppression caused by extensive radiation fields the approached of adding supra-diaphragmatic radiotherapy is now some-what uncommon.

34.8.6   STAGES IIC, III AND IV SEMINOMA

The mainstay of treatment is with com-bination chemotherapy, again using the standard BEP regimen first developed for the treatment of testicular non-seminoma. Since the indications for chemotherapy of semi-noma are less common there is scant informa-tion from prospective randomized trials about alternative treatments. However, the early literature of germ cell tumour chemotherapy did not indicate the efficacy of bleomycin, and reports from some centres have suggested that single agent chemo-therapy based on platinum or a platinum ana-logue may lead to a similar cure rate to combination chemotherapy but with lower toxicity (Horwich *et al.*, 1992).

The response of seminoma following 4 cycles of chemotherapy can be difficult to determine since CT scans frequently reveal residual masses at the site of previous malignancy. In many cases surgical exploration has revealed that these are masses of fibrosis rather than residual active cancer and the excellent prognosis after combination chemotherapy encourages monitoring rather than attempting resection of these masses. If single agent carboplatin has been employed as a chemotherapy regimen there is evidence to suggest that low dose adjuvant radiotherapy to the residual mass may reduce the recurrence rate (Horwich *et al.*, 1992).

34.8.7 SALVAGE CHEMOTHERAPY

Patients who have failed a standard platinum based combination chemotherapy regimen have a poor prognosis with overall survival of approximately 20–30% (Horwich 1993). The optimal treatment is with a combination of chemotherapy and a local treatment modality such as radiation or surgery and best results are obtained where this approach is feasible. Otherwise interest is now focused internationally on the role of high dose chemotherapy with haemopoietic stem cell support in which the principal drugs given in high dose are carboplatin, etoposide and in some centres an alkylating agent, either cyclophosphamide or ifosfamide. There are numerous reports of long term remission, though this occurs in a minority of treated patients and the role of high dose chemotherapy in germ cell tumours has not yet been firmly established.

34.9 OTHER TESTICULAR TUMOURS

Testicular lymphoma is most commonly seen in the context of widespread dissemination, but occasionally appears to be primarily arising within a testis. This group in general have a rather poorer prognosis than extranodal non-Hodgkin's lymphoma at other sites and careful staging including a lumbar puncture to determine meningeal disease is indicated. The principles of treatment are similar to those discussed in Chapter 19, but in patients with good general health adjuvant chemotherapy is indicated following the diagnostic orchidectomy.

Rare tumours of the testis include gonadal stromal tumours which may produce hormones. For a full discussion see Hamilton and Horwich (1988); this review also includes paratesticular tumours including rhabdomyosarcoma and mesothelioma.

34.10 CONCLUSIONS

Testicular germ cell tumours present in young adult males and are highly curable. This places a particular responsibility on the oncologist to ensure correct deployment of surgery, radiotherapy and chemotherapy to ensure that the patient can be cured with the minimum risk of long term morbidity. The development of cisplatin based chemotherapy has led to one of the most dramatic improvements in prognosis of any malignancy during the past 20 years. The effectiveness of treatment and the availability of sensitive tumour markers have lead to the description of germ cell tumours as the model of a curable malignancy.

REFERENCES

Bajorin, D.F., Sarosdy, M.F., Pfister, D.G. *et al.* (1993) Randomized Trial of Etoposide and Cisplatin versus Etoposide and Carboplatin in patients with good-risk germ cell tumours: A Multi-institutional Study. *Journal of Clinical Oncology*, **11**(4), 598–606.

Berthelsen, J.G., Skakkebaek, N.E., Von der Maase, H. and Sorensen, B.L. (1982) Screening for carcinoma *in situ* of the contralateral testis in patients with germinal testicular cancer. *British Medical Journal*, **285**, 1683–6.

Childs, W.J., Goldstraw, P., Nicholls, J.E. *et al.* (1993) Primary malignant mediastinal germ cell tumours: improved prognosis with platinum-based chemotherapy and surgery. *British Journal of Cancer*, **67**, 1098–101.

Chilvers, C.E.D., Saunders, M., Bliss, J.M. *et al.* (1989) Influence of delay in diagnosis on prognosis in testicular teratoma. *British Journal of Cancer*, **59**, 126–8.

Davies, J.M. (1981) Testicular cancer in England and Wales: some epidemiological aspects. *Lancet*, **i**, 928–32.

Dearnaley, D.P., Horwich, A., A'Hern, R. *et al.* (1991) Combination chemotherapy with bleomycin, etoposide and cisplatin (BEP) for metastatic testicular teratoma: long-term follow-up. *European Journal of Cancer*, **27**, 684–91.

Donohue, R.E., Mani, J.H., Whitesel, J.A. *et al.* (1990) Intraoperative and early complications of staging pelvic lymph node dissection in prostatic adenocarcinoma. *Urology*, **35**, 223–7.

Forman, D., Oliver, R.T.D., Brett, A.R. *et al.* (1992) Familial testicular cancer: a report of the UK family register, estimation of risk and an HLA Class 1 sib-pair analysis. *British Journal of Cancer*, **65**, 255–62.

Freedman, L.S., Parkinson, M.C., Jones, W.G. *et al.* (1987) Histopathology in the prediction of relapse of patients with stage I testicular teratoma treated by orchidectomy alone. *Lancet*, **ii**, 294–98.

Hamilton, C.H. and Horwich, A. (1988) Rare tumours of the testis and paratesticular tissues, in *Uncommon Cancer* (eds C.J. Williams, J.G.G. Krikorian, M.R. Green and D. Raghavan), John Wiley, Chichester, pp. 225–48.

Hamilton, C.R., Horwich, A., Easton, D. and Peckham, M.J. (1986) Radiotherapy for stage I seminoma testis: results of treatment and complications. *Radiotherapy and Oncology*, **6**, 115–20.

Hendry, W.F., A'Hern, R.P., Hetherington, J.W. *et al.* (1993) Para-aortic lymphadenectomy after chemotherapy for metastatic non-seminomatous germ cell tumours: prognostic value and therapeutic benefit. *British Journal of Urology*, **71**, 208–13.

Horwich, A. (1991) Current controversies in the management of testicular cancer. *European Journal of Cancer*, **27**, 322–6.

Horwich, A. (1993) Editorial: current issues in the management of clinical stage I testicular teratoma. *European Journal of Cancer*, **29A**, 933–4.

Horwich, A., A'Hern, R.A., Gildersleve, J. and Dearnaley, D.P. (1993a) Prognostic factor analysis of conventional dose salvage therapy of patients with metastatic non seminomatous germ

cell cancer. *Proceedings of the American Society of Clinical Oncology*, **12**, 232.

Horwich, A., Brada, M.J., Nicholls, J. *et al.* (1989a) Intensive induction chemotherapy for poor risk non-seminomatous germ cell tumours. *European Journal of Cancer and Clinical Oncology*, **25**, 177–84.

Horwich, A., Dearnaley, D.P., A'Hern, R. *et al.* (1992) The activity of single-agent carboplatin in advanced seminoma. *European Journal of Cancer*, **28A**, 1307–10.

Horwich, A., Wilson, C., Cornes, P. *et al.* (1993b) Increasing the dose intensity of chemotherapy in poor-prognosis metastatic non-seminoma. *European Urology*, **23**, 219–22.

Lewis, C.R., Fosså, S.D., Mead, G. *et al.* (1991) BOP/VIP – a new platinum-intensive chemotherapy regimen for poor prognosis germ cell tumours. *Annals of Oncology*, **1**, 203–11.

Loehrer, P.J., Elson, P., Johnson, D.H. *et al.* (1991) A randomized trial of cisplatin (P) plus etoposide (E) with or without bleomycin (B) in favorable prognosis disseminated germ cell tumours (GCT): an ECOG Study. *Proceeding, Annual Meeting of the American Society of Clinical Oncology*, **10**, 169.

Mason, M.D. (1991) Tumour markers, in *Testicular Cancer – Clinical Investigation and Management*, (ed. A. Horwich), Chapman & Hall Medical, London, pp. 33–50.

McKendrick, J.J., Theaker, J. and Mead, G.M. (1991) Nonseminomatous germ cell tumor with very high serum human ·chorionic gonadotropin. *Cancer*, **67**(3), 684–9.

Mead, G.M., Stenning, S.P., Parkinson, M.C. *et al.* (1992) The Second Medical Research Council Study of prognostic factors in nonseminomatous germ cell tumours. *Journal of Clinical Oncology*, **10**, (1), 85–94.

Mostofi, F.K. and Sobin, L.H. (1977) *Histological typing of testicular tumours*. World Health Organization, Geneva.

Newlands, E.S., Bagshawe, K.D., Begent, R.H.J. *et al.* (1986) Current optimum management of anaplastic germ cell tumours of the testis and other sites. *British Journal of Urology*, **58**, 307–14.

Peckham, M.J., Barrett, A., Husband, J.E. and Hendry, W.F. (1982) Orchidectomy alone in testicular stage I non-seminomatous germ-cell tumours. *Lancet*, **ii**, 678–80.

Peckham, M.J., Horwich, A., Easton, D.F. and Hendry, W.F. (1988) The management of advanced testicular teratoma. *British Journal of Urology*, **62**, 63–8.

Pugh, R.C.B. and Cameron, K.M. (1976) Teratoma in *Pathology of the Testis*, (eds R.C.B. Pugh), Blackwell Scientific Publications, London, pp. 199–244.

Ray, B., Steven, I., Hajdu, S.I. and Whitemore, W.F., Jr. (1974) Distribution of retroperitoneal lymph node metastases in testicular germinal tumours. *Cancer*, **33**, 340–8.

Schottenfeld, D., Warshauer, M.E. and Sherlock, S. (1980) The epidemiology of testicular cancer in young adults. *American Journal of Epidemiology*, **112**, 232–46.

Senturia, Y.D., Peckham, C.S. and Peckham, M.J. (1985) Children fathered by men treated for testicular cancer. *Lancet*, **ii**, 766–9.

Stoter, G., Kaye, S., Sleyfer, D. *et al.* (1986) Preliminary results of BEP (Bleomycin, Etoposide, Cisplatin) versus an alternating regimen of BEP and PVB (Cisplatin, Vinblastine, Bleomycin) in high volume metastatic (HVM) testicular non-seminomas. *Proceedings of the American Society of Clinical Oncology*, **5**, 106.

Von der Maase, H., Rorth, M., Walbom-Jorgensen, S. *et al.* (1986) Carcinoma *in situ* of contralateral testis in patients with testicular germ cell cancer: study of 27 cases in 500 patients. *British Medical Journal*, **293**, 1398–401.

Williams, S.D., Birch, R. and Einhorn, L.H. (1987) Disseminated germ cell tumours: chemotherapy with Cisplatin plus Bleomycin plus either Vinblastine or Etoposide. A trial of the Southeastern Cancer Study Group. *New England Journal of Medicine*, **316**, 1435–40.

Williams, S.D., Stablein, D.M., Einhorn, L.H. *et al.* (1987) Immediate adjuvant chemotherapy versus observation with treatment at relapse in pathological stage II testicular cancer. *New England Journal of Medicine*, **317**, 1433–8.

RENAL CELL CARCINOMA

Christopher R.J. Woodhouse and Martin Gore

35.1 INTRODUCTION

Adenocarcinoma is the commonest and most important tumour of the renal parenchyma. It accounts for about 3% of all malignant tumours in England and Wales. Although it has been given a number of other names in the past, it should now be called renal cell carcinoma or adenocarcinoma of the kidney. In particular, the term 'hypernephroma' should never be used.

It should be distinguished from transitional cell carcinoma of the renal pelvis which behaves in the same manner as bladder carcinoma, and is rare accounting for only 7% of all renal neoplasms.

35.2 AETIOLOGY AND EPIDEMIOLOGY

No definite aetiological factors have been identified. In males smoking of cigarettes increases the risk of developing renal carcinoma fivefold. The incidence is higher in men than women, but after the menopause, the incidence between the sexes becomes similar.

Minor variations in incidence have been reported in different races and countries. Higher than average death rates are seen in Denmark, Norway, Scotland and New Zealand. Low rates are seen in Ireland, Italy, Japan, Spain and Venezuela (Case, 1964). It is difficult to see any link between these countries that could account for the differences in incidence.

The rare congenital syndrome of von Hippel–Lindau predisposes to neoplasms of the renal parenchyma. Although they are usually adenocarcinomas, the behaviour of the tumours is relatively benign which is fortunate as they tend to be multiple and bilateral. The other features of this syndrome are angiomatosis of the retina, angioblastic tumours or cysts of the cerebellum or medulla oblongata.

Patients on dialysis may develop renal cysts which can undergo malignant degeneration. The cysts that do not become malignant will disappear after a successful renal transplant (Ishikawa *et al.*, 1980, 1983).

Simple cysts that are commonly found incidentally during urological investigation seldom cause symptoms and are almost never malignant.

35.3 PATHOLOGY

The gross appearance of a renal carcinoma is of a lobulated mass arising from the parenchyma. It distorts the calyces. In early stage disease it is confined by the capsule (which may be considerably stretched without being invaded) and by the walls of the collecting system. As it grows it may invade both of these structures. It also characteristically grows into the renal veins. From there it may extend into the inferior vena cava and eventually into the hepatic veins and right atrium. In the early stages of vascular invasion the tumour floats as a thrombus anchored only by its attachment to the main renal mass. Later it becomes adherent to, or may even invade, the vein endothelium.

The cut surface shows areas of solid tumour interspersed with cystic and necrotic areas and haemorrhage. Microscopy reflects the gross appearance. The tumour may be made up of a variety of different cell types, most commonly large, clear cells with big nuclei and prominent nucleoli.

Chemical and histochemical studies of cholesterol in normal and neoplastic renal tissue gave the early clue that the cell of origin was in the proximal or distal convoluted tubule (Leary, 1950). Later, electron microscopy studies of the brush border seen in tumour cells indicated that the proximal convoluted tubule was nearly always the primary site (Seljelid and Ericsson, 1965; Syrjanen and Hjelt, 1978).

Although this evidence has been accepted for many years, recent studies have re-opened the debate. Epithelial membrane antigen that is found only in the distal convoluted tubule has been identified by immunohistochemistry in 31 of 33 consecutive renal carcinomas (Fleming *et al.*, 1985).

Collecting duct carcinomas are a rare subgroup. They present in an advanced stage in patients about 10 years younger than for tubular carcinomas. They may be mistaken for invasive transitional cell carcinomas (Dimopoulos *et al.*, 1993)

It has been suggested that small, solid adenomatous tumours of the kidney should be called adenomas. They are a common incidental finding at post-mortem (Reese and Winstanley, 1958). It was arbitarily suggested that adenomas under 3 cm in diameter were benign. However, histologically these small tumours are indistinguishable from low grade carcinomas and have the same surface antigens (Wallace and Nairn, 1972). If a small biopsy is given to the pathologist without knowledge of the original tumour size, it can only be labelled carcinoma.

In autopsies of 16 294 patients, 235 unsuspected renal carcinomas were found. The number with metastases increased with the size of the primary. Even in the 82 primaries under 3 cm in diameter, three had metastases (Hellsten *et al.*, 1982). When such small tumours are found, radical nephrectomy remains the correct treatment (Licht and Novick, 1993).

Oncocytomas are tumours composed of cells with bizarre appearance and poor glandular differentiation. At presentation they are usually large. On investigation there is no reliable difference in appearance from true carcinoma. Even on biopsy a preoperative diagnosis is not certain because there can be oncocytic areas within a carcinoma or an oncocytoma may be associated with a carcinoma (Mostofi, 1979). Most oncocytomas are benign but a few less well differentiated ones may metastasize (Lieber and Kovach, 1981; Lewi and Fleming, 1984).

Metastatic spread occurs through the blood stream to the lungs, bone and liver. Invasion of the renal veins is associated with remote metastases in 75% of cases (Hellsten *et al.*, 1982).

Lymphatic spread follows an unusual pattern: it may be via the hilar nodes and then in a regular way to the mediastinal nodes. In other cases the spread is through the retroperitoneal lymphatics so that supraclavicular or pelvic nodes may be positive while the local nodes are clear (Hulten *et al.*, 1969). This curious spread may be due to the fact that the cortex of the kidney has lymphatic connections with the perinephric fat (Yoffey and Courtice, 1970).

Lymphatic and blood borne spread proceed independently. In a post-mortem series, 34% of patients with negative hilar nodes had metastases elsewhere (Saitoh, 1981).

It is characteristic of renal carcinoma that metastases may occur up to 25 years after nephrectomy. In a series from the Institute of Urology, 51 of 147 patients were thought to be free of tumour 5 years after radical nephrectomy. By the tenth year, ten of the 51 had died of metastatic disease (Woodhouse *et al.*, 1985). In another series, 11% of patients disease free at 10 years developed metastases in the next 14 years (McNichols *et al.*, 1981).

35.4 PRESENTATION

The majority of patients present with renal pain and haematuria. A classic triad is described, consisting of these two symptoms with a palpable renal mass. In practice, the triad is rare (Table 35.1).

Uncommon presentations include all of the syndromes of systemic disturbance (Table 35.2). These paraneoplastic syndromes are caused by biologically active substances which have effects remote from the primary or secondary tumour. Although only a few patients present entirely with these syndromes, a further group have generalized paraneoplastic symptoms at the time of a more conventional presentation. In addition, up to 50% of patients have measurable biochemical abnormalities without symptoms. As the same substances are produced by metastases they may be useful as tumour markers (for detailed review see Woodhouse, 1987).

A presentation that is becoming more common is the incidental finding of a small renal mass usually on ultrasound. In series from the USA the proportion of cases in this category rose from less than 10% between

1946 and 1955 to 25% between 1976 and 1985 (Thompson and Peek, 1988). The cancers so found are usually small and the prognosis after nephrectomy is much better than in those presenting with symptoms.

35.5 INVESTIGATION

In the patient presenting with symptoms, the first investigation is likely to be an intravenous urogram (IVU). Renal tumours are seen as space occupying lesions. Solid lesions can be distinguished from cystic ones by ultrasound. Solid lesions are virtually always cancers and so there is seldom any indication for biopsy. Angiomyolipoma has a characteristic appearance on both ultrasound and CT and is the only solid lesion that would not be treated by nephrectomy.

Ultrasound will also give useful staging information. Involvement of the renal vein and inferior vena cava may be seen. Sometimes hilar nodes or invasion of adjacent structures are identified, though further imaging would be required for confirmation. Liver metastases are usually visible on ultrasound.

In some cases, a combination of IVU and ultrasound will give all the necessary information about the abdomen to plan surgery. However, if there is any suggestion of venous involvement or invasion of extrarenal structures, more precise definition is required.

Table 35.1 Presentation of renal adenocarcinoma in 147 cases at the Institute of Urology, London

Presentation	Cases (no.)	Cases (%)
'Classic triad'	3	
Haematuria alone	57	
Pain alone	16	81.6
Mass alone	5	
Any two of classic triad	39	
Paraneoplastic syndromes	10	6.8
Varicocele	4	
Microscopic haematuria	1	11.6
Chance finding	12	

From Woodhouse *et al.*, 1985.

Table 35.2   Paraneoplastic syndromes found in renal adenocarcinoma

Clinical feature	Laboratory findings
Endocrine and biochemical	
Hypertension	Raised renal vein renin
Erythrocytosis	Raised red blood cell count
	Normal arterial O_2 tension
Hypercalcaemia syndromes	Raised serum calcium
	Variable serum phosphate
Hepatosplenomegaly (Stauffer's syndrome)	Abnormal liver function tests
Gastrointestinal syndromes	All very rare: raised –
	Gonadotrophins
	Placental lactogens
	Prolactin
	Enteroglucagon
	Insulin
	Adrenocorticoids
	Prostaglandins
Non-specific effects of malignancy	
Pyrexia	Non-white cell pyrogen
	Raised ESR
Anaemia	Normocytic
	Hypochromic
	Decreased iron binding capacity
Amyloidosis	Renal failure
Neuromyopathy	None

Conventional CT will usually define the local invasion and renal vein involvement. If the inferior vena cava is involved, CT may be insufficient to define the upper and lower extents. In the past, venograms were essential for such definition. Recently, it has been suggested that MRI may give the same information more easily.

In all cases there must be a careful search for metastases. The lungs are notorious as a site of small metastases and they may not be seen on plain chest X-ray; CT scan or whole chest tomograms are essential. Most cases require a bone scan.

35.6   TREATMENT

There are few controlled trials of treatment and none which address the question of best first line treatment for localized renal adeno-carcinoma. Surgical treatment is based on opinions formed over many years and series with retrospective controls. It is generally accepted that surgery is the only possible cure and for most surgeons this means radical nephrectomy.

Radiotherapy does not have a part to play in the management of the primary renal cancer except in rare circumstances. In trials it has been found not to prolong survival whether given before or after radical nephrectomy. However it may reduce local recurrence (Rafla, 1970; van der werf Messing, 1973). Occasionally a large and inoperable carcinoma may be palliated by local radiotherapy.

35.6.1   RADICAL NEPHRECTOMY

The standard treatment for carcinoma of the kidney is radical nephrectomy. In an early description of the technique, Robson *et al.*

(1969) described three features that distinguished it from simple nephrectomy: removal of the perinephric fat with Gerota's fascia, removal of the adrenal and ligation of the artery and vein before mobilization of the kidney. This operation has been continued, largely unchanged, ever since (Zingg, 1993).

There are three possible approaches. The author prefers a transverse abdominal incision, dividing both recti. This allows a thorough laparotomy, sampling of the hilar nodes and a wide exposure of the kidney. An approach laterally, above the 12th rib is more traditional. Alternatively, an approach may be made posteriorly, dividing the necks of the lowest three ribs (Nagamatsu incision). All the incisions may be extended up into the chest if necessary.

35.6.2 SIMPLE NEPHRECTOMY VS RADICAL NEPHRECTOMY

In simple nephrectomy the perinephric fat and the ipsilateral adrenal are not removed. It has been shown that perinephric fat contains microscopic tumour in up to 45% of cases (Robson *et al.*, 1969). The renal cortex is drained by lymphatics that freely anastomose with those of the perirenal fat so that peripheral tumours, in particular, are likely to have local spread (Yoffey and Courtice, 1970). As the perinephric fat has no function and is easy to remove there is no case for leaving it behind.

The ipsilateral adrenal is a slightly more difficult problem. The adrenal contains metastases in 19% of cases but is the solitary site in only 2% (Saitoh, 1981). Presumably only this last 2% will be saved by unilateral adrenalectomy. It therefore comes as no surprise to find that there was no difference in survival, in a retrospective series, when the adrenal was left behind (Robey and Schellhammer, 1986). Even so, a general recommendation cannot be made. The adrenal may be very close to the kidney and separation may compromise the integrity of the

cancer field, especially in upper pole tumours. In the absence of a prospective trial it can only be said that the ipsilateral adrenal does not always have to be removed.

Lymphadenectomy with radical nephrectomy has been discussed extensively in the literature. In a review article Marshall and Powell (1982) concluded that there was inadequate evidence to allow the surgeon to dispense with regional lymphadenectomy. This is a reasonable conclusion but presupposes that the surgeon is in the habit of doing a lymphadenectomy: if he is not, is the evidence strong enough to make him start?

The theoretical evidence seems weak. The kidney is drained by lymphatics that flow to the renal hilum and thence to the paracaval and para-aortic nodes. In a post-mortem series the regional nodes contained metastases in 66% of cases but were the sole site in only 12% (Saitoh, 1981). In patients that had nephrectomies with regional lymphadenectomy, the incidence of nodal metastases was 12%, 28% and 34% in histological grades I, II and III (Skinner and de Kernion, 1978).

Unfortunately the lymphatic spread does not always occur in an orderly manner to the local and then remote nodes. The occurrence of 'skip nodes' and the independent nature of blood borne and lymphatic spread have already been mentioned.

Lymphadenectomy is strongly advocated by Robson and by Skinner (Robson *et al.*, 1969; Skinner *et al.*, 1972; Skinner and de Kernion, 1978). In Robson's series the 10 year survival was 38% with nodal metastases. Skinner and de Kernion give a 40% 5 year survival for grade III lesions. They also point out that the 5 year survival in their series was better in each grade compared to a retrospective simple nephrectomy series by a percentage approximately equal to the incidence of positive nodes (Table 35.3).

The difficulty in assessing these claims is, first, that the number of patients followed for 5–10 years is small and, secondly, that factors other than lymphadenectomy are involved.

Table 35.3   The incidence of local nodal involvement and its impact on 5 year survival

	Histological grade		
	I	*II*	*III*
Incidence of positive nodes (%)	12	28	34
5 year survival after simple nephrectomy (%)	77	31	8
5 year survival after radical nephrectomy and lymphadenectomy (%)	87	64	40

From Skinner and de Kernian, 1978.

Robson attributes his excellent results to radical (as opposed to simple) nephrectomy, early ligation of the renal vessels and lymphadenectomy. In addition his patients were very carefully investigated before operation, including a mediastinoscopy, so that patients with small volume but extensive disease were not included.

There are few other series that give both the nodal status and the 10 year survival but where they do, figures range from 0 to 38% (Middleton and Presto, 1973; Marshall and Powell, 1982).

Although it is possible to remove a kidney by a laparoscopic approach, authors feel that the risk of breaching the cancer field makes it inappropriate for the treatment of even the smallest renal neoplasm.

In conclusion, the treatment of choice for renal adenocarcinoma is radical nephrectomy. There is no theoretical and little clinical reason to perform regional lymphadenectomy as well.

35.6.3   SUBTOTAL NEPHRECTOMY

In patients with tumours bilaterally, in solitary kidneys or with very poor renal function, three options exist:

1. Do nothing.
2. Perform radical surgery and accept dialysis.
3. Do a partial nephrectomy or enucleate the tumour.

Doctors must always consider the possibility of offering no active treatment. However, the prognosis without surgery is poor. Non-surgical treatment or no treatment for tumours in a solitary kidney leads to the death of 75% of patients at 2 years; in those with synchronous bilateral disease all may be expected to die in less than 5 months (Wickham, 1975).

Radical surgery which will make the patient anephric is a major step. The management of dialysis is difficult because of the sudden change from normal to renal failure haemodynamics. When it has become apparent that there are no metastases, renal transplantation can be considered. The results in the published series are not promising and this option should only be used for carefully selected patients. Transplantation should be delayed for at least 15 months (Penn, 1977).

Partial nephrectomy is a good operation when it can be done. When the contralateral kidney has been removed for benign disease, a 78% 5 year survival is possible (Wickham *et al.*, 1975). Often, however, the tumour is not in an appropriate position.

In tumours that are less than 7 cm in diameter there is a pseudocapsule of compressed renal tissue that allows enucleation (Marburger *et al.*, 1981).

The theoretical basis for this operation has been investigated by Marshall *et al.* Standard radical nephrectomy was performed on 16 patients. The tumour was then enucleated from the kidney and the clearance of the cancer assessed histologically. The findings were then compared with the radiologist's opinion of the feasibility of enucleation as judged by CT scan. Seven of 16 patients would not have been cured by enucleation because there was residual tumour in the kidney (six cases) or perinephric fat (one case). All well differentiated and some moderately differentiated cancers could be completely enucleated but no poorly differentiated ones could. The size of the tumour was unhelpful in prediction. Neither radiologist nor urologist could consistently predict whether enucleation would be possible (Marshall *et al.*, 1986).

In practice, enucleation has some worthwhile results. Renal cooling or intra-arterial inosine may be used (Wickham *et al.*, 1978; Jaeger *et al.*, 1985) but are not always necessary (Novick *et al.*, 1986). In very difficult cases bench surgery and autotransplantation can be used but the complication rate is high: 43% for bench surgery against 17% for surgery *in situ* (Marburger *et al.*, 1981). The best results are found in well differentiated carcinomas and the multiple tumours of the von Hippel–Lindau syndrome where a 90% 3 year survival rate has been reported (Novick *et al.*, 1986). In a broader selection of patients a 50% 5 year survival rate was reported which is not very different from that following radical nephrectomy (Marburger *et al.*, 1981).

At the other end of the scale are the tumours less than 3 cm in diameter. These are not benign tumours and should not be undertreated. It is the authors' view, shared by many others (Licht and Novick, 1993), that they should be treated by radical nephrectomy. Some have advocated partial nephrectomy. In a series of 28 small peripheral tumours treated by local excision, all are disease free, though the length of follow-up was not given and five were said to have been benign (Bazeed *et al.*, 1986).

35.6.4 SURGERY FOR CAVAL INVOLVEMENT

One of the characteristic features of renal carcinoma is extension along the renal vein and into the vena cava. In a few patients the tumour embolus may extend into the heart. It is surprising how seldom this causes symptoms or signs. No nephrectomy for renal cancer should be done without assessment of the venous system.

Although a caval tumour, presumably, exfoliates tumour cells into the circulation, it is not associated with a particularly poor prognosis: up to a third of patients may have no distant metastases (Hellsten *et al.*, 1982).

If no distant metastases are found every effort should be made to remove the primary and the extension *en bloc*. For this to be done the cava and all its tributaries above and below the embolus must be controlled. When the tumour extends above the diaphragm cardiopulmonary bypass is essential. In earlier patients the inferior vena cava was resected (Lome and Bush, 1972; Skinner and de Kernion, 1978), but it is now known that the tumour can be extracted and the vessels left intact.

Such surgery has a significant morbidity and mortality and careful selection is essential (Marshall and Reitz, 1986). Three of 25 patients did not leave hospital in one series (Pritchett *et al.*, 1986). In particular, the search for metastases must be meticulous. The median survival of patients with distant metastases was 9 months while those with caval involvement alone had a median survival of 29 months and a 5 year survival of 23% (Giuliani *et al.*, 1986). A few long term survivors, up to 20 years, have been reported (Skinner *et al.*, 1972). Where complete tumour clearance is achieved a 5 year survival of 36% has been recorded though no patient with extension above the hepatic veins survived more than 45 months (Pritchett *et al.*, 1986).

Although such major surgery would normally only be justified as a cure, occasional patients may require it for palliation. In Pritchett's series three patients presented with symptoms due to the caval extension and 'many others' were judged to have been able to leave hospital alive because of palliative caval clearance (Pritchett *et al.*, 1986).

35.6.5 SURGERY IN THE PRESENCE OF METASTASES

The natural history of renal carcinoma allows two different situations to be considered: resectable metastases and multiple, non-resectable metastases.

About a third of patients with renal carcinoma present with metastases, a figure that obviously increases with increasing diligence and better technology. Experience in oncology firmly dictates that surgery alone cannot cure patients with metastatic disease. Why, then, is there so much enthusiasm for removing renal primaries in the face of multiple metastases?

The answer lies in the possibility of spontaneous regression of the metastases combined with the knowledge that surgery is the only possible cure. The world literature from 1928 has been reviewed in two papers and 67 cases have been identified where metastases have regressed (Freed *et al.*, 1977; Fairlamb, 1981). In the first 51 patients, 38 cases of regression occurred after nephrectomy and four after renal radiotherapy. In seven the metastases only appeared after the nephrectomy and subsequently regressed and in two regression occurred although no treatment was undertaken. In only 12 was follow-up 5 years or more. In 45 the lung was the only site of known metastases. Although renal carcinoma may be the commonest soft tissue tumour to exhibit regression, it is still a very rare phenomenon.

In considering this information a number of points about spontaneous regression must be taken into account. However incomplete the literature, spontaneous regression is rare and certainly has an incidence lower than the operative mortality. Secondly, regression does not mean a cure, only a change in the X-ray appearances which may be temporary. Not all radiological metastases have had histological confirmation. Thirdly, regression may be seen in some metastases while others are progressing. Fourthly, the reviews have shown that some regressions have occurred unrelated to surgical treatment. On this basis, nephrectomy should not be performed in the hope of spontaneous regression.

Clinical practice also militates against nephrectomy in the presence of unresectable metastases. In 93 patients from the MD Anderson Hospital presenting in this way, 43 had nephrectomies and 50 did not. Median survival was 11.3 months with surgery and 7.9 months without. It was concluded that surgery did not alter the natural history of the disease and that there was no difference in the quality of life between the two groups. The only patients whose survival was slightly improved had bone as the only site of metastasis and had a median survival of 16.1 months. No cases of spontaneous regression were seen (Johnson *et al.*, 1975).

It seems clear that nephrectomy should not be performed in the presence of unresectable metastases. Where the primary is causing local symptoms every effort should be made to control them by other means, especially by embolization. Generalized symptoms, especially the paraneoplastic syndromes, are unlikely to be helped by nephrectomy unless the metastases are of very small volume.

Different values apply to the 1–3% of patients presenting with one or more resectable metastases. In this group, usually with a solitary pulmonary metastasis, nephrectomy and resection of the secondary can have a 35% 5 year survival (Tolia and Whitmore, 1975). Not surprisingly, the smaller the number of metastases, the longer the survival, though repeat operations for local recurrence do seem to have some benefit (Dernevik *et al.*, 1985). It remains a moot point whether these operations are more than palliative: although 6 and 8 year survivors are recorded, all the deaths in Dernevik's series were from carcinomatosis. Such patients are only exhibiting the prolonged natural history that is well known.

35.6.6   EMBOLIZATION OF THE TUMOUR

Interventional radiologists have no difficulty in embolizing the renal arteries and several have advocated the procedure as treatment for renal adenocarcinoma. A number of questions arise.

(a)   Is the tumour infarcted?

Small renal carcinomas derive their blood supply from the surrounding kidney. On angiography a single supplying artery can often be identified. Large tumours have an extensive blood supply from extrarenal collaterals.

In 49 kidneys removed 4–8 days after embolization, 70% had viable tumour on histology which was attributed to collateral circulation seen at angiography (Kaisary *et al.*, 1984). Teasdale *et al.* found that none of 24 kidneys were completely infarcted and eight had escaped completely (Teasdale *et al.*, 1982). In another series of six patients embolized with sodium tetradecyl sulphate, histology showed 'extensive renal infarcts in all patients' (not necessarily the same as complete infarction of all tumour) (Konchanin *et al.*, 1987). The apparently viable tumour might not have survived, but on this evidence it seems unlikely that complete infarction is possible consistently.

(b)   What good does it do?

Embolization may make surgery easier, reduce blood loss and operating time, reduce the liberation of tumour cells into the circulation and make removal of very large tumours possible (McDonald, 1982).

It is difficult to test such possibilities. The tumour volume has been measured before and after embolization. Twenty-seven tumours had a mean preoperative volume of 908 ml. Twenty-seven per cent showed no change in volume and 73% had a mean 33% decrease in volume (Mebust *et al.*, 1984). The operative advantage may depend on the delay between embolization and nephrectomy. When nephrectomy is done within 24 hours of embolization a decrease in blood loss and operating time has been shown (Singsaas *et al.*, 1979), but when delayed for longer it has not (Kaisary *et al.*, 1984; Mebust *et al.*, 1984). Wallace *et al.* found that previously unrecognized collateral vessels developed within 72 hours of embolization (Wallace *et al.*, 1981). It is probably only in very large tumours that embolization and immediate nephrectomy is advantageous (Pontonnier *et al.*, 1980; Mebust *et al.*, 1984). Limitation of tumour cell embolus might be helpful but feasibility has not been tested. Kaisary *et al.* did not find that embolization altered the clinical pattern of metastases (Kaisary *et al.*, 1984).

(c)   What are the complications?

Renal embolization has a significant complication rate and mortality. Nearly all patients have pain (which may be severe), fever, leucocytosis and paralytic ileus (Mebust *et al.*, 1984). Accidental embolization of other organs, sometimes through a renal arteriovenous fistula, accounts for most other complications. Mortality ranges from 4% to 7% (Barth *et al.*, 1981; Teasdale *et al.*, 1982; Mebust *et al.*, 1984).

(d)   What is its role?

In spite of enthusiasm in the 1980s, it is now clear that embolization does not alter the survival in renal carcinoma. It has no role in the primary management of most cases.

In palliation it is probably at least as effective as nephrectomy for local renal symptoms and may allow the identification of the rare patient who will exhibit regression of metastases following treatment of the primary (Kaisary *et al.*, 1984). As an adjunct to surgery it has very limited value except in large tumours.

35.6.7 TREATMENT OF METASTASES

When deciding about treatment for metastatic disease, it is important to remember that, at present, there is no cure. Treatment is palliative and must not be given as an alternative to telling the patient the truth, nor must it be more unpleasant than the symptoms to be treated. Present cytotoxic chemotherapy regimens are ineffective.

(a) Hormone therapy

Medroxyprogesterone acetate (MPA) has been the standard treatment for disseminated renal carcinoma since Bloom reported a 16% response rate (Bloom, 1971). However, recent review of Bloom's data and a literature review shows that the response rate is nearer to 10% (Harris, 1983). Median duration of remission is 3 months (range 2–24). Nonetheless, this drug still has a place as it generally improves patients' well-being even when the objective response is limited.

(b) Radiotherapy

Radiotherapy can be used very effectively to treat the pain of bone metastases. The response rate is 70–80%. In weight bearing bones with large lytic lesions, preliminary internal fixation is indicated. Occasionally locally painful and inoperable primary renal tumours may shrink sufficiently with radiotherapy so that symptoms are relieved.

(c) Biological response modifiers

Interferons

The interferons are a group of proteins classified as alpha, beta and gamma. They have a wide variety of biological actions including antiviral and immunoregulatory activity and an enhancing effect on the cytotoxicity of a variety of leucocytes. Alpha interferon has an antiproliferative effect on normal and malignant cells and is active in renal cell carcinoma.

In 56 published studies of alpha interferon, the overall response rate is 15% of 1112 patients with 2% achieving complete remission (Horoszewicz and Murphy, 1989). The time taken to achieve response is long (1–11 months). The duration of remission is 1–17 months with occasional long term responders up to 31 months (Buzaid *et al.*, 1987; Muss *et al.*, 1987).

Later work has concentrated on defining regimens and identifying patients most likely to respond. Current regimens usually start at low dose (less than 5 MU per day), given 3 times a week subcutaneously. The dose is slowly increased to 10–18 MU per dose depending on the side-effects. In responders treatment is continued until relapse occurs.

No patient should be excluded from interferon treatment if systemic therapy is indicated. However, patients with a good performance status and pulmonary metastases have the best response rates.

Alpha-interferon has been used in combination with cytotoxic chemotherapy, steroids, hormones, aspirin, tumour necrosis factor and other interferons with little improvement in the results.

Most patients have flu-like symptoms which usually abate after a few weeks of treatment. Other common side-effects include nausea, vomiting, anorexia and weight loss. Dose modification may be required if the side-effects continue.

Interleukin-2

Interleukin-2 (IL-2) is a cytokine. It has a variety of effects including stimulation of macrophage cytotoxicity, stimulation of B-cell growth and differentiation, and the production of other cytokines.

When given alone in bolus doses, IL-2 produces an overall response rate of 22% (Rosenberg *et al.*, 1989). These results are improved when IL-2 is combined with lymphokine activated killer cells (LAK). Results are very dependent on dose and regimen but may reach 33% overall response rate, 16% with complete response (Linehan *et al.*, 1989).

The side-effects of such therapy are severe. Nausea, vomiting, diarrhoea, hypotension, fevers and fluid retention are common. Cardiac dysrrhythmias, pulmonary oedema, myocardial infarction and encephalopathy are seen occasionally. There is a treatment related death rate of about 1%.

Although IL-2 shows activity in metastatic disease, its expense and toxicity, especially when combined with LAK, limit its use. Combination with other agents and different dose schedules is under investigation.

REFERENCES

Barth, K.H., White, R.I. and Marshall, F.F. (1981) Quantification of arteriovenous shunting in renal cell carcinoma. *Journal of Urology*, **125**, 161–6.

Bazeed, M.A., Scharfe, T., Becht, E. *et al.* (1986) Conservative surgery of renal cell carcinoma. *European Urology*, **12**, 238–43.

Bloom, H.J.G. (1971) Medroxyprogesterone acetate (provera) in the treatment of metastatic renal cancer. *British Journal of Cancer*, **25**, 250–65.

Buzaid, A.C., Robertone, A., Kisala, C. and Salmon S.E. (1987) Phase II study of interferon alpha 2a, recombinant (roferon A) in metastatic renal cell carcinoma. *Journal of Clinical Oncology*, **5**, 1083.

Case, R.A.M. (1964) The mortality from cancer of the kidney in England and Wales with data from other countries for comparison, in *Monographs on Neoplastic Disease, Volume V, Tumours of the Kidney and Ureter*, (ed. E. Riches), E. and S. Livingstone, London pp. 3–35.

Dernevik, L., Berggren, H., Larsson, S. and Roberts, D. (1985) Surgical removal of pulmonary metastases from renal cell carcinoma. *Scandinavian Journal of Urology and Nephrology*, **19**, 133–7.

Dimopoulos, M.A., Logothetis, C.J., Markowitz, A. *et al.* (1993) Collecting duct carcinoma of the kidney. *British Journal of Urology*, **71**, 388–91.

Fairlamb, D.J. (1981) Spontaneous regression of metastases of renal cancer. *Cancer*, **47**, 2102–6.

Fleming, S., Lindop, G.P.M. and Gibson, A.A.M. (1985) The distribution of epithelial membrane antigen in the kidney and its tumours. *Histopathology*, **9**, 729–39.

Freed, S.Z., Halperin, J.P. and Gordon, M. (1977) Idiopathic regression of metastases from renal cell carcinoma. *Journal of Urology*, **118**, 538–42.

Giuliani, L., Giberti, C., Martorana, G. and Rovida, S. (1986) Surgical management of renal cell carcinoma with vena cava tumor thrombus. *European Urology*, **12**, 145–50.

Harris, D.T. (1983) Hormonal therapy and chemotherapy of renal cell carcinoma. *Seminars in Oncology*, **10**, 422–30.

Hellsten, S., Berge, T., Linell, F. and Wehlin, L. (1982) Clinically unrecognised renal cell carcinoma: an autopsy study, in *Renal Tumours, Proceedings of the 1st International Conference on Kidney Tumours*, (eds R. Kuss, G.P. Murphy, S. Khoury and J.P. Karr), Alan Liss, New York, pp. 273–5.

Horoszewicz, J.S. and Murphy, G.P. (1989) An assessment of the current use of human interferons in therapy of urological cancers. *Journal of Urology*, **142**, 1173–80.

Hulten, L., Rosenkrantz, M., Sleman, T., Wahlquist, L. and Ahren, Ch. (1969) Occurrence and localisation of lymph node metastases in renal carcinoma. *Scandinavian Journal of Urology and Nephrology*, **3**, 129–33.

Ishikawa, I., Saito, Y., Onouch, Z. *et al.* (1980) Development of acquired cystic disease and adenocarcinoma of the kidney in glomerulonephritic haemo-dialysis patients. *Clinical Nephrology*, **14**, 1–6.

Ishikawa, I., Yuri, T., Kitada, H. and Shinoda, A. (1983) Regression of acquired cystic disease of the kidney after successful renal transplantation. *American Journal of Nephrology*, **3**, 310–14.

Jaeger, N., Weissbach, L. and Vahlensieck, W. (1985) Value of enucleation of tumor in solitary kidneys. *European Urology*, **11**, 369–73.

Johnson, D.E., Kaesler, K.E. and Samuels, M.L. (1975) Is nephrectomy justified in patients with metastatic renal carcinoma? *Journal of Urology*, **114**, 27–9.

Kaisary, A.V., Williams, G. and Riddle, P.R. (1984) The role of preoperative embolisation in renal cell carcinoma. *Journal of Urology*, **131**, 641–6.

Konchanin, R.P., Cho, K.J. and Grossman, H.B. (1987) Preoperative devascularisation of advanced renal adenocarcinoma using a sclerosing agent. *Journal of Urology*, **137**, 199–201.

Leary, T. (1950) Crystalline ester cholesterol in adult cortical renal tumours. *Archives of Pathology*, **50**, 151–78.

Lewi, H. and Fleming, S. (1984) Renal oncocytoma. Paper presented at the 7th Edinburgh Urological Festival, Edinburgh.

Licht, M.R. and Novick, A.C. (1993) Nephron sparing surgery for renal cell carcinoma. *Journal of Urology*, **149**, 1–7.

Lieber, M.M. and Kovach, J.S. (1981) Soft agar clonogenic assay for primary human renal carcinoma – *in vitro* chemotherapeutic drug sensitivity testing. *Investigative Urology*, **19**, 111–14.

Linehan, W.M., Shipley, W.U. and Longo, D.L. (1989) Cancer of the kidney and ureter, in *Cancer: principles and practice of oncology*, 3rd edn, (eds V.T. deVita, S. Hellman and S.A. Rosenberg), J.B. Lippincott, Philadelphia, pp. 994–1021.

Lome, L.G. and Bush, I.M. (1972) Resection of the vena cava for renal cell carcinoma: an experimental study. *Journal of Urology*, **107**, 717–19.

McDonald, M.W. (1982) Current therapy for renal cell carcinoma. *Journal of Urology*, **127**, 211–17.

McNichols, D.W., Segua, J.W. and de Weerd, J.H. (1981) Renal cell carcinoma: longterm survival and late recurrence. *Journal of Urology*, **126**, 17–23.

Marburger, M, Pugh, R.C.B., Auvert, J. *et al.* (1981) Conservative surgery of renal carcinoma: the EIRSS experience. *British Journal of Urology*, **53**, 528–32.

Marshall, F.F. and Powell, K.C. (1982) Lymphadenectomy for renal cell carcinoma: anatomical and therapeutic considerations. *Journal of Urology*, **128**, 677–81.

Marshall, F.F. and Reitz, B.A. (1986) Technique for removal of renal cell carcinoma with suprahepatic vena caval tumor thrombus. *Urologic Clinics of North America*, **13**, 551–7.

Marshall, F.F., Taxy, J.B., Fishman, E.K. and Chang, R. (1986) The feasibility of surgical enucleation for renal cell carcinoma. *Journal of Urology*, **135**, 231–4.

Mebust, W.K., Weigel, J.W., Lee, K.R. *et al.* (1984) Renal cell carcinoma – angioinfarction. *Journal of Urology*, **131**, 231–5.

Middleton, R.G. and Presto, A.J. (1973) Radical thoracoabdominal nephrectomy for renal cell carcinoma. *Journal of Urology*, **110**, 36–7.

Mostofi, F.K. (1979) Tumours of the renal parenchyma, in *Kidney Disease – Present Status*, International Academy of Pathology Monograph, vol. 20, (ed. J. Churg), Williams and Wilkins, Baltimore, pp. 356–412

Muss, H.B., Costanzi, J.J., Leavitt, R. *et al.* (1987) Recombinant alpha interferon in renal cell carcinoma: a randomized trial of two routes of administration. *Journal of Clinical Oncology*, **5**, 1083.

Novick, A.C., Zincke, H., Neves, R.J. and Topley, H.M. (1986) Surgical enucleation for renal cell carcinoma. *Journal of Urology*, **135**, 235–8.

Penn, I. (1977) Transplantation in patients with primary renal malignancies. *Transplantation*, **24**, 424–34.

Pontonnier, F., Plante, P., Mourlan, D. and Vidal, R. (1980) Embolisation renale dans le traitement des tumeurs du rein. *Annals of Urology*, **14**, 243–7.

Pritchett, T.R., Lieskovsky, G. and Skinner, D.G. (1986) Extension of renal cell carcinoma into the vena cava: clinical review and surgical approach. *Journal of Urology*, **135**, 460–4.

Rafla, L.P. (1970) Renal cell carcinoma; natural history and results of treatment. *Cancer*, **25**, 26–40.

Reese, A.J.M. and Winstanley, D.P. (1958) The small tumour-like lesions of the kidney. *British Journal of Cancer*, **12**, 507–16.

Robey, E.L. and Schellhammer, P.F. (1986) The adrenal gland and renal cell carcinoma: is ipsilateral adrenalectomy a necessary component of radical nephrectomy? *Journal of Urology*, **135**, 453–5.

Robson, C.J., Churchill, B.M. and Anderson, W. (1969) The results of radical nephrectomy for renal cell carcinoma. *Journal of Urology*, **101**, 297–301.

Rosenberg, S.A., Lotze, M.T., Yang, J.C. *et al.* (1989) Experience with the use of high dose interleukin-2 in the treatment of 652 cancer patients. *Annals of Surgery*, **210**, 474–85.

Saitoh, H. (1981) Distant metastasis of renal adenocarcinoma. *Cancer*, **48**, 1487–91.

Seljelid, R. and Ericsson, J.L.E. (1965) Electron microscopic observations on specialisations of the cell surface in renal clear cell carcinoma. *Laboratory Investigation*, **14**, 435–47.

Singsaas, M.W., Chopp, R.T. and Mendez, R. (1979) Preoperative renal embolisation as adjunct to radical nephrectomy. *Urology*, **14**, 1–5.

Skinner, D.G., Colvin, R.B., Vermillion, C.D. *et al.* (1971) Diagnosis and management of renal cell carcinoma. *Cancer*, **28**, 1165–77.

Skinner D.G., Pfister, R.F. and Colvin, R. (1972) Extension of renal cell carcinoma into the vena cava: the rationale for aggressive surgical management. *Journal of Urology*, **107**, 711–16.

Skinner, D.G. and de Kernion, J.B. (1978) Clinical manifestations and treatment of renal parenchymal tumours, in *Genitourinary Cancer*, W.B. Saunders, Philadelphia, pp. 107–3.

Syrjanen, K. and Hjelt L. (1978) Ultra structural characteristics in relation to the light microscopic grading. *Scandinavian Journal of Urology and Nephrology*, **12**, 57–65.

Teasdale, C., Kirk, D., Jeans, W.D. *et al.* (1982) Arterial embolisation in renal carcinoma: a useful procedure? *British Journal of Urology*, **54**, 616–19.

Thompson, I.M. and Peek, M. (1988) Improvement in survival of patients with renal cell carcinoma – the role of the serendipitously detected tumour. *Journal of Urology*, **25**, 487–90.

Tolia, B.M. and Whitmore, W.F. (1975) Solitary metastasis from renal cell carcinoma. *Journal of Urology*, **114**, 836–8.

van der werf Messing, B. (1973) Carcinoma of the kidney. *Cancer*, **32**, 1056–61.

Wallace, A.C. and Nairn, R.C. (1972) Renal tubular antigens in kidney tumours. *Cancer*, **29**, 977–81.

Wallace, S., Chuang, V.P., Swanson, D. *et al.* (1981) Embolisation of renal carcinoma. *Radiology*, **138**, 563–7.

Wickham, J.E.A. (1975) Conservative renal surgery for adeno carcinoma. The place of bench surgery. *British Journal of Urology*, **47**, 25–36.

Wickham, J.E.A., Fernando, A.R., Hendry, W.F. *et al.* (1978) Inosine: clinical results of ischaemic renal surgery. *British Journal of Urology*, **50**, 465–8.

Woodhouse, C.R.J. (1987) Renal carcinoma, in *Scientific Basis of Urology*, (ed. A.R. Mundy), Churchill Livingstone, Edinburgh, pp. 311–25.

Woodhouse, C.R.J., Hendry, W.F. and Bloom, H.J.G. (1985) Renal carcinoma, in *Textbook of Genito Urinary Surgery*, (eds H.N. Whitfield and W.F. Hendry), Churchill Livingstone, Edinburgh, pp. 945–61.

Yoffey, J.M. and Courtice, F.C. (1970) Lymph flow from regional lymphatics, in *Lymphatics, Lymph and the Lymphomyeloid Complex*, Academic Press, London, pp. 236–50.

Zingg, E.J. (1993) Operations for renal tumour, in *Rob and Smiths Operative Surgery – Genito-urinary surgery*, 5th edn, (ed. H.N. Whitfield), Butterworth-Heinemann, Oxford, pp. 68–89.

EARLY BREAST CANCER

36

Nigel P.M. Sacks and Meron E. Pitcher

36.1 INCIDENCE

The lifetime incidence of breast cancer in the UK is 1 in 12, with an estimated 26 000 new cases per year and 17 000 deaths from the disease annually. Internationally, the highest rates are found in Western Europe, North America and Australia, with much lower rates in China, Japan and in most parts of the Third World (Table 36.1).

36.2 AETIOLOGY

The aetiology of breast cancer is essentially unknown although several risk factors are well established. A family history of breast cancer, especially if of early onset or bilateral in first degree relatives, is highly significant. Approximately 15% of those with breast cancer will have a positive family history, and it has recently been shown that a small percentage of these may be due to the inheritance of a 'cancer-predisposing gene' (Eeles and Ponder, 1992). Typical features are of a large number of affected cases within the one family, an association with other cancers (especially of endometrium, ovary and colon), early onset (before age 50) and bilateral disease. A number of Li–Fraumeni syndrome families, who develop sarcomas, brain tumours, leukaemia, adrenocortical tumours and early onset breast cancers, have been found to express a mutant form of p53, a tumour suppressor gene on the short arm of chromosome 17p.

Endocrine factors are clearly implicated (Table 36.2), as early menarche (< 12 years) and late menopause are associated with an increased risk; early pregnancy (< 20 years is protective and increasing age of first full term pregnancy increases the risk of subsequent breast cancer. Recently a study by Kalache *et al.* (1993) has suggested that age at last full term pregnancy may be more important. Use of the oral contraceptive pill does not appear to increase the risk except in nulliparous women with prolonged usage (McPherson *et al.*, 1987). Hormone replacement therapy with unopposed oestrogen may marginally increase the risk after 10 years use, although the evidence is inconclusive (Van Leeuwen and Rookus, 1989; Steinberg *et al.*, 1991),

Table 36.1 Age standardized incidence and mortality from breast cancer (1988) per 100 000 women

Country	Incidence	Mortality
USA	70–90	33.5
Sweden	60.7	18.1
UK	55.0	53.4
Australia	50.2	28.4
Japan	22.0	9.2

Modified from Parkin, 1989.

Table 36.2   Risk factors for the development of breast cancer

	High risk	*Low risk*	*Relative risk*
Age at 1st full term pregnancy	> 30	< 20	2–4
Age at menarche	Early	Late	1–1.9
Age at menopause	Late	Early	1–1.9
Family history premenopausal bilateral breast cancer	Yes	No	> 4
Past history breast cancer	Yes	No	> 4
Any 1st degree relative with breast cancer	Yes	No	2–4
Biopsy showing atypical hyperplasia	Yes	No	> 4

Modified from Kelsey and Berkowitz, 1988.

but there is little information about the breast cancer incidence in women on prolonged combined oestrogen-progesterone HRT (Nachtigall *et al.*, 1992).

Previous benign breast disease is not a proven risk factor, unless the previous biopsy showed hyperplasia with atypia, papillomatosis or lobular carcinoma-*in-situ* (LCIS). Ionizing radiation, in survivors of atomic bomb explosions, and fluoroscopy for TB have been associated with increased risk. Diagnostic X-rays are rarely of sufficient cumulative dose to constitute a risk (Evans *et al.*, 1986). Obesity is a frequent co-existent problem and postmenopausal women who are overweight are at higher risk (Kushi *et al.*, 1992), however it has not been possible to establish a consistent link between dietary fat intake and breast cancer nor dietary fibre and breast cancer risk (Willett *et al.*, 1992).

The Royal Marsden Hospital is actively recruiting women at high risk of breast cancer into a randomized prevention study giving them tamoxifen or placebo for 5 years and several other centres overseas have started similar prevention programmes (Powles *et al.*, 1990).

36.3   PATHOLOGY

The commonest type (70%) of breast cancer is invasive ductal carcinoma (Table 36.3). Macroscopically it feels hard and is gritty to

Table 36.3   Histological types of invasive breast cancer

Ductal (not otherwise specified, NOS)	70%
Lobular	15%
Tubular	5%
Medullary	
Mucinous	10%
Adenoid cystic	

cut. Microscopically it can have a variable appearance with glands, sheets of cells or islands of cells and there may be associated pre-invasive or *in situ* carcinoma. Grading into poor, moderate and well differentiated tumours on the basis of tubule formation, nuclear pleomorphism and mitotic count has prognostic significance but is subject to observer variability (Gilchrist *et al.*, 1985).

Invasive lobular carcinoma (10–15%) lacks the intense stromal response that gives ductal cancers their hardness and this can make them both difficult to feel and to see on mammography. It has a tendency to diffuse infiltration which can make it macroscopically ill defined; it may be multicentric or bilateral and is often (60%) associated with *in situ* lobular carcinoma.

Tubular carcinomas are macroscopically well defined, and microscopically have prominent tubule formation which must comprise at least 75% of the tumour. They are well differentiated and have an excellent prognosis.

Medullary carcinomas are also circumscribed, contain a uniform population of cells with poorly differentiated nuclei, and with a prominent lymphocytic infiltrate, are of low grade and have a better prognosis. Mucinous or colloid carcinomas, especially in the pure form, are also a low grade malignancy. These 'special' types of breast cancer, tubular, medullary and colloid, are commonly screen detected and have a good prognosis.

In situ carcinoma of the breast may be ductal, lobular or mixed and by definition there is a proliferation of abnormal epithelial cells which do not invade the basement membrane. Ductal carcinoma *in situ* (DCIS) may form a palpable mass in the breast but is more commonly found as a result of mammographic screening. Histologically DCIS shows a heterogeneous pattern and within a single case, several architectural subtypes may be found. The comedo subtype has a solid growth pattern with large pleomorphic cells and central necrosis and is associated with frequent overexpression of the C-*erb*B2 oncogene. The cribriform and micropapillary subtypes usually have smaller, more evenly placed hyperchromatic cells. Accurate correlation between histological appearance and clinical behaviour are still imperfect. DCIS is regarded as premalignant on the basis of its frequent association with invasive carcinoma (45%) (Schnitt *et al.*, 1984); retrospective studies have shown a high incidence of invasive carcinoma developing at the site of previous biopsy for DCIS (Rosen *et al.*, 1980; Page *et al.*, 1982).

LCIS is usually an incidental finding as it is typically impalpable and undetectable mammographically. It is usually diagnosed premenopausally, multicentric foci may be present in up to 90% of cases and contralateral LCIS is found in 25% when a mirror image biopsy is performed (Rosen *et al.*, 1979). It is generally regarded as a risk factor (relative risk increased 10 fold) rather than a premalignant condition because invasive cancer, when it develops, can occur in either breast with equal frequency and be of either ductal or lobular type. Approximately 25% of women with LCIS will develop invasive breast cancer within 20 years from diagnosis, giving an estimated cumulative annual risk of 1% per year.

Breast cancer commonly metastasizes to ipsilateral axillary nodes and tumour deposits are found in up to 50% of symptomatic cases at presentation. Internal mammary nodes are rarely involved in isolation and disease in the supraclavicular lymph node group indicates advanced local disease.

Common sites for distant metastasis for ductal carcinoma are bone, lung, liver and brain. Lobular carcinoma may spread to atypical sites such as the meninges or the serosal surfaces of pleura and peritoneum.

36.4 PRESENTATION

Most patients with breast cancer present with a lump in the breast. Less commonly localized discomfort, nipple discharge, skin deformity, an axillary node mass or Paget's disease of the nipple may be the presenting features. With the advent of mammographic screening asymptomatic cancers are being increasingly diagnosed.

Breast lumps in premenopausal women are most commonly due to benign disease. Fibroadenomas are smooth, regular, mobile swellings most common in the 20–30 year old age group. Breast cysts may be solitary or multiple, and typically present as a hard, mobile, often painful lump of recent onset; these are often seen in women in their forties and are rare after the menopause. Carcinomas can mimic benign breast disease but classically they feel hard and irregular. They may cause localized skin dimpling or oedema, retraction of the nipple, and in advanced stages can ulcerate through the skin or invade pectoralis major and/or the chest wall.

Localized breast discomfort or a 'pricking pain' can be a symptom of breast cancer (McKinna *et al.*, 1992). Nipple discharge is a rare presenting feature of carcinoma but a blood stained or serous discharge, particularly from a single duct or segment of the breast, warrants investigation and duct exploration.

Screening mammography can detect impalpable and asymptomatic cancers. Those detected by screening are more likely to be node negative (65%), small (50% < 15 mm) and more likely to be of a special good prognostic type, well differentiated or *in situ* cancers. Population screening of women over 50 has consistently been shown to reduce their breast cancer mortality at 10 years follow-up by up to 30% although screening younger women has failed to show a significant reduction in mortality (Day, 1991).

36.5   INVESTIGATIONS

36.5.1   MAMMOGRAPHY

Mammography can detect the majority of breast cancers (Figure 36.1) although some 10% of clinically diagnosable cancers will not be seen, i.e. a normal mammogram does not exclude breast cancer. Abnormalities are most easily detected in the atrophic postmenopausal breast, but can still be found in the denser breasts of premenopausal women, although with less sensitivity (Bennett *et al.*, 1991; Yelland *et al.*, 1991).

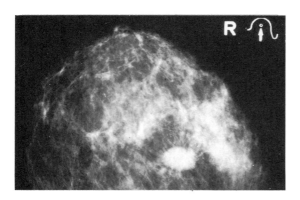

Figure 36.1 Mammogram showing an impalpable screen-detected carcinoma (biopsy proven).

The typical radiological features of a breast cancer include:

1. A mass of high density with peripheral spiculations
2. Architectural distortion
3. Irregular clumped, linear or branching calcification
4. Parenchymal asymmetry present on more than one view.

In women with a diagnosis of breast cancer, mammography is essential to establish the extent of the disease, the presence or absence of multifocality or a contralateral cancer.

36.5.2   ULTRASOUND

Ultrasound, although not useful as a screening tool, can be helpful in the diagnosis of breast cancer.

Cancers are typically seen as solid, irregular and vascular; peripheral enhancement and distal shadowing may be present. Ultrasound is not as sensitive or specific as mammography but it is particularly useful in younger women whose dense breasts can make mammographic interpretation difficult. Ultrasound can categorize palpable masses which are indeterminate mammographically or mammographic lesions which are impalpable. Ultrasound guided fine needle aspiration cytology improves accuracy of technique.

36.5.3   FINE NEEDLE ASPIRATION CYTOLOGY

Fine needle aspiration cytology not only provides a minimally invasive method of accurately establishing the diagnosis in the majority of breast cancer cases but also allows the definitive treatment of cancer as a planned operation. The technique is simple and easily learnt. For palpable masses the skin is swabbed, the lesion immobilized with one hand while the other guides a 23 gauge needle on a syringe into the lump. Negative pressure is applied and the needle repositioned within the lump several times before releasing the negative pressure and with-drawing the needle. If solid the contents of the needle are smeared on a glass slide and allowed to dry. If cystic and there is no resid-ual mass the fluid should be discarded unless it is blood stained. If the lesion is impalpable then aspiration cytology can be performed under ultrasound control or using a mammo-graphic stereotactic grid.

Our cytopathologist reports the specimen as follows:

Category	Definition	Risk of carcinoma (Powles *et al.*, 1991)
C0	No cells	12%
C1	Inadequate sample	3%
C2	Benign	7%
C3	Atypical cells, probably benign	80%
C4	Suspicious of malignancy	92%
C5	Malignant	100%

The most common cause of a false-negative diagnosis is missing the lesion or an acellular aspirate. Tubular or lobular carcinomas can be hard to diagnose and *in situ* carcinomas cannot be distinguished from invasive carci-nomas by cytology alone.

36.5.4   CORE BIOPSY

Tru-cut or core biopsy performed under local anaesthetic can preoperatively accurately confirm the diagnosis, especially if cytology is unavailable; its use has been made easier by the biopsy gun.

36.5.5   LOCALIZATION BIOPSY

Impalpable mammographically suspicious lesions often require localization biopsy for histological diagnosis. After confirming the abnormality on craniocaudal and lateral mammograms, the skin is marked and under local anaesthetic a hollow needle is placed ad-jacent to the abnormality. Its site adjacent to the area of interest is confirmed and either a hook-wire is introduced at that site or a dye injected along the track to enable the surgeon to accurately excise that area. Confirmation that the radiological abnormality has been excised by specimen X-ray is essential before this diagnostic operation is considered complete.

36.6   STAGING

We do not routinely screen patients for the presence of occult metastatic disease. This is because in patients with operable breast cancer the yield is very low (< 1%) and treat-ment in metastatic disease is for symptom control only as it does not prolong and may even shorten survival. Occasionally a decision about local treatment to the breast would be influenced by the presence of metastases (e.g. large or locally advanced primary or bulky axillary nodes) and under these circum-stances we perform full blood count liver function tests, liver ultrasound, chest X-ray and a bone scan.

The TNM (Tumour Nodes Metastasis) classification for breast cancer has been widely used (Table 36.4) but it has several limitations when applied to breast cancer (Barr and Baum, 1992).

Although staging classifications are important for comparing results between centres for practical purposes of patient management, breast cancer can be staged as being:

1. Confined to the breast
2. Having pathologically involved ipsilateral nodes
3. Being locally advanced
4. Having metastatic disease.

Table 36.4   TNM (Tumour Node Metastasis) classification for breast cancer

T1	Tumour < 2 cm
	a. Without fixation to underlying pectoralis fascia or muscle
	b. Fixed to pectoralis fascia or muscle
T2	Tumour between 2 and 5 cm – a and b
T3	Tumour > 5 cm
T4	Tumour of any size fixed to chest wall (i.e. ribs, intercostal muscles, serratus anterior) or skin
	a. Chest wall
	b. Oedema, ulceration of the skin of the breast or satellite skin nodules
	c. a and b
	d. Inflammatory
	Skin dimpling or nipple retraction does not affect classification
N0	Nodes impalpable
N1	Mobile nodes
	a. Clinically uninvolved
	b. Clinically involved
N2	Nodes involved and fixed
N3	Supraclavicular or infraclavicular nodes or arm oedema
M0	No distant metastases
MI	Metastases present

Stage I	T1	N0/NIa	M0
Stage II	T0	NIb	M0
	T1	N0, Ia, Ib	M0
	T2	N0, Ia, Ib	M0
Stage III	T1	N2	M0
	T2	N2	M0
	T3	N0/1/2	M0
Stage IV	T4	any N/M	
	Any T N3	Any M	
	Any T/N	M1	

36.7   PROGNOSTIC FACTORS

The most important prognostic factor in breast cancer is the presence of and the number of involved axillary nodes, with survival decreasing with increasing number of involved nodes. Haagensen's experience with Halstead mastectomy alone (Haagensen and Bodian, 1984) showed that patients with between one and three involved axillary nodes had a 10 year survival rate of 44–70%; between four and seven nodes 36–43% and those with eight or more nodes 16–19%. Similar results have been reported from the Milan group (Cascinelli *et al.*, 1987).

The number of involved nodes increases with the size of the tumour but it has been shown that the size of the primary tumour is also an important independent prognostic factor. Those patients with histologically negative axillary nodes and tumours 1 cm or less in diameter had a 14% chance of recurrence at 20 years whereas those with tumours of 1–2 cm had a 31% chance of recurrence (Fisher *et al.*, 1969).

Histological grade is another very useful prognostic factor. If tumours are graded into three grades on the basis of tubule formation, nuclear pleomorphism and mitotic count then the survival is closely related to degree of differentiation. On this basis Elston and Ellis (1991) reported the 16 year survival in grade I tumours to be 90%, 55% in grade II and 48% in grade III. However, concordance of histological grade between observers has proved to be a problem (Gilchrist *et al.*, 1985).

Oestrogen and progesterone receptors are nuclear and cytosolic proteins which bind and transfer the appropriate steroid molecule into the nucleus to exert its specific effect. Receptor levels can be determined on fresh biopsies by enzyme linked immunochemical assay and immunoradiometric assay. Oestrogen receptor positive tumours (50% total) are more common in the elderly, are more likely to respond to hormone manipulation, especially if they are also progesterone receptor positive, and may have a better prognosis than hormone receptor negative tumours, of which only 10% will respond to hormone manipulation.

Indices of rapid tumour proliferation include S phase fraction, thymidine labelling index, tumour ploidy and Ki67 immunostaining. The protein product of the oncogene C-*erb*B2, epidermal growth factor receptor and cathepsin D are also associated with a worse prognosis, possibly independent of nodal status. These tumour parameters are still largely experimental and we do not use them routinely as yet for clinical decision making.

36.8 MANAGEMENT

36.8.1 LOBULAR CARCINOMA *IN-SITU* (LCIS)

Women with LCIS have an increased risk of developing breast cancer, estimated at 1–3% annually or a lifetime risk of 17–31%. If cancer develops, it is as likely to be ductal as lobular and may occur in either breast in any quadrant. Wide local excision is inappropriate as the condition is usually multifocal. To be curative, mastectomy with or without immediate reconstruction should be bilateral, but we would consider this to be overtreatment in the majority of cases. LCIS is best regarded as a marker of increased risk of breast cancer; patients should be observed clinically, with the addition of regular mammography. The use of tamoxifen in this group of patients is

currently the subject of a randomized clinical trial (EORTC) and the presence of LCIS is an eligibility criterion for the Royal Marsden Hospital tamoxifen prevention trial.

36.8.2 DUCTAL CARCINOMA *IN-SITU* (DCIS)

The management of DCIS currently is controversial and is likely to remain so until the results of the current UK CCCR trial are available (Table 36.5). Total mastectomy, the traditional treatment for extensive DCIS, is certainly effective. It treats any multifocal disease or occult invasion but may represent overtreatment for many women with localized DCIS as the prognosis with all types of treatment has been shown to be excellent.

Treatment by excision alone does have a high local recurrence rate, up to 63% at 9 year follow-up in an early Royal Marsden series (Price *et al.*, 1990) with half the reported recurrences occurring as invasive disease. Lower rates of recurrence (10%) have been possible using strict criteria for breast conservation (Lagios *et al.*, 1989); these are that the DCIS must have been mammographically detected, less than 25 mm in maximal dimension and adequately excised on both histological and mammographic criteria. Radiotherapy does seem to provide some protection against local recurrence, giving overall recurrence rates of about 10% with half recurring as invasive cancer (Solin *et al.*, 1991), although radiotherapy is not without risks and survival is not affected. Treatment of the axilla is not indicated because the incidence of involved nodes (from unrecognized microinvasive disease) is so low (< 2%) that one cannot justify the associated morbidity.

The role of tamoxifen and radiotherapy is currently under study in the UK CCCR/DCIS trial. As the incidence of contralateral invasive cancers is lowered in breast cancer patients on adjuvant tamoxifen, part of this effect may be due to an action on *in situ* disease.

Table 36.5   Reduction in recurrences and mortality in randomized trials of adjuvant ovarian ablation, tamoxifen and chemotherapy

Type of therapy	Reduction in risk of recurrence (% ± SE)	Reduction in risk of mortality (% ± SE)
Oophorectomy alone	30 ± 9	28 ± 9
Oophorectomy and chemotherapy	21 ± 9	19 ± 11
Tamoxifen		
< 50 years old	12 ± 4	6 ± 5*
50–59 years old	28 ± 3	19 ± 4
60–69 years old	29 ± 3	17 ± 4
> 70 years old	28 ± 5	21 ± 6
ER negative [†]	13 ± 4	11 ± 5
ER positive	32 ± 3	21 ± 3
Prolonged polychemotherapy		
< 50 years old	36 ± 5	25 ± 6
50–59 years old	29 ± 5	13 ± 7
60–69 years old	20 ± 5	10 ± 6

Source The Early Breast Triallists' Collaborative Group, 1992.
[*] Not significant; all others highly significant.
[†] Negative < 10 fmol/mg, positive > 10 fmol/mg.

36.8.3   INVASIVE CARCINOMA OF THE BREAST

Our treatment for early invasive breast cancer is generally multidisciplinary with a combination of surgery, radiotherapy and chemotherapy (Sacks and Baum, 1993). We define early breast cancer as that which is potentially curable by surgery. This excludes those with obvious distant metastases, or locally advanced cases with inflammatory breast cancer, muscle or chest wall fixation, extensive skin ulceration or oedema, arm oedema or fixed axillary nodes.

The halsteadian theory of centripetal dissemination of breast cancer, growing locally, then spreading to regional lymphatics and ultimately by the blood to form distant metastases was the rationale behind the radical mastectomy. By removing the breast, pectoralis major and axillary lymph nodes, it was hoped that distant metastases could be prevented. Despite such disfiguring surgery, many women still developed metastatic disease although local tumour control was excellent. Treatment of tumours at an earlier stage should, according to this theory, reduce overall mortality, there being a critical size of cancer that would be curable by surgery alone. This may well be true for DCIS, *in situ* carcinomas with minimal invasion and for certain small or well differentiated special type carcinomas. However, some breast cancers, which are clinically and even mammographically occult, present with axillary or distant metastases and 30% of women with node negative cancers eventually relapse.

The prime role of surgery now is to provide optimal tumour control in the breast and axilla. In achieving this a large proportion of women will achieve a personal cure, i.e. lifelong palliation, dying of another cause. Adjuvant chemotherapy or hormone therapy is usually given in addition to treat undetectable micro-metastases which are presumed to be the cause of later distant relapse (see below).

36.9 SURGERY

Lumpectomy or simple excision of the primary tumour in the absence of radiotherapy is associated with a high incidence of local recurrence. Rates vary from 15% to 40% (Greening *et al.*, 1988) with follow-up of 3–10 years and in the NSABPB-06 study (Fisher *et al.*, 1989) women with tumours of 4 cm or less in diameter who had clear histological margins and who did not have breast radiotherapy had a 39% incidence of recurrence in the treated breast at 8 years follow-up; this was reduced to 10% by the use of postoperative irradiation to the breast. This study required only minimal excision margins, preoperative mammography was not required, and 10% had histologically involved margins. A Swedish study of 381 carefully selected patients with unifocal tumours up to 2.0 cm in diameter treated by excision of the tumour, pectoral fascia and axillary node dissection, had much lower rates of local recurrence after a 3 year follow-up period. For inclusion in this study pathologically the disease had to be unifocal, with no *in situ* disease closer than 20 mm from the tumour edge, have histologically clear margins and pathologically negative nodes. Local recurrence was 2.9% with the use of radiotherapy and 7.6% without; overall and distant disease free survival were not significantly different in either group (Uppsala-Orebro Breast Cancer Study Group, 1990).

With the demonstration that wider excision reduces local recurrence this technique was extended to that termed a quadrantectomy – excising the breast lump down to and including the pectoralis fascia with a wider margin of surrounding normal breast. Quadrantectomy aims for a 2–3 cm clearance by resection of the quadrant of the breast centred on the cancer and is our preferred technique for breast conservation, whereas wide local excision aims for a 1 cm margin. Veronesi's study from Milan (Veronesi *et al.*, 1990a) reported a breast recurrence rate of 3% at 10 years (11/352) in women with cancers less than 2 cm in diameter treated by quadrantectomy axillary dissection and radiotherapy (QUART). Comparing a 1 cm margin and quadrantectomy (both followed by radiotherapy) for tumours < 2.5 cm, they reported local recurrence rates of 7% and 2% respectively at 5 years (Veronesi *et al.*, 1990b) with equivalent survival.

Modified radical mastectomy (MRM) provides no better local control than that obtained with complete local excision of the tumour supplemented by radiotherapy to the breast for cancers up to 4 cm in size. The NSABPB-06 study (Fisher *et al.*, 1989) comparing women who underwent MRM with those treated by lumpectomy axillary dissection and radiotherapy showed that the disease free survival (58 ± 2.6% and 54 ± 2.4%), distant disease free survival (65 ± 2.6% and 62 ± 2.3%) and overall survival (17 ± 2.6% and 71 ± 2.4%) at 8 years follow-up to be the same. Similarly Veronesi's study showed no significant difference in outcome between women treated by Halstead mastectomy or the QUART regimen.

Mastectomy however still has a definite role in the treatment of breast cancer: as the primary treatment of multifocal tumours; those which are centrally situated; those which are large relative to the breast size or where there is extensive adjacent *in situ* disease (EIC). Mastectomy is often necessary if the cancer recurs in a previously conserved breast, especially if the breast has been irradiated. Some patients when given a choice prefer mastectomy to breast conservation, but there is no definite evidence that more conservative approaches to breast resection are associated with a significantly lower incidence of psychosexual morbidity (Fallowfield *et al.*, 1990). Reconstruction of the breast with a submuscular tissue expander or a myocutaneous flap (latissimus dorsi or rectus abdominis) can be performed at the same time with excellent results, minimal morbidity and no interference with subsequent treatment or follow-up.

The axilla is the principal site of regional metastatic disease with up to 50% of women with operable breast cancer having nodal metastases at presentation (Henderson, 1990). Clinical assessment of the axilla is unreliable with false-negative and -positive rates of 25–30%. Imaging the axillary nodes remains in experimental stages although there have been some promising results with radiolabelled monoclonal antibodies (Tjandra *et al.*, 1989). Uncontrolled axillary disease causes great distress with arm swelling, pain and loss of function because of brachial plexus involvement and it should be prevented if at all possible.

Management of the axilla in patients with operable breast cancer is controversial (Sacks *et al.*, 1992). A well performed axillary dissection is effective in preventing axillary relapse (< 2%), and provides valuable prognostic information which may greatly influence decisions about the indication and type of adjuvant systemic therapy.

Axillary radiotherapy is also effective at preventing axillary relapse, but the pathological staging information from the nodes is lost and it is not as effective when there is obvious axillary disease. Both surgery and radiotherapy to the axilla are not without side-effects: arm swelling and shoulder stiffness can occur with either and brachial plexus neuropathy and tumour induction are fortunately rare complications of irradiation. Objective difference in limb volume occurs in up to 25% after treatment of the axilla with surgery or radiotherapy (Kissin *et al.*, 1986), although symptomatic swelling is much less common. The combination of axillary clearance and radiotherapy is associated with a very high (40%) incidence of late arm swelling.

Axillary sampling is practised in some centres and its advocates state that this method (biopsy of at least four axillary nodes) can reliably stage the axilla and enable considered decisions to be made about further axillary treatment (i.e. radiotherapy if the sample is positive) or the need for adjuvant systemic therapy. We do not recommend sampling because an adequate number of nodes is not consistently obtained, residual axillary disease may be left which can cause uncontrolled local symptoms, there is no good evidence that lesser surgery is associated with fewer complications and we believe the combination of axillary surgery and radiotherapy should be avoided.

36.10 RADIOTHERAPY

In patients with early breast cancer radiotherapy is used to reduce the rate of local recurrence in the breast following breast conserving surgery. Factors which are associated with higher local recurrence rates include involved histological margins, large primary tumour, involved axillary nodes, the presence of extensive *in situ* disease and young age. Radiation does not influence survival but as discussed above it does reduce recurrence rate in the treated breast four fold. However some women will never recur locally, and it can be asked whether it is justifiable to submit all women treated by conservative surgery to radiation. Radiotherapy can make the detection of local recurrence more difficult and makes further successful conservative surgery unlikely. Possible long term side-effects, such as myocardial infarction in left sided cancers (Rutquist and Johansson, 1990), and the very rare radiation induced second tumours and sarcomas must be considered.

Our standard treatment policy at present dictates that women treated conservatively should have the breast irradiated with 50 Gy fractionated over 5 weeks with a boost to the tumour bed. Clinical trials of women considered at low risk of recurrence (clear margins, node negative disease and without extensive *in situ* disease) are in progress and will hopefully define a group of patients who can avoid irradiation.

We do not use prophylactic chest wall radiotherapy routinely following mastectomy as it has no impact on survival, although it is indicated in patients adjudged to be at very high risk of chest wall recurrence, e.g. those with positive axillary nodes, muscle invasion, incomplete excision margins or locally advanced tumours.

36.11 ADJUVANT TREATMENT

Treatment confined to the primary tumour will fail to affect any subclinical micrometastases already present at the time of diagnosis. The rationale of adjuvant therapy is to alter the natural history of these metastases, thus increasing both disease free and overall survival.

Both hormonal manipulation and systemic chemotherapy have been subject to intensive study and the following summary is based largely on the 10 year meta-analysis of 75 000 women in 133 randomized adjuvant therapy trials by the EBTCG (Early Breast Triallists Collaborative Group, 1992).

36.11.1 ADJUVANT HORMONAL TREATMENT

(a). Tamoxifen

Tamoxifen had originally been regarded as a pure antioestrogen but it is now known that it as significant agonist properties and minimal side-effects, consisting of hot flushes and vaginal discharge in a minority of patients. Not only does tamoxifen reduce serum cholesterol levels (Bruning *et al.*, 1988) but it also prevents bone demineralization (Fentiman *et al.*, 1988). By stimulating production of tumour suppressor cytokines such as insulin like growth factor I and transforming growth factor beta (TGFbeta), it has been shown that its mechanism of action may not be only via the oestrogen receptor (Colletta *et al.*, 1990).

In the overview meta-analysis all women randomized to adjuvant tamoxifen regardless of age, nodal or menopausal status benefited

by increased disease free and overall survival compared with controls at 10 years, with 58.5% randomized to tamoxifen alive compared with 52.6% of controls, a reduction in the odds of death of 17% (Figure 36.2). As the rate of relapse and death is greater for node positive than node negative women the benefits of adjuvant tamoxifen are larger, with an absolute survival benefit over controls of 8% at 10 years for node positive patients compared with 3.5% for node negative.

The benefit of adjuvant tamoxifen is most noticeable for women older than 50, especially for recurrence free survival. Subset analysis showed that the advantage was not solely confined to those with oestrogen receptor positive tumours as those whose tumours were oestrogen receptor negative still experienced a significant benefit. In addition, those

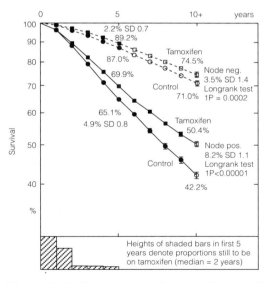

Figure 36.2, Ten-year survival in all tamoxifen trials for all 29 892 women randomized, subdivided by nodal status (13 910 node negative, 16 982 node positive, by axillary dissection or sampling). (Reproduced from EBTCG, *Lancet*, 1992, **339**, with permission.) Key – actuarial survival estimate and SD: ■ ⬜, allocated tamoxifen; ● ⬤, allocated control.

on adjuvant tamoxifen had a 30% reduction in the incidence of subsequent contralateral breast cancer (2.0% control vs 1.3% tamoxifen). The optimum dose and duration of its use is still being determined. We currently use 20 mg/day for at least 2 years with patients randomized at that stage to stop or continue to 5 years.

(b)   Ovarian ablation

Permanent ovarian ablation can be achieved by surgery or radiotherapy and was also shown by the EBCTG to increase the odds of recurrence free survival and overall survival in women under 50 years of age by 30%. At 15 years 42.3% of controls were alive without recurrence, compared with 52.9% of those treated by ovarian ablation. The effect was greater for node positive women, but still reached statistical significance in the node negative group. There was no significant benefit in women older than 50 and it was not possible to study the independent effect of menopausal status.

Surgical and radiation induced castration are permanent whereas luteinizing hormone-releasing hormone (LHRH) agonists inhibit gonadotrophic secretion by the pituitary and result in a fall of plasma oestrogens to castration levels which is reversible on stopping treatment. These agents are currently the subject of further adjuvant clinical trials.

(c)   Adjuvant chemotherapy

In common with the use of cytotoxic chemotherapy in metastatic breast cancer, single agent chemotherapy is less effective then multiple agents, and a prolonged course of treatment (for 6 months) is more effective than single dose or perioperative chemotherapy. However in contrast to experience with metastatic disease, chemotherapy seemed more effective in younger patients (< 50 years) and it provided the same degree of

benefit to that obtained with tamoxifen in those over 50.

In the overview meta-analysis prolonged polychemotherapy was shown to increase recurrence free survival, so that at 10 years 44% are alive and disease free compared with 35.6% of controls, with overall survival of 51.3% in those treated compared with 45.0% for controls (Figure 36.3).

At all ages the benefits of chemotherapy are greater for axillary node positive women and as the risk of relapse and death is higher, the absolute benefit is greater. Overall survival is 46.6% for node positive patients compared with 39.8% for controls. The greater effect is seen in younger women (under 50 years) but even women in their fifties and sixties obtained a significant reduction in the odds of recurrence and death.

Six monthly courses of cyclophosphamide, methotrexate and 5-fluorouracil (CMF) is the

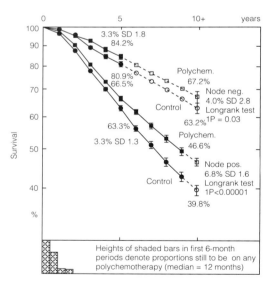

Figure 36.3, Ten-year survival in polychemotherapy trials, subdivided by nodal status (as in Figure 36.2, above). (Reproduced from EBTCG, *Lancet*, 1992, **339**, with permission.) Key – actuarial survival estimate and SD: ■ ⯆, allocated cytotoxic; ● ♀, allocated control.

combination most frequently used and studied. It is generally well tolerated but 10–50% of patients will experience some degree of myelosuppression, nausea, vomiting, alopecia and/or premature ovarian failure. In fact, such drug induced amenorrhoea has been associated with superior disease free survival in some trials leading to speculation that the effects of adjuvant chemotherapy may be related to ovarian suppression.

Node negative patients obtain a very small absolute survival advantage with adjuvant chemotherapy (67.2% vs 63.2% at 10 years). The use of tumour related prognostic factors mentioned above (such as size, differentiation and tumour markers) may help identify the subgroup of node negative women with a poor prognosis who may be more likely to benefit from such treatment, or, conversely, those with such a good prognosis that chemotherapy could be avoided.

36.12 PRIMARY MEDICAL THERAPY (NEOADJUVANT THERAPY)

Initial chemotherapy or endocrine therapy is our routine induction treatment for locally advanced or inflammatory tumours but it has also recently been used experimentally as initial treatment for patients with operable breast cancer. This may enable tumours which would otherwise necessitate mastectomy to be treated more conservatively and enables use of the primary tumour as a marker of response to the treatment. This approach has aroused considerable interest and its exact place is currently the focus of several prospective randomized studies.

Tamoxifen has been used as primary therapy in elderly women for some time, as an alternative to surgery with good response rates, especially in oestrogen receptor positive tumours. However the results of a recent randomized trial showed that surgery as the first treatment followed by adjuvant tamoxifen was associated with less treatment failures than initial tamoxifen therapy alone, so we would advise excision in all but the most frail patients (Bates *et al.*, 1991).

Women with large tumours have a poorer prognosis and although mastectomy usually provides good local control it does not influence the subsequent development of distant metastases. At the Royal Marsden Hospital women who would otherwise require mastectomy or have a locally advanced tumour at presentation are offered initial primary medical treatment with chemotherapy (CMF, or epirubicin, cisplatinum phosphamide and infusional 5FU), and to date we have seen at least a partial clinical response in 95% of patients enabling more conservative surgery to be followed by local radiotherapy. The effect on local recurrence and survival is as yet unknown.

REFERENCES

Barr, L.C. and Baum, M. (1992) Time to abandon TNM staging of breast cancer? *Lancet*, **339**, 915–7.

Bates, T., Riley, D.L., Houghton, J. *et al.* (1991) Breast cancer in elderly women: a cancer research campaign trial comparing treatment with Tamoxifen and optimal surgery with Tamoxifen alone. *British Journal of Surgery*, **73**, 591–4.

Bennett, I.C., Freitas, R. and Fentiman, I.S. (1991) Diagnosis of breast cancer in young women. *Australian and New Zealand Journal of Surgery*, **61**, 284–9.

Bruning, P.F., Bonfrer, J.M.G., Hart, A.A.M. *et al.* (1988) Tamoxifen serum lipoproteins and cardiovascular risk. *British Journal of Cancer*, **58**, 497–99.

Cascinelli, N., Greco, M., Bufalino, R. *et al.* (1987) Prognosis of breast cancer with axillary node metastases after surgical treatment only. *European Journal of Cancer and Clinical Oncology*, **23**, 795–9.

Colletta, A.A., Wakefield, L.M., Howell, F.U. *et al.* (1990) Antioestrogens induce the secretion of active transforming growth factor beta from human fibroblasts. *British Journal of Cancer*, **62**, 405–9.

Day, N.E. (1991) Screening for breast cancer. *British Medical Bulletin*, **47**, 400–15.

Devita, V.T., Hellman, S. and Rosenberg, S.A. (1993) *Cancer: principals and practice of oncology*, 4th edn, Lippincott, Philadelphia.

'The Early Breast Triallists' Collaborative Group (1992) Systemic treatment of early breast cancer by hormonal, cytotoxic or immune therapy. *Lancet*, **339**, 1–15, 71–85.

Eeles, R.A. and Ponder, B.A.J. (1992) Familial breast cancer. *RSM Current Medical Literature Breast and Prostate Cancer*, **5**, (3), 67–70.

Elston, C.W. and Ellis, I.O. (1991) Pathological prognostic factors in breast cancer. The value of histological grade in breast cancer. Experience from a large study with long-term follow up. *Histopathology*, **19**, 403–10.

Evans, J.S., Wennberg, J.E. and McNeil, B.J. (1986) The influence of diagnostic radiography on the incidence of breast cancer and leukaemia. *New England Journal of Medicine*, **315**, 810–15.

Fallowfield, L.J., Hall, A., Maguire, G.P. and Baum, M. (1990) Psychiatric morbidity in breast cancer clinical trials (meeting abstract). *British Journal of Cancer*, **62** (suppl 12), 6.

Fentiman, I.S., Caletti, M., Rodin, A. *et al.* (1988) Bone mineral content of women receiving Tamoxifen for mastalgia. *British Journal of Cancer*, **60**, 262–4.

Fisher, B., Flack, N.H., Bross, D.J. *et al.* (1969) Cancer of the breast; size of neoplasm and prognosis. *Cancer*, **24**, 107–80.

Fisher, B., Redmand, C., Poisson, R. *et al.* (1989) Eight year results of a randomized clinical trial comparing total mastectomy to lumpectomy with or without radiation in the treatment of breast cancer. *New England Journal of Medicine*, **320**, 822–8.

Gilchrist, K.W., Kalish, L., Gould, V.E. *et al.* (1985) Interobserver reproducability of histopathological features in Stage II breast cancer. *Breast Cancer Research and Treatments*, **14**, 91–9.

Greening, W.P., Montgomery, A.W., Gordon, A.B. *et al.* (1988) Quadratic excision and axillary node dissection without radiotherapy: the long-term results of a selective policy in the treatment of stage 1 breast cancer. *European Journal of Surgical Oncology*, **14**, 221–5.

Haagensen, C.D., and Bodian, C. (1984) Personal experience with Halsted's radical mastectomy. *Annals of Surgery*, **199**, 443–50.

Henderson, I.C. (1990) The treatment of metastatic breast carcinoma with adjuvant systemic therapy. *Annals of Oncology*, **1**, 9–11.

Kalache, A., Maguire, A. and Thompson, S.G. (1993) Age at last full term pregnancy and risk of breast cancer. *Lancet*, **341**, 33–6.

Kelsey, J.L. and Berkowitz, G.S. (1988) Breast cancer epidemiology. *Cancer Research*, **48**, 5615–23.

Kushi, L.H., Sellars, T.A., Potter, J.D. *et al.* (1992) Dietary fat and post-menopausal breast cancer. *Journal of the National Cancer Institute*, **84**, 1092–9.

Lagios, M.D., Margolin, F.R., Westdahl, P.R. *et al.* (1989) Mammographically detected duct carcinoma *in situ*. *Cancer*, **63**, 618–24.

McGee, J.O.D., Isaacson, P.G. and Wright, N.A. (1992) Oxford *Textbook of Pathology*, Oxford University Press, Oxford.

McKinna, J.A., Davey, J.B., Walsh, G.A. *et al.* (1992) The early diagnosis of breast cancer – a 20 year experience at the Royal Marsden Hospital. *European Journal of Cancer*, **28A**, 911–16.

McPherson, K., Vessey, N., Neil, A. *et al.* (1987) Early oral contraceptive use and breast cancer: results of another case control study. *British Journal of Cancer*, **56**, 653–60.

Nachtigall, M.J., Smilen, S.W., Nachtigall, R.D. *et al.* (1992) Incidence of breast cancer in a 22-year study of women receiving oestrogen-progestin replacement therapy. *Obstetrics and Gynecology*, **80**, 827–30.

NHSBSP (1992) Cytology Sub-group of the National Co-ordinating Committee for Breast Screening Pathology. Guidelines for Cytology Procedures and Reporting in Breast Cancer Screening. Publication 22.

Page, D.L., Dupont, W.D., Rogers, L.W. *et al.* (1982) Intra ductal carcinoma of the breast: follow up after biopsy only. *Cancer*, **49**, 751–8.

Parkin, D.M. (1989) Cancers of the breast, endometrium, and ovary: geographic correlations. *European Journal of Cancer and Clinical Oncology*, **25**, 1917–25.

Powles, T.J., Tillyer, C.R., Jones, A.L. *et al.* (1990) Prevention of breast cancer with tamoxifen. *European Journal of Cancer*, **26**, 680–4.

Powles, T.J., Trott, P.A., Cherryman, G. *et al.* (1991) Fine needle aspiration cytodiagnosis as a prerequisite for primary medical treatment of breast cancer. *Cytopathology*, **2**, 7–12.

Price, P., Sinnett, H.D., Gusterson, B. *et al.* (1990) Duct carcinoma *in situ*: predictors of local recurrence and progression in patients treated by surgery alone. *British Journal of Cancer*, **61**, 869–72.

Rosen, P.P., Senie, R.T., Farr, G.H. *et al.* (1979) Epidemiology of breast carcinoma: age, menstrual status and exogenous hormone usage in patients with lobular carcinoma *in situ*. *Surgery*, **85**, 219–24.

Rosen, P.P., Brown, D.W. and Kinne, D.E. (1980) Clinical significance of pre-invasive breast carcinoma. *Cancer*, **46**, 919–25.

Rutquist, L.E. and Johansson, H. (1990) Mortality by laterality of the primary tumour among 55 000 breast cancer patients from the Swedish Cancer Registry. *British Journal of Cancer*, **61**, 866–8.

Sacks, N.P.M., Barr, L.C., Allen, S.M. and Baum, M. (1992) The role of axillary dissection in operable breast cancer. *Breast*, **1**, 41–9.

Sacks, N.P.M. and Baum, M. (1993) Primary management of carcinoma of the breast. *Lancet*, **342**, 1402–8.

Schnitt, S.J., Connolly, J.L., Harris, J.R. *et al.* (1984) Pathological predictors of early local recurrence in stage I and II breast cancer treated by primary radiation treatment. *Cancer*, **53**, 1049–57.

Solin, L.J., Recht, A., Fourqet, A. *et al.* (1991) Ten year results of breast conserving surgery and definitive irradiation for intraductal carcinoma (ductal carcinoma *in situ*) of the breast. *Cancer*, **68**, 2337–44.

Steinberg, K.K., Thacker, S.B. *et al.* (1991) Meta-analysis of the effect of oestrogen replacement therapy on the risk of breast cancer. *Journal of the American Medical Association*, **265**, 1985–90.

Tjandra, J.J., Sacks, N.P.M., Russell, I.S. *et al.* (1989) Immunolymphoscintography for the detection of lymph node metastases from breast cancer. *Cancer Research*, **49**, 1600–8.

Uppsala-Orebro Breast Cancer Study Group (1990) Sector resection with or without post operative radiotherapy for stage I breast cancer: a randomized trial. *Journal of the National Cancer Institute*, **82**, 277–82.

Van Leeuwen, F.E. and Rookus, M.A. (1989) The role of exogenous hormones in the epidemiology of breast, ovarian and endometrial cancer. *European Journal of Cancer and Clinical Oncology*, **25**, 1961–72.

Veronesi, U., Vanfi, A., Salvidori, *et al.* (1990a) Breast conservation as the treatment of choice in small breast cancer: long-term results of a randomized trial. *European Journal of Cancer*, **26**, 668–70.

Veronesi, U., Volterrani, F., Luini, A. *et al.* (1990b) Quadrantectomy versus lumpectomy for small size breast cancer. *European Journal of Cancer*, **26**, 671–3.

Willett, W.C., Hunter, D.J., Stampfer, M.J. *et al.* (1992) Dietary fat and fibre in relation to risk of breast cancer. An 8 year follow up. *Journal of the American Medical Association*, **240**, 2037–44.

Yelland, A., Graham, M.D., Trott, P.A. *et al.* (1991) Diagnosing breast carcinoma in young women. *British Medical Journal*, **302**, 618–20.

ADVANCED BREAST CANCER

Alison L. Jones and Trevor J. Powles

37.1 INTRODUCTION

Metastatic and locally advanced breast cancer are incurable but the natural history is very variable and ranges from months to many years. In general patients with mainly soft tissue disease have a longer median survival (20 months) than those with mainly bone metastases (15 months) or visceral metastases (7–8 months). Overall systematic treatment does not influence median survival, although there may be some subgroups of patients who benefit from chemotherapy, e.g. younger patients with rapidly progressive visceral disease. The survival from diagnosis of first metastasis is similar irrespective of whether the patient responds or has stable disease. Patients who fail to respond to systemic treatment may have an inferior prognosis but this is probably due to biological determinants.

37.2 OPTIONS FOR MANAGEMENT

The main aim of therapy for patients with metastatic breast cancer is palliation of disease related symptoms. While radiotherapy may be useful for specific local problems such as bone pain, spinal cord compression and cerebral metastases, metastatic breast cancer requires a systemic approach and the main treatment options lie between endocrine therapy and chemotherapy. Chemotherapy gives a higher objective response rate than endocrine therapy but there is no convincing evidence that it confers a survival benefit even if used early in the course of metastatic disease. This is partly because there are no prospective trials which address the question of survival and in most studies comparing endocrine therapy and chemotherapy patients cross over to the alternative therapy on progression. Although studies which use chemotherapy as first line treatment for metastatic disease may show an apparent superior survival for chemotherapy, this usually reflects a 'lead-time' bias and survival rates in trials should be assessed from first metastasis.

Our policy is to use non-toxic treatment as treatment of choice. This usually involves endocrine therapy as first line treatment, reserving chemotherapy for patients who fail to respond to endocrine therapy or those who present with life threatening visceral disease (e.g. symptomatic pulmonary or hepatic metastases).

37.2.1 ENDOCRINE THERAPY

(a) Tamoxifen

Tamoxifen is the treatment of first choice for postmenopausal women with advanced breast cancer. The overall objective response rate based on 5353 patients in 86 clinical trials was 34%, with disease stabilization in a further 19% of patients. The median duration of response varied between 2 and in excess of 24 months (Litherland and Jackson, 1988). There is no evidence in controlled studies to suggest that increasing the dose of tamoxifen above 20 mg/day improves the response rate. The likelihood of response to tamoxifen (or

Table 37.1   Factors determining response to endocrine therapy in advanced breast cancer

Higher chance of response	*Lower chance of response*
ER +ve	ER–ve
Progesterone receptor (PR) +ve	
Long DFI > 2 yr	Short DFI < 1 yr
Predominantly soft tissue and/or bone disease	Visceral (lung/liver) and CNS disease
Single site of disease	Multiple disease sites

ER, oestrogen receptor; PR, progesterone receptor;
DFI, disease free interval.

other endocrine agents) can be predicted by a number of factors (Table 37.1).

Tamoxifen competes with oestradiol for binding with oestrogen receptor which is a nuclear receptor (Figure 37.1). The tamoxifen–receptor complex can induce a variety of biological responses from oestrogen blockade to oestrogen agonist activity. There is increasing evidence that tamoxifen may exert some of its antitumour activity in breast cancer through growth inhibitory factors such as transforming growth factor beta (Knabbe *et al.*, 1987). This may in part explain the activity of tamoxifen in oestrogen receptor (ER) negative tumours. Patients with ER-positive tumours have a 46% chance of response,

although 12% of patients with ER-negative tumours will also respond to endocrine therapy (Litherland and Jackson, 1988). In practice all patients presenting with metastatic disease are given a trial of endocrine therapy, irrespective of initial ER status, unless there are clinical indications to use chemotherapy.

The response rate to tamoxifen in postmenopausal women increases with age, probably because of a higher number of ER-positive tumours. The role of tamoxifen and the endocrine changes it induces in premenopausal women has been reviewed in detail (Sunderland and Osborne, 1991). Tamoxifen causes a marked increase in circulatory oestrogen levels in premenopausal women with no change or a slight increase in gonadatrophins. This is in contrast to postmenopausal women in whom there is no change in oestrogen levels and a reduction in gonadotrophins on tamoxifen. The response rates in Phase II trials are between 20% and 45% (i.e. similar to ovarian ablation) and tamoxifen is often used as first line therapy in premenopausal women.

Tamoxifen has a low incidence of acute side-effects and this has been confirmed in prospective placebo controlled trials of tamoxifen as a chemopreventative agent in women at high risk of breast cancer (Powles *et al.*, 1990). Tamoxifen does however cause menstrual irregularity, hot flushes and vaginal discharge. This and other studies also indicate that tamoxifen is not a pure antioestrogen but

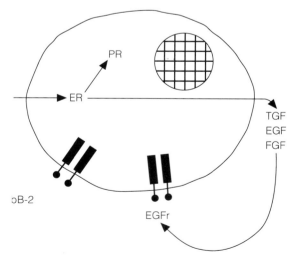

Figure 37.1   Mechanisms of action of tamoxifen.

has oestrogen agonist activity on other organ systems such as coagulation and lipid metabolism with a significant reduction in plasma cholesterol. One prospective study has indicated that ocular toxicity from tamoxifen at conventional dose may be higher than previously realized, with 4/63 patients developing reversible impairment of visual acuity (Pavlidis *et al.*, 1992).

Approximately 40% of patients with ER-positive tumours fail to respond to tamoxifen and nearly all responding patients will relapse at some time while taking the drug. The reasons for tamoxifen resistance are not clear but may involve molecular events including changes in the oestrogen receptor which facilitate hormonal escape (Johnston *et al.*, 1992). Another possibility is altered metabolism of tamoxifen in tumour cells. It is important to recognize that patients who have had a response to tamoxifen may well respond to further endocrine therapy at relapse.

The oestrogen agonist activity of tamoxifen has led to some concerns about a theoretical risk of primary liver and endometrial tumours. New pure antioestrogens are under development which do not have oestrogen agonist activity. One such drug, toremifene, had response rates of 21–68% in Phase II trials

but only 3% in patients who failed prior tamoxifen (Valavaara, 1990). These drugs may allow further investigation of oestrogen deprivation in breast cancer but do not have clear advantages yet over tamoxifen.

37.2.2 SECOND LINE ENDOCRINE THERAPY

The choice of second line endocrine therapy in postmenopausal women lies between an aromatase inhibitor and progestogens.

(a) Aromatase inhibitors

Oestrogen biosynthesis requires conversion of the weak androgen androstenedione to oestrone by the aromatase enzyme system which involves three separate steroid hydroxylations using an aromatase specific cytochrome P-450. In premenopausal women aromatase activity is regulated by granulosa cells in the ovary. In postmenopausal women aromatase activity is non-ovarian and largely found in subcutaneous fat. Oestrone is converted to biologically active oestradiol by 17β hydroxysteroid dehydrogenase. Plasma levels of oestradiol in postmenopausal women are 10–30 pg/ml although tissue levels may be higher (Figure 37.2). Another source of biologically active oestrogen is from the relatively

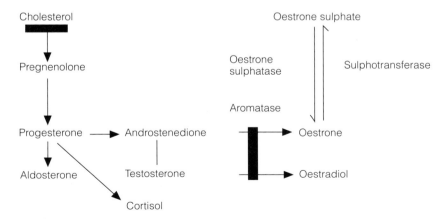

Figure 37.2 Steroid synthesis in postmenopausal women and action of aromatase inhibitors. ■, Action of aminoglutethimide.

inactive conjugate oestrone sulphate by the steroid sulphatase system (Figure 37.2).

Aminoglutethimide (AG) is a non-steroidal drug which acts as a non-specific inhibitor of cytochrome P-450 mediated steroid hydroxylations and inhibits peripheral aromatization reducing oestradiol levels to approximately 30% of pretreatment values (Figure 37.2). The overall response rate to AG is 30% with a median duration of response of 13 months. This is comparable with tamoxifen and in randomized trials both drugs have similar efficacy (Smith *et al.*, 1982). When used as second line endocrine therapy the response rate to AG was 38% in patients who had previously responded to tamoxifen but only 19% in those who had progressed on other endocrine therapy (Harris *et al.*, 1982).

At higher doses (1000 mg/day) AG inhibits other cytochrome P-450 mediated steroid hydroxylase systems and inhibits the initial step of cholesterol side-chain cleavage to 5-pregnenolone in steroidogenesis. This means that AG should be given with hydrocortisone replacement, usually 20 mg orally twice a day. AG also inhibits thyroxine synthesis and although most patients have a compensatory rise in TSH, only 5% require thyroxine replacement. There is no clear evidence for a dose–response relationship and AG is often prescribed at 500 mg daily which reduces the need for steroid replacement. There are a number of other side-effects with AG (Table 37.2) which lead to cessation of treatment in 8–15% of patients. These side-effects usually diminish with continued therapy, possibly because AG accelerates its own metabolism.

The lack of specificity of aminoglutethimide has resulted in interest in development of new, more selective aromatase inhibitors with a lower level of side-effects. One such drug, 4-hydroxyandrostenedione (4-OHA), is a suicide inhibitor of aromatase and competes with androstenedione for the active binding site of aromatase. The enzyme interacts with 4-OHA to yield reactive alkylating species which bind covalently to and irreversibly inhibit the enzyme. A deep intramuscular injection of 4-OHA 250 mg every 2 weeks causes effective oestrogen suppression without significant endocrine or other side-effects and has a response rate of 30%.

Table 37.2   Toxicity of aminoglutethimide in 213 patients

Side-effect	Patients	
	No.	*%*
Drowsiness	80	33
Rash	48	23
Nausea	32	15
Ataxia	9	4
Depression	9	4
Visual disturbance	2	
'Flu/diarrhoea	2	
Electrolyte imbalance	1	
Transient agranulocytosis	1	
Stevens–Johnson syndrome	1	
Headache	2	
Sore mouth	2	
Tinnitus	1	
Cramps	8	

From Harris *et al.*, 1982.

Other new oral aromatase inhibitors are also under development and are undergoing comparison with progestogens to establish response rates, toxicity and quality of life which will influence eventual recommendations for second line endocrine treatment.

(b) Progestogens

Progestogens are also useful in the treatment of metastatic breast cancer. Their antitumour effects may be mediated through a variety of mechanisms, including indirect effects on the pituitary/adrenal and pituitary/ovarian axes and direct effects on the progesterone receptor which result in intracellular events with inhibition of ER synthesis and reduced sensitivity of the cell to oestradiol.

The synthetic progestogens in common use are medroxyprogesterone acetate (MPA) and megestrol acetate (MA). They have equivalent activity to tamoxifen as first line therapy with an overall response rate of 30% in pre- and post-menopausal women. Non-randomized trials have suggested a dose–response relationship for progestogens but this has not been universally confirmed in randomized trials. The most common side-effect is weight gain which may be marked (> 20 kg) in 8% of patients, although lesser degrees of weight gain may be perceived as an advantage by cachetic patients. Other side-effects are dose dependent (Table 37.3) and in view of the lack of convincing evidence for higher doses, progestogens are prescribed at moderate dose: MA 160 mg and MPA 400 mg daily (daily in divided doses).

(c) Luteinizing hormone-releasing hormone (LHRH) analogues

LHRH stimulates pituitary gonadotrophin secretion which promotes peripheral release of oestrogens by the ovaries. LHRH analogues have been developed with greater potency and a longer half-life than LHRH, which cause a brief surge in gonadotrophin secretion followed by downregulation of receptors and inhibition of gonadotrophin secretion. This results in a fall in plasma oestrogens to castration levels although the effect is reversible when the drug is stopped. This may be important in non-responding women who have unpleasant menopausal symptoms. Most clinical studies use monthly depot preparations given by subcutaneous injection. The response rate in Phase II trials in premenopausal women was approximately 30%. The activity of these drugs is equivalent to that of surgical ovarian ablation without the psychological and operative morbidity. These drugs remain expensive, particularly

Table 37.3   Side-effects of progestogens

Side-effect	%
Weight gain	55
(> 20 kg)	8
Tremors	12
Sweats	12
Vaginal spotting	10
'Moon face'	8
Muscular cramps	5
Sterile abscess (i.m. injection)	7
Gastrointestinal (nausea/indigestion)	4

Notes:
Plus rash, depression, sleep disturbance, hypertension.
Caution in patients with diabetes and/or ischaemic heart disease.

for long term use, and any advantage over tamoxifen would need confirmation in a prospective trial. At present tamoxifen remains first line endocrine treatment of choice in premenopausal women (Smith, 1991; Sunderland and Osbourne, 1991).

(d)   Combination endocrine therapy

There has been interest in the use of endocrine therapies in combination to increase response rates. In one study tamoxifen was combined with MPA based on data showing increased expression of PR receptors in the presence of tamoxifen but there was no improvement in survival in the combination arm (Beltran *et al.*, 1991). The combination of tamoxifen, AG, MPA and danzol had a high response rate but no difference in survival compared with single agent endocrine therapy. This may be partly because of increased clearance of tamoxifen due to hepatic enzyme induction by aminoglutethimide. At present it is general policy to use endocrine agents sequentially rather than in combination.

37.2.3   CHEMOTHERAPY

A number of factors contribute to the likelihood of a response to chemotherapy however many lose significance in multivariate analysis. Pre- and post-menopausal patients have similar response rates although some randomized trials suggest that younger women (less than 35 years) may have an inferior survival. Performance status, as with most solid tumours, is an important predictor of response and similarly patients with lower volume of metastatic disease do better. Patients with ER-positive disease have shown higher responses in all studies in which this has been examined. The influence of prior adjuvant chemotherapy on subsequent response in metastatic disease remains an area of controversy.

(a)   Single agent

A wide variety of cytotoxic drugs are active in breast cancer (Table 37.4) and the anthracyclines remain amongst the most active single agents. Doxorubicin at standard doses, 50–75 mg/m^2, every 3 weeks, gives response rates

Table 37.4   Single agent cytotoxic drugs in advanced breast cancer

Drug	No. of Patients	Response (%)
Doxorubicin	182	43
Cyclophosphamide	594	36
Mitoxantrone	134	35
5-Fluorouracil	667	28
Methotrexate	76	26
Thiotepa	139	25
Melphalan	91	25
Mitomycin C	307	22
Vincristine	12	8
Cisplatin*	–	50
Epirubicin*	–	60
Carboplatin	34	35

From Henderson *et al.*, 1987.
*Powles and Smith, 1991.

of up to 60% in untreated patients although the response rate falls to 30% in patients receiving doxorubicin as second line chemotherapy. Doxorubicin causes alopecia and dose dependent mucositis and moderate emesis. Alopecia may be reduced by scalp cooling during infusion and problems of myelosuppression and emesis may be reduced by careful use of antiemetics and possibly haemopoietic growth factors, but although response is dose related dose escalation is limited by stomatitis and skin toxicity. In addition, doxorubicin is cardiotoxic and the total cumulative dose is limited to 450 mg/m^2. There is no evidence that drug scheduling (e.g. weekly treatments) affects response, although more frequent scheduling may be associated with a poorer quality of life (Richards *et al.*, 1992).

Epirubicin is an analogue of doxorubicin which has a maximum tolerated dose of 120 mg/m^2 and achieves response rates of over 65%. In a randomized study epirubicin 75 mg/m^2 had an equivalent response rate (60%) to doxorubicin but with less cardiotoxicity (Brambilla *et al.*, 1986). Epirubicin is eliminated more rapidly that doxorubicin and can be used more safely in patients with hepatic dysfunction from liver metastases in whom doxorubicin would cause prolonged myelosuppression.

Mitoxantrone is a synthetic anthracenedione with structural similarities to anthracyclines but without the amino sugar moiety. In randomized trials in previously treated and untreated patients the response rate with mitoxantrone 10–14 mg/m^2 intravenously every 3 weeks is slightly lower than doxorubicin (Henderson *et al.*, 1989), however toxicity, in particular emesis and alopecia, are much reduced. Myelosuppression is dose limiting. Mitoxantrone is often favoured in older and frail patients who may have pre-existing cardiac problems.

5-Fluorouracil (5FU) has a response rate of only 25% in breast cancer and is generally used in combination regimens. When admin-

istered by continuous infusion in doses of 200–300 mg/m^2/24 h, using an ambulatory pump and a chronic indwelling venous catheter, the response rate is increased up to 50% with responses seen even in patients refractory to bolus 5FU. Myelosuppression is uncommon with this scheduling although diarrhoea and cutaneous toxicity with plantar-palmar erythema are seen.

Cisplatin is an active drug in previously untreated patients with response rates up to 54%, although activity is lower in previously treated patients. The toxicity of cisplatin is high for its routine use in palliative chemotherapy, however its less toxic analogue carboplatin appears to have an inferior response rate in non-randomized studies.

(b) Combination chemotherapy

There is continued debate about the use of single agent versus combination chemotherapy in patients with advanced breast cancer. In general, the response rates with standard combination regimens such as CMF (cyclophosphamide, methotrexate, 5-fluorouracil), CAF (cyclophosphamide, adriamycin, 5-fluorouracil) and 3M (mitomycin, mitoxantrone, methotrexate) at moderate doses are higher (approximately 50–60%) than single agent treatment. There is no convincing evidence that higher response rates translate into improved survival and this is an important issue when considering the role of high dose chemotherapy. The median duration of response is 9–12 months with combination chemotherapy.

CMF is the most commonly used regimen and is generally given as the classical regimen with oral cyclophosphamide for 14 days and methotrexate and 5FU on days 1 and 8 of a 28 day cycle. In a randomized trial this was superior to a regimen giving all three drugs intravenously in terms of response rates and survival (Engelsman *et al.*, 1991). Although some randomized trials suggest superiority for doxorubicin containing regimens in terms of response and median survival, the evidence is not conclusive and minor advantages have to be weighed against toxicity in advanced disease. Epirubicin and mitoxantrone have been introduced into combination regimens to maintain therapeutic activity with lower toxicity. One such regimen, 3M (mitomycin C, mitoxantrene, methotrexate), has equivalent activity to CMF and VAC with response rates of approximately 50% in randomized trials (Jodrell *et al.*, 1991; Powles and Smith, 1991).

(c) Duration of chemotherapy

In a randomized trial combination chemotherapy given for 3 months was compared with the same regimen given until relapse (Coates *et al.*, 1987). The short duration treatment had a significantly shorter progression-free interval, a trend to shorter survival and poorer quality of life than continuous therapy. In other studies which also suggest improved progression-free survival in responding patients randomized to chemotherapy beyond 6 months, any benefit in terms of longer progression-free survival had to be balanced against increased toxicity in the maintenance arm (Muss *et al.*, 1991).

In practice most patients receive chemotherapy for approximately 6 months provided there is continuing evidence of response or disease stabilization at each course without unacceptable treatment-related toxicity.

(d) Second line chemotherapy

Patients who have been treated with chemotherapy for metastatic breast cancer have approximately 30% chance of responding to second line chemotherapy. Increasing number of patients now receive adjuvant chemotherapy for early breast cancer but there is no consensus on whether these patients have an inferior response rate to that of chemotherapy naive patients.

(e) Intensive chemotherapy

It has been argued from analysis of actual doses of drugs delivered that there is a correlation between dose intensity and outcome in metastatic disease (Hryniuk *et al.*, 1988). This has been challenged on the basis of some of the assumptions made; however, dose intensity remains an important issue in treatment. This raises the question of high dose chemotherapy with autologous bone marrow support or peripheral blood stem cell rescue. In early Phase II studies in patients with measurable disease there were high response rates with a complete remission rate of up to 60%. The median duration of response was low with most patients relapsing within 1 year although there may be a small 'tail' of long term survivors (Peters *et al.*, 1986). Most recurrences involved sites of bulk disease and further studies are evaluating high dose treatment as consolidation after induction therapy with standard regimens such as CAF. Another strategy is to irradiate sites of bulk disease before high dose treatment in an attempt to consolidate minimal residual disease. Randomized studies are underway to evaluate the role of high dose chemotherapy and this should be regarded as standard therapy outside a clinical trial.

(f) New drugs

New drugs are continually evaluated in metastatic breast cancer. These include analogues of anthracyclines and more recently anthrapyrazoles which have been developed in an attempt to maintain the antitumour activity of doxorubicin but with less potential for free radical formation and hence less cardiotoxicity (Jones and Smith, 1993). Other drugs are navelbine, a vinca alkaloid with an oral formulation (Jones and Smith, 1993), taxol (Holmes *et al.*, 1991) and related compounds. In a Phase II study of taxol 250 mg/m^2 by 24 h infusion every 21 days there were 12 responses (48%) in 25 patients who had received prior chemotherapy and this drug is under evaluation with doxorubicin (Holmes *et al.*, 1991).

There is an increasing trend to evaluate Phase II drugs before conventional chemotherapy in metastatic breast cancer to avoid the problems of missing drug activity because of the development of multidrug resistance with previous treatment and also because many patients with metastatic breast cancer may not be fit enough for second line chemotherapy. There is no evidence that this approach confers an inferior survival even if some of the Phase II drugs show low activity (Ahmann *et al.*, 1987).

37.3 LOCALLY ADVANCED AND INFLAMMATORY BREAST CANCER

Locally advanced inoperable breast cancer includes approximately 10% of all patients at presentation with inflammatory breast cancer as a subgroup, accounting for 1–5% of breast cancers. Inflammatory cancer is characterized by induration of the skin with an erysipeloid margin. The prognosis for locally advanced disease is poor with surgery ± radiotherapy and current data suggests that induction chemotherapy may improve disease free survival and also overall survival for inflammatory cancer (Jaiyesimi *et al.*, 1992). The choice of regimens is similar to that for metastatic disease. The optimal local treatment (radiotherapy ± surgery) following chemotherapy remains an area for research.

More intensive regimens and high dose treatment are of particular interest in these patients as any impact on the natural history of the disease will become apparent in a relatively short time period.

37.4 SPECIFIC PROBLEMS

37.4.1 BONE METASTASES

Bone is the first site of recurrence in 40% of patients with advanced breast cancer and may result in significant morbidity and mor-

tality. Clinical problems include bone pain, pathological fracture and hypercalcaemia. These results from an imbalance between bone formation and resorption usually with accelerated bone loss due to unopposed bone resorption (uncoupling). The major cellular mechanism is an increase in number and/or activity of osteoclasts with skeletal lesions induced by paracrine factors from osteoclasts. Hypercalcaemia in breast cancer is nearly always associated with osteolytic metastases, although there may be a humoral component with parathyroid hormone releasing peptide (PTHrP) which causes both a generalized increase in bone resorption and increased tubular resorption of calcium in approximately one-third of patients.

The development of hypercalcaemia or progressive bone disease is an indication for systemic treatment. Patients usually also require specific treatment of hypercalcaemia to relieve distressing symptoms and to facilitate systemic treatment. Serum calcium levels above 3.25 mmol/l require urgent treatment with intravenous fluids to correct dehydration using central venous monitoring in severe cases. Fluid replacement alone causes a transient fall in serum calcium but patients require additional therapy to maintain normal calcium levels. This can be achieved using bisphosphonates. These drugs are pyrophosphate analogues and are potent inhibitors of osteoclast bone resorption. Several bisphosphonates have been used in clinical practice including pamidronate and clodronate. Our practice is to use pamidronate 30–60 mg intravenously over 6 hours according to serum calcium level. This may be repeated every 2–3 weeks. Oral bisphosphonates can also be used, although oral pamidronate has dose limiting gastrointestinal toxicity. Other drugs including calcitonin are sometimes used although in the treatment of hypercalcaemia the duration of action is shorter.

Painful bone metastases often respond to local radiotherapy and a single fraction (8 Gy) usually provides effective relief. Pathological fractures and incipient fractures are best managed by internal fixation followed by radiotherapy. A recent double blind controlled trial of oral clodronate in patients with bone metastases from breast cancer indicates that clodronate has a beneficial effect on skeletal morbidity with a reduction in hypercalcaemic episodes, vertebral fractures and deformity (Patterson *et al.*, 1992). Similar results have been obtained with pamidronate (Van Holfen–Verzantvoort *et al.*, 1991). It has been suggested that the expression of PTH-P in primary breast cancer specimens may predict for subsequent development of bone metastases (Bundred *et al.*, 1992). This could identify patients at high risk of developing bone metastases who could benefit from prophylactic bisphosphonate therapy.

37.4.2   PLEURAL EFFUSIONS

Although up to 50% of patients with metastatic breast cancer will develop a pleural effusion during their disease, this is rare as a single first site of relapse occurring in < 10% of patients and should therefore be confirmed by cytology or biopsy. Pleural effusions, unless causing significant dyspnoea, can be managed· by systemic therapy. It should be remembered that any effusion acts as a 'third space' and may prolong the half-life of drugs such as methotrexate and this, together with dyspnoea, may be an indication for drainage. Thoracocentesis is preferred to repeated aspiration and when the pleural cavity is dry installation of bleomycin or tetracycline can be used to achieve a chemical pleurodesis.

Minor pericardial effusions can also be managed by systemic treatment but larger or symptomatic effusions require drainage. Recurrent symptomatic pericardial effusions may be managed surgically by a pleural–pericardial window.

37.4.3   CEREBRAL AND MENINGEAL METASTASES

Brain metastases are also rare as first site of relapse but autopsy studies suggest an incidence of 9–25%. Standard treatment is with short term high dose cortisteroids and whole brain irradiation, although solitary lesions may be considered for a stereotactic approach. If the patient has metastatic disease elsewhere which require treatment, systemic chemotherapy can be used as initial treatment with careful monitoring of CNS disease, holding radiotherapy in reserve.

Patients with meningeal disease may present with headache and/or local neurological deficits. Diagnosis can be made by MRI and/or cytology of cerebrospinal fluid (CSF), although 10% of patients will have persistently negative CSF. Patients are usually treated by intrathecal methotrexate twice weekly for 3 weeks and maintenance treatment for 6 months provided there is clinical improvement. Radiotherapy is reserved to treat specific local neurological dysfunction.

37.5   QUALITY OF LIFE

Table 37.5 shows the symptomatic relief of 100 consecutive patients treated with chemotherapy at the Royal Marsden Hospital and demonstrates that tumour related symptoms are significantly improved in most patients. As well as the relief of specific cancer related symptoms, assessment of quality of life is being given increasing attention in advanced breast cancer and a number of methods have been developed which allow reliable and valid measurement of aspects of quality of life affected by the disease and its treatment. These include linear analogue self-assessment (LASA) scales which measure specific parameters, e.g. physical well-being, mood, pain, etc., on a scale from very poor to normal and a variety of quality of life questionnaires. These assessments have usually been used to compare different treatments (Coates *et al.*,

Table 37.5 Symptom relief after chemotherapy in advanced breast cancer (100 patients)

Symptom	Patients (no.)	Symptom relief (%)
Bone pain	63	48 (13)
Malaise/anorexia	52	65 (38)
Dyspnoea	44	61 (27)
Soft tissue discomfort	33	63 (55)

Royal Marsden Hospital data.
Figures in parentheses are percentage with complete relief.

1987) but may also be independent predictors of survival (Coates *et al.*, 1992). Overall it appears that the beneficial effects of chemotherapy in control of disease outweigh the treatment related side-effects resulting in improved quality of life. Any prospective trial in advanced breast cancer should include formal quality of life assessments as an end point.

37.6 CONCLUSIONS

The natural history of advanced breast cancer is extremely variable and many patients with indolent disease may have good quality of life for many years with sequential endocrine treatment. Chemotherapy for advanced disease remains controversial in terms of timing, selection of drug(s) and dose intensity, however there is no convincing evidence from randomized trials that chemotherapy affects survival for the majority of patients. It is important to remember however that chemotherapy used appropriately can provide palliative benefit and significant improvement in quality of life for many patients and the development of new drugs and schedules may improve the outlook in advanced disease. Even when specific anticancer therapies have failed, supportive care may minimize disease related symptoms.

The indentification of active agents in advanced breast cancer is important and may allow improved control of micrometastatic disease early in treatment as adjuvant therapy when there is potential to influence the course of the disease.

REFERENCES

Ahmann, D.L., Schaid, D.J., Bisel, H.F. *et al.* (1987) The effect of initial chemotherapy in advanced breast cancer: polychemotherapy vs single drug. *Journal of Clinical Oncology*, **5**, 1928–31.

Beltran, M., Alonso, M.C., Ojeda, M.B. *et al.* (1991) Alternating sequential endocrine therapy: tamoxifen and medroxyprogesterone acetate versus tamoxifen in postmenopausal advanced breast cancer patients. *Annals of Oncology*, **2**, 495–9.

Brambilla, C., Rossi, A., Bonfante, B. *et al.* (1988) Phase II study of doxorubicin versus epirubicin in advanced breast cancer. *Cancer Treatment Report*, **70**, 261.

Bundred, N.J., Walker, R.A., Ratcliffe, W.A. *et al.* (1992). Parathyroid hormone related protein and skeletal morbidity in breast cancer. *European Journal of Cancer*, **28**, 690–2.

Coates, A., Gebski, V., Bishop, J.F. *et al.* (1987) Improving the quality of life during chemotherapy for advanced breast cancer, a comparison of intermittent and continous treatmant strategies. *New England Journal of Medicine*, **317**, 1490–5.

Coates, A., Gebski, V., Signorini, D. *et al.* (1992). Prognostic value of quality-of-life scores during chemotherapy for advanced breast cancer. *Journal of Clinical Oncology*, **10**, 1833–8.

Engelsman, E., Klijn, J.C.M., Rubens, R.D. *et al.* (1991) 'Classical' CMF versus a 3-weekly intravenous CMF schedule in postmenopausal patients with advanced breast cancer. *European Journal of Cancer*, **27**, 966–70.

Harris, A.L., Powles, T.J. Smith, I.E. *et al.* (1982) Aminoglutethimide in the treatment of advanced postmenopausal breast cancer. *Cancer Research*, **42**, 3405–8.

Henderson, I.C. (1987) Chemotherapy for advanced disease, *Breast Diseases*, (eds J.R. Harris, S. Hellman, I.C. Henderson and D.W. Kinne), Lippincott, Philadelphia, pp. 428–79.

Henderson, I.C., Hayes, D.R. and Gelman, R. (1989). Dose response in the treatment of breast cancer: a critical review. *Journal of Clinical Oncology*, **6**, 1501–15.

Holmes, F.A., Wathers, R.S., Theriault, R.L. *et al.* (1991) Phase II trial of taxol, an active drug in the treatment of metastatic breast cancer. *Journal of the National Cancer Institute*, **83**, 1797–1805.

Hrynuik, W.M., Levine, M.N. and Levin, L. (1988) Analysis of dose intensity for chemotherapy in early (Stage II) and advanced breast cancer. *Monographs of the National Cancer Institute*, **1**, 87–94.

Jaiyesimi, I.A., Buzdar, A.U. and Hortobagyi, G. (1992) Inflammatory breast cancer: a review. *Journal of Clinical Oncology*, **10**, 1014–25.

Jodrell, D.I., Smith, I.E., Mansi, J.L. *et al.* (1991) A randomised comparative trial of mitoxantrone/methotrexate/mitomycin C (MMM) and cyclophosphamide/methotrexate/5FU (CMF) in the treatment of advanced breast cancer. *British Journal of Cancer*, **63**, 794–8.

Johnston, S.R.D., Dowsett, M. and Smith, I.E. (1992) Towards a molecular basis for tamoxifen resistance in breast cancer. *Annals of Oncology*, **3**, 503–11.

Jones, A.L. and Smith, I.E. (1993) Navelbine and the anthrapyrazoles. *Clinics in Haematology and Oncology*, (in press).

Knabbe, C., Lippman, M.E., Wakefield, L.M. *et al.* (1987) Evidence that transforming growth factor beta is a hormonally regulated negative growth factor in human breast cancer cells. *Cell*, **48**, 417–28.

Litherland, S. and Jackson, I.M. (1988) Antioestrogens in the management of hormone-dependent cancer. *Cancer Treatment Reports*, **15**, 183–94.

Muss, H.B., Case, D.L., Richards, F. *et al.* (1991) Interrupted versus continuous chemotherapy in patients with metastatic breast cancer. *New England Journal of Medicine*, **325**, 1342–8.

Patterson, A.H.G., Powles, T.J., Kanis, J.A. *et al.* (1992) Double-blind controlled trial of oral clodronate in patients with bone metastases from breast cancer. *Journal of Clinical Oncology*, **11**, 59–65.

Pavlidis, N.A., Petis, C. Biassoulis, E. *et al.* (1992) Clear evidence that long-term tamoxifen can induce ocular toxicity. *Cancer*, **69**, 2961–4.

Peters, W.P., Shpall, E.J., Jones, R.B. *et al.* (1986) High-dose combination cyclophosphamide, cisplatin and carmustine with bone marrow support as initial treatment for metastatic breast cancer. *Journal of Clinical Oncology*, **6**, 1368–76.

Powles, T.J., Tilly, C.J., Jones, A.L. *et al.* (1990) Prevention of breast cancer using tamoxifen – an update on the Royal Marsden Hospital pilot programme. *European Journal of Cancer*, **26**, 680–84.

Powles, T.J. and Smith, I.E. (eds) (1991) *Medical Management of Breast Cancer*, Martin Dunitz, London.

Richards, M.A., Hopwood, P., Ramirez, A.J. *et al.* (1992) Doxorubicin in advanced breast cancer: influence of schedule on response, survival and quality of life. *European Journal of Cancer*, **28A**, 1023–8.

Smith, I.E. (1991) LHRH analogues in breast cancer: clever but do we need them? *British Journal of Cancer*, **63**, 15–16.

Smith, I.E., Harris, A.L., Morgan, M. *et al.* (1982) Tamoxifen versus aminoglutethimide versus combined tamoxifen and aminoglutethimide in the treatment of advanced breast cancer. *Cancer Research*, **42**, 3430–3.

Sunderland, C.M. and Osbourne, C.K. (1991) Tamoxifen in premenopausal patients with metastatic breast cancer: a review. *Journal of Clinical Oncology*, **9**, 1283–97.

Valavaara, R. (1990). Phase II trials with toremifene in advanced breast cancer: a review. *Breast Cancer Research and Treatment*, **16**, 531–5.

Van Holfen-Verzantvoort, A.T.M., Zwinderman, A.H., Aaronson, N.K. *et al.* (1991) The effect of supportive pamidronate treatment on aspects of quality of life in patients with advanced breast cancer. *European Journal of Cancer*, **27**, 544–9.

HEAD AND NECK CANCER

J.M. Henk and Peter Rhys Evans

The term 'head and neck cancer' is usually applied to malignant tumours of the upper air and food passages and associated structures. Skin, central nervous system and thyroid tumours are not included. The major anatomical sites are the nasal cavity, paranasal sinuses, nasopharynx, oral cavity, oropharynx, hypopharynx, larynx and salivary glands.

38.1 EPIDEMIOLOGY AND AETIOLOGY

Approximately half a million cases of head and neck cancer occur annually worldwide (Parkin *et al.*, 1988). The UK has one of the lowest incidences in the world; about 5000 per annum are registered which accounts for less than 3% of all malignancies. Most cases occur in the middle-aged and elderly with a considerable male predominance.

The most important risk factors are alcohol and tobacco. A number of carcinogens can act locally on the mucosa of the upper aerodigestive tract, of which tobacco, either smoked or chewed, is by far the commonest. Others include nickel, wood dust, aromatic hydrocarbons and textile fibres. There is probably a genetic preponderance in some ethnic groups, especially nasopharyngeal carcinoma in South China. Other genetic factors are emerging, e.g. congenital predisposition to mutagen induced chromosome fragility has been demonstrated in some individuals. In some cases viruses may have an aetiological role, for example Epstein–Barr virus (EBV), herpes simplex and human papilloma virus.

Multiple primary tumours are common in the head and neck, presumably because all the mucosal surfaces are exposed to the same carcinogens. Dysplastic changes in the mucosa often precede the development of carcinoma. These appear clinically either as white (leucoplakia) or red (erythroplakia) patches. The genetic basis of carcinogenesis in head and neck cancer is not yet known. Frequent findings in squamous cell carcinoma are deletions of chromosomes 3p and 18q, and also p53 mutations, but no changes specific to squamous cell carcinoma have been found.

38.2 PATHOLOGY

The vast majority of head and neck cancers are squamous cell carcinomas arising from the mucosal surfaces. They are usually moderately or well differentiated. Anaplastic carcinomas arising from the epithelium are sometimes seen, especially in the nasopharynx where there is a typical histological appearance, often with a lymphoid stroma, formerly called 'lympho-epithelioma', but this term is now obsolete and has been replaced by the term 'undifferentiated carcinoma of nasopharyngeal type (UCNT)'. Similar tumours are sometimes seen in the tonsillar fossa. A wide variety of histological types of tumour can arise in the salivary glands, the commonest being adenoid-cystic carcinoma, muco-epidermoid carcinoma, acinic cell carcinoma, and various types of ductal and terminal duct adenocarcinoma.

Similar tumour types, especially adenoid-cystic carcinoma, can arise in minor salivary glands anywhere in the head and neck mucosa. The lymphoid tissue in the naso-pharynx, tonsil and base of tongue, known as Waldeyer's ring, is the occasional site of origin of malignant lymphoma. Rare malignant tumours include mucosal melanoma, aesthesioneuroblastoma and sarcoma.

38.3 NATURAL HISTORY

Head and neck cancers typically arise as superficial mucosal tumours which if untreated eventually enlarge and infiltrate deeper tissues. Lymphatic spread occurs initially to the first group of lymph nodes in the neck draining the tumour bearing site. Nodes lower in the neck are not normally involved until the first station nodes contain metastases large enough to be palpable. Blood borne metastases occur at a relatively late stage in the disease and are quite rare in the absence of extensive lymph node involvement. Less than 10% of head and neck cancer patients die of distant metastases in the absence of loco-regional recurrence. Post-mortem studies demonstrate that 30–40% of patients dying of head and neck cancer do in fact have blood borne metastases, but in the majority of such cases locoregional disease at the primary site or in the neck dominates the clinical picture and is the major cause of death.

In contrast to many other cancers, therefore, head and neck cancer tends to spread in an orderly stepwise manner. Accordingly, early diagnosis and successful local radical treatment can significantly influence the course of the disease and the prognosis.

38.4 DIAGNOSIS AND STAGING

Symptoms and signs vary with the primary site of the tumour. A very small lesion of a vocal cord, for example, presents early as persistent hoarseness, whereas a carcinoma of the maxillary antrum or of the pyriform fossa may grow to a large size before giving rise to symptoms.

A thorough physical examination of the upper air and food passages and of the neck is the first essential step. If cancer is suspected an examination under anaesthetic and biopsy must be carried out. Radiological assessment using either CT or MRI helps to determine the extent of the primary tumour and may detect lymph node involvement which is not palpable on clinical examination. A chest X-ray is advisable in all cases, as pulmonary metastases or a synchronous lung primary are occasionally found. Staging of UCNT, but not other tumour types, should include isotope bone scan and liver ultrasound. The Union Internationale Contre le Cancer (UICC) TNM system has different T specifications for each primary site. Therefore patients with the same T stage cannot be considered collectively, e.g. a T2 carcinoma of the vocal cord has an excellent prognosis, whereas a T2 carcinoma of the hypopharynx carries a 50% mortality.

38.5 BASIC PRINCIPLES OF MANAGEMENT

The patient with head and neck cancer is best managed by a multidisciplinary team. A unit treating head and neck cancer should contain representatives of the specialties of ear, nose and throat surgery, plastic and reconstructive surgery, oral and maxillofacial surgery, radiotherapy and medical oncology. The services of specialized nurses, speech therapists, dietitians, dental hygienists and physiotherapists are also very important. A patient with newly diagnosed head and neck cancer should ideally be seen and discussed at a multidisciplinary combined clinic where a policy of treatment is decided.

Most head and neck cancer patients are suitable for an attempt at locally curative treatment. Some patients may be incurable at presentation because of their extensive local disease, or the presence of distant metastases, but such patients are a small minority at least in the UK.

If curative treatment is deemed possible, the first and most fundamental decision to be made is between the alternative policies of either elective surgery, or radical radiotherapy keeping surgery in reserve for a proven residual or recurrent tumour. If the former is chosen radiotherapy may also be given as an adjuvant treatment, either pre- or postoperatively. Chemotherapy may also be used as an adjuvant to either radiotherapy or surgery, but its role in increasing the probability of cure is not well established (see below).

The aim of radical radiotherapy is to eliminate all malignant cells within the volume of tissue irradiated, so avoiding the necessity for surgery. If radiotherapy fails then salvage surgery is often possible. However, operating on patients after failure of radical radiotherapy is more difficult and carries a higher complication rate than elective surgery. Assessment of whether or not salvage surgery is necessary should be delayed until at least 6 weeks have elapsed after the end of the course of radiotherapy to allow time for the normal tissues to heal and tumour cells killed by radiation to disappear. Before 6 weeks both clinical and histological assessment of residual disease may be misleading (Suit *et al.*, 1965). If there is no evidence of residual tumour 6 weeks after radical radiotherapy careful follow-up is necessary so that any recurrence can be diagnosed early thereby giving salvage surgery the best chance of success.

Elective surgery aims to remove the entire tumour and so should not be attempted unless it is anticipated that a macroscopically complete removal of all disease can be achieved. Radiotherapy should be given after surgery whenever histological findings suggest a high likelihood of local recurrence; these include tumour at or very close to the resection margins, perineural infiltration, or lymph node involvement either multiple or with extracapsular extension. Preoperative radiotherapy is now rarely used for head and neck cancer. It has theoretical biological advantages over postoperative radiotherapy which have been confirmed in animal experiments, but in head and neck cancer it has considerable practical drawbacks. A large controlled trial by the RTOG group in the USA, (Tupchong *et al.*, 1991) compared pre- and postoperative radiotherapy at what are probably optimal dosages, i.e. 50 Gy in 25 fractions for preoperative radiotherapy and 60 Gy in 30 fractions for postoperative radiotherapy. There was a small but statistically significant advantage for postoperative radiotherapy in this study.

The choice between the policies of elective surgery or radical radiotherapy depend on a number of factors including the histology, site and stage of the tumour, and the general condition of the patient including his ability to attend for follow-up. With tumours of high radiosensitivity such as lymphoma or undifferentiated carcinoma of nasopharyngeal type, local cure rates by radiotherapy are very high so there is no need for surgery, even in easily operable tumours. On the other hand mucous and salivary gland tumours have a relatively low radiosensitivity and should always be excised whenever possible. Squamous cell carcinoma is of intermediate sensitivity, so the decision depends mainly on the site and stage of the disease. A small tumour which can be excised without producing any significant cosmetic or functional defect, for example a T1 tumour of the anterior third of the tongue, is best treated surgically. In other sites surgical excision may cause some functional defect and the outcome of radical radiotherapy is superior, e.g. most early laryngeal carcinomas. In the case of some intermediate stage tumours the relative merits of surgery or radiotherapy are highly controversial, e.g. T3 carcinoma of the larynx and T2 carcinoma of the oral cavity. Advanced stage tumours with deep infiltration are relatively rarely cured by radiotherapy and so a policy of surgery and postoperative radiotherapy usually gives the patient the best chance of cure accepting that there will be some functional disability as a result of the treatment. This particularly applies to tumours invading bone or cartilage. It is difficult to eliminate malignant cells from these tissues by radiotherapy because of hypoxia, and even if the tumour is eliminated the tissues do not heal well, leaving necrotic and chronically infected areas which are the source of considerable morbidity. Accordingly tumours involving bone or cartilage are normally treated surgically. Some large tumours may be unresectable either because of inaccessibility, e.g. carcinoma of the nasopharynx, or because of very advanced stage. These very advanced tumours can only be treated by radical radiotherapy but the chances of a cure are very low.

The general medical condition of the patient must be taken into account when deciding between surgery or radiotherapy. Some patients may be medically unfit to undergo major surgery. Age is sometimes quoted as a contraindication to surgery but the elderly often also tolerate radiotherapy badly and surgery may be preferable. An important factor which must be taken into account is the likely ability or willingness of the patient to attend for follow-up if radical radiotherapy is given. In intermediate stage disease a policy of radical radiotherapy is likely to give the same survival rates as elective surgery only if the patient can be carefully followed up and salvage surgery instituted at the first signs of recurrence.

38.6 PRINCIPLES OF SURGERY

Surgical treatment of head and neck cancers, together with radiotherapy, remain the two main curative options, and therapeutic management of each individual case must be clearly discussed to obtain optimal results. Surgical treatments for head and neck cancer include radical ablation with or without reconstruction, palliative operations and adjunctive minor procedures.

Where limited disease is present there has been an increasing trend towards conservation operations with optimal functional and cosmetic preservation. For instance, in surgery of the floor of the mouth marginal or segmental mandibulectomy is now often possible instead of full thickness resection of the mandible. Similarly, in carcinoma of the larynx, the development of conservation surgery has permitted safe excision of tumours with preservation of laryngeal function, even for some early radiation failures. The introduction of the 'conservation' or functional neck dissection by Bocca in 1967 (discussed below) was also an important landmark in reducing unnecessary morbidity in surgical treatment of neck disease (Bocca and Pignataro, 1967).

38.6.1 RADICAL SURGERY

The purpose of radical surgery, whether this is carried out as the initial treatment or for recurrence after radiotherapy, is to excise the tumour completely with as safe a margin of surrounding tissue as possible together with any lymph node metastases. Surgery still offers the best chance of successful loco-regional control of many head and neck cancers. For more advanced disease post-operative radiotherapy will increase the chances of success.

The majority of head and neck tumours are squamous cell carcinomas and local spread has certain characteristics which have to be taken into account during planning of the surgery. Local spread is by direct invasion along tissue planes, but the extent may vary considerably according to the site, the degree of differentiation, and whether previous radiotherapy has been given.

Vocal cord carcinomas are often well demarcated and a margin of 3–4 mm is usually adequate. Tumours of the tongue infiltrate along muscle bundles and ideally a 2 cm margin of clearance around the palpable tumour mass is advisable. In the hypopharynx, tumours may spread submucosally or there may be field change, and a 2–3 cm clearance is preferable. Following previous radiotherapy, however, the margins of tumour are less distinct because of fibrosis, so frozen section control at the time of resection is advisable to ensure complete excision.

In the head and neck margins of excision may be limited by natural anatomical barriers and by the presence of vital neurovascular structures whose resection would produce unacceptable risks of postoperative morbidity and mortality. Before contemplating surgery, the general medical status of the patient and suitability for radical surgery should be considered carefully. Preliminary CT scan is helpful to determine the extent of the tumour and presence of possible cervical metastases.

A temporary tracheostomy is often required as a precaution for resections of the oral cavity and pharynx or if there is a significant risk of damage to the vagus or the recurrent laryngeal nerve. Provision must also be made for postoperative feeding, either via a small bore nasogastric tube, a pharyngostomy tube, gastrostomy or jejunostomy.

Cosmetic incisions are planned according to the extent of the resection and whether a neck dissection is being carried out at the same time, and whether a skin flap is being used for reconstruction. The vascularity of the skin can be seriously impaired by previous radiotherapy or surgery which can lead to postoperative complications such as marginal necrosis or fistula formation.

38.6.2 RECONSTRUCTION IN HEAD AND NECK SURGERY

Although long term survival in squamous carcinoma of the head and neck has not improved appreciably in the past 30 years, the most significant advance has been in the functional rehabilitation of the patient. During the 1950s and 1960s the deltopectoral flap (Bakamjian, 1965) was used for reconstruction in many cases, but this often involved multistage operations and many patients died from recurrence before the final reconstruction had been completed.

The advent of the pectoralis major and latissimus dorsi myocutaneous flaps in the 1970s and 1980s allowed immediate one-stage reconstruction (Ariyan, 1979) with satisfactory functional and cosmetic results, as well as reducing hospital inpatient time and postoperative morbidity. More recently during the last decade, free tissue flaps, e.g. from the forearm or jejunum, (Mühlbauer *et al.*, 1982) have given even more versatility to reconstructive options.

In laryngeal cancer, total laryngectomy no longer carries with it the dreaded disability of loss of speech since the introduction of the tracheo-oesophageal valve which gives satisfactory speech to 80–90% of patients.

38.7 PRINCIPLES OF RADIOTHERAPY

Brachytherapy where appropriate gives higher tumour control rates than external beam, but in the head and neck is applicable to only a few sites, especially the oral cavity. Consequently most head and neck radiotherapy is given by external beam. Most radiotherapists treat with 5 fractions a week over periods from 3 to 8 weeks. The most popular regimen is 2 Gy per day, 5 days per week to a total dose of 66–70 Gy. Three or 4 week schedules using fraction sizes from 2.5 to 3.3 Gy remain popular in some centres. Although it has been widely believed that longer fractionation schemes give a better therapeutic ratio between tumour cure and late normal tissue damage, the few controlled trials which have been done to compare shorter and longer treatment regimens have failed to confirm this, no significant differences having been demonstrated between 3 and 6 week treatment times.

In general, shorter treatment times have the advantage of economy and convenience and are less taxing on the patient. However they tend to cause more severe acute mucositis;

when the area of mucosa irradiated is large this may lead to greater difficulty in maintaining nutrition. Late normal tissue effects are certainly related to fraction size. The central nervous system is especially vulnerable to large dose fractions so it is advisable to use small fractions where the tumour is close to the optic nerve, brain stem or spinal cord. The author's policy is to treat over 3–4 weeks using fraction sizes of 2.75–3.1 Gy where the treatment volume is small and confined to the primary tumour, but to use 2 Gy fractions for large volumes or where central nervous system tissue is at risk.

Probably small fraction sizes of 2 Gy or less do provide a better therapeutic ratio than larger fractions. On the other hand squamous cell carcinoma tends to repopulate fast during treatment so short overall times should be preferable. The ideal of short times and small fractions can only be achieved by hyperfractionation, i.e. more than one fraction per day. A variety of hyperfractionation strategies are being investigated in head and neck squamous cell carcinoma. These include simple hyperfractionation using 2 fractions of 1.2 Gy, twice daily, (Horiot *et al.*, 1990), accelerated regimes such as 'CHART' using 1.5 Gy 3 times per day over 12 consecutive days to a total dose of 54 Gy (Dische and Saunders, 1990), and the concomitant boost technique (Ang *et al.*, 1990). All of these show promise of better local control, but gains are likely to be small until methods of predictive testing of tumour cell sensitivity, kinetics and oxygenation permit the design of optimum fractionation schedules for individual tumours.

Other strategies to improve the results of radiotherapy include synchronous chemotherapy (see below) and measures designed to overcome the problems of radioresistant hypoxic tumour cells. Irradiation in high pressure oxygen has shown some benefit but the technique is too cumbersome for routine use (Henk, 1981). Drugs which selectively sensitize hypoxic cells have been developed; these are mainly nitro-imidazole compounds, e.g. misonidazole. These substances have proved to be too toxic to be administered at effective dosage. Another approach to the problem of the hypoxic cell is the use of fast neutron therapy which is less oxygen dependent than photon therapy. It is now rarely used because of the high incidence of severe late normal tissue effects, although some authorities still recommend it for the treatment of inoperable salivary gland tumours (Griffin *et al.*, 1989).

38.7.1 SIDE-EFFECTS OF RADIOTHERAPY

The major acute side-effect of radiotherapy is mucositis. The severity of mucositis depends on the size of the volume irradiated and the dose of radiation administered per day. It can be exacerbated by continued smoking and alcohol intake. There is considerable individual variation in the severity of mucositis which may be related to genetic differences in DNA repair. Mucositis is treated with local analgesics; aspirin is very effective as a mouth wash for the oral cavity, a gargle for the oropharynx or combined in lemon mucilage for the hypopharynx. Sucralfate suspension is useful for providing a protective coating over ulcerated areas. The pain of mucositis interferes with nutrition and it is important to maintain an adequate calorie intake and hydration. The services of a dietitian are invaluable in such patients. Some patients will need liquid food supplements and if adequate intake is not possible the patient should be provided with a fine bore nasogastric tube until normal swallowing is restored. Superadded candida infection is quite common; it should be managed initially with local antifungal agents, i.e. nystatin or amphotericin; if it does not respond to local agents it should be treated with systemic fluconazole. Taste loss is common especially if any part of the tongue or salivary apparatus is in the radiation fields. This adds to problems with nutrition and may last for several months after the end of radiotherapy.

Mucous and salivary gland tissue is particularly vulnerable to radiation and secretion from glands in the radiation field ceases within a few days of starting treatment. This leads to dryness of the irradiated mucosa and if all the salivary glands are irradiated, as for example in the case of carcinoma of the nasopharynx, the mouth becomes very dry. Some degree of dryness is permanent. The mouth should be kept clean using a simple mouth wash, avoiding antiseptic compounds which tend to be irritant. If tenacious mucus in the mouth is a problem, sodium bicarbonate or hydrogen peroxide should be used as a mouth wash. With the exception of dryness, acute radiation changes heal within a few weeks of completing the course of treatment.

Late normal tissue effects are of more serious consequence but should be infrequent if careful attention is paid to dosage and technique. Late effects include necrosis of soft tissue, bone and cartilage, and fibrosis of subcutaneous and pharyngeal tissues.

Dental care in the patient receiving radiotherapy to the head and neck is of great importance. The mandible is particularly at risk from osteoradionecrosis because of its relatively poor blood supply. A combination of a high dose of radiation and trauma especially from dental extraction can precipitate necrosis. In a patient in whom any part of the mandible is in the high dose treatment volume the teeth should be assessed before starting treatment. Teeth should be preserved where ever possible for the life-time of the patient, but if there are any teeth which are not salvageable they should be extracted before treatment begins, as postradiotherapy extraction is more likely to cause osteoradionecrosis than preradiotherapy extraction. If osteoradionecrosis occurs it should be treated conservatively in the first instance with scrupulous oral hygiene and long term administration of tetracycline to control super-added infection. Sequestra should be allowed to separate spontaneously. Hyperbaric oxygen, if available, is useful in trouble-

some cases (Hart and Mainous, 1976). If conservative measures fail surgery may be necessary with excision of the necrotic area of bone and restoration of mucosal cover by the introduction of a vascularized flap.

In a patient with a dry mouth the teeth are particularly at risk of marginal caries. In order to prevent loss of teeth careful attention to oral hygiene is essential with topical application of fluoride.

38.8 CHEMOTHERAPY

Mucous gland tumours with their low growth fraction are generally insensitive to cytotoxic drugs. Squamous carcinomas on the other hand have a high growth fraction and high cell loss factor so that they often respond, but are not curable by chemotherapy. The drugs most active against squamous cell carcinomas of the head and neck are methotrexate, cisplatin, carboplatin, bleomycin and fluorouracil, especially when given by continuous infusion. Other drugs with some activity include vinca alkaloids, cyclophosphamide and hydroxyurea. Combinations of drugs are more effective than single agents. The regimen most often used and regarded as the most effective consists of cisplatin $100 \text{ mg}/m^2$ followed by a 5 day continuous infusion of fluorouracil $1 \text{ g}/m^2$ per day, repeated at 3 weekly intervals provided that renal function is adequate (Kish *et al.*, 1982).

Reported response rates to chemotherapy vary considerably. A number of factors influence the probability of a response, especially previous treatment. Tumours recurring after radiotherapy and surgery are much less likely to respond to chemotherapy than untreated tumours. Other factors which militate against good response to chemotherapy are performance status (greater than 2) and very extensive disease, especially involvement of bone. In previously untreated disease a partial response of up to 80% to the cisplatin and fluorouracil combination is usual, with a proportion of complete responses (Rooney *et al.*, 1985). In recurrent disease response to the same regimen has been reported as anything between 11% and 79% (Urba and Forastiere, 1989).

Chemotherapy may be used either as part of combined treatment for locoregional disease or as palliative treatment for recurrence or metastases. There are three approaches to the use of chemotherapy as part of combined treatment.

1. 'Neoadjuvant' or 'induction' chemotherapy administered before local treatment, which aims to decrease the size of the tumour and thereby increase the chance of cure by subsequent surgery or radiotherapy.
2. 'Adjuvant' chemotherapy after locoregional treatment, which aims to eradicate microscopic residual tumour or micrometastases which are presumed to remain after the local treatment.
3. 'Concomitant' or 'synchronous' chemotherapy given at the same time as radiotherapy with the aim of enhancing the effect of radiation on the local disease and possibly at the same time eliminating micrometastases.

The high response rates to neoadjuvant chemotherapy suggest that cure rates should be improved, and indeed responders to induction chemotherapy have a better prognosis than non-responders. Unfortunately a number of controlled trials have failed to show any survival advantage, so it is likely that a good response to chemotherapy serves only to identify patients with curable disease rather than actually to contribute to cure. An overview of trials has revealed a slightly worse survival in patients given neoadjuvant chemotherapy (Stell and Rawson, 1990). There could be three reasons for this:

1. There are some instances of fatal chemotherapy toxicity.
2. In non-responders chemotherapy will delay effective local treatment.

3. Chemotherapy may stimulate more rapid cell division in the tumour cells which survive the chemotherapy, so diminishing the chances of a radiotherapy cure.

Tumours which respond well to induction chemotherapy usually prove subsequently to be radiocurable. Induction chemotherapy has been used in the USA as a predictive test to select patients with advanced laryngeal carcinoma for radical radiotherapy or elective surgery (Department of Veteran Affairs Laryngeal Study Group, 1991). However, most tumours respond, and it is not clear whether survival rates are higher than from a policy of radical radiotherapy and salvage surgery for all patients.

Adjuvant chemotherapy has not been used very much in head and neck cancer and the few studies done are largely negative. However in one study patients who responded to induction chemotherapy were randomized to adjuvant or no subsequent chemotherapy; the patients receiving the adjuvant chemotherapy had a longer median survival (Ervin *et al.*, 1987). In a study in oral cancer in India immediate postoperative adjuvant methotrexate was shown to improve survival rates, and this approach warrants further study (Rao *et al.*, 1991).

Concomitant chemotherapy and radiotherapy has been the subject of many studies. Drugs have been used either for their additive effect in the hope that this will be greater on tumour than on dose-limiting normal tissues, e.g. cisplatin, fluorouracil (Lo *et al.*, 1976), bleomycin (Fu *et al.*, 1987), or because the drugs may be expected to be selectively more toxic to a radioresistant population of cells, e.g. methotrexate (Gupta *et al.*, 1987) and hydroxyurea (Richards and Chambers, 1973) on cells in S phase of the mitotic cycle, or mitomycin C (Weissberg *et al.*, 1989) on hypoxic cells. Most studies of concomitant chemotherapy have shown an increase in local tumour control at the expense of greatly increased mucositis, and in some cases increased late radiation toxicity has also been observed (Peters *et al.*, 1988). It is not yet clear whether concomitant cytotoxic drugs have any advantages over higher dose or more accelerated radiotherapy schedules.

38.9 CHEMOPREVENTION

In cured head and neck cancer patients second primary tumours develop at a rate of about 3% per annum (Cooper *et al.*, 1989). There is now interest in the use of drugs to inhibit carcinogenesis in these patients.

Vitamin A and related compounds, known collectively as 'retinoids', have been shown to reverse dysplastic changes in oral epithelium of patients manifesting leucoplakia in about two-thirds of cases. These substances have been tested as adjuvant treatment after surgery with or without radiotherapy for head and neck cancer. In one placebo-controlled study isotretinoin had no effect on the rate of recurrence of the original tumours but significantly reduced the incidence of secondary primary tumours (Hong *et al.*, 1990). Further studies are in progress testing the chemopreventative action of both retinoids and also antioxidants, e.g. *N*-acetylcysteine (de Vries *et al.*, 1991).

38.10 MANAGEMENT OF CERVICAL LYMPH NODES

The management of cervical lymph node metastases depends on the stage of the disease and the site of the primary.

38.10.1 PATIENTS WITH NO CLINICAL EVIDENCE OF LYMPH NODE METASTASES (STAGE N0)

A proportion of patients who have no clinically or radiologically detectable lymph node metastases will nevertheless have micrometastases in nodes. The likelihood of micrometastases depends on the site, stage and histology of the primary tumour. The less well differentiated the primary tumour the greater the likelihood of lymph node metastases and in undifferentiated carcinoma of nasopharyngeal type the incidence is over 80%. Tumours of the nasopharynx, oropharynx, supraglottis and hypopharynx have a high incidence whereas tumours of the paranasal sinuses, lip and glottis have a low incidence. In the case of the oral cavity the incidence is strongly dependent on the size of the primary tumour, being low with tumours under 2 cm diameter and higher with larger tumours.

There has been much controversy for many years over whether elective nodal treatment improves survival, especially in the case of oral cavity carcinoma. An advantage for elective neck dissection has been claimed from retrospective reviews (Piedbois *et al.*, 1991) but only small prospective randomized trials have been done and these have failed to show any advantage over a watch and wait policy (Vandenbrouck *et al.*, 1980). There is similarly conflicting evidence of the value of elective neck irradiation. Radiotherapy and neck dissection are equally effective at eradicating micrometastases and therefore management of the neck depends on the management of the primary tumour. If treatment of the primary is surgical an elective neck dissection is usually performed, whereas if the primary is treated by radical radiotherapy elective neck irradiation is done at the same time. The dosage for elective neck irradiation need not be as large as that given to the primary tumour. There is good evidence that 50 Gy in 25 fractions will control over 90% of subclinical lymph node metastases (Mendenhall *et al.*, 1980).

The authors' policy is to give elective lymph node treatment except in those cases where the risk of micrometastases is considered to be less than 20%, which in practice includes carcinoma of the glottis, paranasal sinuses, lip, and early oral cavity carcinomas.

38.10.2   UNILATERAL LYMPH NODE METASTASES (STAGES N1, N2A, N2B)

A lymph node metastasis may be found at the time of initial diagnosis, or may appear at follow-up after treatment of the primary. It is usually possible to diagnose lymph node metastases with some degree of confidence on clinical and radiological grounds, although sometimes a swelling in the neck may prove to be an enlarged submandibular salivary gland or a reactive lymph node. Therefore fine needle aspiration biopsy is advisable to confirm the diagnosis. Open biopsy should be avoided if at all possible and in cases of real doubt the whole node should be excised for histology.

In general lymph node metastases are better treated surgically than by a policy of radical radiotherapy and salvage surgery. This is not because lymph node metastases are inherently more radioresistant than the primaries from which they are derived, as is sometimes claimed. The problem with radical radiotherapy of lymph node metastases is the difficulty in diagnosing recurrence and the very poor results of salvage surgery, which is in contrast to the quite good results of salvage surgery for recurrent primary tumours.

38.10.3   SURGICAL MANAGEMENT OF THE NECK

Where there are palpable nodes present, a radical neck dissection (Crile, 1906) is usually preferable, incorporating resection of the whole of the lymph node field on that side of the neck (levels I–V),[*] together with the sternomastoid muscle, the accessory nerve and the internal jugular vein.

In some patients the nodes may be small and mobile, or may only be demonstrable on CT scan, in which case some form of functional neck dissection may be considered. Selective preservation of the accessory nerve, the internal jugular vein or the sternomastoid muscle can be considered but should only be undertaken by an experienced and competent surgeon.

In N0 necks where there are no demonstrable node metastases but a high risk of microscopic deposits, a partial functional neck dissection of the local draining nodes may be undertaken. For instance, in floor of mouth and tongue tumours a supra-omohyoid neck dissection can be considered incorporating the submandibular triangle, and upper and middle deep cervical chain nodes (levels 1–3) including the jugulo-omohyoid nodes. A suprahyoid dissection is dangerous because metastases may spread directly to the omohyoid nodes and if these are not resected, there is a high incidence of later recurrence in the lower part of the neck. Ideally, frozen section of the resected nodes should be undertaken and the neck dissection completed if any are positive.

Postoperative radiotherapy to the neck is indicated if there are multiple metastatic nodes, if there is perineural or vascular invasion or if there is extracapsular extension of tumour.

One other way of combining surgery and radiotherapy is the use of afterloaded iridium wire implants. Some patients who have had radical dose irradiation to the neck develop recurrence at the same site despite adequate control elsewhere. The recurrence may appear inoperable; it may have invaded skin or be closely applied to the carotid artery, or may be giving rise to severe pain. Some form of palliative procedure may be indicated to relieve symptoms and in these situations a radical neck dissection may be combined with insertion of plastic tubes at operation across the bed of the neck dissection at the site where the metastases had been excised. Radioactive iridium wires are then inserted postoperatively for a period of 3–4 days to

---

[*] Level I   = submandibular nodes.
   Level II   = upper deep cervical nodes.
   Level III   = midcervical nodes.
   Level IV   = lower deep cervical nodes.
   Level V   = posterior triangle nodes.

give up to 60 Gy localized to the site at risk. Using this technique a local control rate of 60% at 2 years has been achieved. Reconstruction of the overlying skin is essential with some form of skin or myocutaneous flap in order to avoid skin necrosis.

38.11 CARCINOMA OF THE NASOPHARYNX

38.11.1 INCIDENCE AND AETIOLOGY

Carcinoma of the nasopharynx has its highest incidence in South East Asia where in some parts it is the most frequently occurring neoplasm. Other ethnic groups with a high incidence are Eskimos and inhabitants of North and East Central Africa. The tumour is very rare in the UK, with an incidence of 0.1 per 100 000 per annum. This compares with an incidence of between 10 and 20 per 100 000 in Hong Kong for example.

There is a male to female preponderance of approximately 2 to 1. The peak incidence is in the fifth decade in South East Asia, whereas in Africa a bimodal age distribution is seen with peaks in the third and sixth decades. The tumour is occasionally seen in children and adolescents. In the UK, despite its rarity, it is the commonest epithelial head and neck tumour of children and adolescents.

The aetiology is multifactorial. The ethnic incidences indicate that genetic factors predominate. Environmental factors in Hong Kong which have been associated with a significant increase in risk are the administration of salted fish at weaning, and living in smoky atmospheres. The tumour is associated with EBV, but the precise aetiological role is unclear.

38.11.2 PATHOLOGY

The official World Health Organization classification is as follows:

1. **Keratinizing carcinoma** – clear histological evidence of squamous differentiation.

2. **Non-keratinizing carcinoma** – an epithelial growth pattern is seen but no evidence of squamous differentiation can be seen on light microscopy.
3. **Undifferentiated carcinoma of nasopharyngeal type (UCNT)** – the cells have a syncitial appearance on light microscopy, but electron microscopy shows evidence of epithelial origin.

Types 2 and 3 have similar behaviour. Either may show a lymphoid infiltrate, hence the old term 'lympho-epithelioma'. These types always predominate where there is a high incidence of the disease; e.g. they together comprise 97% of nasopharyngeal carcinoma in Hong Kong. They invariably have EBV DNA detectable in the cell nucleus, whereas type 1 often does not (Hording *et al.*, 1993).

38.11.3 BEHAVIOUR

All types spread locally to adjacent structures taking lines of least resistance. The routes of spread are important in planning target volumes for radiotherapy. Superiorly the base of skull is invaded but usually at a late stage; the weakest barrier to upward spread is provided by the foramen lacerum immediately lateral to the basisphenoid bone. The tumour thereby enters the floor of the temporal fossa in the cavernous sinus, affecting in turn the 6th, 5th and 3rd cranial nerves. Laterally the tumour enters the parapharyngeal space through the lateral wall of the nasopharynx. Upward and lateral spread through the sphenopalatine foramen leads to involvement of the pterygoid fossa and posterior part of the orbit. Direct spread anteriorly into the nasal fossa and inferiorly into the oropharynx may occur.

Lymphatic spread occurs at a relatively early stage especially in histological types 2 and 3. One of the first nodes to be involved is the lateral pharyngeal, which may affect the lower four cranial nerves as they emerge from the skull base. The first nodes to become palpable in the neck are frequently at the apex of the posterior triangle in the submastoid region. The upper deep cervical nodes are also commonly affected and subsequently all node groups in the neck can become involved.

Types 2 and 3 are the most likely of all epithelial head and neck tumours to give rise to blood borne metastases. These are seen especially in patients who also have extensive lymph node involvement in the neck. The principal sites of distant metastasis in order of frequency are bone, lung and liver.

38.11.4   PRESENTATION

Approximately 70% of cases have lymph nodes palpable in the neck at the time of presentation, and a lump in the neck is often the first symptom. The commonest presentation is with ear symptoms resulting from serous otitis media consequent upon eustachian tube obstruction. Nasal symptoms, i.e. obstruction and epistaxis, are relatively less common. Occasionally cranial nerve palsies are the presenting symptoms.

38.11.5   DIAGNOSIS

When nasopharyngeal carcinoma is suspected the nasopharynx should be examined, usually by fibre-optic naso-endoscopy as mirror examination is not always satisfactory. If a tumour is seen, an examination under anaesthetic and biopsy is needed. Imaging with CT or MRI is necessary to demonstrate the extent of the tumour. In undifferentiated carcinoma, especially where there is lymph node involvement, an isotope bone scan should be performed.

Nearly all cases of histological types 2 and 3 carcinoma have elevated serum antibodies to EBV. The most specific for nasopharyngeal carcinoma is the viral capsid antigen (VCA) IgA titre. A titre greater than 1 in 10 is strongly suggestive of nasopharyngeal carci-

noma. This test is used for screening high risk populations.

38.11.6   TREATMENT

In all patients in whom no blood borne metastases can be detected radiotherapy is the treatment of choice.

For the first phase of treatment the tumour and all potential routes of spread are covered to a dose of 50 Gy in 25 fractions in 5 weeks. At the primary site these include the entire nasopharynx, the posterior half of the nasal fossa, the soft palate, the adjacent parapharyngeal space, the adjacent part of the base of skull, i.e. that formed by the greater wing of the sphenoid and sphenoid sinus, and the posterior half of the orbit. In a patient with no lymph node involvement the upper half of the neck is irradiated in the case of squamous cell carcinoma and the whole neck in the case of undifferentiated carcinoma. A boost is given to areas of gross tumour, 14 Gy in 5 fractions in the case of undifferentiated carcinoma and 20 Gy in 10 fractions in the case of squamous carcinoma. Care must be taken to avoid exceeding the tolerance dose of vulnerable nearby structures. The dose to the spinal cord, brain stem and hypothalamus should not exceed 40 Gy and that to the retina and optic nerve should not exceed 50 Gy.

As the lateral fields used to treat the nasopharynx inevitably pass through both parotid glands the major side-effect of radiotherapy is severe dryness of the mouth, which is usually permanent.

UCNT is the most chemosensitive of the epithelial head and neck tumours. A variety of regimens have been used to treat recurrent and metastatic disease with a high response rate. At the Royal Marsden the cisplatin and fluorouracil infusion combination is used (see above). There have been many studies of the use of chemotherapy in a neoadjuvant manner before radiotherapy. Overall no survival benefit has yet been demonstrated and the results of controlled clinical trials to date are disappointing, despite some claims of prolonged survival in patients with advanced nodal stage disease (Bachouchi *et al.*, 1990). Several series have suggested improved survival in children with nasopharyngeal carcinoma treated with chemotherapy plus radiotherapy, compared with historical controls treated with radiotherapy alone, but again there is no evidence as yet from randomized studies (Ingersoll *et al.*, 1990).

Local recurrences of UCNT often do well with retreatment, especially if they occur more than 2 years after the initial treatment. Some of these late recurrences may in fact be new primaries. Where it is possible, local excision of the tumour via a Le Fort I maxillotomy approach combined with brachytherapy is giving encouraging results. A second course of external radiotherapy may be curative, but is associated with a high morbidity.

38.11.7 PROGNOSIS

Overall reported 5 year survival rates average around 65% for histological types 2 and 3 and 40% for histological type 1. With the former, ultimate failure at the primary site occurs in only about 10% of cases; lymph node failure is particularly rare, nearly all fatal cases having distant metastases. With type 1 the major cause of death is failure at the primary site. Unfavourable prognostic features include involvement of the base of skull and nodes in the lower half of the neck (Sham and Choy, 1990).

38.12 CARCINOMA OF THE OROPHARYNX

38.12.1 INCIDENCE AND AETIOLOGY

Carcinoma of the oropharynx is relatively rare in the UK with an incidence of approximately 0.8 per 100 000 per annum. The highest incidence is in France where it is more that 10 times as common as in the UK. There is also a relatively high incidence in the USA where it is commoner in the black than the white population. Where the disease is common the male/female ratio tends to be about 10 to 1, whereas in areas with a lower incidence there is a less strong male preponderance. For example the ratio in the UK is 2.5 to 1.

There is a strong correlation between smoking and alcohol intake but no other aetiological factors have been demonstrated.

38.12.2 PATHOLOGY

The vast majority of tumours are squamous carcinoma, usually poorly differentiated. Undifferentiated carcinoma of nasopharyngeal type occasionally occurs in the tonsil.

Lymph node involvement is common. Tonsillar carcinoma metastasizes initially to the upper deep cervical lymph nodes on the same side. Contralateral lymph node involvement is uncommon, occurring in about 15% of cases who also have ipsilateral nodal involvement. Carcinoma of the base of tongue metastasizes initially in most instances to the midcervical nodes and lymph node involvement is frequently bilateral. Lymph node involvement from soft palate carcinoma is also frequently bilateral to upper deep cervical and retropharyngeal lymph nodes.

38.12.3 PRESENTATION AND DIAGNOSIS

Tumours in this area often give minimal symptoms at an early stage so that presentation is frequently late. The usual symptoms are a feeling of discomfort in the throat especially on swallowing and pain radiating to the ear. It is not unusual for a lump in the neck to be the presenting symptom. For some reason metastases from carcinoma of the tonsil tend readily to become cystic; the so-called carcinoma in a brachial cyst nearly always turns out to be a lymph node metastasis from a tonsillar primary. Examination under anaesthetic and biopsy is necessary to establish the diagnosis.

38.12.4 TREATMENT

Most oropharyngeal carcinomas are best treated by radiotherapy. In general radiotherapy gives local control rates and survival rates as good as those of surgery, but with better functional outcomes. An exception is large infiltrating tumours of the base of the tongue; these have a poor prognosis however treated but in a patient fit for the procedure surgical removal and reconstruction offer the best chance of survival. Surgery in such a case however often involves total glossectomy and sometimes partial or total laryngectomy. Access for surgery to the oropharynx may be difficult and a mandibulotomy is sometimes necessary, and in cases where there is deep invasion from the tonsil, resection of the ascending ramus of the mandible is usually required. Reconstruction of the oropharynx depends on the extent of resection. For tumours on the lateral aspect of the tongue base excision includes hemiglossectomy and often resection of the tonsillar fossa or lateral pharyngeal wall. In these cases a free radial forearm flap is most suitable as this can be accurately contoured to the shape of the defect. For larger tumours involving the centre of the tongue base a total glossectomy is necessary and reconstruction in this case is best carried out with a latissimus dorsi flap which does give additional bulk to the oropharynx which is more helpful for rehabilitation of speech.

Brachytherapy is used for treatment of base of tongue tumours in some centres; this technique is not used in this institution as it carries a risk of complications, especially haemorrhage, and the evidence of superior results over external radiotherapy is not convincing.

In a patient with unilateral nodal metastases radiotherapy to the primary is usually followed by a neck dissection.

Because of the high incidence of lymph node involvement elective nodal irradiation is advisable in all cases. In the case of T1 or T2 carcinoma of the tonsil without palpable lymph nodes the radiation volume can be confined to the primary site and the first station, i.e. upper deep cervical, lymph nodes on the same side. Irradiation of both sides of the neck in such a case is unnecessary and results in increased morbidity especially xerostomia. For carcinoma of the soft palate, base of tongue and posterior pharyngeal wall, the first station nodes on both sides of the neck must be included in the treatment volume. In any patient with lymph node involvement the entire cervical lymphatic system on both sides of the neck should be irradiated.

38.12.5 PROGNOSIS

The prognosis is influenced by the site of the primary tumour within the oropharynx, stage of the disease and performance status. Tonsillar carcinoma has a better prognosis than carcinoma at any of the other sites within the oropharynx.

Local control rates by radiotherapy for T1 and T2 tumours of the tonsil exceed 80% in most series; rates for the base of tongue are usually 10% or 15% lower. Control rates between 50% and 75% have been reported for T3 tumours but the results of T4 tumours are very poor. Survival rates are usually considerably lower than the local control rates, mainly because of deaths from other diseases and distant metastases. Overall 5 year survival rates for all stages combined are about 40%.

38.13 CARCINOMA OF THE ORAL CAVITY

38.13.1 INCIDENCE AND AETIOLOGY

Worldwide, oral cavity cancer is estimated to represent about 8% of all malignancy in men and 4% in women. The incidence in the UK is relatively low where it represents less than 1% of all cancers. The incidence in men fell by a factor of 10 between 1930 and 1970, while remaining almost constant in women. The reasons for this change have never been satisfactorily explained.

The parts of the world with the highest incidence are the Indian subcontinent and France. In most populations there is a steeply rising incidence after the age of 40, before which oral cancer is rare. Known aetiological factors include smoking, alcohol, tobacco and betel chewing, and nutritional deficiencies. Certain infections, e.g. chronic candidiasis, syphilis, human papilloma virus and herpes simplex, have been suggested as causative factors but their precise role is not clear. Similarly the role of dental sepsis and trauma, although often quoted as a cause of cancer, is by no means established.

38.13.2 PATHOLOGY

The vast majority of oral cavity malignancies are squamous carcinomas often well differentiated. Tumours can also arise from minor salivary glands, where the same histological types occur as in major salivary glands, of which adenoid cystic carcinoma is the commonest.

Some squamous carcinomas arise on areas of pre-existing dysplasia. This usually manifests itself as a white patch (leucoplakia) or as a red patch (erythroplakia). The former may represent either hyperkeratosis, which is not premalignant, or dysplasia which is, so biopsy is necessary. Erythroplakia is more likely to be premalignant.

Squamous cell carcinoma of the oral cavity spreads by local infiltration and via lymphatics. The first station lymph nodes are the first to be involved, usually either submandibular or upper deep cervical; however anterior midline lesions occasionally spread by so-called 'fast pathways' to the lower deep cervical nodes. The incidence of lymph node metastases is strongly correlated with the size of the primary tumour. There is also a correlation with histology, poorly differentiated carcinoma being more likely to give rise to lymph node metastases than well differentiated. Distant metastases are relatively rare and are only seen in patients with extensive lymph node involvement.

38.13.3 PRESENTATION AND DIAGNOSIS

Oral cancer characteristically presents as a swelling or ulcer on the oral mucosa which is usually painless initially. As deep infiltration into muscle or bone occurs the lesion becomes painful. On clinical examination it may appear indurated and craggy or exophytic with a cauliflower appearance. As prognosis depends on stage at first treatment it is important that general medical and dental practitioners are aware of the possibility of a carcinoma when a patient complains of a lesion in the mouth.

The diagnosis must be established by biopsy. If excision biopsy of a small lesion is performed it must be preceded by an accurate record of the position and limits of the lesion. A radiotherapist should not be presented with a patient who has no visible or palpable abnormality in the mouth but is accompanied by a report of an oral carcinoma incompletely excised.

38.13.4 TREATMENT

Small lesions and areas of premalignant change which can easily be removed without any deformity, e.g. a small lesion on the anterior third of the tongue, are best treated by surgery which is quicker and simpler than radiotherapy. Advanced stage T3 and T4 tumours which generally do badly with radical radiotherapy should be treated surgically whenever possible, usually combined with postoperative radiotherapy.

The management of intermediate stage lesions, including more posteriorly situated T1 and most T2 tumours, is more controversial. Surgery is now the more popular treatment, but can often result in some functional defect. Radical radiotherapy can give

comparable cure rates provided brachytherapy is used, and if successful often results
in less residual disability than surgery. In our
unit radiotherapy is often preferred for these
intermediate stage tumours subject to the
criteria outlined previously.

38.13.5   SURGERY

Premalignant lesions and small tumours up
to about a 1 cm in diameter situated on the
anterior part of the tongue are best excised
using a laser and left to epithelialize spontaneously. Larger lesions requires resection
and reconstruction. After hemiglossectomy a
free radial forearm flap is ideal for reconstruction as a piece of skin can be introduced with
its own artery and vein which can be anastomosed to vessels in the neck; it can be made
to conform well to the contours of the structures within the mouth. This allows good
mobility of the tongue with only minimal
disturbance of speech. A neck dissection is
performed at the same time as the hemiglossectomy. If there is no clinical evidence of
nodal involvement a supra-omohyoid dissection removing nodes from levels 1, 2, and
3 is sufficient. This also facilitates access to
branches of the external carotid artery for the
free flap anastomosis.

Tumours of the floor of the mouth adjacent
to bone and tumours of the inferior alveolus
are best treated surgically, although brachytherapy is an alternative treatment for smaller
tumours of the floor of mouth which do not
encroach near the bone. Invasion of the
mandible tends to be late, usually through the
dental roots at the apex of the alveolus. For
early lesions a partial thickness resection of
the mandible can be carried out with flap
reconstruction. In more advanced cases
where there is obvious invasion of the mandible a segment of mandible must be excised.
Reconstruction of the mandible is necessary
particularly of the anterior arch in order to
avoid severe deformity. At present the most
successful reconstruction method for the

mandible is the free fibular graft. This can be
contoured to the defect by multiple osteo-
tomies and can be used incorporating an
overlying skin graft to replace the mucosa.

38.13.6   RADIOTHERAPY

It is well established that local control rates
are higher with brachytherapy or combined
brachytherapy and external beam than with
external beam alone. (Wallner *et al.*, 1986). All
tumours selected for radical radiotherapy
which are sufficiently accessible and not
involving the periosteum should receive
brachytherapy at least as part of the
treatment.

Iridium-192 hairpins are used to implant
lesions of the tongue and floor of mouth.
Buccal mucosa lesions are implanted using
iridium-192 wire inserted percutaneously via
plastic tubes. T1 tumours are generally
treated by implant alone because of the relatively low incidence of lymph node metastases. T2 tumours because of the greater
likelihood of occult nodal metastases are
treated by combined external beam and
implant; the primary receives 40 Gy from
external beam and 35 Gy from an implant,
while the neck receives 50 Gy from external
beam. For technical details see Henk and
Langdon (1994).

38.13.7   PROGNOSIS

Survival rates have changed very little over
the past 30 years despite claims of improvement in local control from better surgical
technique. Local control rates are over 80%
for T1 and T2 tumours by either surgery or
brachytherapy; however 5 year survival rates
are only about 80% for T1N0 and 60% for
T2N0, because of an appreciable mortality
from nodal disease, distant metastases,
second primary tumours and intercurrent
illness. In patients presenting with nodal
involvement or T3 or T4 primaries 5 year
survival rates remain below 40%.

38.14 CARCINOMA OF THE LARYNX

The frequent sites of origin of carcinoma in the larynx are the vocal cord (glottic), and the supraglottic region where tumours can arise from any part from the tip of the epiglottis to the laryngeal ventricle. Tumours arising from the larynx below the vocal cord (subglottic) are rare.

38.14.1 INCIDENCE AND AETIOLOGY

The worldwide incidence of laryngeal cancer is more evenly spread than that of many other head and neck sites. However, the relative incidence of glottic and supraglottic cancer varies in different parts of the world. In the UK glottic cancer is far commoner than supraglottic. France, Spain, Italy, Poland and many other countries have a higher incidence of supraglottic cancer.

The incidence of supraglottic carcinoma is strongly related to alcohol intake and smoking, but glottic cancer although commoner in smokers is less strongly correlated with tobacco and alcohol.

38.14.2 PATHOLOGY

Epithelial dysplasia is quite common especially on the vocal cord in smokers. Dysplasia may progress to *in situ* and subsequently to invasive squamous carcinoma in a proportion of cases. Dysplasia is less common in the supraglottis but when it occurs is more likely to be associated with invasive carcinoma.

The majority of malignant laryngeal tumours are squamous carcinomas mostly well or moderately differentiated. Mucous gland tumours and small cell carcinoma similar to that seen in the lung occur rarely.

38.14.3 BEHAVIOUR

The vocal cord is a relatively avascular structure with limited lymphatic drainage. Carcinoma usually grows slowly and invades adjacent parts of the larynx eventually, e.g. the anterior commissure, ventricle and subglottis. It is usually at a late stage before deep infiltration of muscle, fixing the vocal cord, and cartilage occurs. Advanced disease if untreated will eventually give rise to airway obstruction. Nodal metastases occur infrequently and only when the subglottic or supraglottic region becomes involved.

The supraglottis on the other hand is highly vascular and has a rich lymphatic drainage. Supraglottic carcinoma therefore can give rise to lymphatic metastases at an early stage, and surprisingly the risk of lymph node metastases seems independent of the size of the primary tumour. About one-third of patients have involved lymph nodes palpable at presentation; histological evidence of lymph node involvement is found in about 70% of patients who undergo surgery.

38.14.4 PRESENTATION AND DIAGNOSIS

Glottic carcinoma presents as persistent hoarseness at a very early stage. If the significance of this symptom is recognized lesions of no more than 2 mm in size can be diagnosed and treated. If persistent hoarseness is not investigated for many months stridor and airway obstruction eventually supervene.

Supraglottic carcinoma on the other hand gives to rise to very few symptoms in the early stages. The first symptom is often just a vague discomfort on swallowing. Later there may be pain radiating to the ear. Hoarseness will occur if there is involvement of the ventricular band or vocal cord but this is often a late symptom. A lump in the neck may be the first sign of the disease.

The diagnosis must be established by endoscopy and biopsy. Imaging is probably unnecessary if endoscopy shows a very small lesion confined to the vocal cord, but all other cases should have a CT scan to demonstrate the extent of the primary tumour, and cartilage invasion and lymph node involvement.

38.14.5   TREATMENT

T1 and T2 tumours are best treated by radical radiotherapy and careful follow-up. In some units partial laryngeal surgery is preferred to radiotherapy but the voice quality is not usually as good as after successful radiotherapy and there may be swallowing difficulties. Patients with laryngeal cancer in the UK often have associated chronic obstructive airways disease and are therefore unable to tolerate the small amount of aspiration which is inevitable in the early stages after partial laryngeal surgery.

The management of more advanced laryngeal carcinoma is more controversial. The chance of tumour control by radiotherapy in T3 tumours is about 60% on average. After radiotherapy the larynx often does not return completely to normal. There may be persistent oedema and limitation of movement but no obvious tumour visible, so that it is difficult to diagnose persistent or recurrent tumour. Many laryngologists take the view that recurrence after radiotherapy tends to be diagnosed too late and that salvage laryngectomy has a higher rate of both morbidity and failure than immediate laryngectomy. Accordingly they prefer the latter, believing it to give a higher survival rate. Nevertheless, there has not been a controlled trial comparing immediate laryngectomy with radical radiotherapy and salvage surgery in advanced laryngeal carcinoma. Retrospective reviews such as those of Marshall *et al.* (1972) have shown no difference in survival rates between the two policies, and if a policy of radical radiotherapy is used at least half the survivors retain the larynx.

Our policy is to treat advanced laryngeal carcinoma with radical radiotherapy with three exceptions. These are:

1. **Invasion of cartilage** because tumour invading cartilage is hypoxic and relatively radioresistant; even if the tumour is eliminated the damaged cartilage fails to heal well resulting in chronic oedema and pain and infection in the larynx.

2. **Airway obstruction** necessitating tracheostomy, because a preliminary tracheostomy probably facilitates spread of the disease and there is a risk of stomal recurrence worsening the prognosis. An exception is if the obstruction is due to proliferative exophytic tumour which can be partly removed by laser or diathermy excision providing a good airway without recourse to tracheostomy.

3. A patient who is **unlikely to attend regularly for follow-up.**

Operable lymph nodes should be treated surgically but there is debate whether the presence of lymph node metastases is an indication for surgical treatment of the primary. There is conflicting evidence on whether or not lymph node involvement is associated with a lower rate of tumour control by radiotherapy stage for stage. Our policy in a patient with a supraglottic tumour and mobile unilateral lymph nodes is to treat the primary tumour by radiotherapy and at the same time giving a preoperative dose of 50 Gy in 5 weeks to the nodes. Six weeks after the end of treatment the primary site is assessed and if it is clear a neck dissection is performed preserving the larynx.

Early recurrent T1 and T2 carcinomas of the glottis can be salvaged by vertical partial hemilaryngectomy. Supraglottic recurrences however are best treated with total laryngectomy because there is a high incidence of overspill and pulmonary complications following supraglottic salvage laryngectomy.

Following total laryngectomy voice restoration has undergone a major change in the last 10 years since the advent of the tracheo-oesophageal voice prosthesis. At the time of the laryngectomy a small fistula is made through the posterior tracheal wall into the oesophagus just below the mucocutaneous junction. A 14 FG catheter is inserted through the fistula into the oesophagus and used for postoperative feeding. When the neck is healed and swallowing has been established the catheter is removed and replaced immediately with a small silicone valve. The one that we have been using with success at the Royal Marsden Hospital is the Blom Singer valve which is a one way valve allowing air to pass from the trachea into the oesophagus and the vocal tract but it prevents any food or fluid flowing back into the trachea. The success rate in achieving a good quality voice is in the region of 80–90% even in patients who have a total pharyngolaryngectomy with reconstruction.

In patients with recurrent unilateral tumour which is too extensive for a vertical hemilaryngectomy, a near total laryngectomy may be feasible, provided that careful frozen section clearance is obtained at operation. This technique may also be used for primary surgical treatment of T3 or transglottic tumours where radiotherapy is not suitable. At operation, the side of the larynx with the tumour is excised under frozen section control. The remnant portion of the contralateral vocal cord and false cord, which still has its sensory and motor nerve innervation from the recurrent laryngeal nerve, is then reconstructed in a tubular fashion. This provides a tracheopharyngeal speech fistula with minimal problems of leakage. The tracheostomy is permanent but no prosthesis is required.

38.14.6 PROGNOSIS

Death from early glottic carcinoma is extremely rare. Local control by radiotherapy in our unit is over 90% for T1 and 80% for T2. The overall survival for T3 glottic carcinoma is about 60%; the local control by radiotherapy in the patients selected as described above is 70%. Supraglottic carcinoma has a worse prognosis because of the high incidence of nodal metastases. For T1 and T2 tumours without nodal involvement local control by radiotherapy is at least 75% in

most reported series with a 5 year survival of between 60% and 70%, most patients dying of other causes. Overall the 5 year survival of patients presenting with nodal disease is about 40%.

38.15 CARCINOMA OF THE HYPOPHARYNX

Carcinoma of the three sites of the hypopharynx have different aetiologies and natural history and therefore will be considered separately.

38.15.1 PYRIFORM FOSSA

Carcinoma of the pyriform fossa is very similar in incidence and aetiology to supraglottic carcinoma. It also tends to present with vague symptoms of discomfort on swallowing, progressing to dysphagia and pain radiating to the ear. Hoarseness and respiratory obstruction occur at a late stage.

Nodal involvement is very common and in many cases a lump in the neck is the first symptom. Lymphatics pass to the upper end of the deep cervical chain so that there is a predilection for nodal metastases to become fixed to the base of the skull.

T1 and T2 tumours without nodal involvement can be treated either by radical radiotherapy or partial laryngectomy with similar survival rates. The former is preferred in the UK for the same reason as in the case of laryngeal carcinoma. However very few are diagnosed at an early stage. Surgery is the better treatment if there is cartilage involvement or unilateral operable nodal metastases. Very advanced disease unsuitable for surgery is also often treated by radical radiotherapy but results are poor and especially in an elderly patient it may be better to offer only palliative care.

The overall survival rate is low, mainly because of late presentation and a high death rate from other smoking and alcohol related diseases. Most large series quote 5 year survival rates of 20% for node positive and 40%

for node negative patients. These figures seem largely independent of the method of treatment (Shah *et al.*, 1976; Bataini *et al.*, 1981).

38.15.2   POSTCRICOID CARCINOMA

Carcinoma of the postcricoid region differs in incidence and aetiology from most other head and neck cancers. It is commoner in women than men and has its highest incidence in northern latitudes in western countries, e.g. Scotland, Northern England, Wales, Scandinavia and Canada. About 50% of the cases are associated with iron deficiency anaemia and mucosal atrophy (Paterson–Kelly syndrome).

The tumour spreads circumferentially to surround the hypopharynx at the oesophageal junction. It can spread down the oesophagus by direct mucosal extension or via submucosal lymphatics. Lymph node involvement is common; the first involved nodes may be in the superior mediastinum or high in the neck as in the case of pyriform fossa carcinoma.

Postcricoid carcinoma presents as worsening dysphagia. Unfortunately it is often diagnosed at a late stage because the patient frequently has a history of some difficulty in swallowing over a period of many years because of the Paterson–Kelly syndrome or a postcricoid web, and therefore the early symptoms of the disease go unrecognized.

Except for T1N0 stage disease surgery gives higher local control rates than radical radiotherapy and holds out a better chance of restoring swallowing. However many patients are elderly and present at an advanced stage. If there is mediastinal node involvement or bilateral neck node involvement it is best not to attempt radical treatment.

The overall 5 year survival rate is about 10%, ranging from 45% for stage T1 to less than 5% for T3 and T4.

38.15.3   POSTERIOR PHARYNGEAL WALL

The posterior wall is the least common site for carcinoma in the hypopharynx. Tumours at this site are sometimes associated with the Paterson–Kelly syndrome but most are not. Dysphagia is the presenting symptom.

It is difficult to obtain adequate surgical clearance of a posterior pharyngeal wall tumour. Results of radical radiotherapy seem generally comparable to those of surgery with a lower morbidity. Five year survival is about 33%.

38.15.4   SURGERY FOR HYPOPHARYNGEAL TUMOURS

Surgery involves a total pharyngolaryngo-oesophagectomy with neck dissection in most cases. Reconstruction of the hypopharynx can be carried out with stomach pull up or colon transposition but these methods carry a mortality of 10–15%. More recently the free jejunum graft has been used with success in reconstruction of the pharyngeal defect and this has a much lower morbidity. Skin flap reconstruction, either with a latissimus dorsi pedicled flap or a free radial forearm flap, can give excellent results and morbidity from these reconstructions is minimal. They have the additional advantage of tolerating postoperative radiotherapy better than stomach or colon.

Voice restoration using a Blom Singer valve can be carried out at a secondary stage a few months after the patient has recovered from the pharyngectomy.

38.16   CARCINOMA OF PARANASAL SINUSES

Tumours of the paranasal sinuses are relatively uncommon. They occur most frequently in the maxillary antrum, and rather less frequently in the ethmoid sinus. Tumours of the frontal and sphenoid sinuses are very rare. The majority are well differentiated squamous cell carcinoma, especially in the maxillary antrum. Anaplastic and transitional cell types occur more often in the ethmoid sinus. Some cases are associated with exposure to carcinogens, e.g. in the nickel smelting and furniture industries, but in most cases there is no known aetiological factor.

Presentation is characteristically late as no symptoms occur until the tumour spreads beyond the sinus of origin. Carcinoma of the maxillary antrum may present as swelling of the cheek from anterior extension, dental symptoms or a lump in the palate from inferior extension, or nasal symptoms from medial extension. Involvement of the pterygoid fossa or orbit may occur and is sometimes responsible for the presenting symptoms. Ethmoid sinus carcinoma will present either with nasal symptoms or with proptosis because of extension into the orbit. Lymph node involvement is relatively uncommon, occurring in less than 25% of cases. The first nodes involved may be the facial, submandibular or lateral pharyngeal.

The diagnosis must be established by biopsy. The maxillary antrum is best biopsied via a nasal antrostomy which also establishes drainage. CT or MRI are necessary to define the extent of tumour prior to treatment.

As paranasal sinus tumours are usually large at presentation combined treatment is necessary with surgery and postoperative radiotherapy. A possible exception is anaplastic carcinoma of the ethmoid sinus where control rates by radiotherapy alone are high. Maxillary antral carcinoma is treated by maxillectomy which leaves a large cavity in communication with the oral cavity. This is best closed by a prosthesis consisting of an obturator and denture, although some surgeons favour reconstruction. Five year survival rates for paranasal sinus carcinoma in the UK average around 30%.

38.17 OTHER HEAD AND NECK SITES

A variety of tumour types can occur in the nasal fossa. These include squamous cell carcinoma, mucous gland tumours, plasmacytoma and lymphoma. The condition formally known as midline or Stewart's granuloma is now known to be a variety of T-cell lymphoma which tends to remain localized but be associated with considerable tissue destruction. Early squamous cell carcinomas are treated by radiotherapy alone; larger tumours require combined treatment.

Aesthesioneuroblastoma is a rare tumour arising from olfactory epithelium. It tends to be slow growing with a propensity for local recurrence and rarely metastasizes to nodes or via the blood stream. Treatment is by surgical excision and postoperative radiotherapy.

Carcinoma of the middle ear is also rare. It usually arises in a patient with a long history of chronic suppurative otitis media. It tends to present late when there is considerable destruction of the petrous bone and severe pain. The optimum treatment is by temporal bone resection and postoperative radiotherapy, although in many cases the disease is too advanced for this to be possible. The prognosis is generally rather poor with 5 year survival rates of around 25% on average.

REFERENCES

Ang, K.K., Peters, L.J., Weber, R.S. *et al.* (1990) Concomitant boost radiotherapy schedules in the treatment of carcinoma of the oropharynx and nasopharynx. *International Journal of Radiation Oncology, Biology, Physics*, **19**, 1339–45.

Ariyan, S. (1979) The pectoralis myocutaneous flap. *Plastic and Reconstructive Surgery*, **63**, 73–81.

Bachouchi, M., Cvitkovic, E., Azli, N. *et al.* (1990) High complete response in advanced nasopharyngeal carcinoma with bleomycin, epirubicin and cisplatin before radiotherapy. *Journal of the National Cancer Institute*, **82**, 616–20.

Bakamjian, V.Y. (1965) A two-staged method of pharyngoesophageal reconstruction using a primary pectoral skin flap. *Plastic and Reconstructive Surgery*, **36**, 173–81.

Bataini, P., Brugere, J., Bernier, J. *et al.* (1981) Results of radiotherapeutic treatment of carcinoma of the pyriform sinus: experience of the

Institut Curie. *International Journal of Radiation Oncology, Biology, Physics*, **8**, 1271–86.

Bocca, E. and Pignataro, O. (1967) A conservative technique in radical neck dissection. *Annals of Otology, Rhinology and Laryngology*, **76**, 975–87.

Cooper, J.S., Pajak, T.F., Rubin, P. *et al*. (1989) Second malignancies in patients who have head and neck cancer: incidence, effect on survival and implications based on the RTOG experience. *International Journal of Radiation Oncology, Biology, Physics*, **17**, 449–56.

Crile, G. (1906) Excision of cancer of the head and neck with special reference to the plan of dissection based on 132 operations. *Journal of the American Medical Association*, **47**, 1780–6.

Department of Veteran Affairs Laryngeal Study Group (1991) Induction chemotherapy plus radiation compared with surgery plus radiation in patients with advanced laryngeal cancer. *New England Journal of Medicine*, **324**, 1685–90.

de Vries, N., van Zandwijk, N. and Pastorino, U. (1991) The Euroscan Study. *British Journal of Cancer*, **64**, 985–9.

Dische, S. and Saunders, M.I. (1990) The rationale for continuous, hyperfractionated, accelerated radiotherapy (CHART). *International Journal of Radiation Oncology, Biology, Physics*, **19**, 1317–20.

Ervin, T.J., Clarke, J.R., Weichselbaum, R.R. *et al*. (1987) An analysis of induction and adjuvant chemotherapy in the multi-disciplinary treatment of squamous cell carcinoma of the head and neck. *Journal of Clinical Oncology*, **5**, 10–20.

Fu, K.K., Kosmidis, P., Beer, M. *et al*. (1987) Combined radiotherapy and chemotherapy with bleomycin and methotrexate for advanced inoperable head and neck cancer: update of a Northern California Oncology Group randomized trial. *Journal of Clinical Oncology*, **5**, 1410–8.

Griffin, T.W., Pajak, T.F., Laramore, G.E., *et al*. (1989) Neutron vs photon irradiation of inoperable salivary gland tumours: results of an RTOG-MRC cooperative randomized study. *International Journal of Radiation Oncology, Biology, Physics*, **15**, 1085–90.

Gupta, N.K., Pointon, R.C.S. and Wilkinson, P.M. (1987) A randomised clinical trial to contrast radiotherapy with radiotherapy and methotrexate given synchronously in head and neck cancer. *Clinical Radiology*, **38**, 575–81.

Hart, G.B. and Mainous, E.G. (1976) The treatment of radiation necrosis with hyperbaric oxygen. *Cancer*, **37**, 2580–5.

Henk, J.M. (1981) Does hyperbaric oxygen have a future in radiation therapy? *International Journal of Radiation Oncology, Biology, Physics*, **7**, 1125–8.

Henk, J.M. and Langdon, J.D. (1994) *Malignant Tumours of the Mouth, Jaws and Salivary Glands*, Edward Arnold, London.

Hong, W.K., Lippman, S.M., Itri, L.M. *et al*. (1990) Prevention of second primary tumours with isotretinoin in squamous-cell carcinoma of the head and neck. *New England Journal of Medicine*, **315**, 1501–5.

Hording, U., Nielsen, H.W., Albeck, H. and Daugaard, S. (1993) Nasopharyngeal carcinona: histopathological types and association with Epstein–Barr virus. *European Journal of Cancer*, **29B**, 137–40.

Horiot, J.C., le Fur, R., N'Guyen, T. *et al*. (1990) Hyperfractionated compared with conventional radiotherapy in oropharyngeal carcinoma: an EORTC randomised trial. *European Journal of Cancer*, **26**, 779–80.

Ingersoll, L., Woo, S.Y., Donaldson, S.S. *et al*. (1990) Nasopharyngeal carcinoma in the young: a combined MD Anderson and Stanford experience. *International Journal of Radiation Oncology, Biology, Physics*, **19**, 881–7.

Kish, J.A., Drelichman, A., Jacobs, J. *et al*. (1982) Clinical trial of cisplatin and 5-fluorouracil infusion as initial treatment of advanced squamous carcinoma of the head and neck. *Cancer Treatment Reports*, **66**, 471–4.

Lo, T.C., Wiley, A.L., Ansfield, F.J. *et al*. (1976) Combined radiation therapy and 5-fluorouracil for advanced squamous cell carcinoma of the oral cavity and oropharynx: a randomized study. *American Journal of Roentgenology*, **126**, 229–35.

Marshall, H.F., Mark, A. and Bryce, D.P. (1972) The management of advanced laryngeal cancer. *Journal of Laryngology and Otology*, **86**, 309–15.

Mendenhall, W.M., Million, R.R. and Cassisi, N.J. (1980) Elective neck irradiation in squamous cell carcinoma of the head and neck. *Head and Neck Surgery*, **3**, 15–20.

Mühlbauer, W., Herndl, E. and Stock, W. (1982) The forearm flap. *Plastic and Reconstructive Surgery*, **70**, 336–44.

Parkin, D.M., Laara, E. and Muir, C.S. (1988) Estimates of the worldwide frequency of sixteen major cancers in 1980. *International Journal of Cancer*, **41**, 1184–97.

Piedbois, P., Mazeron, J.J., Haddad, E. *et al*. (1991) Stage I–II squamous carcinoma of the oral cavity treated by iridium-192: is elective neck dissection indicated? *Radiotherapy and Oncology*, **21**, 100–6.

Peters, L.J., Harrison, M.L., Dimery, I.W. *et al.* (1988) Acute and late toxicity associated with sequential bleomycin-containing chemotherapy regimes and radiation therapy in the treatment of carcinoma of the nasopharynx. *International Journal of Radiation Oncology, Biology, Physics*, **14**, 623–33.

Rao, R.S., Parikh, D.M., Parikh, H.K. *et al.* (1991) Perioperative chemotherapy in oral cancer. *Journal of Surgical Oncology*, **47**, 21–6.

Richards, G.J. and Chambers, R.G. (1973) Hydroxyurea in the treatment of neoplasms of the head and neck. A resurvey. *American Journal of Surgery*, **128**, 513–8.

Rooney, M., Kish, J., Jacobs, J. *et al.* (1985) Improved complete response rate and survival in advanced head and neck cancer after three-course induction therapy with 120-hour 5-FU infusion and cisplatin. *Cancer*, **55**, 1123–8.

Shah, J.P., Shaha, A.R., Spiro, R.H. and Strong, E.W. (1976) Carcinoma of the hypopharynx. *American Journal of Surgery*, **132**, 439–43.

Sham, J.S.T. and Choy, D. (1990) Prognostic factors of nasopharyngeal carcinoma: a review of 759 patients. *British Journal of Radiology*, **63**, 51–8.

Stell, P.M. and Rawson, N.S.B. (1990) Adjuvant chemotherapy in head and neck cancer. *British Journal of Cancer*, **61**, 779–87.

Suit, H.D., Lindberg, R. and Fletcher, G.H. (1965) Prognostic significance of extent of tumour regression at completion of radiation therapy. *Radiology*, **84**, 1100–7.

Tupchong, L., Scott, C.B., Blitzer, P.H. *et al.* (1991) Randomized study of preoperative versus postoperative radiation therapy in advanced head and neck carcinoma: long-term follow-up of RTOG study 73-03. *International Journal of Radiation Oncology, Biology, Physics*, **20**, 21–8.

Urba, S.G. and Forastiere, A.A. (1989) Systemic therapy of head and neck cancer: most effective agents, areas of promise. *Oncology*, **3**, 79–98.

Vandenbrouck, C., Sancho–Garnier, H., Chassagne, D. *et al.* (1980) Elective versus therapeutic radical neck dissection in epidermoid carcinoma of the oral cavity: results of a randomised clinical trial. *Cancer*, **46**, 386–90.

Wallner, P.E., Hanks, G.E., Kramer, S. and McLean, C.J. (1986) Patterns of care study: analysis of outcome survey data – anterior two-thirds of tongue and floor of mouth. *American Journal of Clinical Oncology*, **9**, 50–7.

Weissberg, J.B., Son, Y.H., Papac, R.J. *et al.* (1989) Randomized clinical trial of mitomycin C as an adjunct to radiotherapy in head and neck cancer. *International Journal of Radiation Oncology, Biology, Physics*, **17**, 3–9.

THYROID CANCER

Clive Harmer

39.1 INTRODUCTION

The fascination of cancer arising in the thyroid gland is attributable to the variety of distinct tumour types. Within each tumour type there is a wide spectrum of natural history resulting from different rates of growth and biological aggressiveness. The therapist must be alert to these differences so that, in any individual patient, treatment can be tailored to be vigorous enough to eradicate tumour but not excessive so as to cause unnecessary morbidity.

The well differentiated papillary and follicular carcinomas are the most common. Surgery provides the definitive treatment, comprising total (or near-total) thyroidectomy, together with excision of adjacent lymph nodes when involved, or a modified block dissection if there is extensive lymphatic involvement. Ablation of residual normal thyroid tissue with radioactive iodine usually follows as this will permit subsequent whole body ^{131}I scanning to exclude the presence of residual or metastatic disease. Normally such patients have an excellent prognosis and can be followed simply with serial serum thyroglobulin estimations. Occasionally therapeutic radioactive iodine is necessary to eradicate metastatic disease.

The anaplastic carcinomas present a very different clinical picture as they grow and metastasize rapidly. They are usually inoperable at presentation and the cells have lost their ability to concentrate iodine. Their prognosis is terrible, with palliative external beam radiotherapy providing the only worthwhile treatment.

Medullary carcinoma of the thyroid is quite different again as it arises from the parafollicular or C cells. Total thyroidectomy must be undertaken as these tumours are frequently multifocal; a central compartment resection is ideally undertaken together with a formal block dissection if lymph node disease is found to be present. External beam radiotherapy is often required. These tumours may be inherited, sometimes forming part of the multiple endocrine neoplasia (type II) syndrome. They produce the tumour marker calcitonin.

The rarest group of thyroid cancer is the lymphomas. Like the anaplastic carcinomas, they typically present with explosive rapidity but, unlike the former, are exquisitely radioresponsive. The additional use of chemotherapy becomes necessary when they are of advanced stage or demonstrate poor prognostic features. Finally, the thyroid may be involved in spread from an adjacent squamous cancer of the neck or may be the site of distant metastasis from a primary tumour such as the lung or breast.

39.2 INCIDENCE AND AETIOLOGY

In the UK thyroid cancer is designated a rare tumour as there are only 800 new cases registered per year from a population of 56.6 million. In England and Wales there are approximately 200 female and 70 male deaths attributed to thyroid cancer annually.

A sex ratio of nearly 3 : 1 is what we recognize as typical of this condition, both at diagnosis and death (Waterhouse, 1991). In most countries it accounts for about 1% of all cancers. Worldwide, incidence rates vary considerably, ranging from 15 per 100 000 women in the islands of Iceland and Hawaii down to only 1 per 100 000 in the British Isles where the incidence is nearly the lowest recorded.

Papillary carcinoma occurs more commonly in iodine rich areas such as islands where fish is an important component of the diet. Follicular carcinoma is the opposite, appearing more commonly in low iodine, endemic goitre areas, presumably induced when thyroid stimulating hormone (TSH) concentration is high. Anaplastic carcinoma is almost exclusively a disease of the elderly, typically presenting from a goitre known to have been present for many years. It may also arise from a pre-existing differentiated carcinoma, including those not treated with either radioactive iodine or external beam radiotherapy. Medullary carcinoma arises from the calcitonin producing parafollicular or C cells; most are sporadic but 10–20% are familial. There is a relationship between C-cell hyperplasia and the risk of familial medullary carcinoma. Lymphoma of the thyroid is strongly associated with Hashimoto's thyroiditis and high titres of thyroid auto-antibodies.

Radiation is known to induce thyroid cancer, typically of papillary type. This has been documented amongst survivors of atomic bombs and also follows low dose radiotherapy which was previously employed in children for the treatment of an enlarged thymus. However high dose radiotherapy given to the thyroid in adults, e.g. in the treatment of laryngeal cancer, is not associated with an increased incidence of thyroid carcinoma; neither has therapeutic radioactive iodine in the treatment of thyrotoxicosis ever been documented as carcinogenic (despite prolonged follow-up of such patients, including children).

39.3 HISTOPATHOLOGY

Goitre simply means enlargement of the thyroid gland and the vast majority of goitres are benign. Multinodular goitre is the commonest, often requiring no treatment. Most causes of thyroid gland enlargement are not due to tumours but are caused by nodules or cysts or hyperplasia. The only common benign tumour is the follicular adenoma.

Although papillary carcinoma has such a characteristic appearance under the microscope, it arises from the follicular cells. It is characterized by complex branching papillae arranged on a fibrovascular stalk with the epithelium typically comprising a single layer. The tumour cells are cuboidal with a homogeneous cytoplasm surrounding a central ovoid nucleus. The nuclear chromatin is often dispersed in fine grains giving a 'ground glass' appearance. Mitoses are extremely rare but the cells show positive immunocytochemical staining with thyroglobulin. They are very slow growing and may contain laminated calcified psammoma bodies. The latter may be visible on plain X-ray as a fine stippled calcification similar to that caused by breast adenocarcinoma on mammography. Papillary tumours are typically well differentiated and easily recognized on fine needle aspiration cytology. The World Health Organization has decreed that whenever any recognizable papillary structure is present within a tumour, it shall be designated a papillary carcinoma. They therefore comprise 60% of all thyroid cancer and there exists no benign counterpart.

In contrast, follicular carcinoma (15–20% of all malignant tumours) may be extremely difficult to diagnose when well differentiated as the appearance is similar to both normal thyroid and the benign follicular adenoma; even metastases may appear histologically identical to normal thyroid tissue. Invasion of the capsule or of blood vessels are often the only features which denote malignancy and it follows that fine needle aspiration cytology is unreliable for diagnosis. It is thyroglobulin positive and has been defined as the malignant tumour of follicular cell origin lacking the diagnostic features of papillary carcinoma. When less than well differentiated, diagnosis is much easier as it takes on a solid growth pattern to become either moderately or poorly differentiated. A rare variant where the cells are plump and intensely eosinophilic is designated Hurthle cell carcinoma; the curious feature about this tumour is that, although it expresses thyroglobulin and is typically well differentiated, it has never been shown to be capable of taking up radioactive iodine.

It must be emphasized that the majority of these well differentiated thyroid tumours demonstrate a mixture of papillary and follicular areas but will be designated papillary carcinoma. The pure follicular tumours tend not to produce lymph node metastases or to extend through the intrathyroidal lymphatic system. By contrast, the papillary tumours often present clinically with a lymph node metastasis and disseminate widely through the intrathyroidal lymphatics, giving the false appearance of multicentricity. However there is a continuous spectrum blurring these two distinct entities; for instance, an apparently pure follicular primary tumour may be associated with papillary lymph node metastasis.

Anaplastic carcinoma comprises 10% of all thyroid malignancies and also arises from the follicular cells. There is a spectrum of histological appearance that merges with poorly differentiated follicular carcinoma. Variants include giant cell, small cell and spindle cell types; there may even be a squamous metaplastic component but pure squamous cell carcinoma is excessively rare. There may be weak staining for thyroglobulin.

Medullary carcinoma comprises 5–10% of all cancers and is identified immunocytochemically by calcitonin staining granules. It is composed of round or polygonal cells with eosinophilic cytoplasm arranged in a solid closely packed pattern. Although these tumours arise from the parafollicular or C cells, residual follicles can often be seen so that they may be mistaken for follicular carcinoma; such a wrong diagnosis could lead to incorrect treatment with ^{131}I. Careful review of the histopathology is mandatory in every patient with thyroid cancer. A characteristic feature of medullary carcinoma is the presence of amyloid thought to be chemically related to the precursor of calcitonin (the previously invaluable congo red stain to demonstrate amyloid has been superseded by the use of immunocytochemistry). Nests of tumour cells may become calcified and this will be visible on plain X-ray as a very coarse appearance, quite unlike the fine stippling of papillary carcinoma and reminiscent of tuberculous calcification (Figure 39.1).

Primary lymphoma of the thyroid comprises only 5% of all malignant thyroid tumours. The vast majority are non-Hodgkin's lymphomas. They may be nodular but are usually diffuse. They are usually large cell but may be small cell or mixed. Immunocytochemistry is necessary to distinguish them from the small cell variant of anaplastic carcinoma; that is most important as clinical presentation may be identical but treatment is quite different. The adjacent thyroid typically demonstrates lymphocytic thyroiditis. A significant number of these tumours display mucosa associated lymphoid tissue (MALT) characteristics which seem to be associated with a less aggressive natural history, with the corollary that treatment can be less intensive.

39.4 CLINICAL PRESENTATION

Papillary carcinoma typically presents in the young female with very slowly enlarging cervical lymphadenopathy. The primary tumour may have gone unnoticed and remain occult on investigation. The lung is the only common site of distant metastasis. The incidence of lung involvement at

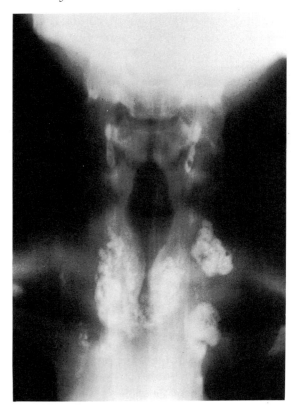

Figure 39.1 This young Irish girl presented with bilateral cervical lymphadenopathy which had been mistaken for tuberculosis. The anteroposterior tomograph of the neck shows extensive coarse calcification within medullary carcinoma. There is bilateral tumour within the thyroid resulting in gross subglottic narrowing as well as in bilateral cervical lymph nodes.

presentation is 5–10% in adults rising to 15–20% in children.

Follicular carcinoma is also three times more common in females than males, although it tends to present in middle life, typically without lymph node enlargement. Again it is a slow growing tumour with a time-course spanning a number of years, although this becomes proportionately less with the moderately differentiated and poorly differentiated types. Distant metastases are present at diagnosis in 14% of patients, most

commonly in the lung. However this is a tumour which may present as a bone metastasis from an unknown primary; pathological fracture, vertebral collapse or even paraplegia may be the first symptom.

The anaplastic tumours typically present in old age and again there is a marked predominance in females. They produce a rapidly enlarging goitre which causes dysphagia and may compress the trachea to result in stridor. The primary mass rapidly becomes fixed due to extraglandular extension. Lymph node metastases soon become visible and are frequently bilateral, merging with the primary tumour to form a collar of tumour which also extends retrosternally (Figure 39.2). Confluent lymphadenopathy may extend down the paratracheal gutter as far as the carina. Hilar lymphadenopathy often follows and pulmonary metastases soon become evident. Early spread also develops in the bones and liver leading to rapid demise.

Medullary carcinoma has its highest incidence between the ages of 40 and 70 but, unlike other thyroid tumours, has an equal sex incidence. It presents with a nondescript thyroid mass, frequently associated with unilateral lymphadenopathy and not infrequently with bilateral lymph node disease. Its tempo is variable but comparable to the moderately differentiated follicular tumours. Like them, metastases arise in the lung and skeleton but also in the liver. Less than 20% of patients have an inherited predisposition to this tumour; the pattern of inheritance is autosomal dominant, with incomplete penetrance. The responsible gene has recently been identified on chromosome 10. Inherited medullary thyroid carcinoma may occur as the only abnormality but is more usually part of the multiple endocrine neoplasia type IIA syndrome, with phaeochromocytoma (which may be bilateral) and parathyroid hyperplasia or adenoma. These other features may develop subsequent to diagnosis of the thyroid tumour or may antedate it. Investigation of family members may reveal medullary cancer in asymptomatic rela-

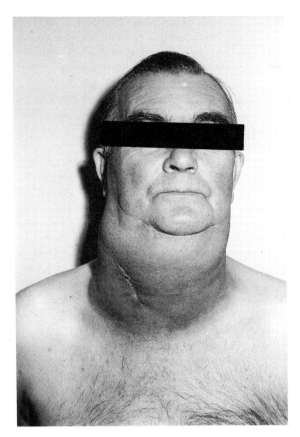

Figure 39.2   A collar of tumour is the typical presentation for anaplastic carcinoma. This patient demonstrates confluent primary and metastatic tumour in bilateral cervical lymph nodes extending from the upper deep cervical regions into the superior mediastinum. More typically the patient would be elderly and female.

tives, including the children. In the rare multiple endocrine neoplasia type IIB syndrome, mucosal neuromas may be visible (involving the tongue, oral mucosa and conjunctiva) with a marfanoid habitus. Prostaglandin secretion can cause intractable diarrhoea which may be the presenting symptom, treated for years prior to discovery of the thyroid cancer.

Primary lymphoma of the thyroid presents typically with early stage disease as a firm painless enlargement, with or without lymph-adenopathy in the neck. B symptoms are rarely present. Involvement of the thyroid by generalized lymphoma is more frequent. In the Royal Marsden Hospital study of 46 cases of primary lymphoma confined to the neck there were 43 females and only three males, with a median age at diagnosis of 66 years and a range from 17 to 86 (Tupchong *et al.*, 1986). Seventy four per cent presented with a history of < 3 months. Symptoms of local compression (stridor and dysphagia) were prominent and associated with a marked adverse effect on survival; stridor and hoarseness often coexisted. Pain was uncommon and usually accompanied a very short history. Only 4% presented with superior vena caval obstruction. A mass greater than 6 cm was typically present, usually affecting only one lobe but with diffuse involvement in 24%. This was often fixed, with an ill defined edge indicative of extracapsular spread, identical to the presentation of anaplastic carcinoma. One characteristic scenario at presentation was a patient with known hypothyroidism due to Hashimoto's thyroiditis who subsequently developed a progressive goitre despite treatment with thyroxine.

Clinically the differential diagnosis of any thyroid tumour from a benign nodule may be difficult in the euthyroid patient; in thyrotoxicosis malignancy is rare. Between 4% and 7% of the entire population have palpable nodules and half of the remainder have nodules at autopsy (Mazzaferri, 1993). Solitary nodules are clinically three times more common than multiple nodules although at autopsy the reverse is true. Physical characteristics are poor predictors of malignancy although the following are suspicious: nodules at the extremes of age, male sex, hard consistency, fixation, size greater than 4 cm, a new nodule or rapid growth, and a nodule which is solitary. The incidence of cancer in patients with obstructive symptoms is about 10% and in those patients with vocal cord palsy the incidence is less than 40%. These figures simply reflect the fact that thyroid cancer is rare and benign nodules are common. Fine needle aspiration cytology should be performed whenever there is clinical suspicion, including the dominant nodule if present in a multinodular goitre.

39.5   INVESTIGATIONS AND STAGING

Patients with well differentiated papillary or follicular carcinoma are usually referred when the diagnosis has been made following excision of a nodule or lymph node. The single most important investigation is for the histology to be confirmed. The patient should be discussed with the referring surgeon and a copy of his operation details obtained as well as a copy of the histology report to determine the size of tumour (and the margins of clearance) for staging, as shown in Table 39.1. Completion thyroidectomy may have been performed but if not, is usually requested. Palpation of the neck is usually adequate to exclude residual lymphadenopathy. Haematology, liver function tests, blood urea, serum calcium and a chest X-ray should be performed. It is also worthwhile measuring the thyroglobulin level as it could be argued that, if unrecordable, there can remain neither normal residual thyroid nor tumour, in which case the iodine ablation dose could be replaced by a diagnostic dose of only 200 MBq ^{131}I. Replacement thyroid hormone should not have been given yet, so there is no point in measuring the thyroxine level or TSH. CT of the neck is required only if further surgery is contemplated.

The anaplastic carcinomas are usually referred following biopsy only, as definitive surgery is impossible due to the extent of locoregional disease. There is usually some urgency to commence radiotherapy so the initial investigations comprise haematology, biochemistry and chest X-ray only. CT may be of help in identifying the extent of retrosternal disease and planning for irradiation. If tomography is requested it is worth including the whole thorax which may reveal asymptomatic pulmonary metastases. A clinical (as opposed to pathological) staging can thereby be derived, according to the same criteria as used for the well differentiated carcinomas. CT of the liver and an isotope bone scan complete the metastatic screen as soon as obstructive symptoms have been controlled.

Table 39.1   TNM clinical classification for carcinoma of all histological types

T – Primary tumour

T1	≤ 1 cm in greatest dimension
T2	> 1–4 cm in greatest dimension
T3	> 4 cm in greatest dimension
T4	Tumour of any size extending beyond the thyroid capsule

All categories may be subdivided: (a) solitary tumour, (b) multifocal

N – Regional lymph nodes

N0	No regional lymph node metastasis
N1	Regional lymph node metastasis
	N1a in ipsilateral cervical lymph node(s)
	N1b in bilateral, midline or contralateral cervical or mediastinal lymph node(s)

M – Distant metastases

pTNM Pathological classification
The pT, pN and pM categories correspond to the T, N and M categories.

Adapted from Hermanek, 1987.

Medullary carcinoma is much more complex although staging is the same. At the initial consultation it is worth undertaking haematology, biochemistry, a chest X-ray, serum calcitonin and a CEA. Although calcitonin is highly specific, levels can fluctuate widely and serial CEA levels may prove more reliable during follow-up (Palmer *et al.*, 1984). Hopefully the postoperative calcitonin will have fallen to negligible levels indicating complete surgical eradication of disease. It is then necessary to take a detailed family history in order to exclude the possibility of a familial tumour. However, a negative family history is not reliable in excluding familial disease such that first degree relatives should be screened for occult tumour using a pentagastrin stimulation test and any positive can be considered for total thyroidectomy (Ponder *et al.*, 1988); systematic screening of the families of a series of 39 patients with apparently sporadic tumour detected seven new cases in four families. A normal serum calcium is adequate to exclude parathyroid adenoma or hyperplasia. Phaeochromocytoma should be excluded by measuring the blood pressure, CT of the adrenals and a 24 hour urinary estimation of catecholamines.

The all too frequent problem is that the postoperative calcitonin level fails to fall to an unmeasurable level (although may be much lower than it had been preoperatively). Such patients are often asymptomatic with no clinically detectable abnormality. It must be assumed that residual tumour is present at some site in the body and a determined search should ensue to document its location with a view to excision. The most likely sites of residual tumour are: within residual thyroid tissue, lymphadenopathy in the neck or superior mediastinum, or metastases in lungs, liver or bone. Such a patient should therefore be referred for CT of the neck, mediastinum, thorax and liver plus a bone scan. When these results are negative a whole body DMSA scan may document the site of disease. Occasionally it is necessary to measure calcitonin levels from the neck, mediastinum, and abdomen by selective venous catheterization.

Patients with compressive symptoms from thyroid lymphoma demand urgent treatment such that haematology, biochemistry and a chest X-ray are all that is possible at their first attendance. However full lymphoma staging should follow as soon as possible comprising CT of the neck, mediastinum, thorax, abdomen and pelvis, plus a bone marrow aspirate and trephine. Staging is the same as for other non-Hodgkin's lymphomas. The thyroid represents an extranodal site so that patients with local disease only are designated I$_E$. When lymph nodes in the neck are also involved the stage becomes II$_E$. Stages III and IV are occasionally encountered but B symptoms are rarely present.

39.6 PROGNOSTIC FACTORS

Prognostic factors for the well differentiated carcinomas are illustrated in Table 39.2. The anaplastic cancers have a dismal prognosis, with the average interval from time of first symptom to death being only 6 months. Metastatic disease rapidly evolves, even if not apparent at presentation. Just occasionally, thyroidectomy is performed for what was assumed to be a benign condition and histology reveals anaplastic carcinoma; the diagnosis is thus made incidentally and such patients may be cured.

The tempo of disease in medullary carcinoma of the thyroid is extremely variable with survival ranging from a few months to 30 years. Occasionally an elderly patient may die from an unrelated cause with tumour which has never demanded treatment. There is some evidence to suggest that the tempo within a given family has a consistent biological behaviour. The overall 5 and 10 year survival rates are 75% and 50% respectively, although patients with the MEN IIA syndrome may demonstrate a more indolent course resulting in a 10 year survival of up to

Table 39.2 Prognostic factors for differentiated carcinoma

Variable	Hazard ratio	P value
Age		
< 30	1.00	
30–39	4.5	
40–49	14.9	$P < 0.001^*$
50–59	25.9	
> 60	34.1	
Grade		
I, II	1.00	
III	2.81	$P < 0.01$
Stage		
T1, T2	1.00	
T3	1.78	$P < 0.001^*$
T4	3.13	
Metastases		
None	1.00	$P < 0.001$
Lung only	3.41	
Other	10.1	

Adapted from O'Connell, 1992.
Derived by multivariate analysis using Cox's regression model for 649 patients treated at the Royal Marsden Hospital between 1949 and 1991.
* P value for trend; other P values refer to tests for heterogeneity.

90%, especially when diagnosed only by investigation of a relative of a known patient. The worst prognosis is seen in the MEN IIB syndrome. Extent of disease is most important: tumour localized to the thyroid carries a better prognosis than disease associated with lymph node metastases and metastatic disease is almost invariably fatal. Diarrhoea is of bad prognostic significance, usually related to size and extent of tumour, although not invariably present.

In the Royal Marsden Hospital series of 46 patients with primary lymphoma of the thyroid (Tupchong *et al.*, 1986), 91% had high grade histology, with diffuse large cell lymphoma being the most common (78%). The crude overall 5 year survival rate was 40%, with 30% surviving beyond 10 years. Disease free and overall survival were virtually identical indicating the ineffectiveness of salvage therapy. The important prognostic factors were: size of tumour, fixation, extracapsular extension and retrosternal involvement. Those patients with MALT characteristics

demonstrate a more indolent course and superior outcome. Patients with either stage III or IV disease fair very badly.

39.7 TREATMENT AND FOLLOW-UP

39.7.1 WELL DIFFERENTIATED PAPILLARY AND FOLLICULAR CARCINOMA

Surgery is the potentially curative treatment both for initial disease and also for locoregional recurrence. The extent of the operative procedure remains controversial but the minimum requirement is complete extirpation of all macroscopic disease including resection of adjacent muscle should this be infiltrated. Routine resection of uninvolved cervical lymph nodes is not necessary but all involved nodes should be removed and, if extensively invaded, a modified (functional) neck dissection is required. The recurrent laryngeal nerves must be identified and avoided. At least one parathyroid gland should be preserved as the necessity for lifelong calcium supplements also represents a significant morbidity.

If only partial removal of the thyroid has been performed, completion thyroidectomy is usually advised. The advantages of total or near-total thyroidectomy are as follows. Of 80 patients subjected to whole organ serial sectioning, 87.5% extended either into the isthmus, the opposite lobe, or the pericapsular lymph nodes of the opposite lobe (Russell *et al.*, 1963). In a more recent series, the 20 year locoregional recurrence rate of 25% following unilateral lobectomy contrasted with only 6% after bilateral lobar resection (Hay *et al.*, 1992). Half the patients who die of thyroid cancer do so as a result of central neck disease (Clark, 1982).

The above advantages of total thyroidectomy apply predominantly to papillary tumours. Advantages applicable equally to papillary and follicular carcinoma include the following. Any residual tumour has the potential to transform to anaplastic carcinoma. Residual tumour may not have the ability to concentrate ^{131}I. Whole body scanning with iodine to detect metastases is reliable only after total thyroidectomy or radioactive ablation; surgical ablation of normal residual thyroid is quicker than repeated administrations of iodine and avoids unnecessary whole body radiation. Finally, thyroglobulin monitoring for follow-up is more reliable after all normal thyroid tissue has been removed.

Exceptions to this aggressive surgical policy include patients undergoing subtotal thyroidectomy for multinodular goitre when the diagnosis of cancer is an incidental finding and young female patients with a primary tumour measuring < 1 cm (possibly < 2 cm). For patients with such an excellent prognosis, lifelong suppression of TSH is all that is required.

39.7.2 RADIOACTIVE IODINE: ABLATION AND TREATMENT

The concept that well differentiated thyroid cancer runs a benign course and rarely results in death is obsolete. Disease progression is slow and throughout the first 15 years after treatment the initial mode of therapy may not influence survival. However, after 15 years survival curves diverge significantly in groups of patients matched for age, sex and histology treated radically or non-radically (Savoie *et al.*, 1985). Death from thyroid cancer may occur as long as 40 years after initial treatment (Powell and Harmer, 1990). These facts support the rationale for the aggressive surgical policy described above and the routine use of radioactive iodine ablation described below (Figure 39.3). Possible prevention of local recurrence and metastases by optimal treatment of the initial disease must be the ideal, provided that it does not result in significant morbidity.

Following total or near-total thyroidectomy, a single dose of 3000 MBq ^{131}I is all that is required to achieve ablation or destruction of residual normal thyroid, some of which almost invariably remains. This is best achieved 3 weeks after the operation and prior to the commencement of replacement thyroid hormone. Admission to a specially designed and protected room in an isotope suite is mandatory with expert support provided by physics staff. An existing pregnancy must be excluded and the dose should be given within 10 days of the beginning of the last menstrual period, according to the 10 day rule. Patients of both sex should be advised against conception for the ensuing year. All nursing procedures are minimized to reduce the possibility of radioactive contamination of staff.

A liberal intake of fluids encourages rapid renal excretion of surplus radioactivity and thereby results in a low total body burden of radiation. Frequent micturition should be advised to reduce radiation to the bladder and other pelvic organs. There is some physiological concentration of iodine within salivary tissue so this should be stimulated with lemon drops or bitter sweets. Iodine-rich foods should have been avoided for 3 weeks

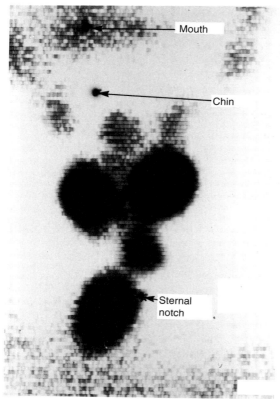

Mouth

Chin

Sternal notch

Figure 39.3 Six months previously this young female patient had undergone near total thyroidectomy for papillary carcinoma arising in the right lobe following which diagnostic ^{131}I scanning revealed uptake only within a small focus of residual normal thyroid just to the left of the midline. She then received 60 Gy external beam irradiation to the neck together with TSH suppressive thyroxine. On referral she was asymptomatic with no clinically detectable abnormality. According to protocol she was given ablation ^{131}I. The scan shows localization as before within the left sided normal thyroid remnant but in addition there are two intense areas of localization in the right side of her neck as well as several other foci of uptake, all indicative of metastatic carcinoma in lymph nodes. Such a scenario is not unusual; it vindicates the routine use of ablation ^{131}I and demonstrates the futility of routine external beam radiotherapy.

before admission, as should iodine-rich contrast media used for radiological investigations. Scans of the neck and whole body are

obtained after 3 days when the patient is usually permitted to return home, subject to the total body radioactive level having fallen below the permitted level. Replacement thyroid hormone is commenced in the form of triiodothyronine 20 μg three times a day. Blood needs to be taken on the 6th day after iodine for a protein bound ^{131}I level.

Three months later the neck and whole body scans must be repeated as ablation films cannot be relied on to reveal metastatic tumour. Provided that there are no adverse features, these can be performed as an outpatient procedure using a diagnostic dose of 200 MBq ^{131}I. Hopefully, the whole body scan will show only physiological concentration of iodine in the bladder and colon; the neck view will be either completely clear or possibly show a ghost like remnant of uptake within normal residual thyroid. A new site of uptake indicates metastatic cancer. Triiodothyronine is discontinued for 10 days prior to iodine administration and, on the day, the TSH level should be > 33 mU/l to ensure maximum uptake.

In patients with known inoperable residual or metastatic tumour and those whose diagnostic scan shows abnormal uptake, therapeutic doses of 5500 MBq ^{131}I are required every 6 months until all tumour has been eradicated, as shown in Figure 39.4. Outpatient attendances between therapy doses permit clinical evaluation, blood sampling to ensure the T3 level is not excessive but that TSH is totally suppressed, and serial thyroglobulin assays. When all treatment has been completed, triiodothyronine is replaced by thyroxine at an average single daily dose of 0.2 mg.

Early morbidity from ^{131}I therapy is minimal and pulmonary fibrosis does not occur at these dose levels. In a 25 year follow-up of 40 children treated with a mean total dose of 7400 MBq and maximum dose of 26 GBq, there was no decreased fertility or abnormal birth history (Sarker *et al.*, 1976). In a review of Pochin's early work (Edmonds and Smith, 1986) a small but significant excess

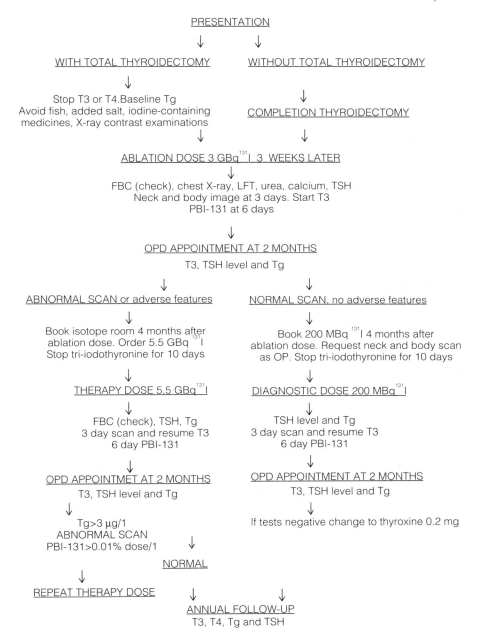

PRESENTATION

↓   ↓

WITH TOTAL THYROIDECTOMY   WITHOUT TOTAL THYROIDECTOMY

↓

Stop T3 or T4.Baseline Tg
Avoid fish, added salt, iodine-containing   ↓
medicines, X-ray contrast examinations   COMPLETION THYROIDECTOMY

↓   ↓

ABLATION DOSE 3 GBq ^{131}I 3 WEEKS LATER

↓

FBC (check), chest X-ray, LFT, urea, calcium, TSH
Neck and body image at 3 days. Start T3
PBI-131 at 6 days

↓

OPD APPOINTMENT AT 2 MONTHS
T3, TSH level and Tg

↓   ↓

ABNORMAL SCAN or adverse features   NORMAL SCAN, no adverse features

↓   ↓

Book isotope room 4 months after   Book 200 MBq ^{131}I 4 months after
ablation dose. Order 5.5 GBq ^{131}I   ablation dose. Request neck and body scan
Stop tri-iodothyronine for 10 days   as OP. Stop tri-iodothyronine for 10 days

↓   ↓

THERAPY DOSE 5.5 GBq ^{131}I   DIAGNOSTIC DOSE 200 MBq ^{131}I

↓   ↓

FBC (check), TSH, Tg   TSH level and Tg
3 day scan and resume T3   3 day scan and resume T3
6 day PBI-131   6 day PBI-131

↓   ↓

OPD APPOINTMET AT 2 MONTHS   OPD APPOINTMENT AT 2 MONTHS
T3, TSH level and Tg   T3, TSH level and Tg

↓   ↓

Tg>3 µg/1   If tests negative change to thyroxine 0.2 mg
ABNORMAL SCAN
PBI-131>0.01% dose/1   ↓

↓   NORMAL

↓   ↓   ↓
REPEAT THERAPY DOSE   ANNUAL FOLLOW-UP
T3, T4, Tg and TSH

Figure 39.4   Protocol for differentiated thyroid carcinoma.

of deaths from leukaemia and cancer of the bladder was found. The latter can be minimized by liberal hydration at the time of iodine administration and the former occurred only in patients repeatedly treated when bone marrow was invaded by tumour, which would also be contrary to current practice. Treatment with high activity ^{131}I should always be at the lowest level for effective control. Initial completion thyroidectomy and consideration of the surgical alternatives for persistent or recurrent tumour are crucial to achieve this objective, together with avoidance of repeated iodine administrations when dosimetry indicates a likely subtherapeutic outcome (Harmer, 1991).

The impact of therapy in 576 patients with papillary carcinoma demonstrated a significantly lower rate of recurrence ($P < 0.001$) and mortality ($P < 0.01$) when ^{131}I and thyroid hormone were given postoperatively, compared with thyroid hormone alone or no adjunctive therapy (Mazzaferri *et al.*, 1977). In a similar study of 214 patients with follicular carcinoma, the cumulative recurrence rate at 17 years was only 6% in those who received ^{131}I in addition to thyroid hormone, contrasted with 12% in patients treated postoperatively with hormone only (Young *et al.*, 1980).

Eighty per cent of well differentiated carcinomas will concentrate ^{131}I; the likelihood of such uptake and of an effective response to therapy does not differ substantially whether the tumour is predominantly papillary or follicular (Pochin, 1971). However, the ability to trap iodine is related to age. In patients with pulmonary metastases from papillary carcinoma uptake was present in 87% of those aged < 50 years but in only 21% of patients aged > 50 (Charbord *et al.*, 1977). With the follicular tumours, advancing age and decreasing histological differentiation are both associated with less iodine avidity. Patients with inoperable metastatic disease which does not concentrate iodine have a significantly worse prognosis than those who do uptake and must be relegated to third line treatment with external beam irradiation or chemotherapy.

Even when metastatic tumour can be seen to be concentrating ^{131}I, outcome may not be favourable (Brown *et al.*, 1984). This Royal Marsden Hospital series also demonstrated that site of metastases was related to outcome: when confined to the lungs 54% of patients were free of disease 10 years after iodine treat-

ment but no patient with skeletal involvement survived for this long. External beam radiotherapy may reduce the uptake of iodine by metastases and therefore should not precede therapeutic [131]I. Treatment with radioactive iodine has been described as a radiotherapeutic utopia (Harmer, 1979); no other solid tumour is curable with a radioactive drug once it has become widely disseminated.

Potential morbidity makes it imperative that excessive treatment with iodine should not be pursued in the absence of demonstrable benefit; scanning systems are so sensitive that the practical difficulty lies in knowing when to withhold further therapy. An indirect method of quantifying a positive scan is to measure the protein bound [131]I. The percentage of the administered dose per litre which is organically bound in plasma at 6 days after the dose (in the absence of normal thyroid) is proportional to the remaining amount of functioning tumour and the progress of its destruction can be monitored during consecutive treatments. When this figure is < 0.01% neither residual thyroid nor functioning tumour can be present (Harmer, *et al.*, 1977).

Measurement of the absorbed dose delivered by ^{131}I in tumour is now possible, in contrast to simple knowledge of the total dose of radioactivity empirically administered. This can be achieved using a specially designated dual-headed whole-body scanner together with tracer dose [124]I positron emission tomography (to estimate functioning tumour mass, Flower *et al.*, 1989). The true absorbed dose in thyroid remnants, regional lymphadenopathy and bone metastases has been measured; a dose–response relationship has been demonstrated (O'Connell, 1992).

39.7.3 EXTERNAL BEAM RADIOTHERAPY IN THE TREATMENT OF WELL DIFFERENTIATED CARCINOMA

External beam radiotherapy may play a valuable role but should be reserved for patients whose initial, recurrent or metastatic disease is both surgically unresectable and demonstrated not to take up iodine to any worthwhile degree. A dose of 60 Gy delivered by megavoltage photons over 6 weeks in daily fractions is the most that the oesophagus will tolerate. Irradiation after incomplete surgery is effective (Tubiana *et al.*, 1985): the actuarial probability of local recurrence was 11% at 5 years contrasted with 23% for patients treated by surgery alone (although the irradiated patients had larger and more extensive tumours). Occasionally, initial radiotherapy will render an inoperable tumour operable.

For treatment of the thyroid bed an antero-oblique wedged pair of portals is applied in the same way as is used for treatment of early glottic cancer; if necessary the volume can be extended posteriorly to include para-oesophageal disease. Occasionally the volume must extend into the superior mediastinum to encompass paratracheal nodes, in which case the antero-oblique wedged pair must diverge caudally, similar to the technique used for postcricoid carcinoma. When it is necessary to treat the lateral compartments of the neck and deep cervical chains, it must be remembered that adequate dose must be given down to the level of the suprasternal notch such that the shoulders preclude use of lateral portals. Anterior and undercouched fields must therefore be employed, as described below for the treatment of anaplastic carcinoma.

Metastatic disease represents a further indication for external beam radiotherapy, although higher doses than are usually employed for palliation will be required. Pain resulting from bone metastases can readily be relieved and occasionally a lung or mediastinal metastasis may demand symptom control. The results of chemotherapy are disappointing.

39.7.4 FOLLOW-UP AND SURVIVAL OF PATIENTS WITH WELL DIFFERENTIATED CARCINOMA

Annual follow-up is adequate for patients with papillary and follicular carcinoma as the tempo of disease is so slow but must be lifelong. Repeat whole body scans are unnecessary because thyroglobulin is such a reliable tumour marker, measured with the patient on replacement thyroid hormone (Black *et al.*, 1981); concordance values approach 100%. Routine chest X-ray is not necessary provided the thyroglobulin remains undetectable. A progressively rising thyroglobulin in an asymptomatic patient demands investigation with a view to further surgery, or ^{131}I therapy if inoperable.

Outcome in 649 patients treated at the Royal Marsden Hospital between 1949 and 1991 (O'Connell, 1992) demonstrated a significant survival advantage for females compared with males ($P < 0.01$). Patients with papillary histology had a better survival than those with follicular carcinoma, the 15 year survival rates being 71% and 50% respectively ($P < 0.005$). Patients with histological grade I or II (papillary and follicular) had a significantly better survival than those with poorly differentiated tumours. Age was the single most important prognostic factor. The actuarial survival rates at 15 years were: 90% for patients < 40 years of age, 70% for patients aged between 40 and 59, and < 20% for patients aged > 60. For patients aged > 45 at the time of diagnosis, more advanced disease as reflected by TNM designation resulted in progressively impaired probability of survival. The initial surgical procedure was also significant with the 15 year actuarial survival being 75% in those patients who had undergone near-total thyroidectomy but 35% when only enucleation or biopsy had been performed.

Analysis of 113 patients treated by megavoltage external beam irradiation with curative intent demonstrated overall survival rates of 85% at 5 years, 60% at 10 years, and 15% at 15 years, when probable or definite microscopic residual disease had been present. For gross residual disease the 5 year survival was only 27%. Of these 113 patients, 62 have subsequently died, although 20 of the deaths were due to unrelated causes and 15 due to distant metastases; 15 were attributed to local disease and 12 patients died with both local and distant tumour.

39.7.5 TREATMENT OF ANAPLASTIC CARCINOMA

These tumours are almost invariably inoperable at presentation and do not take up radioactive iodine. TSH suppression has little impact such that the only worthwhile treatment is external beam radiotherapy. Although it does not prolong survival, there is usually some shrinkage of the primary mass and adjacent confluent lymphadenopathy if high dose treatment is given. Stridor resulting from obstruction (often at a level too low for tracheostomy) can be relieved and patients unable to swallow their own saliva can have deglutition returned to normal.

Wide field radiotherapy extends from the tips of the mastoids down to the carina with lateral extensions encompassing both sides of the neck and supraclavicular fossae (Harmer, 1977). Using anterior and undercouched portals, lead is inserted to protect the sub-apical portions of both lungs and the central portion of the mandible with the neck maximally extended. The larynx goes unprotected as does the greater length of the spinal cord and oesophagus up to the Phase I midplane dose of 40 Gy in 4 weeks with daily treatment (Figure 39.5). Only then should midline lead be introduced into the undercouched field throughout its length and the Phase II mid plane dose taken to 50 Gy in 5 weeks (by which time the spinal cord dose will be at the limit of tolerance of 45 Gy). Phase III is optional, dependent on response, the patient's general condition and side-effects of the treatment so far delivered; it is not indicated if extensive metastases are present. However an additional 10 Gy can be given during a sixth week of treatment by whatever portal arrangement can encompass residual tumour without adding to the cord dose.

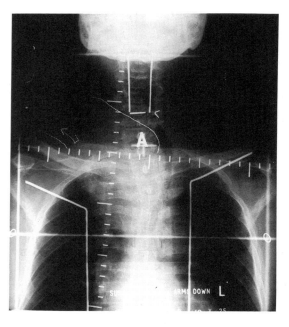

Figure 39.5 Simulator planning film demonstrating the Phase I volume required for anaplastic carcinoma. Lead protects the adjacent lungs and there is midline shielding superiorly. The two headed arrow indicates the biopsy scar and the single arrow demonstrates the larynx which is grossly displaced to the left by the massive right sided tumour.

A brisk cutaneous erythema is invariable as is severe oesophagitis. Full supportive nursing care is required for these patients, with particular attention to oral hygiene, adequate hydration and dietary intake. Pain resulting from bone metastases can readily be relieved with single large fraction external beam treatment.

Although radiotherapy usually achieves symptom control, almost all patients are dead within 6 months from widespread metastases and inanition. An effective systemic agent is therefore urgently required. In the Royal Marsden Hospital series of 29 patients with advanced thyroid cancer of all histologies, sequential chemotherapy was given to assess the benefit of different single agents, resulting in a total of 60 evaluable drug exposures

(Hoskin and Harmer, 1987). Out of 18 evaluable courses of treatment for anaplastic carcinoma, only three showed a response. Combination drug treatment has not been shown to be superior and many patients are never well enough to tolerate additional side-effects.

39.7.6 TREATMENT OF MEDULLARY THYROID CARCINOMA

Surgery provides the potentially curative treatment, comprising total thyroidectomy plus a central compartment lymph node dissection (Figure 39.6). In the majority of patients, the diagnosis is made by the pathologist only after an initial surgical procedure such as lobectomy or excision of a cervical lymph node. Completion thyroidectomy should always be recommended as these tumours may be genuinely multifocal and residual C-cell hyperplasia may have the potential of malignant transformation. Once the diagnosis is known, phaeochromocytoma should be excluded; if present it should be removed prior to further neck surgery. When involvement of the cervical nodes is detected at the time of surgery, a thorough ipsilateral modified neck dissection should be undertaken. Superior mediastinal disease can usually be removed from above but if necessary the sternum should be split for thorough eradication.

Hopefully the postoperative calcitonin level will fall to an undetectable level. All too often however it remains elevated, although lower than before. Residual tumour must then be assumed and reinvestigation instituted in order to document its site, the most likely being in the thyroid bed or adjacent lymph node areas. Further surgery should always be contemplated and may require a microdissection (Tissel, 1986). If surgery proves impossible or if the site of disease cannot be determined, a diagnostic whole body mIBG scan is undertaken as this isotope is occasionally taken up by tumour. If positive a thera-peutic dose of ^{131}I-labelled mIBG can be given, as is used in the treatment of neuroblastoma and paraganglioma (Ball *et al.*, 1991), although such treatment is rarely as effective as the use of ^{131}I for well differentiated cancer.

Medullary carcinoma is not particularly radioresponsive, but with high doses in the order of 60 Gy over 6 weeks, small foci of residual tumour can be eradicated, so external beam radiotherapy is indicated when surgical excision is impossible or incomplete. Radiotherapy can also achieve a significant decrease in locoregional recurrence in patients treated solely on account of a persistently high postoperative calcitonin level (Schlumberger *et al.*, 1991). The volume irradiated must be generous, extending from the hyoid to the carina in order to encompass the middle and lower deep cervical lymph node chains in both sides of the neck, the paratracheal nodes, and those in the anterior mediastinum. The usual field arrangement therefore comprises anterior plus undercouched portals, as described for the treatment of anaplastic carcinoma. Postoperative radiotherapy should always be given if block dissection reveals extensive nodal disease or extracapsular nodal invasion, although may be avoided when the postoperative calcitonin becomes undetectable. In patients presenting with inoperable primary or nodal disease, high dose irradiation may render surgery possible or, at least, will provide local control. Radiotherapy is also of considerable palliative benefit in relieving the pain of bone metastases.

Metastatic medullary carcinoma is often asymptomatic and may remain indolent for years. The use of chemotherapy should be contemplated only when metastatic disease is unresectable, progressive and symptomatic. A less toxic agent can be selected initially, escalating to the more toxic drugs only when the previous agent has failed or when a previously responsive tumour develops resistance. Active drugs include etoposide,

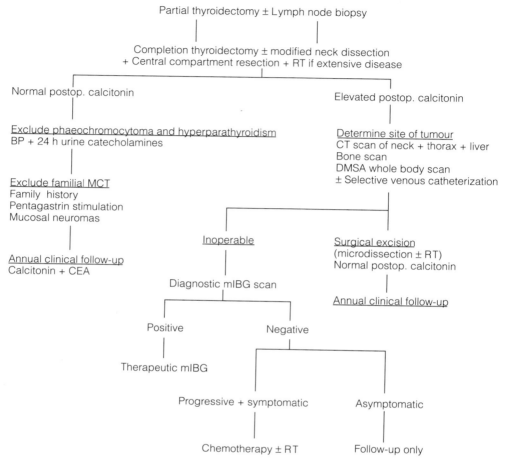

Figure 39.6 Care plan for medullary thyroid carcinoma.

carboplatin, cisplatin and doxorubicin. The partial response rate to chemotherapy and especially to doxorubicin is significantly higher than for other thyroid tumours, being > 60%, contrasted with < 20% for the well differentiated and anaplastic types (Hoskin and Harmer, 1987).

Routine follow-up is accomplished by 6-monthly clinical evaluation together with serial monitoring of calcitonin and CEA. No additional investigations are required provided the calcitonin remains undetectable. However, in familial cases it is worth checking the blood pressure regularly as well as the serum calcium, with formal re-investigation to exclude the development of phaeochromocytoma every 2 years. Lifelong maintenance thyroxine in physiological dose will be required, although there is no necessity to monitor thyroid function regularly once the patient has been rendered euthyroid, neither is there benefit from achieving TSH suppression.

39.7.7 TREATMENT OF LYMPHOMA

It is essential to differentiate between lymphoma and anaplastic carcinoma as treatment and prognosis are so different. The minimum surgery required therefore is a generous biopsy; resection of the isthmus is usefully undertaken if there is tracheal obstruction. In the Royal Marsden Hospital series, patients who had undergone total macroscopic removal of all lymphoma demonstrated the highest rate of local control and survival, so this option should always be considered (Tupchong *et al.*, 1986).

Treatment principles are similar to those for other lymphomas (Chapter 19). For stages I and II disease moderate dose radiotherapy should always be delivered: 40 Gy over 4 weeks usually achieves local control even in patients with unresectable disease. Anterior and undercouched portals are utilized as described for anaplastic carcinoma. The superior mediastinum should always be included but there is no evidence that treatment below the level of the carina is beneficial. A dramatic response is usually visible, often within 24 hours, but occasionally less responsive disease may demand Phase II dosage up to 50 Gy or more via a planned volume which excludes further dose to the spinal cord.

With a median survival time of 15 months and the majority of deaths due to widespread disease, there is a strong inclination towards the use of adjuvant combination chemotherapy for stages I and II disease. Initial chemotherapy using the same drugs as for other high grade non-Hodgkin's lymphomas is the preferred treatment at some centres, with irradiation to areas of initial bulk disease being given later. Patients with adverse prognostic features including stridor, dysphagia, gross residual tumour after surgery, and those with mediastinal involvement should therefore be considered for this approach. However some patients with these adverse features have been successfully treated with radiotherapy alone and identification of MALT features may be the way to select patients for locoregional treatment alone. Patients with stages III or IV disease at presentation should be treated with definitive chemotherapy and irradiation used only if there persists bulk disease at the primary site. Follow-up is the same as for any patient with lymphoma.

39.8 DIRECTIONS OF CURRENT CLINICAL RESEARCH

The exciting advance over the last decade has been the development of the ability to calculate the absorbed radiation dose in recurrent or metastatic tumour which concentrates radioiodine. This has permitted the construction of dose–response curves to determine the tumoricidal dose for differentiated thyroid carcinoma and so enable precise prescription of further ^{131}I therapy. In turn this will maximize tumour kill but minimize patient morbidity, staff exposure, and the expense of ineffective therapy. Dose–response data explain, for the first time, the spectrum of clinical response when patients are treated with fixed administered doses of radioiodine. These techniques must be both refined and simplified for reliable and widespread use.

For anaplastic cancer, both physical and biological optimization of external beam radiotherapy is required to improve the poor control of locoregional disease. Accelerated irradiation may be of value in such rapidly growing tumours and, although initial results are promising, normal tissue morbidity is unacceptable. Conformal planning therefore appears to have a role and this is being investigated in association with the use of the multileaf collimator. The most important advance in the treatment of these tumours would be the discovery of a drug effective against metastatic disease. In the meantime dose escalation studies of presently available chemotherapeutic agents are underway.

Improved chemotherapy is also required for metastatic medullary carcinoma. In familial cases the main impact for the future will follow early detection of apparently uninvolved relatives with effective surgical treatment before metastases develop.

Location of the responsible gene on chromosome 10 has now been identified such that genetic counselling is possible.

For the thyroid lymphomas it has never been clear which patients require adjuvant chemotherapy in addition to locoregional irradiation, as the majority are of high grade. Present analysis is attempting to correlate MALT appearance with local control and survival, with the hope that the subgroup requiring initial drug treatment may be identified.

REFERENCES

Ball, A.B.S., Tait, D.M., Fisher, C. *et al.* (1991) Treatment of metastatic para-aortic paraganglioma by surgery, radiotherapy and I-131 m IBG. *European Journal of Surgical Oncology*, **17**, 543–6.

Black, E.G., Cassoni, A., Gimlette, T.M.D. *et al.*(1981) Serum thyroglobulin in thyroid cancer. *Lancet*, **ii**, 443–5.

Brown, A.P., Greening, W.P., McCready, V.R. *et al.* (1984) Radioiodine treatment of metastatic thyroid carcinoma: The Royal Marsden Hospital experience. *British Journal of Radiology*, **57**, 323–7.

Charbord, P., L'Heritier, C., Cukersztein, W. *et al.* (1977) Radioiodine treatment in differentiated thyroid carcinomas. Treatment of first local recurrences and of bone and lung metastases. *Annals of Radiology*, **20**, 783–6.

Clark. O.H. (1982) Treatment of choice for patients with differentiated thyroid cancer. *Annals of Surgery*, **196**, 361–8.

Edmonds, C.J. and Smith, T. (1986) The long-term hazards of the treatment of thyroid cancer with radioiodine. *British Journal of Radiology*, **59**, 45–51.

Flower, M.A., Schlesinger, T., Hinton, P.J. *et al.* (1989) Radiation dose assessment in radioiodine therapy. 2. Practical implementation using quantitative scanning and PET, with initial results on thyroid carcinoma. *Radiotherapy and Oncology*, **15**, 345–57.

Harmer, C.L. (1977) External beam therapy for thyroid cancer. *Annals of Radiology*, **20**, 791–800.

Harmer, C. (1979) Unsealed radioactive isotopes in treatment. *Nursing Times*, 20-27 December, 41–44.

Harmer, C. (1991) Multidisciplinary management ·of thyroid neoplasms, in *Head and Neck Oncology for the General Surgeon*, (eds P.E. Preece, R.D.

Rosen and A.G.D. Maran), W.B. Saunders, London, pp. 55–90.

Harmer, C.L., Tyrell, C.J. and McCready, V.R. (1977) Uptake of isotope in residual normal thyroid tissue following I-131 ablation for carcinoma, Book of abstracts: XIV Congresso International de Radiologica, Rio de Janeiro, p. 562.

Hay, I.D., Bergstralh, E.J., Ebdersold, J.R. *et al.* (1992) Papilliary thyroid carcinoma ≤ 1.5 cm diameter: Woolner's 'occult' tumour revisited (Abstr.). *Journal of Endocrinological Investigation*, **15**, (Suppl. 2), 32.

Hermanek, P. and Sobin, L.H. (eds) (1987) *TNM Classification of Malignant Tumours*, Springer-Verlag, London, pp. 33–4.

Hoskin, P.J. and Harmer, C.L. (1987) Chemotherapy for thyroid cancer. *Radiotherapy and Oncology*, **10**, 187–94.

Mazzaferri, E.L. (1993) Management of a solitary thyroid nodule. *New England Journal of Medicine*, **328**, 553–9.

Mazzaferri, E.L., Young, R.L., Oertel, J.E. *et al.* (1977) Papillary thyroid carcinoma: the impact of therapy in 576 patients. *Medicine*, **56**, 171–96.

O'Connell, M.E. (1992) MD thesis accepted by the University of London. Treatment outcome and radioiodine dose response in differentiated thyroid carcinoma.

Palmer, B.V., Harmer, C.L. and Shaw, H.J. (1984) Calcitonin and carcino-embryonic antigen in the follow-up of patients with medullary carcinoma of the thyroid. *British Journal of Surgery*, **71**, 101–4.

Pochin, E.E. (1971) Radioiodine therapy of thyroid cancer. *Seminars in Nuclear Medicine* **4**, 503–15.

Ponder, B.A.J., Finer, N., Coffey, R. *et al.* (1988) Family screening in medullary thyroid carcinoma presenting without a family history. *Quarterly Journal of Medicine. New Series 67*, **252**, 299–308.

Powell, S. and Harmer, C.L. (1990) Death from thyroid cancer after forty years: rationale for initial intensive treatment. *European Journal of Surgical Oncology*, **16**, 457–61.

Russell, W.O., Ibanez, M.L., Clark, L.R. and White, E.C. (1963) Thyroid carcinoma: classification, intraglandular dissemination and clinicopathological study based upon whole organ sections of 80 glands. *Cancer*, **16**, 1425–60.

Sarker, S.D., Beierwaltes, W.H., Gill, S.P. and Cowley, B.J. (1976) Subsequent fertility and birth histories of children and adolescents treated with I-131 for thyroid cancer. *Journal of Nuclear Medicine*, **17**, 460–4.

Savoie, J.C., Massin, J.P., Leger, A.F. *et al.* (1985) Outcome of differentiated thyroid cancer after long-term follow-up: 1000 cases, in *Thyroid Cancer,* (eds C.Jaffiol and G. Milhaud), Elsevier Science, The Netherlands, pp. 209–17.

Schlumberger, M., Gardet, P., de Vathaire, F. *et al.* (1991) External radiotherapy *and chemotherapy in MTC patients, in Medullary Thyroid Carcinoma,* vol. 211, (eds C. Calmettes and J.M. Guliana), Colloque INSERM, John Libbey Eurotext Ltd, pp. 213–20.

Tissel, L.E., Hansson, G., Jansson, S. and Salander, H. (1986) Reoperation in the treatment of asymptomatic metastasizing medullary thyroid carcinoma. *Surgery,* **99**, 60–6.

Tubiana, M., Haddad, E., Schlumberger, M. *et al.* (1985) External radiotherapy in thyroid cancers. *Cancer,* **55**, 2062–71.

Tupchong, L., Hughes, F. and Harmer, C.L. (1986) Primary lymphoma of the thyroid: clinical features, prognostic factors, and results of treatment. *International Journal of Radiation Oncology, Biology, Physics,* **12**, 1813–21.

Waterhouse, J.A.H. (1991) Epidemiology of thyroid cancer, in *Head and Neck Oncology for the General Surgeon* (eds P.E. Preece, R.D. Rosen, and A.G.D. Maran), W.B. Saunders, London, pp. 1–10.

Young, R.L., Mazzaferri, E.L., Rahe, A.J. and Dorfman, S.G. (1980) Pure follicular thyroid carcinoma: impact of therapy in 214 patients. *Journal of Nuclear Medicine,* **21**, 733–7.

SMALL CELL LUNG CANCER

Paul A. Ellis and Ian E. Smith

40.1 INTRODUCTION

Small cell lung cancer (SCLC) comprises around 20–25% of all cases of lung cancer and has been recognized as a distinct clinico-pathological entity for over two decades. It differs markedly from other histological sub-types of lung cancer, both in its biological behaviour and in its responsiveness to chemotherapy and radiotherapy. More than any other subtype, SCLC is particularly asso-ciated with cigarette smoking; only three of the last 500 patients referred to our unit were life-time non-smokers. Its natural history is characterized by a highly aggressive clinical course and a propensity for early widespread dissemination. It is thus best thought of as a 'systemic' disease with chemotherapy the cornerstone of modern treatment.

40.2 HISTOPATHOLOGICAL CLASSIFICATION

The 1981 WHO classification divided SCLC into three subtypes as follows:

1. Oat cell
2. Intermediate type
3. Combined oat cell type (with squamous or adenocarcinoma).

The oat cell subtype consists of small round hyperchromatic cells with scanty cytoplasm while the intermediate subtype consists of fusiform or polygonal cells with granular chromatin, inconspicuous nucleoli and modest amounts of cytoplasm. This classi-fication has a number of problems including poor interobserver concordance and lack of clinicopathological correlation. It also fails to recognize the previously described subtype of small cell/large cell (SC/LC). A new classification taking these findings into account has therefore been proposed by the International Association for the Study of Lung Cancer, redefining the subtype of SCLC in an attempt to make it more clinically relevant (Table 40.1) (Yesner, 1985).

Cells with small cell carcinoma histology (excluding SC/LC) are typically found to have neurosecretory granules on electron microscopy, raising the possibility that SCLC

Table 40.1 Classification of small cell lung cancer

Small cell lung carcinoma	Combines previous, WHO subtypes 'oat cell' and 'intermediate type'
Small cell/large cell carcinoma	Containing subpopulation of cells resembling large cell carcinoma
Combined small cell carcinoma	With a substantial component of squamous or adenocarcinoma cells or both

From Yesner, 1985.

is derived from neuroendocrine cells. While the pathological diagnosis of SCLC is based primarily on morphology, immunohisto-chemical staining for neuroendocrine differ-entiation markers such as chromogranin A and neurone specific enolase (NSE) may be useful in cases where the diagnosis is not clear or the tissue specimen poor.

40.3 TUMOUR BIOLOGY

The past decade has seen rapid progress in our understanding of the biological proper-ties of SCLC. A major factor here has been the development of techniques for establishing *in vitro* cell lines from human SCLC (Carney *et al.*, 1985). This has led to the identification of a number of different biomarkers and growth factors secreted by SCLC cells; the identification of surface antigens on the cell surface and the development of monoclonal antibodies to these; the development of pro-grammes for *in vitro* testing of drug sensitiv-ity; and the elucidation of some of the genetic events leading to the transformation of SCLC cells.

SCLC cell lines can be subclassified into two major subgroups:

1. 'Classic' SCLC cell lines (approximately 70%)
2. 'Variant' cell lines.

Classic cell lines express elevated levels of L-dopa decarboxylase (DDC), bombesin/ gastrin releasing peptide (BLI/GRP), neurone specific enolase (NSE) and creatine kinase BB (CK-BB); have a relatively long doubling time; are radiosensitive; and have the morphological characteristics of the WHO intermediate cell type of SCLC. Variant cell lines have low levels of DDC, lack BLI/GRP, but continue to secrete NSE and CK-BB; have more rapid growth than classic lines; are more radioresistant; and morphologically more closely resemble the SC/LC variant of SCLC (Table 40.2) (Carney and De Leij, 1988).

SCLC cells produce a number of bio-markers including the hormones adreno-corticotrophin (ACTH), calcitonin, vasopressin (ADH), GRP and neurophysins, the enzymes CK-BB and NSE, and the tumour antigen carcinoembryonic antigen (CEA). Some of these including NSE and CEA have been shown to correlate inversely with prognosis.

Studies of SCLC cells have identified the secretion of several growth factors that may function as autocrine growth factors for these cells. The peptide hormone bombesin and its related peptide gastrin releasing peptide GRP (BLI/GRP) have been found to be potent mitogens for SCLC cells (Cutita *et al.*, 1985), as has another growth factor, insulin like growth factor 1 (IGF-1) (Macaulay *et al.*, 1988). The elucidation of these factors and their mechanism of action raises the possibility of developing specific growth factor antagonists for therapeutic strategies in the treatment of SCLC.

Two recent international workshops have classified the surface antigens on SCLC cell lines and fresh tissue (Souhami *et al.*, 1991). These workshops have allowed the sub-grouping of monoclonal antibodies into dif-ferent clusters according to their pattern of reactivity with SCLC cell lines and normal tissue. The largest number of antibodies of SCLC have been found to react with cluster 1 antigen, a 145 kDa molecule recently identified as the neural cell adhesion mole-cule (NCAM). The use of surface antigens as targets for monoclonal antibodies raises the possibility of tumour localization and deliv-ery of therapy at an early stage in the devel-opment of SCLC, and preclinical and clinical studies investigating this approach are currently being undertaken.

Attempts have been made to carry out *in vitro* chemosensitivity assays on SCLC cell lines. Recently prospective trials have been reported correlating results of *in vitro* drug sensitivity testing with response to chemo-therapy and survival in patients with SCLC (Tsai *et al.*, 1990). SCLC cell lines have also

Table 40.2 Biological properties of small cell lung cancer cell lines

Characteristic	SCLC	
	Classic	*Variant*
Growth morphology	Suspension	Suspension
Cytology	SCLC	SCLC
Colony forming efficiency	2%	13%
Doubling time	72 hour	32 hour
Dense core granules	+	−
DDC (L-dopa decarboxylase)	++	−
BLI/GRP (Bombesin/Gastrin releasing peptide)	++	−
NSE (Neurone specific enolase)	++	+
CK BB (Creatine Kinase BB)	++	++
Neurotensin	++	−
Peptide hormones	++	+/−
BLI receptors	+	−
EGF receptors (Epidermal Growth Factor)	−	−
HLA/B_2 microglobulin	Low/Absent	Low/Absent
Chromosome 3_p Deletion	+	+
Intermediate cell filaments	Cytokeratins	Cytokeratins
Leu-7 antigen	+	+
Radiation sensitivity	Sensitive	Resistant
C-*myc* amplification	−	+
N-*myc* amplification	+/−	+/−
L-*myc* amplification	+/−	−

Carney, 1988.

been used to evaluate drug resistance mechanisms, and to screen new compounds for clinical trials.

Developments in molecular biology have enabled the identification of some of the genetic changes associated with the development of SCLC and perhaps lung cancer in general. The most frequently recognized abnormality is a deletion on the short arm of chromosome 3 {3p(14-23)} which is found in approximately 90% of cases of SCLC (Whang-Peng *et al.*, 1982). This was originally thought to be specific for SCLC but has recently been reported in approximately 50% of patients with non-small cell lung cancer (NSCLC). The 3p(14-23) deletion appears to be an important early event in the development of lung cancer and suggests the deletion of an antioncogene. Other sites of loss of heterozygosity include 13q and 17p, shown to be due to mutations in the retinoblastoma (RB) gene

and the p53 gene respectively. The RB gene and its product are altered in nearly all cases of SCLC and approximately 10–30% of cases of NSCLC, while the p53 gene appears mutant in almost 100% of SCLC cases and approximately 50% of NSCLC.

Amplification and overexpression of the c-*myc* oncogene have been reported in a number of studies on SCLC cells lines and in fresh tumour tissue. It is commoner in previously treated patients than at initial presentation (Brennan *et al.*, 1991). This has pointed to the amplification of c-*myc* as a relatively late event in the pathogenesis of SCLC, perhaps contributing to the more aggressive behaviour observed at relapse. Amplification of n-*myc* and L-*myc* has also been reported, although their significance is not yet clear. Amplification of the *ras* oncogenes, important in NSCLC, does not normally occur in SCLC.

It is hoped some of these developments in the biology of SCLC may lead to novel and more effective approaches to therapy in the next few years.

40.4   NATURAL HISTORY AND CLINICAL FEATURES

There are no specific symptoms and signs which differentiate SCLC from other types of lung cancer, but its clinical course is usually much more abrupt in onset and aggressive in nature. The asymptomatic, 'chance' diagnosis of SCLC with a peripheral nodule on chest radiograph is a rare event. The great majority of patients are symptomatic at presentation with tumours that arise centrally in proximal large bronchi, and most have local and regional mediastinal lymph node involvement. Common presenting symptoms include haemoptysis, wheeze, dyspnoea, cough and chest pain. Superior vena caval obstruction (SVCO), hoarseness secondary to recurrent laryngeal nerve palsy and dysphagia are also frequent findings (Table 40.3). Approximately 60% of patients have overt metastatic disease at diagnosis with common sites including liver, adrenals, bone marrow, bone and brain. Patients with widespread disease also frequently complain of consitutional symptoms including anorexia, weight loss and fatigue.

Table 40.3   SCLC: symptoms at presentation (Royal Marsden Hospital series – unpublished data, 200 patients)

Symptom	% Occurrence
Malaise	66
Pain	53
Cough	77
Dyspnoea	70
Haemoptysis	7
Dysphagia	6
Hoarseness	10
SVCO*	10

* Superior Vena Caval Obstruction.

Paraneoplastic syndromes commonly occur with SCLC, and occasionally may be the first manifestation of the disease. By far the most common is the syndrome of inappropriate ADH secretion (SIADH). Although occurring in as many as 10% of patients, the presence of SIADH does not appear to correlate with stage of disease, or prognosis. More rarely, ectopic ACTH secretion is associated with SCLC. Because of its rapid onset, this seldom presents with Cushing's syndrome; patients are much more likely to have severe metabolic disturbance including hypokalaemia or hyperglycaemia. The Eaton–Lambert or myasthenia-like syndrome is commonly linked with SCLC (but in the authors' experience is very rare). It is characterized by muscle weakness and fatigue, usually most pronounced in the pelvic girdle and thighs. In contrast to true myasthenia gravis, muscle strength improves with exercise and there is a poor response to edrophonium (Tensilon). A number of other neurological syndromes may also occur, including limbic encephalitis, visual retinopathy, subacute cerebellar degeneration, necrotizing myelopathy, and subacute sensory or sensorimotor neuropathy.

40.5   STAGING

Many staging system have been proposed for SCLC but the one that has stood the test of time is a simple two stage system introduced by the Veterans Administration Lung Cancer Study Group (Mountain, 1978). This is an effective, reliable anatomical staging method that correlates with prognosis. It was originally based on radiotherapy considerations (now redundant): limited disease is defined as disease confined to one hemithorax with or without ipsilateral mediastinal or supraclavicular lymphadenopathy, while extensive disease covers any disease spread outside this defined area. More recently a consensus report has recommended the inclusion of contralateral mediastinal and supraclavicular nodes and ipsilateral pleural effusion independent of cytology in the 'limited disease' category, as these patients have a prognosis superior to patients with distant disease.

Standard staging investigations include patient history and examination, full blood count, serum biochemistry including albumin, liver function tests and LDH, cytological or histological documentation of SCLC, and chest X-ray. CT scanning of chest and upper abdomen (to stage liver and adrenals) is useful in the setting of a clinical trial allowing uniform groups of patients to be studied. Outside this setting and depending on local resources, chest X-ray and ultrasound of the upper abdomen can provide almost as much information. The role of bone marrow sampling is controversial. Some authors argue for bilateral marrows but current opinion is that this is unnecessary, as bone marrow involvement as the only site of disease is rare (less than 2%) and not of prognostic significance. CT scanning of the brain is positive in only a minority of asymptomatic patients and is unnecessary as a routine.

40.6 PROGNOSTIC FACTORS IN SCLC

Traditionally, stage of disease and performance status have been seen as the most important prognostic factors in SCLC. In addition, within the Extensive Disease category, number of sites of metastatic disease has provided further discrimination: patients with only one metastatic site have a better prognosis that those with multiple sites, and have a survival approaching that of Limited Disease (Abrams *et al.*, 1988). Other clinical factors of prognostic significance include weight loss and sex; most but not all studies show that females do better than males, independent of other variables. A number of laboratory variables have been found to correlate with worse prognosis including high serum LDH, low albumin (Alb), high alkaline phosphatase (ALP) and low serum sodium. Raised

biomarkers NSE and CEA also correlate inversely with prognosis.

Various groups have recently carried out multivariate analysis of clinical and laboratory parameters in large numbers of patients with SCLC to try to identify simple prognostic indices which might complement or even replace the standard LD/ED (Limited Disease/Extensive Disease) staging system. Our group (Vincent *et al.*, 1987) found that a simple combination of PS (Performance Status), serum albumin and alanine transaminase (ALT) could define three groups of good, medium and poor prognostic significance with better definition than LD and ED (Figure 40.1). Subsequently, a large British study analysing over 4000 patients found PS, alkaline phosphatase and stage of disease to be the most important factors followed by AST and LDH (Rawson and Peto, 1990). The South West Oncology Group studied over 2500 patients and found LDH to be the most significant prognostic factor, and has developed a simple staging system based on distant disease, LDH, age less than 70 years, and gender (Albain *et al.*, 1990). While each group has identified a slightly different set of prognostic factors, the general principle remains that prognostic assessment of patients with SCLC can be most effectively established with a combination of PS and two or three simple biochemical parameters.

40.7 TREATMENT

The median survival of untreated patients with small cell lung cancer ranges from as little as 6 to only 17 weeks (Mountain, 1978). Furthermore, less than 0.5% of all patients survive 5 years following surgical treatment alone. It was appreciated many years ago that small cell lung cancer was markedly responsive to radiotherapy but long term results with this treatment are not much better than with surgery. These results starkly illustrate the systemic nature of small cell lung cancer even

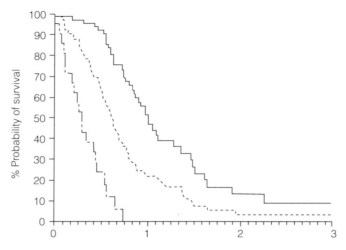

Figure 40.1 Survival. Prognostic subgroups based on performance status, serum albumin and alanine transaminase. Good Prognosis (————): albumin ≥ 36 g/l, normal alanine transaminase, PS = 0/1. Medium prognosis (-------), up to two of: albumin 30–35 g/l, elevated alanine transaminase, PS = 2. Poor prognosis (--------): all others. (Figure reproduced from Vincent *et al.* 1987, with permission.)

at the time of initial diagnosis when the disease might appear clinically localized.

40.7.1   CHEMOTHERAPY

Small cell lung cancer is markedly more responsive to chemotherapy than non-small cell and indeed this is probably the most chemosensitive of all of the so-called common solid cancers. Early trials demonstrated that the use of chemotherapy prolonged median survival compared with local treatment alone. Modern combination chemotherapy regimens achieve a high response rate for both LD and ED patients. For patients with limited disease, response rates of 80–90%, complete remission rates of around 50% and a median survival of 15–18 months are regularly reported; comparative figures for patients with extensive disease are around 50–60%, with complete remission rates of 10–30% and median survival of 7–12 months. There is considerable debate about the long term achievements of combination chemotherapy. Some individual series report 2 year survival rates of 30% or more for patients with limited disease

(McCracken *et al.*, 1990). In contrast, data from larger studies and randomized trials suggest only 5–10% of patients with limited disease are alive at 5 years and probably cured, and very few patients with extensive disease achieve long term survival (Johnson, 1990a; Souhami, 1990).

A whole range of different treatment strategies have been investigated over the last 10 years to try to improve results. These include alternating chemotherapy, maintenance treatment and high dose chemotherapy with autologous bone marrow transplantation. Frustratingly, none of these approaches have so far shown significant benefit over standard treatment.

(a)   Single agent studies

The first evidence for the effectiveness for chemotherapy in SCLC came in the late 1960s with a report that three courses of cyclophosphamide improved survival, compared with radiotherapy alone (Green *et al.*, 1969). Following this a number of active drugs have been identified with response rates of greater than 30%:

1. Cyclophosphamide
2. Doxorubicin
3. Etoposide
4. Teniposide
5. Cisplatin
6. Carboplatin
7. Vincristine
8. Methotrexate
9. Ifosfamide.

In recent years, carboplatin and etoposide have proved particularly active with response rates of 60% and 60–80% respectively in previously untreated patients (Smith *et al.*, 1985a; Clark *et al.*, 1990). Curiously cisplatin, a very effective agent in combination regimens, is reported in most single agent studies as having a response rate of only 13–20%, which almost certainly reflects the fact that this drug was assessed almost exclusively in previously treated patients. Single agent chemotherapy has in general been superseded by combination chemotherapy, but oral etoposide may be useful as palliative therapy in certain groups of patients, including the elderly and those of poor performance status (Clark *et al.*, 1990; Johnson, 1990b).

(b) Combination chemotherapy

Combination chemotherapy is superior to single agent therapy in most studies in terms of both response rate and duration, although few randomized controlled trials have been performed. No one combination chemotherapy regimen has been consistently shown to be superior to others, and commonly used regimens include CAV (cyclophosphamide, adriamycin and vincristine), ACE (adriamycin, cyclophosphamide and etoposide) and EP (etoposide, cisplatin) (Table 40.4).

The combination of cisplatin with etoposide is particularly popular in USA. It has been shown to be highly synergistic in animal models and unlike other regimens has produced impressive responses as a salvage regimen in relapsed patients (Evans *et al.*, 1985). When compared with CAV in two randomized trials the response rate for EP was slightly higher in one trial but neither demonstrated any survival difference (Fukuoka *et al.*, 1991; Roth *et al.*, 1992).

The cisplatin analogue, carboplatin, has also been tested in combination with other agents. We carried out an early study in combination with etoposide and found favourable response rates and modest toxicity; duration of response was disappointingly short, however (Smith *et al.*, 1987). Subsequently we

Table 40.4 Common combination chemotherapy regimens in small cell lung cancer

CAV	Cyclophosphamide	750 mg/m^2	i.v. day 1	q 21 days
	Adriamycin	40 mg/m^2	i.v. day 1	
	Vincristine	1.4 mg/m^2 (max. 2 mg)	i.v. day 1	
ACE	Adriamycin	40 mg/m^2	i.v. day 1	q 21 days
	Cyclophosphamide	750 mg/m^2	i.v. day 1	
	Etoposide	100 mg/m^2	i.v. days 1–3	
		(or 100 mg/m^2	i.v. day 1	
		+ 200 mg/m^2		
		orally days 2 + 3)		
EP	Etoposide	100 mg/m^2	i.v. days 1–3	q 21 days
	CisPlatin	25 mg/m^2	i.v. days 1–3	

found a more intensive regimen of carbo-platin, etoposide and ifosfamide to be very active with high response rates and a median survival of 18 months in LD but with significant toxicity (Smith *et al.*, 1990). Carboplatin based combination chemother-apy has also been assessed as simple palli-ative treatment for patients with advanced disease in poor PS. A combination of CVM (carboplatin, vinblastine and methotrexate) was compared with ACE with no significant difference in response rates or survival between the two groups, but significantly less symptomatic (alopecia in particular) and haematological toxicity in the CVM arm (Jones *et al.*, 1991).

(c)   Alternating therapy

Although combination chemotherapy regi-mens produce high response rates most pa-tients relapse with disease that subsequently proves drug resistant. Several groups have therefore explored the strategy of alternating chemotherapy, testing the Goldman–Goldie hypothesis that rapid alternation of non-cross resistant regimens might improve tumour cell kill. Early studies failed to demonstrate any benefit for this approach but interest was rekindled by a trial demonstrating better sur-vival for CAV alternating with EP than for CAV alone (Evans *et al.*, 1987). Unfortunately two further trials comparing CAV alternating with EP versus the two regimens alone have failed to demonstrate a survival benefit for the alternating approach (Fukuoka *et al.*, 1991; Roth *et al.*, 1992). The overall conclusion from these trials and others is that alternating chemotherapy holds no advantage over stan-dard regimens.

(d)   Dose intensity/high dose therapy

Another strategy in the treatment of SCLC has been the exploration of the effect of dose intensity. Current standard combination chemotherapy regimens are designed to produce moderately severe mylosuppression (nadir leucopenia 1000–1500 cells/mm^3 or thrombocytopenia 50 000 to 100 000 platelets/mm^3) in the majority of patients. In general, patients on these regimens do not require frequent admission to hospital between cycles. Higher doses of CAV (Johnson *et al.*, 1987) and EP (Ihde *et al.* 1991) were com-pared with standard doses in randomized trials with significantly increased toxicity in the high dose groups but no difference in overall response rates or median survival. The use of growth factors such as granulo-cyte colony stimulating factors (GCSF) to enable intensive chemotherapy to be given on schedule has also been looked at (Crawford *et al.*, 1991). Although the inci-dence of febrile neutropenia episodes is reduced, life threatening myelosuppression still occurs and no obvious benefit in terms of improved survival has thus far been demonstrated.

Very high dose chemotherapy with ABMT (Autologous Bone Marrow Transplantation) as late intensification for patients in remission following standard dose chemotherapy has also been studied (Smith *et al.*, 1985b; Humblet *et al.*, 1987). Although response rates have been shown to be higher with this ap-proach, median and overall survival are little different, and this treatment strategy remains experimental.

(e)   Duration of therapy

For many years there was uncertainty about the optimum duration of therapy for SCLC, and some groups continued treatment for up to 2 years; in practice for most patients this meant being on treatment for the rest of their lives. Recently several trials have demon-strated that shorter courses of treatment produce similar results with less toxicity, with around 6 months of treatment being as effective as more prolonged maintenance therapy and with less morbidity (Byrne *et al.*, 1989).

(f)   Chemotherapy for relapsed disease

The vast majority of patients treated for SCLC eventually relapse. Unfortunately the results of further chemotherapy at this stage are poor. Fit patients who have relapsed off treatment can be offered participation on Phase I and II trials for new agents, whereas patients relapsing on chemotherapy are best treated symptomatically. High response rates can sometimes be achieved but the median response is usually only 2 or 3 months and survival is short. Such treatment can sometimes have useful palliative benefit, but careful patient selection and close monitoring of symptomatic relief are needed.

40.7.2   RADIOTHERAPY IN SCLC

(a)   Thoracic irradiation

For reasons already discussed, thoracic radiotherapy alone is not normally appropriate for SCLC and its role in combination with chemotherapy in the treatment of patients with limited disease has been debated vigorously. Thoracic irradiation certainly reduces local recurrence rates, but this is offset by the increased haematological, pulmonary and oesophageal toxicity compared with chemotherapy alone. Several large randomized prospective trials have recently compared combined modality therapy with chemotherapy alone for LD SCLC. Most but not all have demonstrated a small but significant improvement in overall survival for combined modality treatment. A meta-analysis has confirmed a small benefit for combined modality treatment with a 14% relative reduction in death rate and an absolute increase of 5% in overall survival at 3 years (Pignon *et al.*, 1992).

It was initially thought that the dose of thoracic irradiation needed to control locoregional SCLC could be reduced when given with chemotherapy. Increased local recurrence rates with doses of around 30 Gy, however, have emphasized the need for higher doses in the range of 45–50 Gy for optimal local control. The optimal timing of irradiation remains a problem. There is some evidence pointing to the superior efficacy of concurrent irradiation delivered in conjunction with chemotherapy, compared with that sequentially delivered during a break in chemotherapy or following its completion. The optimum timing of thoracic irradiation needs further investigation in controlled trials.

Thoracic radiotherapy has little if any role to play in patients with extensive disease. Large retrospective reviews and a randomized trial have shown no benefit in this setting and hence it should be reserved for palliation.

(b)   CNS treatment and prophylaxis

Cerebral metastases are common in SCLC. They occur in approximately 10–15% of patients at presentation with a cumulative risk of intracranial relapse after treatment of approximately 50% at 2 years. The poor quality of life and short survival of patients with cerebral metastases has stimulated interest in prophylactic cranial irradiation (PCI) in selected patients, and in particular those with LD who have obtained complete remission with standard therapy. An initial series of randomized trials of PCI all demonstrated a reduced incidence of cranial relapse but no significant improvement in median or overall survival (Bleehan *et al.*, 1983). Some of these however had insufficient numbers of patients to detect a small survival benefit.

If PCI were a completely non-toxic treatment then it could be justified on the basis of reducing potentially debilitating intracranial relapse. The problem is that a number of long term survivors have developed long term neuropsychiatric impairment following PCI, varying from mild impairment of intellectual function to severe dementia and gait disturbance (Frytak *et al.*, 1989). Many factors may predispose to late CNS toxicity including choice of cytotoxic agents, scheduling of drugs in relation to PCI and radiotherapy factors including in particular fraction size. PCI is not therefore without the risk of long term problems and cannot at present be considered part of standard therapy. PCI is currently being further investigated in patients who have achieved complete remission, in a large European multicentre trial.

40.7.3   OVERT CNS DISEASE

Views on the treatment of overt cerebral metastatic disease at presentation have changed in the last few years. Until recently such lesions were treated with steroids and cranial irradiation as it was thought that cytotoxic agents did not adequately penetrate the blood–brain barrier. Several chemotherapy studies have countered this view with an overall response to chemotherapy in the CNS of 76% (Kristensen *et al.*, 1992), similar to results for other sites of metastatic disease. The authors postulate that cerebral metastases at presentation should be treated with chemotherapy alone initially, with cranial irradiation reserved for cases of delayed cerebral disease on treatment. This seems a sensible policy to us, but the issue of whether consolidative cranial irradiation should be given at the end of initial chemotherapy in patients presenting with cerebral metastases remains unclear. Second line chemotherapy for cranial relapse is unimpressive and steroids with cranial irradiation should continue to be used to provide palliation here.

40.7.4   THE ROLE OF SURGICAL RESECTION IN SCLC

The poor results with surgery for SCLC led most clinicians to abandon this approach in the early 1970s, but recently its role has been re-evaluated. The Veterans Administration Lung Study Group reported 5 year survival rates of 25–35% following complete resection

of isolated pulmonary nodules later found to be SCLC (Higgins *et al.*, 1975) and others have confirmed excellent results for surgery followed by adjuvant chemotherapy in small localized TNM stage I and II tumours ranging from 30% to 80% 5 years survival (Karrer *et al.*, 1989; Shepherd *et al.*, 1991). It must be kept in mind however that patients presenting with small localized tumours represent less than 10% of the overall patient population, and patients that have surgery are therefore highly selected. What is not clear is whether the superior outcome of these patients is attributable to the surgery, or to an inherently better prognosis of patients with minimal tumour burden. Patients defined as 'very limited disease' (without evidence of mediastinal involvement) treated with chemoradiotherapy have been found to have median and 5 year survivals compared to those undergoing surgical resection followed by chemoradiotherapy (Shepherd *et al.*, 1984).

Likewise the role of surgery in the resection of residual disease following chemotherapy is controversial. Some studies suggest prolonged disease free survival with this approach, but again this is in a highly selected group with excellent performance status, low levels of co-morbid disease, and by definition responsiveness to induction chemotherapy.

In our view, surgical resection is appropriate in the treatment of the rare patient presenting with an isolated peripheral lung nodule, and there is an argument for subsequent adjuvant chemotherapy here. It has little role at present in the great majority of patients with more advanced disease.

40.8   LONG TERM SURVIVAL

Even with modern treatments the large majority of patients with SCLC ultimately relapse and die of their disease. Encouraging long term results are reported regularly from small single centre studies with all the uncertainty of selection bias, but large series still report overall 5 year survival figures ranging from only 5% to 12% (Johnson, 1990a; Souhami and Law, 1990). Relapses continue to occur between 2 and 5 years but are extremely rare after this stage and patients surviving 5 years are effectively cured.

Second malignancies are a problem, with the risk exceeding that of relapsed SCLC after only 3–4 years of disease free survival (Heyne *et al.*, 1992). By far the most common is the development of non-small cell lung cancer, and any patient presenting with a new solitary pulmonary lesion should be re-evaluated as if they had a new potentially curable malignancy. Predictably, other smoking related malignancies including carcinomas of the head and neck, oesophagus, bladder and pancreas also occur. SCLC survivors also appear to be at risk of acute myeloid leukaemia (AML) or myelodyoplastic syndrome, which is almost certainly chemotherapy related.

40.9 FUTURE PROSPECTS

A lot of current interest is focused on optimal scheduling of chemotherapy, including in particular etoposide. This drug has been shown to be schedule dependent in preclinical studies and in early phase II studies (Cavalli *et al.*, 1978). In an important study Slevin and co-workers (1989) found a significant improvement in response rates and median survival for patients treated with intravenous etoposide over 5 days compared with the same dose as a single injection. This has led to the hypothesis that the cytotoxicity of etoposide may be related to the maintenance of continued low plasma concentrations. Further evidence supporting this hypothesis comes from studies showing the effectiveness of prolonged schedules of oral etoposide in previously treated patients (Johnson, 1990b) and untreated elderly or unfit patients (Clark *et al.*, 1990). We are investigating the efficacy and toxicity of continuous low dose infusional etoposide in the

hope that it may be as active but less toxic than current combination chemotherapy regimens when used in this way.

There is currently a dearth of new agents active in SCLC. Novel drugs currently being tested include taxol and its analogue taxotere, and the campothecins. Preliminary results do not indicate significantly increased efficacy over conventional agents.

New approaches are needed for this disease. The increasing understanding of the biology of SCLC may soon open up new therapeutic options. Autocrine growth factors including gastrin-releasing peptides (GRP) and insulin-like growth factors (IGF-I) and their receptors offer possible targets. We have shown for example that monoclonal antibodies against IGF-I and its major receptor will inhibit *in vitro* human SCLC growth (Macaulay *et al.*, 1988). Likewise we and others have shown that analogues of substance P, a sensory neurotransmitter, inhibit SCLC growth *in vitro* and in xenografts (Langdon *et al.*, 1992). These agents are thought to act at least in part through inhibition of GRP. Biological response modifiers including the interferons are currently being studied, particularly as maintenance treatment in patients with small cell lung cancer who have achieved good response to chemotherapy. In one randomized trial interferon-alpha has been reported as achieving prolonged survival (Mattson *et al.*, 1991). Interferon-gamma has greater immunomodulatory properties than interferon-alpha and is likewise being investigated in randomized trials. First results in one such trial have failed to show survival benefit and a similar but larger trial is currently being carried out by the EORTC.

40.10 CONCLUSIONS

SCLC remains an enigma in modern oncology. It is markedly sensitive both to radiotherapy and to chemotherapy, and modern combination chemotherapy schedules, sometimes with thoracic irradiation, have led to improved survival and effective palliation for the majority of patients. A small proportion of patients achieve long term survival and are probably cured. However, the vast majority of patients still relapse and die of their disease. The initial optimism engendered by treatment successes in the late 1970s and early 1980s has now been tempered by survival figures that have remained static throughout the last decade. Cure therefore remains an elusive goal for most patients and new therapeutic strategies and directions are urgently needed.

REFERENCES

Abrams, J., Doyle, L.A. and Aisner, J. (1988) Staging, prognostic factors and special considerations in small cell lung cancer. *Seminars in Oncology*, **15**, 261–77.

Albain, K.S., Crowley, J.J., Le Blanc, M. *et al.* (1990) Determinants of improved outcome in small cell lung cancer: an analysis of the 2,580-Patient Southwest Oncology Group Database. *Journal of Clinical Oncology*, **8**, 1563–74.

Bleehan, N.M., Bunn, P.A., Cox, J.D. *et al.* (1983) Role of radiation therapy in small cell anaplastic carcinoma of the lung. *Cancer Treatment Reports*, **67**, 11–19.

Brennan, J., O'Connor, T., Makuch, R.W. *et al.* (1991) Myc family DNA amplification in 107 tumours and tumour cell lines from patients with small cell lung cancer treated with different combination chemotherapy regimens. *Cancer Research*, **51**, 1708–12.

Byrne, M.J., Van Hazel, O., Trotter, J. *et al.* (1989) Maintenance chemotherapy in limited small cell lung cancer: a randomised controlled clinical trial. *British Journal of Cancer*, **60**, 413–18.

Carney, D.N. and De Leij, L. (1988) Lung cancer biology. *Seminars in Oncology*, **15**, 199–214.

Carney, D.N., Gazdar, A.F., Bepler, G. *et al.* (1985) Establishment and identification of small cell lung cancer cell lines having classic and variant features. *Cancer Research*, **45**, 2913–23.

Cavalli, F., Sonntag, R.W., Jungi, F. *et al.* (1978) VP16-213 Monotherapy for remission induction of small cell lung cancer: a randomised trial using 3 dosage schedules. *Cancer Treatment Reports*, **62**, 473–5.

Clark, P.I., Cottier, B., Joel, S.P. *et al.* (1990) Prolonged administration of single agent oral etoposide in patients with untreated small cell lung cancer. *Proceedings of the American Society of Clinical Oncology*, **9**, A 874.

Crawford, J., Ozer, H., Stoller, R. *et al.* (1991) Reduction by granulocyte colony-stimulating factor of fever and neutropenia induced by chemotherapy in patients with small cell lung cancer. *New England Journal of Medicine*, **325**, 164–70.

Cutita, F., Carney, D.N., Mulshine, J. *et al.* (1985) Bombesin-like peptides can function as autocrine growth factors in human small cell lung cancer. *Nature*, **316**, 823–4.

Evans, W.K., Osoba, D., Feld, R. *et al.* (1985) Etoposide (VP16) and cisplatin: an effective treatment for relapse in small cell lung cancer; a multicentre randomised clinical trial by the National Cancer Institute of Canada. *Journal of Clinical Oncology*, **3**, 65–71.

Evans, W.K., Feld, R., Murray, N. *et al.* (1987) Superiority of alternating non-cross resistant chemotherapy in extensive small cell lung cancer. *Annals Internal Medicine*, **107**, 45–58.

Frytak, S., Shaw, J.N., O'Neill, B.P. *et al.* (1989) Leucoencephalopathy in small cell lung cancer patients receiving prophylactic cranial irradiation. *American Journal of Clinical Oncology*, **12**, 27–33.

Fukuoka, M., Furuse, K., Saijo, N. *et al.* (1991) Randomised trial of Cyclophosphamide, Doxorubicin, and Vincristine versus Cisplatin and Etoposide versus alternation of these regimens in small cell lung cancer. *Journal of the National Cancer Institute*, **83**, 855–61.

Green, R.A., Humphrey, E., Close, H. *et al.* (1969) Alkylating agents in bronchogenic carcinoma. *American Journal of Medicine*, **46**, 516–25.

Heyne, K.H., Lippman, S.M. and Lee, J.J. (1992) The incidence of second primary tumours in long term survivors of small cell lung cancer *Journal of Clinical Oncology*, **10**, 1519–24.

Higgins, G.A., Shields, T.W. and Keehan, R.J. (1975) The solitary pulmonary nodule. Ten year follow up of the Veterans Administration-Armed Forces Cooperation Study. *Archives of Surgery*, **110**, 570–5.

Humblet, Y., Symann, M., Bosly, A. *et al.* (1987) Late intensification chemotherapy with autologous bone marrow transplantation in selected small cell carcinoma of the lung: a randomised study. *Journal of Clinical Oncology*, **5**, 1864–73.

Ihde, D.C., Mulshine, J.L., Kramer, B.S. *et al.* (1991) Randomised trial of high versus standard dose etoposide and cisplatin in extensive stage small cell lung cancer. *Proceedings of the American Society of Clinical Oncology,* **10**, 240.

Johnson, B.E., Grayson, J., Makuch, R.W. *et al.* (1990a) Ten year survival of patients with small cell lung cancer treated with combination chemotherapy with or without irradiation. *Journal of Clinical Oncology,* **8**, 396–401.

Johnson, D.H., Einhorn, L.H., Birch, R. *et al.* (1987) A randomised comparison of high dose versus conventional dose cyclophosphamide, doxorubicin and vincristine for extensive stage small cell lung cancer: a phase III trial of the Southeastern Cancer Study Group. *Journal of Clinical Oncology,* **5**, 1731–8.

Johnson, D.H., Strupp, J., Greco, F.A. *et al.* (1990b) Prolonged administration of oral Etoposide in previously treated small cell lung cancer (SCLC) patients: a phase II trial. *Proceedings of the American Society of Clinical Oncology,* **9**, 227.

Jones, A.L., Holborn, J. and Ashley, S. (1991) Effective new low toxicity chemotherapy with carboplatin, vinblastine and methotrexate for small cell lung cancer: a randomised trial against Doxorubicin, Cyclophosphamide and Etoposide. *European Journal of Cancer,* **27**, 866–70.

Karrer, K., Shields, T.W., Denck, H. *et al.* (1989) The importance of surgical and multimodality treatment for small cell bronchial carcinoma. *Journal of Thoracic and Cardiovascular Surgery,* **97**, 168–76.

Kristensen, C.A., Kristjansen, P.E.G. and Hansen, H.H. (1992) Systemic chemotherapy of brain metastases from small cell lung cancer: a review. *Journal of Clinical Oncology,* **10**, 1498–502.

Langdon, S., Sethi, T., Ritchie, A. *et al.* (1992) Broad spectrum neuropeptide antagonists inhibit the growth of small cell lung cancer *in vivo. Cancer Research,* **52**, 4554–7.

McCracken, J.D., Janaki, L.M., Crowley, J.J. *et al.* (1990) Concurrent chemotherapy/radiotherapy for limited small cell lung carcinoma: a Southwest Oncology Group study. *Journal of Clinical Oncology,* **8**, 892–8.

Macaulay, V.M., Teale, J.D., Everard, M.J. *et al.* (1988) Somatomedin-C/Insulin-like growth factor-1 is a mitogen for human small cell lung cancer. *British Journal of Cancer,* **57**, 91–3.

Mattson, K., Niiranen, A., Pyrhönen, S. *et al.* (1991) Recombinant interferon gamma treatment in non-small cell lung cancer. Antitumour effect and cardiotoxicity. *Acta Oncologica,* **30**, 607–10.

Mountain, C.F. (1978) Clinical biology of small cell carcinoma. Relationship to surgical therapy. *Seminars in Oncology,* **5**, 272–9.

Pignon, J.P., Arriagada, R., Ihde, D.C. *et al.* (1992) A metaanalysis of thoracic radiotherapy for small cell lung cancer. *New England Journal of Medicine,* **327**, 1618–25.

Rawson, N.S.B. and Peto, J. (1990) An overview of prognostic factors in small cell lung cancer. *British Journal of Cancer,* **61**, 597–604.

Roth, B.J., Johnson, D.H., Einhorn, L.H. *et al.* (1992) Radomised study of Cyclophosphamide, Doxorubicin and Vincristine versus Etoposide and Cisplatin versus alternation of these two regimens in extensive small cell lung cancer: a phase III trial of the Southeastern Cancer Study Group. *Journal of Clinical Oncology,* **10**, 282–91.

Shepherd, F.A., Ginsberg, R.J., Evans, W.K. *et al.* (1984) Very limited small cell lung cancer. Results of non surgical treatment. *Proceedings of the American Society of Clinical Oncology,* **3**, 223.

Shepherd, F.A., Ginsberg, R.J., Feld, R. *et al.* (1991) Surgical treatment for limited cell lung cancer. *Journal Thoracic and Cardiovascular Surgery,* **101**, 385–93.

Slevin, M.L., Clark, P.I., Joel, S.P. *et al.* (1989) A randomised trial to evaluate the effect of schedule on activity of etoposide in small cell lung cancer. *Journal of Clinical Oncology,* **7**, 1333–40.

Smith, I.E., Harland, S.J., Robinson, B.A. *et al.* (1985a) Carboplatin: a very active new cisplatin analog in the treatment of small cell lung cancer. *Cancer Treatment Reports,* **69**, 43–6.

Smith, I.E., Evans, B.D., Harland, S.J. *et al.* (1985b) High dose cyclophosphamide with autologous bone marrow rescue after conventional chemotherapy in the treatment of small cell lung cancer. *Cancer Chemotherapy and Pharmacology,* **14**, 120–4.

Smith, I.E., Evans, B.D., Gore, M.E. *et al.* (1987) Carboplatin and etoposide as first line combination therapy for small cell lung cancer. *Journal of Clinical Oncology,* **5**, 185–9.

Smith, I.E., Perren, T.J., Ashley, S.A. *et al.* (1990) Carboplatin, Etoposide, Ifosfamide as intensive chemotherapy for small cell lung cancer. *Journal of Clinical Oncology,* **8**, 899–905.

Souhami, R.L. and Law, K. (1990) Longevity in small cell lung cancer. *British Journal of Cancer,* **61**, 584–9.

Souhami, R.L., Beverley, P.C.L., Bobrow, L.G. *et al.* (1991) Antigens of lung cancer: results of the Second International Workshop on Lung Cancer

Antigens. *Journal of the National Cancer Institute,* **83,** 609–12.

Tsai, C.M., Ihde, D.C., Kadoyoma, C. *et al.* (1990) Correlation of *in vitro* sensitivity testing of long term small cell lung cancer cell lines with response and survival. *European Journal of Cancer,* **26,** 1148–52.

Vincent, M.D., Ashley, S.E. and Smith, I.E. (1987) Prognostic factors in small cell lung cancer: a simple prognostic index is better than conventional staging. *European Journal of Cancer and Clinical Oncology,* **23,** 1589–99.

Whang-Peng, J., Kao-Shan, C.S., Lee, E.C. *et al.* (1982) Specific chromosome defect associated with human small cell lung cancer: deletion 3p (14–23). *Science,* **215,** 181–82.

Yesner, R. (1985) Classification of lung cancer histology. *New England Journal of Medicine,* **312,** 652–3.

NON-SMALL CELL LUNG CANCER

41

Marjan Jahangiri, Rachael Barton and Peter Goldstraw

Lung cancer is one of the most prevalent cancers in the industrialized world and is a leading cause of cancer death. The major causative factor is tobacco consumption and, therefore, it is potentially preventable. Non-small cell lung cancer (NSCLC) is the term adopted by the World Health Organization (WHO) in 1977 to group together adeno-carcinoma, squamous cell carcinoma and large cell carcinoma. It accounts for approximately 80% of all lung cancers. Because they have a potential for cure by resection, the NSCLC group have major therapeutic interest to the surgeon.

41.1 INCIDENCE

From a trivial health problem at the beginning of this century and a minor one by 1930

(causing fewer than 5 deaths annually per 100 000), lung cancer has now become epidemic. In the UK lung cancer is responsible for 6% of all deaths and a quarter of all cancer deaths, that is, approximately 40 000 deaths per annum. It is the commonest cause of cancer death in men and the second commonest in women after breast cancer. In Scotland, female deaths from lung cancer have exceeded those from breast cancer since 1984. Figure 41.1 shows the mortality trends by age and sex from 1941 to 1991 for men and women in England and Wales. After the large increase in mortality rates in the 1970s, there has been a decline in all male mortality rates and in women under the age of 55.

Similarly, in the USA, lung cancer has long been the leading cancer killer, accounting for 36% of all cancer deaths. By 1986 it had

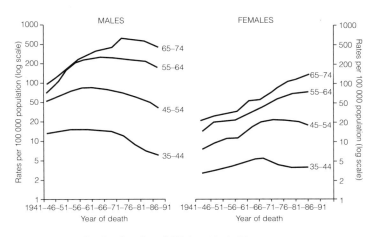

Figure 41.1 Mortality time trends. England and Wales 1941–90.

become the leading killer of women, accounting for 20% of cancer deaths (breast cancer causing 18% of all cancer deaths). With a death rate of 76 per 100 000 per annum (161 000 new lung cancer cases per year, of which approximately 80% will be NSCLC), nearly twice as many will die from lung cancer as will die from all accidents. In most European countries, the most frequent cancer among males is lung cancer. The only exception among EC countries is Portugal, where the frequency of lung cancer is increasing, but it is still lower than stomach cancer.

Overall, more than 150 000 new cases of lung cancer occur in the EEC every year and the number is increasing.

41.2 AETIOLOGY

Cigarette smoking is the predominant factor in the aetiology of lung cancer (Doll and Peto, 1976). Despite antismoking campaigns, there are around 14 million people who smoke in the UK. The latest statistics from the General Household Survey for Great Britain (OPCS Monitor, 1990) show that smoking is most common in the 20–24 year age group for women and in the 20–49 year age group for men. It also appears that most adult smokers have acquired the habit by the time they are 19 years old. Very few 11 and 12 year olds smoke, but by the age of 15, one in four children are regular smokers. The risk of lung cancer is related to the number of cigarettes smoked and it is more dependent on the duration of smoking than consumption. That is, smoking one packet of cigarettes a day for 40 years is eight times more hazardous than smoking two packets a day for 20 years.

The risk can be reduced by giving up smoking and the amount of benefit increases with the time of not smoking. After 10 or more years, an ex-smoker has nearly the same risk as a non-smoker. There is evidence that tar contains the carcinogens that cause lung cancer. Today almost no one smokes high tar cigarettes (18 mg tar/cigarette). It appears that lower tar cigarettes carry a lower risk of lung cancer than higher tar cigarettes.

It is difficult to quantitatively define the role of passive smoking. It is estimated that about a quarter of all lung cancers in non-smokers are due to passive smoking and that in the UK at least 300 people die each year from lung cancer caused by passive smoking (Imperial Cancer Research Fund and Cancer Research Campaign, 1991). The association of lung cancer with asbestos, haematite, uranium, arsenic and other pollutants is well established (Selikoff *et al.*, 1960). If all smoking were to cease today, the impact, in terms of lung cancer mortality, would not be evident for many years. Therefore, secondary prevention by screening to detect asymptomatic 'early' lung cancer is very attractive. Several studies have been conducted to assess the value of screening in asymptomatic patients by using sputum cytology and chest radiographs. In 1971 the National Cancer Institute of the USA initiated three large randomized controlled trials of periodic radiological and cytological screening of asymptomatic, high risk populations for early stage lung cancer. These trials were carried out at the Johns Hopkins Medical Institutions, the Memorial Sloan–Kettering Cancer Center and the Mayo Clinic (Melamed *et al.*, 1984; Fawana *et al.*, 1986). The Johns Hopkins and Memorial trials compared 4 monthly sputum cytology and annual chest X-rays to annual chest X-rays alone. No reduction in lung cancer mortality was demonstrated. However, the Mayo trial compared 4 monthly sputum cytology and chest X-rays with a recommendation that the test be repeated annually. This study demonstrated significant increases in lung cancer detection and resectability in the 4 monthly sputum cytology and chest X-rays with a recommendation that the test be repeated annually. This study demonstrated significant increases in lung cancer detection and resectability in the 4 monthly screened group, but there was no difference in lung cancer mortality. The results of these trials have been widely interpreted as showing no benefit for screening programmes. In reality they only show that more intensive screening programmes have no advantage over annual chest radiographs in the high risk group. It is, however, widely agreed that large scale intensive radiological or cytological screening for lung cancer cannot be advocated as a public health policy.

41.3 PATHOLOGY

NSCLC comprises squamous cell carcinoma, adenocarcinoma and large cell carcinoma. There is a high degree of overlap in histopathology of most of these tumours, especially when they are less differentiated. This is partly due to interobserver variability and partly due to the heterogeneity of the tumours.

Squamous cell carcinomas tend to arise centrally in major bronchi and eventually spread to adjacent hilar nodes. Generally, they disseminate later than other cell types. Slow growth is often a characteristic of squamous cell carcinoma which has a longer volume doubling time, around 90 days, especially when compared with small cell carcinomas, with a doubling time of 30 days (Geddes, 1979). Metaplasia in the bronchial epithelium may progress to dysplasia which, if severe, is classified as carcinoma-*in-situ*, a stage that may last for years before the development of frank invasion. Squamous cancers may present as central bulky masses obstructing a major bronchus and producing atelectasis and infection. The centrally located tumours may invade the peribronchial and hilar lymph nodes by direct invasion rather than by lymphatic spread. The slow growing peripherally located tumours may lead to local chest wall invasion. Histologically, they range from well differentiated squamous cell carcinomas to the poorly differentiated large cell patterns with some residual squamous cell features.

In many areas of the world there is an increase in frequency of adenocarcinoma in both absolute terms and relative to other cell types. This is partly attributed the increasing incidence of lung cancer in women (Wu *et al.*, 1986). Adenocarcinoma is the most frequent type in women. The association with cigarette smoking is less certain. Adenocarcinomas tend to be more peripherally located, can grow very slowly with an average doubling time of 160 days and tend to be smaller at presentation than the other variants of lung cancer. Early metastases, especially to the brain, adrenals and bone, are a feature of adenocarcinoma and cerebral metastases will present in about half of the cases at some time during the course of the disease.

Large cell carcinoma constitutes the remainder of NSCLCs. The cells are usually anaplastic and often lack histological differentiation. They are more often peripheral than central and are generally bulky neoplasms. They tend to spread early and, like adenocarcinoma, have a propensity to metastasize to the adrenals, the brain, the liver.

41.4 CLINICAL PRESENTATION

Only a small number of patients (5–15%) with lung cancer are asymptomatic at the time of initial diagnosis, their tumours being detected on routine chest radiographs. The symptoms of lung cancer can be due to the local effects of the tumour or result from metastasis or the general effects of carcinoma. Rarely lung cancer may present as one of the paraneoplastic syndromes.

The most frequent presentation is the development of a new cough or exacerbation of an already present cough. Haemoptysis is common, but this is usually minor with blood streaking of the sputum; massive haemoptysis is rare. Dull chest pain is a non-specific but common complaint. However, chest pain which is more persistent and severe, and of a localized nature, is often due to invasion of the parietal pleura or chest wall. Dyspnoea may be due to major bronchial obstruction or result from a pleural effusion or paralysis of a hemidiaphragm due to phrenic nerve invasion. Hoarseness is the result of recurrent laryngeal nerve paresis. It is nearly always the left nerve which is damaged because of its long intrathoracic course, and damage may be caused by direct invasion or by metastasis to adjacent lymph nodes. Major bronchial obstruction can cause distal atelectasis and consolidation with fever. Wheezing and stridor may result from partial obstruction. Any smoker who develops a pneumonia which proves resistant to therapy should be suspected of having an underlying lung cancer. Mediastinal extension of the primary tumours or metastases to mediastinal lymph nodes may compress the oesophagus and cause dysphagia or result in the superior vena caval obstruction syndrome, causing facial oedema and distention of superficial vessels of the head and neck. Apical neoplasms, Pancoast's tumours, may invade the brachial plexus causing pain in the distribution of the ulnar nerve or involve the sympathetic chain and stellate ganglion resulting in Horner's syndrome (ipsilaterial exophthalmus, ptosis, miosis and anhidrosis).

Metastatic spread to local and distal lymph nodes is common. Lymph node enlargement in the supraclavicular and cervical regions may be evident on clinical examination. Involvement of axillary lymph nodes is rare except in conjunction with chest wall invasion. Mediastinal lymph node metastasis may be evidenced by involvement of adjacent mediastinal structures – trachea, oesophagus, superior vena cava or phrenic and recurrent laryngeal nerves.

Spread by the vascular route to the liver, central nervous system, adrenals and the skeleton is a common complication of all variants of lung cancer, and it is important to examine for hepatomegaly, search for any neurological defect, enquire as to any personality change and to specially question the patient about any recent bone or joint symptoms which they may rationalize as 'arthritis'

or 'sciatica'. In one-half of cases studied at autopsy no extrathoracic metastasis could be identified. In the remainder, metastases were identified in the liver, adrenals, kidney and bone in about 25% of cases. In a study of 30 patients with adenocarcinoma dying within 30 days of surgery, 43% had extrathoracic metastasis at autopsy. In contrast large cell tumours and squamous carcinomas are more likely to remain restricted to the lung and disseminate fairly late.

In a 30 day postoperative autopsy study, 14% of patients subjected to curative surgery had evidence of extrathoracic metastasis at autopsy. Large cell tumours and adenocarcinomas tend to metastasize to the adrenals, liver, central nervous system and bone marrow. In addition, large cell tumours at autopsy metastasized to the mucosa and submucosa of the small bowel (Mattrews *et al.*, 1983). General malaise, fatigue and weight loss are usually present if specifically asked for. Patients with unexplained weight loss of more than a few kilograms are more likely to be inoperable and have distant metastases. It is estimated that 3–10% of all lung cancer patients develop clinically evident paraneoplastic syndromes. These syndromes are more frequent with small cell lung cancer (SCLC); however, they are also seen in the NSCLC variants. The most common syndrome is hypercalcaemia which is often associated with squamous cell cancer and is caused by a parathormone-like polypeptide. Cushing's syndrome caused by increased secretion of adrenocorticotrophic hormone, diabetes insipidus caused by inappropriate secretion of antidiuretic hormone and, less frequently, a variety of myopathies and neuropathies are seen. Clubbing of the fingers and hypertrophic pulmonary osteoarthropathy are also seen.

41.5 DIAGNOSIS

Whilst the clinical and radiographic features may suggest the diagnosis of lung cancer, every effort should be made to establish a tissue diagnosis prior to treatment. Sputum cytology is more likely to prove positive in patients with larger and more central tumours.

It is valuable to obtain repeated specimens as the positive results increase from 40% with one specimen to 85% after four good samples. Whilst the specificity as to cell type is reliable for squamous cancers, it is less so for other variants of NSCLC (Oswald and Hinsen, 1971).

Fibre-optic bronchoscopy is a valuable staging investigation (see below) and will often provide histological material, especially in central tumours.

Fine needle aspiration biopsy has a high yield for peripheral tumours, but unless such patients are inoperable, tissue diagnosis may be deferred until operation, saving the patient the distress and complications of this procedure, and avoiding the management problems resulting from a negative biopsy which the patient may wrongly interpret as excluding a diagnosis of lung cancer. In patients one suspects to be incurable by dint of mediastinal spread or distant metastases, it is useful, if safe and convenient, to biopsy such sites – by mediastinoscopy for nodes in the superior mediastinum or Fine Needle Aspiration Biopsy (FNAB) of the secondary deposit, hence at once obtaining tissue diagnosis and establishing the extent of disease beyond doubt.

41.6   TREATMENT

The appropriate treatment for an individual patient will depend upon their fitness and the extent or stage of their disease. The formal assessment of fitness will be considered later. The staging process is a stepwise series of tests to identify those patients who remain eligible for curative treatment. Once the disease has been shown to be too extensive for cure there is no purpose in proceeding with further staging tests.

As surgery is the only reliable prospect for cure in lung cancer, staging is considered as part of the preoperative assessment and there is no benefit in the investigation of patients who are demonstrably unfit for operation. An exception might be the occasional patient who, whilst fit enough for surgery, elects to undergo radiotherapy. Unfortunately the great majority of patients are inoperable, and hence incurable at presentation, and for most, evaluation need not proceed to the elaborate tests described in the later steps of the staging process. A flow diagram of pretreatment assessment is shown in Figure 41.2.

41.7   PREOPERATIVE EVALUATION AND STAGING

The preoperative evaluation of patients with lung cancer seeks to ensure that the patient and their tumour are both suitable for surgical treatment.

Patient suitability is an assessment of perioperative risks and postoperative morbidity, based on physical and psychological fitness.

In the history, general fitness should be assessed, and enquiries made into past medical history and medication.

As smoking is a common risk factor for lung cancer and cardiovascular disease, many of the patients in this age group will have overt or covert cardiovascular disease. Measurement of blood pressure and an ECG should be routine. If there is a known history of ischaemic heart disease, a cardiological assessment is necessary and a stress ECG should be considered. Clearly, however, if one is contemplating pulmonary resection an assessment of lung function is critical. Whilst one gains valuable information from the patient's lifestyle and exercise capacity, routine lung function testing should include simple spirometry, measuring forced vital capacity (FVC), forced expiratory volume in 1 second (FEV_1) and the ratio of FEV_1/FVC. The level of lung function necessary for pulmonary resection will depend upon the

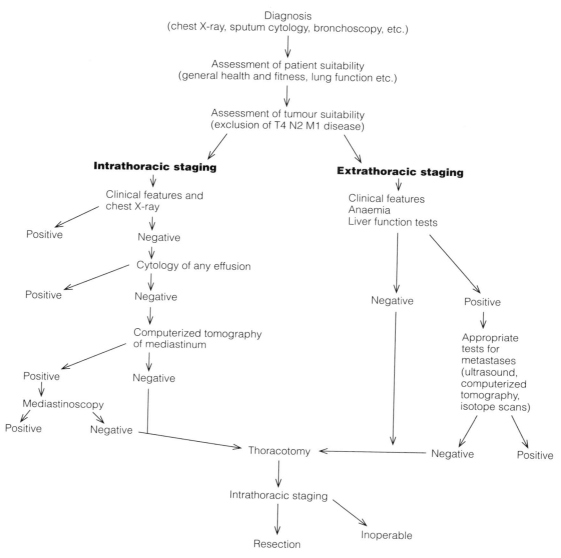

Figure 41.2   Flow diagram to show the steps in preoperative evaluation of a patient with lung cancer.

extent of the proposed resection and the function of the lung tissue to be removed. As a general guide, however, pneumonectomy is feasible if the FEV_1 exceeds 1.5 litres and the FEV_1/FVC ratio is greater than 50%. As lung function falls below these figures, perioperative problems increase. Lung resection is still possible if lung function tests are suboptimal.

Those patients will benefit from preoperative inpatient treatment to improve lung function by physiotherapy, clearance of sputum and treatment of chest infection. In borderline cases, a split-lung technetium perfusion lung scan can be used to predict postoperative pulmonary function. The predicted postoperative FEV_1 is equal to the measured preoperative FEV_1 divided by the percentage of perfusion to the remaining lung. A predicted postoperative FEV_1 > 800 ml has been associated with an operative mortality of approximately 15% in high risk patients whose preoperative FEV_1 was below 2 litres (Mohr and Jett, 1988).

Tumour suitability entails the determination of tumour stage. The most widely used staging system is the TNM system adopted by the American Joint Committee for Cancer Staging and End Results Reporting first published in 1979 and modified in 1986 (Mountain, 1986) (Table 41.1). Increasing numerical subscripts of the T stage indicate progressively more advanced tumours and similarly advancing numerical subscripts in the N category denote more proximal nodal metastases within the thorax and supraclavicular fossa. For example, a 5 cm peripheral cancer without evidence of invasion to surrounding structures and with no nodal and distant metastases would be designated $T_2N_0M_0$ and a tumour invading the chest wall with hilar node metastases but no distant spread would be $T_3N_1N_0$. It should be possible to construct a TNM stage for a patient at the start of the evaluation. However, it is inevitable that this will evolve and become more accurate as the assessment proceeds.

For the purpose of discussion it is easier to consider the staging process as having an intrathoracic and extrathoracic component. In practice these two components and assessment of fitness proceed concurrently.

The updated recommendations for the minimal preoperative staging for NSCLC by the International Association for the Study of Lung Cancer (1993) are given in steps I, II and III, and provide useful and internationally recognized guidelines.

41.7.1 INTRATHORACIC STAGING

A detailed history and examination should seek out those features which suggest extensive mediastinal involvement such as dysphagia, hoarseness or superior vena cava obstruction. The neck should be carefully palpated in all patients by an experienced clinician. Much information may be gained from the chest radiograph.

The T stage may be detected from the chest radiograph, assessing the size of the peripheral tumours, invasion of the chest wall with rib erosion or the presence of an effusion. If an effusion is found it should be aspirated, as positive histology will indicate T_4 disease. Mediastinal involvement may be evident on chest radiograph with enlarged mediastinal glands, N_2 or N_3 states or elevation of the hemidiaphragm indicative of phrenic nerve paresis.

Bronchoscopy is important to obtain diagnosis and also allows some staging assessment of centrally located tumours. Fibre-optic bronchoscopy is often carried out by physicians. If at the initial bronchoscopic examination, the extent of the tumour is close to the limits of resectability, the surgeon will wish to repeat this procedure using the rigid bronchoscope and assessing the proximal extent of the tumour. If this is carried out with mediastinoscopy or immediately prior to thoracotomy the need for an additional general anaesthetic is obviated. Most surgeons in any case undertake their own bronchoscopic evaluation prior to surgery to detect anatomical variants and some technical aspects may be highlighted which can affect the options for resection (Le Roux, 1962). In addition, it may be possible to assess the involvement of subcarinal and paratracheal lymph nodes by transbronchoscopic fine needle aspiration of these, therefore avoiding mediastinoscopy (Wang *et al.*, 1983).

If at this stage the tumour is still suitable for resection, more accurate assessment of the mediastinum is required.

41.7.2 CT SCANNING

In recent years, CT scanning of the mediastinum has become widely used in the pre-

Table 41.1 The revised TNM staging classification for lung cancer (from Mountain, 1986)

Primary tumour (T)

TX	Tumour proved by presence of malignant cells in bronchopulmonary secretions but not visualized roentgenographically or bronchoscopically, or any tumour that cannot be assessed, as in re-treatment staging.
T0	No evidence of primary tumour.
Tis	Carcinoma-*in-situ*
T1	A tumour that is ≤ 3 cm in greatest dimension, surrounded by lung or visceral pleura, and without evidence of invasion proximal to a lobar bronchus at bronchoscopy*
T2	A tumour > 3 cm in greatest dimension, or a tumour of any size that either invades the visceral pleura or has associated atelectasis or obstructive pneumonitis that extends to hilar region. At bronchoscopy, proximal extent of demonstrable tumour must be within a lobar bronchus or at least 2 cm distal to carina. Any associated atelectasis or obstructive pneumonitis must involve less than an entire lung
T3	A tumour of any size with direct extension into the chest wall (including superior sulcus tumours), diaphragm or mediastinal pleura or pericardium without involving the heart, great vessels, trachea, oesophagus or vertebral bodies; or a tumour in the main bronchus within 2 cm of carina without involving it
T4	A tumour of any size with invasion of the mediastinum or involving the heart, great vessels, trachea, oesophagus, vertebral bodies, or carina; or with the presence of malignant pleural effusion+

Nodal involvement (N)

N0	No demonstrable metastatic involvement of regional lymph nodes
N1	Metastatic involvement of lymph nodes in peribronchial or ipsilateral hilar region, or both, including direct extension
N2	Metastatic involvement of ipsilateral mediastinal lymph nodes and subcarinal lymph nodes
N3	Metastatic involvement of contralateral mediastinal lymph nodes, contralateral hilar lymph nodes, or ipsilateral or contralateral scalene or supraclavicular lymph nodes

Distant metastatic involvement (M)

M0	No (known) distant metastatic lesion
M1	Distant metastatic involvement present; specify site(s)

Stage grouping, 1986 (current)

Occult carcinoma	TX	N0	M0
Stage 0	Tis	Carcinoma-*in-situ*	
Stage I	T1	N0	M0
	T2	N0	M0
Stage II	T1	N1	M0
	T2	N1	M0
Stage IIIA	T3	N0	M0
	T3	N1	M0
	T1–3	N2	M0
Stage IIIB	Any T	N3	M0
	T4	Any N	M0
Stage IV	Any T	Any N	M1

* The uncommon superficial tumour of any size with its invasive component limited to the bronchial wall which may extend proximal to the main bronchus is classified as T1.

+ Most pleural effusions associated with lung cancer are due to tumour. There are, however, some few patients in whom cytopathological examination of pleural fluid (on more than one specimen) is negative for tumour, the fluid is non-bloody and is not an exudate. In such cases where these elements and clinical judgement dictate that the effusion is not related to the tumour, the patient should be staged T1, T2 or T3, excluding effusion as a staging element.

operative evaluation of patients with lung cancer. CT scanning will detect lymph nodes larger than 0.5 cm in diameter. This is facilitated with contrast enhancement of the vascular structures. The reported results of the use of CT scanners in NSCLC is shown in Table 41.2.

There is no definite pattern but it appears that as the size criteria used to determine abnormal lymph nodes increases, the sensitivity

Table 41.2 The three steps involved in the staging protocol

Investigation	Patient group	Confirmatory tests
STEP I		
Clinical history to include weight loss and performance status	All patients	As appropriate
Clinical examination	All patients	As appropriate
Chest radiographs PA		
Lateral	All patients	Aspiration of effusion (considered +ve if cytology malignant)
Blood tests Hb Alk. phos. Transaminase LDH Serum calcium	All patients	As per Step II

If still thought suitable for curative therapy proceed to Step II

STEP II		
Bronchoscopy	All patients with central tumours or those in whom central extension is suspected	The features or proximal, extrinsic compression are unreliable and require further evaluation of the mediastinum by CT and/or mediastinal exploration
Bone scan	High risk group*	Skeletal X-rays +/− CT/MRI of bone if dubious +ve result
CT chest and upper abdomen (to lower pole of kidneys, with i.v. contrast enhancement of mediastinal vessels)	All patients if available	Dubious findings confirmed (not necessarily histological)
Liver ultrasound	High risk group* if CT of abdomen not available	
Brain assessment by CT and MRI	Advisable in high risk groups	

If still thought suitable for curative treatment proceed to Step III

Table 41.2 Cont'd

STEP III

a. Bronchoscopy if not previously undertaken

b. Thoracoscopy or video assisted
   thoracoscopy

c. Mediastinal exploration
   - it is recommended that this is
     performed preoperatively by
       - transcarinal aspiration
       - cervical mediastinoscopy

       - additional evaluation of the
         subaortic fossa by left
         anterior mediastinotomy
   - this *must* be performed intraoperatively

       - palpation insufficient
       - careful and extensive
         mediastinal disection
       - separate labelling as per
         Naruke or ATS of excised
         nodes for subsequent histological
         examination (only N1 nodes on
         resection specimen)
       - re-evaluation of T stage

All patients	
If pleural effusion present, cytology −ve but clinical suspicion remains	
Patients in whom CT suggests mediastinal invasion or if CT shows nodes > 1.0 cm	
The above groups with tumours of the left upper lobe and left main bronchus	
All patients, including those whose mediastinum has been assessed preoperatively	

PROCEED WITH RESECTION

Postscript: The Group considered other tests which may be of value but made no recommendations as these tests are not universally available or acceptable and require validation.

*Patients having those non-specific features identified by Hooper *et al.* 1987:

- Unexplained anaemia (HB < 11G%).
- Unexplained weight loss (> 8 lb (3 kg) in 6/12).
- Abnormal alkaline phosphatase, or serum calcium or transaminase.

will fall whilst specificity will improve (Goldstraw, 1986). It is generally accepted that lymph nodes smaller than 1.5 cm in diameter are unlikely to be metastatic. If, therefore, a CT scan of the mediastinum is normal, mediastinal exploration may be omitted and the surgeon can proceed directly to a thoracotomy. However, abnormal mediastinal nodes require further evaluation by mediastinoscopy and, if need be, by left anterior mediastinotomy. The CT scan may also suggest mediastinal invasion by the primary tumour but this also requires confirmation by mediastinoscopy.

41.7.3 MEDIASTINOSCOPY

Cervical mediastinoscopy is an endoscopic evaluation of the superior mediastinal lymph nodes, under general anaesthesia through a short transverse cervical incision, midway between the thyroid cartilage and the suprasternal notch. Dissecting inferiorly into the mediastinum within the pretracheal fascia, lymph nodes on both sides of the trachea and at the main carina are inspected and biopsied. These glands are those most commonly involved by tumours and have a critical impact on the chances of surgical resection

Table 41.3 CT assessment of mediastinal node metastases using 3rd and 4th generation scanners

Nos.	Sensitivity (%)	Specificity (%)	Size criteria for abnormality
42	94	62	0.5–0.6
22	80	76	Any seen
35	86	76	> 1 cm
48	95	68	> 1 cm
42	72	83	> 1 cm
49	95	64	100 mm^2
56	82	100	> 1.5 cm
49	88	94	> 1.5 cm
94	74	80	> 1.5 cm
94	100	100	> 2 cm

and cure (Mannam *et al.*, 1993). Lymph node mapping carried out by Naruke *et al.* (1978) demonstrated that prognosis was significantly affected by involvement of subcarinal lymph nodes, whereas this was not affected if the superior mediastinal, paratracheal, tracheobronchial, pretracheal and the subaortic and para-aortic lymph nodes were involved (Table 41.3).

Mediastinoscopy is important in identifying the presence of N_2 disease preoperatively, as these patients have reduced prospects for resection and long term survival (Goldstraw, 1992). However, tumours of the left upper lobe invading the mediastinum or those which have reached the left main bronchus may invade mediastinal structures or involve nodes which are beyond the reach of the mediastinoscopy. These cannot be assessed by mediastinoscopy and thorough evaluation by left anterior mediastinotomy is necessary (Bowen *et al.*, 1978). Similarly, glands below the carina may be involved by tumours of the lower lobe which cannot be assessed by mediastinoscopy and require assessment by thoracotomy. Mediastinoscopy in experienced hands will reduce the number of 'open and close' thoracotomies and those patients having incomplete resections, whilst ensuring that patients are not inappropriately denied a chance of cure by inaccurate radiographic features suggesting inoperability.

41.7.4 EXTRATHORACIC STAGING

The purpose of this staging is to identify patients with distant metastases. Once again, a careful clinical history and examination can often elicit features of metastases without proceeding to further investigations. Unexplained weight loss (> 3 kg in 6 months), bone pain, personality changes, lymphadenopathy and irregular hepatomegaly suggest the presence of metastases. Simple blood tests including measurement of haemoglobin, alkaline phosphatase, calcium and lactate dehydrogenase are carried out in the early stages of preoperative evaluation. If any abnormalities are detected, further search for metastases using isotope bone scan, ultrasound or CT scanning is indicated. Bone scans provide a valuable assessment of the skeleton, but have a high false-positive yield which are often due to old trauma or degenerative conditions. Skeletal radiographs are useful in confirming or refuting such dubious positive findings. The problem of an isolated hot spot in the absence of other metastases may be resolved by local CT scanning of the bone and/or percutaneous bone biopsy. CT scanning of the brain and abdomen has superseded other investigations and is now widely used as a single test to search for metastases in the brain, liver, adrenals, kidneys and abdominal lymph nodes. In a study of 114 consecutive patients with lung cancer, routine CT of the abdomen and brain before surgery showed that 15 patients (13%) had extrathoracic deposits, although only three of the extrathoracic deposits were isolated metastases (Grant *et al.*, 1988). The presence of an isolated adrenal lesion poses a special difficulty. The prevalence of adrenal metastases detected by CT at presentation in patients with bronchogenic carcinoma ranges from 12% to 32%. In contrast, individual benign adrenal adenomas are found in 0.6% of subjects with non-malignant disease and these are commoner still in the patients with lung cancer. This underlines the importance of differentiating between a benign adrenal adenoma, adrenal hyperplasia and metastatic lesions, especially when the lesion is the only contraindication to surgery. If the CT appearances of the adrenals suggest a metastatic lesion or are equivocal, fine needle aspiration should be performed (Gillams *et al.*, 1992), but often the radiologist can be confident that an enlargement of the adrenal gland is due to benign disease.

41.7.5   INTRAOPERATIVE STAGING

Thoracotomy is now regarded as the final investigation prior to resection. This entails a detailed evaluation to:

1. Obtain histological diagnosis if earlier investigations have failed to do so.
2. Check the T and N stage determined in the earlier stages of evaluation.
3. Decide if complete resection is possible.
4. Decide if such a resection is justified, and if so,
5. Decide upon the extent of the resection.

As part of such intrathoracic staging, routine mediastinal node dissection is performed. All excised nodes from each nodal station are separately labelled according to Naruke's chart (Naruke *et al.*, 1978) and sent for histology.

Despite careful preoperative evaluation we have found 'unexpected N_2 disease' in 26% of our patients at thoracotomy. In this group 85% underwent complete resection with a survival rate of 20.1% at 5 years (Mannam *et al.*, 1993). Furthermore, data from clinical TNM staging (cTN) versus postsurgical pathological TNM staging (pTN) emphasizes the inaccuracy of even careful preoperative staging. In one study it was shown that cTN correlated with pTN in only 46% of cases; whilst cTN was downstaged in 9% of cases it was upstaged in 45% (Fernando and Goldstraw, 1990).

Incomplete resection carries no survival advantage and, therefore, resection is only performed if complete removal of the tumour and involved lymph nodes is feasible. With thorough preoperative evaluation resection is justifiable in 95% of patients undergoing thoracotomy (Goldstraw, 1988).

41.8   PROGNOSTIC FACTORS

The extent of the disease defined by TNM classification and complete resection are thought to be the most important prognostic factors. The prognosis in patients with NSCLC remains very poor, with an overall 5 year survival of approximately 15%. The staging system is used to provide prognostic information. Five year survivals after surgical resection in stages I and II disease are reported to be as high as 70% and 50% respectively (Martini, 1990). Asymptomatic patients or fully mobile symptomatic patients tend to have a better prognosis than the severely symptomatic, non-compliant patients who are reluctant to have surgery. Other significant prognostic factors are reported to be normal lactate dehydrogenase and calcium levels, and a single metastatic site (Albain *et al.*, 1991).

41.9   CURRENT MANAGEMENT

It is generally agreed that in patients with NSCLC surgical resection offers the only chance for cure. However, complete resection is only feasible in patients with stage I, stage II and selected patients with stage IIIa disease. Radiotherapy and chemotherapy are also used in the management of NSCLC. When deciding to use any of these modalities, the risk–benefit ratio in the care of these patients should be considered.

41.9.1 SURGERY

The results of surgical treatment for stage I and II disease are very good and surgery is established management for this group of patients. As far as the surgeon is concerned, stage IIIa disease is a heterogeneous group, subsets of which benefit from resection.

The outcome in highly selected subgroups of stage IIIa disease ($T_3 N_0$) is similar to stage I and stage II disease (Table 41.4). T_3 comprises tumours invading the chest wall, the diaphragm, the mediastinal pleura, the pericardium and tumours within 2 cm from the carina. For each feature designating T_3 status there is enormous variability in its impact on resection; pericardial invasion may entail resection of a fringe of this structure or wide excision with sacrifice of the phrenic nerve and the need for pericardial replacement and diaphragmatic plication.

N_2 disease is a heterogeneous group of patients with varied potential for surgery and prognosis. N_2 disease which evaded detection despite a detailed preoperative assessment by chest radiography, CT scanning, bronchoscopy and mediastinoscopy only to be discovered at thoracotomy seems to have the best prognosis. This 'unexpected N_2 disease' is present in up to 26% of patients undergoing thoracotomy (Mannam *et al.*, 1993). Whenever present, complete mediastinal lymph node dissection is warranted and when feasible 5 year survival of nearly 20% has been achieved (Naruke *et al.*, 1971). Mediastinoscopic findings of N_2 disease is an adverse factor probably influencing survival. These patients have little prospect of complete resection and the small prospects of cure are outweighed by the mortality and morbidity of pulmonary resection.

As for the types of lung resection, it is now generally agreed that there is no survival advantage in undertaking resections greater than that required to remove the tumour and its involved lymph nodes. In 60% of patients resection can be accomplished by lobectomy or bilobectomy, in 35% by pneumonectomy and in the rest by segmentectomy or sleeve resection. Sleeve resection is used to conserve functioning lung tissue when tumours extend into the junction of the upper lobe bronchus with the main and intermediate bronchus. A sleeve of main and distal bronchus with the upper lobe bronchus attached is resected. The cut ends of the main and intermediate bronchus on the right and the main and the lower lobe bronchus on the left are anastomosed.

The results of surgery for advanced stage disease, stage IIIb and stage IV disease are generally poor and do not justify 'open and close' thoracotomies or incomplete resections (Table 41.5). 'Open and close' thoracotomy is associated with 1.5–4.6% mortality (Bowen *et al.*, 1978) and incomplete resection confers no survival advantage.

Pulmonary resection is certain to have an impact on the quality of life. The risk of death following pulmonary resection is influenced by the extent of resection, and the fitness of the patients. The reported mortality rate for lobectomy is 2–3% and for pneumonectomy 6–7% (Roxburgh *et al.*, 1991). The risk for

Table 41.4 Surgical treatment of NSCLC: results of resection (from Mountain, 1986)

Stage	Nos.	5 year survival (%)
$T_1 N_0$	429	69
$T_2 N_0$	436	59
$T_1 N_1$	67	54
$T_2 N_1$	250	40

Table 41.5 Results of surgery in advanced stage NSCLC in reported series.

Stage	5 year survival (%)
$T_3 N_0$	22–50
$T_3 N_1$	8–33
$T_3 N_2$	0–13.5
T_4	8.2–42
N_2	15–30
N_3	0
M_1	7.5

older patients is only slightly higher. Pulmonary resection is associated with loss of lung function; following lobectomy this is often not noticeable. Following pneumonectomy there is usually a 30% reduction in spirometry which in most patients affects life style. Early postoperative pain is now satisfactorily controlled by using a variety of techniques; cryoablation of intercostal nerves, epidural analgesia, opiate infusions and a cocktail of oral analgesia. However, approximately 5% of patients suffer from severe and chronic post-thoracotomy pain. Although it is important to assess quality of life in patients undergoing pulmonary resection, this is only likely to influence decisions regarding surgery in borderline cases when one is considering surgery or high risk cases or patients with advanced disease.

41.9.2 RADIOTHERAPY

The majority of patients with NSCLC will receive thoracic irradiation at some time during the course of their illness. This may be radical radiotherapy in patients with limited disease who are technically or medically inoperable or who choose not to have surgery. Alternatively, radiotherapy has a well defined role as a palliative treatment for advanced, symptomatic disease in those not considered suitable for surgery or for radical radiotherapy.

Most patients with stages I and II disease and some with stage IIIa are suitable for radical therapy, although tumours which lie close to the spinal cord are difficult to treat in this way as the maximum tolerated dose is limited by normal tissue. Patients with severe chronic lung disease and poor lung function should be assessed as carefully prior to a course of radical radiotherapy as they are before surgery, as postradiation fibrosis may result in unacceptable morbidity. Radiotherapy has been given in the pre- and postoperative setting but more commonly is used as a sole treatment or in combination with chemotherapy.

(a)　Preoperative radiotherapy

There have been several non-randomized studies of preoperative radiotherapy suggesting a benefit but two randomized studies in the 1970s showed no survival advantage using doses of 40–50 Gy over 4–6 weeks in the preoperative period (Shields, 1972; Warram and A Collaborative Study, 1975). In the first study (Shields, 1972) there was recognizable tumour in 100% of the resected specimens from the surgery only group but in 75% of the radiotherapy and surgery group. This was not translated into a survival benefit and in addition, postoperative complications were more common in the group receiving radiotherapy. Even with today's sophisticated staging techniques, preoperative radiotherapy has no proven role in the routine treatment of NSCLC.

One area where local control is of paramount importance is in the management of Pancoast's tumours. Symptoms arise from invasion of nerves and chest wall and the disease may remain localized for years before metastases become apparent. Paulson advocates preoperative radiotherapy to a dose of 30 Gy in ten fractions over 12 days followed by radical resection (Paulson, 1979). Pancoast's tumours which are inoperable are taken to a radical dose of 60 Gy in order to prevent progression and severe local symptoms.

(b) Postoperative radiotherapy

Retrospective studies have suggested a benefit for postoperative radiotherapy but two randomized studies in the 1980s showed no survival advantage to a dose of 50–60 Gy to the mediastinum given over 5–6 weeks (Van Houtte *et al.*, 1980; Weisenburger and The Lung Cancer Study Group, 1986). In both studies the rate of local recurrence was lower in the group receiving radiotherapy but there was no survival advantage. In the trial by the Lung Cancer Study Group (Van Houtte *et al.*, 1980), 21 of 108 patients allocated to the surgery only arm had their first site of relapse within the ipsilateral lung or mediastinum compared to 1 of 102 patients receiving radiotherapy and surgery. However, 75% of all relapses were at distant sites suggesting that metastatic disease dominates the clinical picture. There is therefore no role for routine postoperative radiotherapy although some centres will deliver treatment to the mediastinum and bronchial stump in cases where surgical resection has been incomplete.

(c) Radiotherapy alone

Technically or medically inoperable disease confined to the lung or regional lymph nodes is potentially curable with radiotherapy alone. However, in the majority of cases, the disease recurs locally or with distant metastases and the results have improved little over the past 20 years.

A retrospective study of 152 patients with medically inoperable, T_1–T_3 node negative, non-metastatic disease reported 2 year and 5 year actuarial survival rates of 40% and 10% respectively with disease free survival rates of 31% and 15% (Dosoretz *et al.*, 1992). When divided by tumour stage it can be seen that T_1 tumours are more readily controlled than T_2 or T_3 with 55% disease free survival at 2 years

for patients with T_1 disease compared to 20% and 25% for T_2 and T_3 disease respectively. Patients with T_1 tumours are also less likely to show a local component of relapse after radiotherapy than those with T_2 and T_3 tumours. The dose given to the primary and mediastinum in 142 of the 152 patients was 50–70 Gy. In the retrospective analysis a dose response was seen in disease free survival but not in overall survival.

The RTOG set up a trial in 1973 to examine the question of dose in the radical treatment of unresectable NSCLC (Perez *et al.*, 1986). Patients were randomized between three dose levels of 40, 50 or 60 Gy delivered to the primary and mediastinum and a dose response was reported in the rates of complete response (CR) and partial response (PR) of the tumour. A 3 year survival rate of 23% was seen in those achieving CR compared to 10% and 5% respectively for patients with a PR or no response. There was no overall survival advantage for higher dose when comparing all patients treated. A dose response was seen in the rate of intrathoracic failure, with the 60 Gy arm showing a local failure rate at 3 years of 33% compared with 42% and 52% for the 50 Gy and 40 Gy arms respectively. Adenocarcinoma and large cell carcinoma were more likely to relapse with distant metastases than squamous cell carcinoma which had a higher rate of local relapse.

The importance of local control in NSCLC has been stressed by Saunders who made a careful autopsy study of patients who had taken part in a randomized, controlled trial of misonidazole and radical radiotherapy (Saunders *et al.*, 1984). Sixty-one of the 62 patients in the trial had died by the time of the report and autopsies were performed on 42 with very careful examination of the primary and likely metastatic sites. The conclusion was that local tumour was present in 95% and was the primary cause of death in 72% whereas distant metastases were present in 61% and the primary cause of death in only 15%. This suggests that if local control could be improved, there may be a survival benefit and this has in turn led to attempts to improve the efficacy of radical radiotherapy.

There are studies to increase the dose delivered to the primary and mediastinum without exceeding the tolerance of the normal tissues. These include boosting the primary site with brachytherapy or using complex computer controlled planning techniques to produce a tightly defined volume which can be treated using conventional fractionation. An alternative approach is the use of continuous hyperfractionated accelerated radiotherapy (CHART). A multicentre study is comparing such a regimen with a conventional treatment arm of 60 Gy given in 30 fractions over 6 weeks. The CHART arm of the study involves treating the primary tumour and mediastinum in two phases to a total dose of 54 Gy in 36 fractions over 12 days. Three fractions of 1.5 Gy are given each day and the radiotherapy continues without a break over the weekend. The rationale for the CHART regimen stems from radiobiological data, suggesting that the potential doubling time of human NSCLC cells may be as short as 5 days compared to an observed tumour doubling time of 30–120 days (Dische and Saunders, 1990). Theoretically, the effects of repopulation may be avoided if the course of radiotherapy is shortened (accelerated). This requires the use of several fractions per day with time between the fractions for repair of sublethal damage and in the current trial of CHART a gap of 6 hours is allowed (Saunders *et al.*, 1991).

Dose and fractionation remain controversial issues, but, in general, patients who are considered suitable should receive a dose of 64 Gy in 32 fractions over $6^1/_2$ weeks or a biologically equivalent regimen such as 50 Gy in 20 fractions over 4 weeks. The constraints imposed by normal tissue tolerance usually require that the dose is delivered in two phases, the first encompassing the primary tumour, ipsilateral hilum and the mediastinum to a dose of 40–44 Gy and the second, the known sites of disease to 64 Gy.

(d)   Toxicity

The main acute side-effect is oesophagitis which develops towards the end of the treatment period and usually continues for approximately 2 weeks after the radiotherapy is complete. In most cases this responds adequately to measures such as local anaesthetic preparations but in severe cases patients may need opioid analgesia and nasogastric feeding to avoid dehydration and malnutrition. Many patients will experience tiredness and possibly nausea or a change in taste during the treatment but these are rarely severe. Radiation pneumonitis is classified as an acute reaction but usually develops some 6–12 weeks after completion of the radiotherapy. Radiographic changes of pneumonitis are common and coincide with the treatment volume but are usually asymptomatic and resolve without specific intervention. If the radiation fields are large, symptoms and signs of pneumonitis may develop which include cough, shortness of breath and sometimes fever accompanied by fine crackles in the lungs. Therapy is usually with corticosteroids.

Late toxicity is largely pulmonary fibrosis with a gradual loss of lung volume, compliance and diffusion capacity. This manifests as progressive shortness of breath and once the process is underway there is no useful therapy to prevent further deterioration. The only way to avoid radiation fibrosis is to plan treatment volumes to exclude normal lung wherever possible. Radiation myelitis is a risk with radical radiotherapy to the chest but with modern planning it should not arise if cord doses are carefully monitored.

(e)   Palliative radiotherapy

Radiotherapy is a very effective method of palliating local symptoms arising from a carcinoma of the bronchus. Symptomatic improvement in up to 80% of patients has been seen in the management of cough, haemoptysis, chest pain and superior vena cava obstruction. Radiotherapy is also invaluable in the treatment of bony or cerebral metastases.

Traditionally, palliation has been achieved with doses of 30–45 Gy over 2–3 weeks to the primary tumour and mediastinum. The current trend is to move towards shorter regimens in order to reduce the number of visits a sick patient has to make to the hospital and the heavy workload in many departments. Two randomized studies have reported the use of shorter regimens in the palliation of bronchial carcinoma (MRC Lung Cancer Working Party, 1991, 1992). The first compared 30 Gy in 10 fractions over 2 weeks with 17 Gy in 2 fractions 7 days apart in 369 patients with advanced disease (MRC Lung Cancer Working Party, 1991). Toxicity was similar and there was no significant difference in the degree of palliation or in its duration, both arms achieving palliation with a median duration of more than 50% of the patient's remaining lifespan. The second study looked only at patients of poor performance status and found that in those with a WHO performance status of 2 or more, a single fraction of 10 Gy provided equivalent palliation when compared to 17 Gy in 2 fractions and there was significantly less oesophagitis with a single fraction.

An MRC trial of 39 Gy in 13 fractions compared to 17 Gy in 2 fractions in patients with a good performance status is now collecting follow-up data.

41.9.3 CHEMOTHERAPY

Even with effective local control the rates of relapse with distant metastases in NSCLC are disappointingly high. This has led to attempts to improve long term survival rates using systemic chemotherapy agents. Initial studies were non-randomized using single agents or combination chemotherapy in patients with advanced disease. More recently, randomized trials have been carried out

looking for the most effective combination regimen and exploring the possibilities of integrating radiotherapy, surgery and chemotherapy in the radical treatment of NSCLC.

Unlike SCLC, response rates to single agent chemotherapy are low, ranging from 8–10% for 5FU, CCNU, methotrexate and etoposide to 20–27% for mitomycin-C, vinblastine and ifosfamide (Earl and Cullen, 1992). Combinations of drugs with differing side-effect profiles have produced increased response rates in patients with advanced local disease or in those with distant metastases. The most effective combinations have been those including mitomycin-C, ifosfamide and cisplatin with CR rates of approximately 10% and overall response rates of 40–50%. Other commonly used regimens contain ifosfamide, etoposide and cisplatin or etoposide and cisplatin alone with overall response rates of 40–50% and 33% respectively.

There are few randomized trials which assess the benefit of combination chemotherapy in either palliative or radical treatment of NSCLC. It is important in all new studies of systemic therapy given either alone or in combination with other modalities to assess carefully the effect of treatment on quality of life. This is particularly relevant in the case of patients with advanced disease, as the life expectancy of the majority is short and the toxicity of chemotherapy may be considerable.

Two recent meta-analyses have been carried out of all published, randomized trials of combination chemotherapy versus best supportive care in patients with unresectable NSCLC (Grilli *et al.*, 1993; Souquet *et al.*, 1993). Seven randomized trials were included, covering the years 1980–88. All trials randomized patients with advanced disease (stages IIIb–IV) but there were marked differences between the protocols and individual patient data were not available. On meta-analysis, a statistically significant survival advantage was seen in favour of the chemotherapy arm at 3 and 6 months, with a 20% reduction in risk of death, but this had decreased to a non-significant difference of 7% by 1 year of follow-up. The conclusion reached was that combination chemotherapy should be used as a palliative measure in patients with unresectable NSCLC. However, the survival benefit as assessed in this way is small and no data on quality of life were available. Further large, randomized studies are required to assess the impact of combination chemotherapy on overall survival, disease free survival and quality of life before it can be recommended as a standard treatment.

41.9.4   COMBINED MODALITY TREATMENT

The results of radiotherapy alone are disappointing in all but small (T_1 and T_2) node negative tumours. Distant relapse is common and improvements in both local control and systemic therapy are probably required to produce a prolongation of survival. NSCLC is only moderately radiosensitive and the dose delivered is limited by normal tissue tolerance. Therefore, combined modality therapy is an attractive option. It is not, however, a straightforward matter of choosing chemotherapy and radiotherapy regimens which are known to be active and delivering them in an arbitrarily derived sequence, since chemotherapy and radiotherapy interact in a variety of ways both to increase and decrease the therapeutic ratio (Steel and Pekcham, 1979).

(a)   Sequential chemotherapy and radiotherapy

Many studies over the last decade have addressed the question of sequential combined modality chemotherapy and radiotherapy in patients with advanced disease but most have been non-randomized phase II

studies. Several trials have failed to report a survival benefit although response rates range from 27% to 82%. The studies showing a benefit have used chemotherapy before radiotherapy except for one (Trovo *et al.*, 1982) which used a regimen of 45 Gy in 3 weeks followed by cyclophosphamide, adriamycin, methotrexate and procarbazine every 3 weeks for 6 courses. The overall response rate in 64 patients with stage III disease was 62% with a median survival of 12.7 months and acceptable toxicity with no treatment related deaths. Dillman reported a significant survival benefit for combined therapy in a randomized trial using an induction course of vinblastine and cisplatin prior to radiotherapy compared to radiotherapy alone (Dillman *et al.*, 1990). In 155 patients with stage III disease and good performance status, there was an increase in median survival of 4 months and a doubling of 3 year survival to 23%. Interestingly, there was no difference between the groups in frequency of local or distant relapse. Hospitalization for severe infection was more common in the chemotherapy group as was severe weight loss but there were no treatment related deaths. One of the apparently more successful regimens was reported by Wils *et al.* (1984) who used cisplatin, etoposide and adriamycin as two courses given before and four after radical radiotherapy in a randomized trial accruing 33 patients. A dose of 60 Gy was used for the radiotherapy-only control arm and 50 Gy for the combined therapy arm. The overall response rate for combined modality therapy was 82% with 18% CRs compared to a PR rate of 54% with no CRs in the control arm. There was also an improvement in median survival from 5 months in the control arm to 11 months in the arm receiving both chemotherapy and radiotherapy.

There is still a lack of consensus on the most effective way of delivering sequential chemoradiotherapy. In view of this and the problems of balancing side-effects against potential benefits, all patients considered for combined modality therapy should be entered into clinical trials whenever possible and these should include a quality of life assessment.

(b) Concurrent chemotherapy and radiotherapy

The concurrent use of chemotherapy and radiotherapy is complicated by the risk of synergistic toxicity and many regimens have been modified with reduced doses of drugs to take this into account. Several studies have reported response rates of 64–92% achieved without life-threatening toxicity but with doses of drugs lower than if the chemotherapy had been given alone. In studies which have used unmodified doses there has been marked toxicity particularly in the radiation fields with severe pneumonitis and oesophagitis. Umsawasdi reported 10 patients treated with radiotherapy, 50 Gy in 5 weeks and concurrent full dose CT with cyclophosphamide, adriamycin and cisplatin given at 3 weekly intervals (Umsawasdi *et al.*, 1985). Four patients developed severe oesophagitis of whom three developed late complications of either a stricture or fistula.

The early studies were non-randomized phase II studies of single agents such as 5-FU, mitomycin-C, vincristine and actinomycin-D. There have since been randomized trials of bleomycin, hydroxyurea and levamisole, all of which have failed to show a survival advantage in locally advanced NSCLC (Belani, 1993). Much of the recent attention has been directed at cisplatin because of its known properties as a radiation sensitizer. Of four randomized trials comparing single agent cisplatin and radiotherapy to radiotherapy alone, three have shown no significant difference in response rate or median survival (Trovo *et al.*, 1992; Belani,1993). The one trial to show a significant benefit compared weekly cisplatin with daily cisplatin given during radiotherapy and a control arm receiving radiotherapy alone. Only the daily treatment arm showed a survival benefit

Cisplatin-containing combination chemotherapy given concurrently with radiotherapy has been evaluated in several phase II studies. Response rates of up to 58–86% have been seen with a median survival of 7–17 months (Belani, 1993). Drugs used with cisplatin have included etoposide, 5-FU, vinblastine, methotrexate and mitomycin-C with doses of radiotherapy of 50–60 Gy. These trials are not randomized between chemotherapy and no chemotherapy or between different chemotherapy regimens. There is a need for properly conducted, randomized, controlled trials to evaluate the optimum schedule, combination and dose of chemotherapy and radiotherapy in concurrent treatment.

(c) Pre- and postoperative chemoradiotherapy

Most studies of chemotherapy given as an adjuvant treatment after surgery have shown no benefit. Two studies by the Lung Cancer Study Group have demonstrated an improvement in the disease free survival of patients given adjuvant therapy, with a combination of cyclophosphamide, adriamycin and cisplatin (CAP) (Holmes *et al.*, 1986; Lad and Lung Cancer Study Group, 1988). The first study compared CAP combination chemotherapy after complete surgical resection in stages II and III adenocarcinoma and large cell carcinoma with immunotherapy consisting of intrapleural BCG and levamisole. A significant benefit was seen in favour of the chemotherapy arm in terms of disease free survival. The second randomized patients with incompletely resected, locally advanced disease to receive adjuvant therapy with CAP and radiotherapy, or radiotherapy alone. In the group receiving both chemotherapy and radiotherapy there was a significant benefit in terms of disease free survival. A further study by the same Lung Cancer Study Group has looked at the role of adjuvant chemotherapy in the treatment of completely resected stage I NSCLC and has found no benefit. This question is still unanswered but adjuvant chemotherapy is not standard practice and should still be confined to clinical trials.

Neoadjuvant chemoradiotherapy has been used preoperatively in stages IIIA and IIIB NSCLC in the hope of improving resectability. Results vary, but in some series up to 20% of patients have a complete pathological response and 40–80% are able to undergo complete resection. The toxicity of such treatment is considerable and a recent report of 13 patients who underwent resection of locally advanced NSCLC after neoadjuvant chemoradiotherapy warns against its over-enthusiastic use (Fowler *et al.*, 1993). Lobectomy was performed safely in six patients with no undue morbidity whereas three of seven patients undergoing pneumonectomy died, two of adult respiratory distress syndrome and one of a bronchopleural fistula. However, an interim report of a trial by the South West Oncology Group (Rusch *et al.*, 1993) has reported only 6% mortality in 63 patients who had thoracotomy after neoadjuvant chemotherapy and concurrent radiotherapy. In this study 2 year survival figures are encouraging with 40% survival for stages IIIA and IIIB, and this forms a basis for phase III clinical trials in the future.

In summary, the use of combination chemotherapy is expanding as trials begin to show encouraging results. It may be given alone as a palliative treatment in advanced disease or in combination with radiotherapy and surgery in the radical treatment of patients with locally advanced disease. Few randomized trials have been reported and of those which have, few have addressed quality of life issues. Further results are awaited before combination chemotherapy becomes a standard treatment in NSCLC.

REFERENCES

Albain, K.S., Crowley, J.J., LeBlanc, N., and Liningston, R.B. (1991) Survival determinants in extensive-stage non-small cell lung cancer: the Southwest Oncology Group experience. *Journal of Clinical Oncology*, **9,** 1618–26.

Belani, C.P. (1993) Multimodality management of regionally advanced non-small-cell lung cancer. *Seminars in Oncology*, **20**, 302–14.

Bowen, T.E., Zajtchuk, R., Green, D.C. and Brott W.H. (1978) Value of anterior mediastinotomy in bronchogenic carcinoma of the left upper lobe. *Journal of Thoracic and Cardiovascular Surgery*, **76**, 269–71.

Dillman, R.O., Seagren, S.L., Propert, K.J. *et al.* (1990) A randomized trial of induction chemotherapy plus high-dose radiation versus radiation alone in stage III non-small-cell lung cancer. *New England Journal of Medicine*, **323**, 940–5.

Dische, S. and Saunders, M.I. (1990) The rationale for continuous, hyperfractionated, accelerated radiotherapy (CHART). *International Journal of Radiation Oncology, Biology, Physics*, **19**, 1317–20.

Doll, R. and Peto, R. (1976) Mortality in relation to smoking: 20 years observations on male British doctors. *British Medical Journal*, **2**, 1525.

Dosoretz, D.E., Katin, M.J., Blitzer, P.H. *et al.* (1992) Radiation therapy in the management of medically inoperable carcinoma of the lung: results and implications for future treatment strategies. *International Journal of Radiation Oncology, Biology, Physics*, **24**, 3–9.

Earl, H.M. and Cullen, M.H. (1992) Non-small cell carcinoma of the lung, in *Combined Radiotherapy and Chemotherapy in Clinical Oncology*, (ed. A. Horwich), Edward Arnold, London, pp. 102–12.

Fernando, H.C. and Goldstraw, P. (1990) The accuracy of clinical evaluative introthoracic staging in lung cancer as assessed by post-surgical pathologic staging. *Cancer*, **65**, 2503–6.

Fontana, R.S., Sanderson, D.R., Woolner L.B. *et al.* (1986) Lung cancer screening: the Mayo program. *Journal of Occupational Medicine*, **28**, 746–50.

Fowler, W.C., Langer, C.J., Curran, W.J. and Keller, S.M. (1993) Postoperative complications after combined neoadjuvant treatment of lung cancer. *Annals of Thoracic Surgery*, **55**, 986–9.

Geddes, D.M. (1979) The natural history of lung cancer. A review based on notes of tumour growth. *British Journal of Diseases of the Chest*, **73**, 1–17.

Gillams, A., Roberts, C.M., Shaw, P., *et al.* (1992) The value of CT scanning and percutaneous fine needle aspiration of adrenal masses in biopsy-proven lung cancer. *Clinical Radiology,* **46**, 19–22.

Goldstraw, P. (1986) CT scanning in the pre-operative assessment of non-small cell lung cancer, in *Lung Cancer: basic and clinical Aspects,* (ed. H.H. Hansen), Martinus Nijhoff, Boston, pp. 183–99.

Goldstraw, P. (1988) Mediastinal exploration by mediastinoscopy and mediastinotomy. *British Journal of Diseases of the Chest,* **82**, 111–20.

Goldstraw, P. (1992) The practice of cardiothoracic surgeons in the perioperative staging of non-small cell lung cancer. Editorial.*Thorax,* **47**, 1–2.

Goldstraw, P., Rocmans, P., Ball, D. *et al.* (1994) Pre-treatment minimal staging for non-small cell lung cancer: an updated consensus report. *Lung Cancer,* in press.

Grant, D., Edwards, D. and Goldstraw, P. (1988) Computed tomography of the brain, chest and abdomen in the preoperative assessment of non-small cell lung cancer. *Thorax,* **43**, 883–6.

Grilli, R., Oxman, A.D. and Julian, J.A. (1993) Chemotherapy for advanced non-small-cell lung cancer: How much benefit is enough? *Journal of Clinical Oncology,* **11**, 1866–72.

Holmes, E.C., Gail, M. and for Lung Cancer Study Group (1986) Surgical adjuvant therapy for stage II and stage III adenocarcinoma and large-cell undifferentiated carcinoma. *Journal of Clinical Oncology,* **4**, 710–15.

Hooper, R.G., Beechler, C.R. and Johnson, M.C. (1978) Radioisotope scanning in the initial staging of bronchogenic carcinoma. *American Review of Respiratory Disease,* **118**, 279–86.

Imperial Cancer Research Fund and Cancer Research Campaign (1991) *Passive Smoking. A health hazard.* Imperial Cancer Research.

Lad, T. and Lung Cancer Study Group (1988) The benefit of adjuvant treatment for resected local advanced non-small cell lung cancer. *Journal of Clinical Oncology,* **6**, 9–17.

Le Roux, B.T. (1962) The bronchial anatomy of the left upper lobe. *Journal of Thoracic and Cardiovascular Surgery,* **44**, 216–24.

Mannam, G., Goldstraw, P., Kaplan, D. and Michail, P. (1993) Surgical management of non-small cell lung cancer with N_2 disease. Presented at the Annual Meeting of the American Association for Thoracic Surgery, Chicago.

Martini, N. (1990) Surgical treatment of non-small cell lung cancer by stage. *Seminars in Surgical Oncology,* **6**, 248–54.

Mathews, M.J., Mackay, B. and Lukerman, J. (1983) The pathology of non-small cell carcinomas of the lung. *Seminars in Oncology,* **10**, 34–55.

Melamed, M.R., Flehinger, B.J., Zamar, M.B. *et al.* (1984) Screening for early lung cancer. Results of the Memorial Sloan-Kettering study in New York. *Chest,* **86**, 44–53.

Mohr, D.N. and Jett, J.R. (1988) Preoperative evaluation of pulmonary risk factors. *Journal of General Internal Medicine,* **3**, 277–87.

Mountain, C.F. (1986) A new international staging system for lung cancer. *Chest,* **89**, (suppl), 2258–335.

MRC Lung Cancer Working Party (1991) Inoperable non-small-cell lung cancer (NSCLC): a Medical Research Council randomised trial of palliative radiotherapy with two fractions or ten fractions. *British Journal of Cancer,* **63**, 265–70.

MRC Lung Cancer Working Party (1992) A Medical Research Council (MRC) randomised trial of palliative radiotherapy with two fractions or a single fraction in patients with inoperable non-small-cell lung cancer (NSCLC) and poor performance status. *British Journal of Cancer,* **65**, 934–41.

Naruke, T., Suemasu, K. and Ishikawa, S. (1978) Lymph node mapping and curability at various levels of metastasis in resected lung cancer. *Journal of Thoracic and Cardiovascular Surgery,* **76**, 832–9.

Naruke, T. Goya, T., Tsuchikya, R. and Svenasu, K. (1988) The importance of surgery to non-small cell carcinoma of lung with mediastinal lymph node metastasis. *American Thoracic Surgery,* **46**, 603–10.

OPCS Monitor (1990) *Cigarette Smoking 1972 to 1988.* OPCS, London.

Oswald, N.C. and Hinsen, K.F.W. (1971) The diagnosis of primary lung cancer with special reference to sputum cytology.*Thorax,***26**, 623.

Paulson, D. L. (1979) Carcinoma in the superior pulmonary sulcus. *Annals of Thoracic Surgery,* **28**, 3–4.

Perez, C.A., Bauer, M., Edelstein, S. *et al.* (1986) Impact of tumour control on survival in carcinoma of the lung treated with irradiation. *International Journal of Radiation Oncology, Biology, Physics,* **12**, 539–47.

Roxburgh, J.C., Thompson, J.C. and Goldstraw, P. (1991) Hospital mortality and long-term survival after pulmonary resection in the elderly. *Annals of Thoracic Surgery,* **51**, 800–3.

Rusch, V.W. Albain, K.S., Crowley, J.J. *et al.* (1993) Surgical resection of stage IIIA and stage IIIB non-small-cell lung cancer after concurrent induction chemoradiotherapy: a Southwest Oncology Group Trial. *Journal of Thoracic Cardiovascular Surgery*, **105**, 97–104.

Saunders, M.I., Bennett, M.H., Dische, S. and Anderson, P.J. (1984) Primary tumour control after radiotherapy for carcinoma of the bronchus. *International Journal of Radiation Oncology, Biology, Physics*, **10**, 499–501.

Saunders, M.I., Dische, S., Grosch, E.J. *et al.* (1991) Experience with CHART. *International Journal of Radiation Oncology, Biology, Physics*, **21**, 871–8.

Shields, T.W. (1972) Preoperative radiation therapy in the treatment of bronchial carcinoma. *Cancer* **30**, 1388–93.

Selikoff, I., Hamad, E. and Chug, J. (1960) Asbestos exposure, smoking and neoplasia. *Journal of the American Medical Association*, **204**, 106.

Souquet, P.J., Chauvin, F., Boissel, J.P. *et al.* (1993) Polychemotherapy in advanced non small cell lung cancer: a meta-analysis. *Lancet*, **342**, 19–21.

Steel, G.G. and Pekcham, M.J. (1979) Exploitable mechanisms in combined radiotherapy-chemotherapy: the concept of additivity. *International Journal of Radiation Oncology, Biology, Physics*, **5**, 85–91.

Trovo, M.G., Minatel, E., Franchin, G. *et al.* (1992) Radiotherapy versus radiotherapy enhanced by cisplatin in stage III non-small cell lung cancer. *International Journal of Radiation Oncology, Biology, Physics*, **24**, 11–15.

Trovo, M.G., Tirelli, U., De Paoli, A. *et al.* (1982) Combined radiotherapy and chemotherapy with cyclophosphamide, adriamycin, methotrexate, procarbazine (CAMP) in 64 consecutive patients with epidermoid bronchogenic carcinoma, limited disease: a prospective study. *International Journal of Radiation Oncology, Biology, Physics*, **8**, 1051–4.

Umsawasdi, T., Valdivieso, M., Barkley, T.J. *et al.* (1985) Esophageal complications from combined chemoradiotherapy (Cyclophosphamide + Adriamycin + Cisplatin + XRT) in the treatment of non-small cell lung cancer. *International Journal of Radiation Oncology, Biology, Physics*, **11**, 511–19.

Van Houtte, P., Rocmans, P., Smets, P. *et al.* (1980) Postoperative radiation therapy in lung cancer: a controlled trial after resection of curative design. *International Journal of Radiation Oncology, Biology, Physics*, **6**, 983–6.

Wang K.P., Brower R. and Japonik E.F. (1983) Flexible transbronchial needle aspiration for staging bronchogenic carcinomas. *Chest*, **84**, 571–6.

Warram, J. and A Collaborative Study (1975) Preoperative irradiation of cancer of the lung: final report of a Therapeutic Trial. *Cancer*, **36**, 914–25.

Weisenburger, T.H. and The Lung Cancer Study Group (1986) Effects of postoperative mediastinal radiation on completely resected stage II and stage III epidermoid cancer of the lung. *New England Journal of Medicine*, **315**, 1377–81.

Weisenburger, T.H., Gail, M. and The Lung Cancer Study Group (1986) Effects of postoperative mediastinal irradiation on completely resected stage II and stage III epidermoid cancer of the lung. *New England Journal of Medicine*, **315**, 1377–81.

Wils, J.A., Utama, I., Naus, A. and Verschueren, T.A. (1984) Phase II randomized trial of radiotherapy alone vs the sequential use of chemotherapy and radiotherapy in stage III non-small cell lung cancer. Phase II trial of chemotherapy alone in stage IV non-small cell lung cancer. *European Journal of Cancer*, **20**, 911–14.

Wu, A.H., Henderson, B.E., Thomas, D.C. and Mack, T.M. (1986) Secular trends in histologic types of lung cancer. *Journal of the National Cancer Institute*, **77**, 53–6.

COLORECTAL CANCER

Simon M. Allan and Nigel P.M. Sacks

42.1 INTRODUCTION

Cancers of the colon and rectum are very common and are treated in a range of hospitals from district general level to specialist research oncology centres such as at the Royal Marsden. It will be only by basic scientific and clinical research that the static survival figures of the past 20 years will be improved. Current popular reliance on surgical resection alone as the sole method of treatment is now antiquated and should be superseded by multimodality therapy regimens in selected cases. Similarly it is time to abandon the nihilistic approach to patients with metastatic disease as systemic chemotherapy and, in selected cases, hepatic resection are of proven benefit. This chapter outlines the incidence, aetiology, pathology, investigation and management of cancer of the colon and rectum and presents the Royal Marsden's clinical approach to treatment for these cancers.

42.2 INCIDENCE AND AETIOLOGY

Carcinomas of the colon and rectum are currently the second most common cause of deaths due to malignant disease. In the UK, there are approximately 27 000 new cases every year and 19 000 attributable deaths per annum from the disease (Office of Population Censuses and Surveys, 1990; Cancer Research Campaign, 1991). Prognosis is determined by the extent of disease spread at presentation and overall only 40% of patients presenting

with colorectal cancer are estimated to be likely to survive for 5 years; approximately one-third of cases are found on presentation to have liver metastases. Slight improvements is survival have been matched by an increasing disease incidence so that death rates have changed little over the past 40 years.

Colorectal tumours can occur at any age (mean age at diagnosis is 62 years) and there is a noticeable increase in frequency directly related to increasing age from middle age onwards. There is an equal sex distribution for rectal cancers and a minimal preponderance for females with colonic malignancies, although this may well be a reflection of the increasing elderly female population in both the UK and USA.

The aetiology of the disease in the general population appears unclear, with dietary factors championed by some after the landmark observational study by Burkitt (1971) noting reduced colorectal cancer rates in those African populations who have a high dietary fibre intake. The relevance of bile salts and fats, anaerobic colonic micro-organisms and their potential production of mutagens and possible carcinogen production by certain cooking procedures have all been studied as causes in the aetiology of large bowel malignancy without any definite conclusions (reviewed by Weisburger, 1991). In the case of dietary fibre, the African incidence figures are quoted in support of the protective nature of a diet rich in vegetable fibre but the similar low incidence of colorectal cancer in other African tribes to those of the Masai tribe with a diet almost entirely reliant on products derived directly from bovine sources and low in dietary fibre are difficult to explain. Nevertheless, recent overview analysis of 13 case control studies concluded that the intake of dietary fibre rich foods is inversely related to the relative risk of developing colorectal cancers (Howe *et al.*, 1992)

Whilst factors that predispose to increased risk of colorectal cancer have been identified (Table 42.1), less than 10% of the population falls into this subgroup. There does appear to be a familial tendency to colorectal malignancy. A direct inheritance with the Lynch familial syndromes of carcinoma of the colon and a genetic determinant has been identified in some cases with a point mutation on the 5q chromosome postulated as leading to the development of colorectal malignancy. Familial polyposis coli (FAP) and the associated Gardner's syndrome show an invariable risk of malignancy if left untreated, with the presence of the mendelian dominant FAP gene on chromosome 5 (Bodmer *et al.*, 1987) resulting in the development of malignancy from the multiple polyps by early adult life if allowed to follow the natural disease course (Lynch *et al.*, 1991). These patients can be cured by prophylactic proctocolectomy with terminal ileostomy or ileo-anal anastomosis with a pouch.

The fate of sporadic polyps in the large bowel is less clear and is dependent on the histology of the polyp. Metaplastic polyps of the colon are very common and do not represent a premalignant condition. Hamartomatous polyps such as found in those with Peutz–Jeghers syndrome have a reported prevalence of 17% for malignant potential over the age of 30 years (Iwama *et al.*, 1990). True adenomatous polyps, however, do show a malignant potential (Morson, 1974). It is now generally accepted that the majority of adenomas will follow the so-called adenoma–carcinoma sequence eventually becoming overtly malignant and modern molecular biology techniques have confirmed this (Fearon and Vogelstein, 1990). Large bowel adenomas can therefore be considered as truly premalignant conditions and four factors have been shown to be important in the development of carcinomas from preexistent adenomas:

1. Polyp size (malignancy risk if adenoma < 1 cm is 1.3%, 1–2 cm is 9.5% and 46% if size is > 2 cm).

Table 42.1   Risk factors for colorectal cancer

Low risk
Age < 50 years, no family history of early onset colorectal cancer or personal history of high risk diseases

Average risk
Age > 50 years and asymptomatic

High risk
Personal history
   Adenoma or large bowel cancer
   Inflammatory bowel disease
   Breast, ovarian or endometrial cancer
   Previous ureterosigmoidostomy
Family history
   Sporadic colorectal cancer or adenoma
   Familial adenomatous polyposis and associated syndromes
   Hereditary non-polyposis colorectal cancer syndromes

Table 42.2 Risk of further adenomatous polyps and cancer

	Adenoma			Cancer		
Years of observation	5	10	15	5	10	15
Single adenoma (%)	14	33	50	1	2	5
Multiple adenoma (%)	33	67	80	7	12	12

2. Histological type of polyp (St Mark's series showed a malignancy rate of 5% for tubulous adenomas, 22% for tubulovillous and 40% with villous adenomas) (Lockhart-Mummery *et al.*, 1976) (Table 42.2).
3. The degree of epithelial dysplasia shown by the polyp.
4. The absolute number of polyps present throughout the large intestine.

In view of these factors, the presence of any large bowel polyp other than metaplastic polyps must be considered as a predisposing factor for colorectal malignancy and should be removed.

Longstanding inflammatory conditions (ulcerative colitis and Crohn's disease) predispose to colorectal malignancy with up to a 30-fold increase in relative risk. The degree of dysplastic mucosal change, position of the disease, age of onset and extent of the inflammatory condition directly relate to the relative risk of developing colorectal cancer (Kirsner and Shorter, 1988). Patients who have pancolitis for 10 years or more have a greater than 35% chance of developing colorectal malignancy (Ekbom *et al.*, 1990).

The situation in patients suffering from AIDS is unclear; figures from the western areas with high HIV prevalence show that there is an increased risk of malignancy in this population of particularly rectal and anal cancers. However, whether this is in part caused by the altered immunity, repeated local trauma or associated sexually transmitted disease such as viral papillomatosis requires further study (Lorenz *et al.*, 1991).

42.3 PATHOLOGY

The most common malignant tumour of the large intestine is an adenocarcinoma. Carcinoid tumours, lymphomas, sarcomas and malignant melanomas can all occur but are all rare tumours and account for less than 5% of all cases. Seventy per cent of colorectal tumours will be found in the rectosigmoid region, but recently there has been an increased incidence of right sided lesions (Cady *et al.*, 1974; Slater *et al.*, 1984). The rectum is approximately 15 cm long and for the purposes of description is divided into thirds; approximately 45% of all colorectal cancers arising here. The adenocarcinoma will usually have gross features of either an annular constricting ulcer or a polypoid fungating type growth, with the former more common on the left side and the latter in the right colon. Mucoid and undifferentiated tumours are less frequent and account for a further 10% of tumours. In the anal canal, squamous carcinoma accounts for 50% but basal cell and mucoepidermoid carcinomas are also found.

The spread of colorectal cancer is by the blood stream, lymphatics and direct local extension. Blood spread is predominantly to the liver and lungs with the liver being the main site for metastasis due to the portal venous drainage of the large bowel from above the midrectal line. Lymphatic spread follows the blood vessels and passes either upwards through the mesorectum to the para-aortic nodes or in the case of lower rectal and anal tumours, downwards following the blood supply from the perineal and inguinal areas.

Table 42.3   Modified Dukes' staging system for colorectal cancer

Stage	A	Tumour confined to wall of bowel
Stage	B1	Tumour invades muscularis propria but does not involve extramural tissues
Stage	B2	Tumour penetrates through muscularis propria to involve extramural tissues
Stage	C1	Metastases confined to regional lymph nodes
Stage	C2	Metastases present in nodes at mesenteric artery ligature (apical nodes)

There are now numerous pathological classifications of colorectal cancer but at the Royal Marsden, colorectal tumours are staged according to a modification of that first described by the St Mark's Hospital's first pathologist, Cuthbert Dukes (Dukes, 1932). Stage 'A' defined disease confined to the wall of the colon or rectum, 'B' extends through the wall into surrounding fat but with no involvement of the regional lymph nodes and stage 'C' represents involvement of the regional nodes with metastases (Table 42.3). More recent staging systems (Jass *et al.*, 1987) have included new prognostic classifications based on four survival related variables: the number of nodes involved by metastasis, the character of the invasive margin, peritumoural lymphocyte infiltration and the presence or absence of local spread. Despite these newer classifications, Dukes' original system of classification remains both universally recognized and applied.

42.4   PRESENTATION

The clinical manifestations of carcinoma of the colon and rectum are related to the position and extent of the tumour or the presence of systemic metastases. The most common symptom is a recent change in bowel habit; this may be constipation, diarrhoea or indeed the two symptoms alternating with each other. The diarrhoea may have a high mucus content in those rectal polypoid or mucoid tumours that excessively secrete mucus or it may be explosive, intermittent, foul smelling and watery in spurious diarrhoea when obstructed faeces liquidify and leak around the obstructing lesion. The second most common presenting symptom is that of bright rectal bleeding. The exact nature of the rectal blood is dependent on the tumour site and rate of bleeding and it may be frank fresh or altered blood, melaena or remain 'occult' presenting as an iron deficiency anaemia of uncertain cause. The recent onset of bright bleeding or iron deficiency anaemia in patients over the age of 40 should not be ascribed to haemorrhoids without appropriate investigation.

A tumour that is annular and constricting the bowel lumen may present with features of intestinal obstruction and this may be acute, chronic or acute on chronic in nature. The symptoms of the obstruction will be determined by the exact site of the tumour with an ileocaecal tumour presenting as a distal small bowel obstruction whereas a left sided colonic tumour presents with symptoms of colonic obstruction unless the ileocaecal valve is incompetent. Right sided colonic cancers due to their tendency to form proliferative tumours and the distensibility of the caecum often present with anaemia, anorexia, palpable mass and weight loss rather than the more typical obstructive symptoms found with left sided colonic tumours.

Less common presentations of a local nature include free perforation into the peritoneal cavity causing peritonitis, local perforation with the formation of a pericolic abscess or fistulation into surrounding organs such as the small intestine, bladder or vagina. Rarely the effects of metastases are the presenting feature and these may include jaundice, abdominal distension due to ascites or hepatomegaly.

42.5 SCREENING

Despite enormous interest in screening, there is no evidence from randomized control trials that population screening for colorectal cancer is effective in prevention and reducing mortality from the disease (Table 42.4). One of the main problems with the Nottingham trial of faecal occult blood screening was with patient compliance, where only 30% of patients fulfilled the screening protocols (Hardcastle, 1989). Whilst the results of occult blood testing methods have shown some merit, they are not widely employed due to their low positive predictive value and the failure to produce any detectable overall benefit when the extra 'cost' of investigating false positives are taken into consideration. The only currently accepted role for colorectal cancer screening is for surveillance of particular subgroups at especially high risk (Table 42.1). Such screening relies first on detecting occult faecal blood loss by testing for peroxidase activity of haemoglobin in faeces with reagent strips such as Haemoccult and secondly regular colonoscopic follow-up for patients shown to have had previous polyps. Trials of screening using tumour markers such as serum carcinoembryonic antigen levels have been undertaken with limited success. For high risk screening we need genetic markers to accurately predict the individual's risk and equally we also require methods to identify a population subset with particularly low risk of disease that would not require screening at all.

42.6 INVESTIGATIONS

Patients with suspected colorectal malignancy should be investigated to confirm the diagnosis and assess the extent of the disease. Rectal examination and rigid sigmoidoscopy are part of the initial examination of all colorectal patients on presentation. Many of the signs suggestive of malignancy such as bleeding and mucus secretion may be seen and biopsied on sigmoidoscopy which in fact only reliably reveals to the rectosigmoid junction. By using either a flexible fibre-optic sigmoidoscope or preferably a colonoscope the rest of the colon can be directly visualized. At the Royal Marsden, we routinely perform colonoscopy for patients presenting with bright rectal bleeding rather than flexible sigmoidoscopy because it allows both diagnosis, biopsy and therapeutic intervention, although colonoscopy can be replaced by double contrast barium enema when change in bowel habit is the main symptom or facilities for colonoscopy do not exist. The barium enema will usually reveal the tumour as a constant filling defect in the bowel lumen or as a stricture in the bowel contour ('apple core defect'). The problem of differentiating a malignant stricture from that caused by diverticular disease on barium enema examination is not always easy and is why direct

Table 42.4 Screening programmes for colorectal cancer using faecal occult blood tests

Study	Patient number	Compliance (%)	Positive tests (%)	Predictive value (%)
Gilbertsen *et al.*, 1979	23 000	72	2.3	11.3
Winawer *et al.*, 1980	13 127	74	2.5	17.7
Winchester *et al.*, 1980	54 101	26	4.4	4.7
Sontag *et al.*, 1983	13 522	22	4.6	10.3
Cummings *et al.*, 1986	58 943	20	2.3	6.4
Hardcastle *et al.*, 1989	10 253	39	2.4	13.7

Predictive value = number of true positive results/total number of positive results obtained.

visualization by fibre-optic scope is preferred by us so that a definite diagnosis by biopsy can be achieved, thus making the need for a diagnostic laparotomy in the elective situation rare.

On making a diagnosis of colorectal cancer, we perform a full blood count, ESR, liver function tests, urea and electrolytes and a baseline carcinoembryonic antigen (CEA) assay. Liver function tests are a useful screening test for liver metastases although it requires over 65% of the liver to be affected by metastatic disease before significant changes will be noted. The CEA assay is a valuable baseline (in the 5% of patients with CEA positive tumours), especially if used to monitor response to chemotherapy or for surveillance to detect progressive or recurrent disease, and it is also of prognostic significance (Midiri *et al.*, 1983). Unless renal function tests are abnormal, we do not routinely perform radiological investigations of the renal tract. Preoperative colonoscopy or barium enema examination is essential as 5% of all patients have synchronous tumours.

In patients with rectal cancers, particularly for large ones, the extent of transmural penetration can be accurately assessed by an experienced surgeon. A useful adjunct is the use of intrarectal ultrasound as we find that this technique is not only easy to perform but also provides valuable information about tumour size, penetration and nodal involvement (Rifkin and Marks, 1985). Where there is demonstrable extrarectal disease, CT and more recently, MRI may have a role in providing further information about resectability of the tumour and the need for preoperative pelvic radiotherapy.

In all cases, preoperative or operative assessment of the liver is undertaken by ultrasound examination. CT, nuclear medicine scans and direct visualization at laparoscopy may all supplement assessment of the liver. Should liver resection be contemplated for isolated metastases, further assessment by arterial and venous phase angiography and CT portography are undertaken. It may also be necessary to include further radiological studies such as intravenous ureterography and pyelography and/or urethrocystoscopy to inspect the ureters, bladder and prostate for invasion by a locally advanced rectal tumour.

42.7   DIFFERENTIAL DIAGNOSIS

The differential diagnosis depends largely on the predominant presenting symptoms but diverticular disease, colitis (inflammatory or ischaemic) and infective diarrhoea can all produce a similar clinical picture. For this reason, biopsy to prove malignancy is preferable in colorectal disease prior to embarking on treatment. The differential diagnosis in the rectum includes benign conditions such as haemorrhoids and benign polyps, extension from neighbouring malignancies such as prostate or cervix, solitary rectal ulcer and infective causes. Clinical confusion is often caused by a loop of the sigmoid colon felt through the pouch of Douglas (although this often indicates sigmoid obstruction), the normal cervix and even faeces may be confused for a rectal or left iliac fossa mass.

42.8   MANAGEMENT

The mainstay of treatment for colorectal cancer is still surgical. This applies to both potentially curative cases and situations where effective palliation alone is sought. Adjuvant therapy in the form of radiotherapy and or chemotherapy is now being used by us far more often and our indications for adjuvant therapy are discussed in the next section.

42.8.1   SURGERY

Surgical treatment aims for cure but in certain circumstances only palliation from distressing symptoms can be achieved. The decision about the required surgical procedure to be undertaken can often only be decided at laparotomy as current staging procedures are usually less than adequate at complete assessment of tumour extent. Approximately 50% of patients operated on with curative intent survive cancer free at 5 years and this is directly related to stage: 90% for stage A, 70% for stage B and 30% for stage C (Dukes and Bussey, 1958; Rao *et al.*, 1981; McFarlane *et al.*, 1993). More than 80% of patients undergoing palliative resection or diversion are dead within 2 years.

The mode of presentation of the patient will also have significant impact on the management plans (Figure 42.1). There is a distinct difference in the surgical approach when one compares cases that present as an emergency with large bowel obstruction as opposed to those that present electively. Despite recent publications to the contrary (Dorudi *et al.*, 1990), many surgeons are reluctant to perform curative resection with primary anastomosis for emergency obstructed cases for fear of anastomotic failure and complications. The

question of operating on a faecally loaded colon is often given as the reason for defunctioning procedures followed by elective resection. We advocate that in all but the worst complicated cases of perforation and gross faecal contamination of the peritoneum, this conservative approach is outmoded and primary resection with anastomosis should be attempted since the overall mortality figures for this condition are independent of extent or duration of operation (Dorudi *et al.*, 1990). In the few cases unsuitable for this type of surgery, we still believe that simple defunctioning surgery is inadequate treatment as it leaves the primary tumour *in situ* and does not give a histological diagnosis. Such cases should be dealt with by a modified Hartmann's procedure, which entails resection of the tumour and mesentery, closure of the rectal stump and formation of a simple end colostomy as a drainage procedure. This should be followed wherever possible by a reversal procedure where the end colostomy

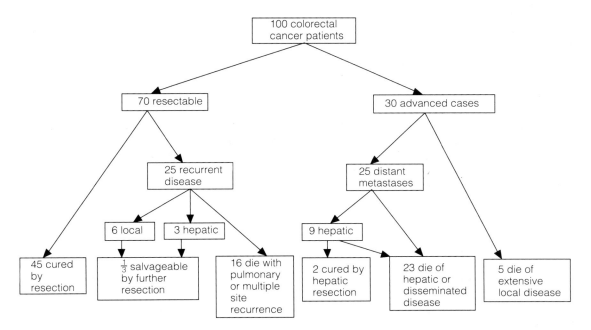

Figure 42.1 Patterns of failure in patients presenting with colorectal cancer.

and the closed rectal stump are rejoined, preferably within 6 months to avoid a potentially temporary stoma becoming permanent as for a variety of clinical reasons up to one-third of all cases never undergo reversal (Whiston *et al.*, 1993). This factor may well influence the operating surgeon to attempt primary anastomosis in those patients who are unlikely to survive a second major operation or in those patients for whom a colostomy would be an intolerable handicap such as the extremely arthritic or blind.

The need for elective preoperative bowel preparation is currently controversial. We favour bowel preparation by oral laxatives (Picolax) on the day before surgery together with oral fluids (intravenous for the elderly) 24 hours prior to operation, routine use of prophylactic antibiotics (cefuroxime and metronidazole) to cover the perioperative period starting with premedication and then for the 24 hours subsequent to surgery and in all cases heparin or heparinoid prophylaxis for deep venous thrombosis is employed.

Surgery of colorectal cancer is based on the following principles:

1. Colorectal cancer spreads to the regional nodes in a predictable pattern.
2. Survival after apparently curative resection is directly related to the stage of the disease.
3. Tumour related factors (but not size) influence long term survival (unlike other solid tumours such as breast) and thus more radical resection improves survival in selected cases.

The surgeon aims to excise the primary tumour including the regional lymph node areas, to obtain optimal local disease control with minimal morbidity and where possible to restore bowel continuity. The exact operation required for each cancer depends entirely on the position of the tumour within the colon and its local extent. At the time of laparotomy attention should be paid to tumour fixity and extent of spread; the presence or absence of enlarged nodes, peritoneal seedlings and liver metastases should be noted and biopsied if not removable. Doubtful areas of excision should also be biopsied. In general, right sided tumours, that is those in the caecum and ascending colon, should be treated by right hemicolectomy, with tumours in the transverse colon treated by extended right or left hemicolectomy. Carcinomas in the splenic flexure or the left side of the colon are both treated surgically by left hemicolectomy with full mobilization of the splenic flexure, although sigmoid colectomy may be performed for those tumours located within the upper and mid sigmoid area of the colon where palliation alone is intended. Provided the anastomosis is not performed under tension and has an adequate blood supply, there is no reason to compromise clearance in order to follow a named operation and sufficient colon should be excised to provide maximal regional nodal clearance. We advocate a single layer interrupted, seromuscular hand sewn anastomosis as the surgical technique of choice for all colonic operations.

The optimal operative management of rectal tumours depends on their position and size as well as the age of the patient. It is important to aim for complete tumour clearance whilst attempting to maintain bowel continuity and sphincter function without compromising the cancer operation. Recent studies of anastomotic and local recurrence have shown that a minimum margin of clearance from the tumour of 2 cm is required and that there is also need to adequately include the mesorectum in the resection so as to reduce the incidence of extrarectal pelvic recurrence which varies widely from 2% to 50% (Heald and Ryall, 1986; McFarlane *et al.*, 1993). The relative position of the tumour from the sphincters plays a vital part in planning the resection technique and wherever possible, limited by the clearance margins and the need to widely excise the mesorectum, the operation should attempt to preserve the anal sphincters and thus colonic continuity. For lower sigmoid or upper and mid rectal tumours anterior resection of the rectum is our operation of choice sewn by hand or in the case of the narrow pelvis with a stapled anastomosis. A lower third rectal cancer can also be dealt with by sphincter saving surgery and colo-anal anastomoses provided the sphincters are competent (rare in the elderly), which requires the anastomosis to be created outside the confines of the pelvis by eversion of the anal and colonic wall through the anal canal. Those lower rectal tumours where this is not possible require abdominoperineal excision of the rectum and end sigmoid colostomy.

In certain cases it becomes apparent that palliation alone is the likely outcome but even in these cases safe excision of the tumour remains our goal as it has been shown that better palliation is provided by removing the tumour mass. Since patients who are deemed suitable for palliative surgery are likely to have a short life expectancy, it is the surgeon's duty to try and ensure that only one operation will be required in this period and if possible the patient can maintain anal continence and optimal quality of life. Recently, laparoscopic tumour resection techniques have been proposed but the exact place of this technique in colorectal cancer patients needs examining and careful evaluation. In extremely old or frail patients, abdominoperineal excision can be avoided by palliative transanal resection or fulguration of lower rectal carcinomas; these procedures are repeatable often without a general anaesthetic.

The general improvements in anaesthetic care and postoperative intensive therapy have improved the corrected survival figures for both elective and emergency colorectal surgery.

42.8.2 RADIOTHERAPY

Radiotherapy has two prime objectives in colorectal cancer. First the prevention of local disease recurrence particularly in the pelvis for rectal tumours (which occurs in about one-third of all patients) and, secondly, to convert 'inoperable' locally advanced rectal tumours to resectability. In the case of adjuvant radiotherapy, this may be given either before or after surgical excision (Table 42.5). There is no detectable difference in the end result which ever order is chosen but it has been shown that preoperative radiotherapy may compromise the vascularity of the surgical anastomosis and makes case selection difficult; we thus prefer postoperative irradiation (40–50 Gy). When given to make a rectal cancer more easily resectable, we feel that providing 6 weeks are allowed to elapse from the completion of moderate dose (40–50 Gy) radiotherapy to the proposed date of surgery no significant adverse affects have been seen from preoperative radiotherapy; if worried one can protect the anastomosis by defunctioning loop colostomy or ileostomy.

Radiotherapy has little role in the management of colonic cancer because of toxicity to the organs surrounding such tumours but it may be used to treat the tumour bed when resection is incomplete or doubtful. Unresectable tumours are not usually suitable for radiotherapy unless bleeding is the predominant problem, as the radiation is likely to cause perforation of the bowel at the site of the disease or marked small bowel toxicity.

We consider that the management of Dukes' stage B rectal tumours should include postoperative radiotherapy to prevent local recurrence if there is direct tumour extension outside the wall (stage B2) or else within the setting of a clinical trial. Dukes' stage C rectal tumours also benefit from postoperative irradiation; the planning of such fields should include the anastomosis, presacral areas and pelvic sidewall as appropriate for the tumour position and extent as determined at surgery. This planning of fields of therapy will ensure that the most likely local recurrence sites are treated and close cooperation between the surgeon and radiotherapist are essential for optimum results.

Table 42.5   Rectal cancer: results of randomized pre- and postoperative radiotherapy trials

Study	Dose (cGy)	5 year survival (%)	
		Radiotherapy	Surgery
Preoperative low dose			
MRC	500	42	38
MRC	2000	40	38
MSKCC	2000	52	59
VASOG	3150	35	35
Stockholm	2500	45	45
Preoperative high dose			
EORTC	3000–4500	69	59
Postoperative radiation			
GITSG	4000–4800	45	51*
NSABP	4600–5100	40	31

Studies: MRC, Medical Research Council; MSKCC, Memorial Sloan Kettering Cancer Center; VASOG, Veterans Association Surgical Oncology Group; EORTC, European Organization & Research and Treatment of Cancer; GITSG, Gastrointestinal Tumour Study Group; NSABP, National Surgical Adjuvant Bowel Project.
*Addition of chemotherapy and radiotherapy increased survival to 60%
($P = 0.005$ surgery alone vs surgery + radiotherapy + chemotherapy)

The main symptom of recurrent rectal cancer following surgery is pain. Radiotherapy provides complete pain relief in approximately half of these patients and partial relief in up to two-thirds.

42.8.3   CHEMOTHERAPY

Chemotherapy for colorectal cancer can be used as an adjunct to surgery or to treat metastatic disease. The results of adjuvant combination chemotherapy for colorectal cancer are shown in Table 42.6; the chemotherapy can be given either alone or in conjunction with radiotherapy. Single agent chemotherapy with 5-fluorouracil (5-FU) has been widely used but with no significant impact on 5 year survival figures for case control matched and randomized series (Grage and Moss, 1981).

Table 42.6   Colorectal cancer: results of randomized adjuvant chemotherapy trials

Study	5 year survival (%)		
	Surgery	S + RT	S + RT + Chemo
Rectum			
GITSG	43	52	59*
NCCTG	–	47	58*
NSABP	43	41	53*
Colon			
GITSG	62	–	59–61
NSABP	59	–	67*
SWOG	52	–	59*

S + RT, Surgery plus radiotherapy; S + RT + Chemo, Surgery plus radiotherapy plus chemotherapy; NCCTG, National Colon Cancer Treatment Group; SWOG, South West Oncology Group; GITSG, Gastrointestinal Tumour Study Group; NSABP, National Surgical Adjuvant Bowel Project.
* Statistically significant compared to controls.

In view of the poor 5 year survival rates (20–50%) for patients with stage B2 and C colorectal cancer, adjuvant systemic therapy has been extensively evaluated over the last 20 years. Single agent 5-FU has not been shown in over 3000 patients to significantly improve disease free or overall survival so several studies aimed at assessing the value of combination chemotherapy have been carried out (reviewed by Kane, 1991). Only one, NSABP C-01, was able to demonstrate improved survival for chemotherapy (67% vs. 59%, $P = 0.05$). Once it became apparent that the regimen was leukaemogenic it was demonstrated that Me-CCNU could be eliminated from the regimen without loss of benefit (GITSG, 1992). More recently several randomized studies have suggested small survival benefits for stage C colorectal cancer patients given adjuvant 5-FU and the immunostimulant levamisole, although the underlying mechanisms of action remain unknown. The exact place of adjuvant radiotherapy and chemotherapy in colorectal cancer patients is currently under investigation in a large multicentred UK committee for clinical cancer research (UKCCCR) trial.

Metastatic colorectal cancer is almost, by definition, incurable. The only exceptions are those patients who achieve long term survival following resection of isolated liver or lung metastases. Therefore the aim of chemotherapy in metastatic disease is palliation of symptoms and prolongation of survival. Single agent 5-FU, which is the most active available agent for colorectal cancer, has been found to be disappointing when evaluated, with response rates of between 3% and 20% and no evidence of improved survival. This can be improved slightly by longer term infusional regimens. The activity of 5-FU can be increased by biochemical modulation with either folinic acid or methotrexate producing response rates of up to 45% (Kohne-Womper *et al.*, 1992). Our standard protocol for metastatic patients is folinic acid 20 mg/ m^2/day i.v. bolus and 5-FU 425 mg/ m^2/day

i.v. bolus, given on 5 consecutive days and repeated from day 29 to day 33 and thereafter repeated until no further response.

In the past physicians have been reluctant to treat patients with asymptomatic disease but two recent studies have shown that early chemotherapy in these patients is superior in terms of survival, duration of asymptomatic period and the time to disease progression by 6–11 months over primary expectancy (NGTATG, 1992; Scheithaeur *et al.*, 1993).

Locally delivered chemotherapy via portal vein or hepatic artery cannulations and infusions have been studied as a means of reducing treatment related toxicity yet still providing adequate treatment to the liver, which is the predominant site of colorectal metastases. Solitary or isolated liver metastases are best dealt with surgically but multiple deposits can be dealt with either by regional infusional techniques or systemic chemotherapy regimens.

42.8.4 LIVER METASTASES

The majority of patients with hepatic colorectal metastases have multiple deposits in both lobes of the liver which renders them surgically irresectable. These patients may derive benefit from various regimens of cytotoxic chemotherapy which can produce partial remissions in up to 50% of these cases (Arbuck, 1989) and approximately 25% of cases will have metastases that are surgically resectable with minimal morbidity and mortality (Iwatsuki *et al.*, 1986). It is exceptional for untreated patients with colorectal metastases to survive more than 3 years from the time of diagnosis. New techniques in liver resection such as ultrasonic aspirators have revolutionized the potential for treating patients with surgically resectable hepatic metastases. The first meta-analysis of series reporting hepatic colorectal metastases resection shows an actuarial 5 year survival of 33% (Hughes *et al.*, 1988). Providing there is no co-morbid or extrahepatic disease, three or fewer metastases are present and all the disease is resected with a margin of at least 1 cm, then the best option for these patients will be achieved (Steele and Ravikumar, 1989) by resection of their isolated liver metastases.

42.8.5   RECURRENT DISEASE AND FOLLOW-UP

The treatment of recurrent disease depends on its site and extent. For metastatic disease the only option is systemic chemotherapy. Patients with local recurrence of colonic or rectal cancer often benefit from further surgical resection and we advocate a second look laparotomy in cases shown to have localized disease on staging tests since there is a chance of being able to complete excision of disease discovered at laparotomy, even if the operation proves to be palliative. For example, an ileo-colonic bypass procedure can be performed as a palliative procedure which often alleviates obstructive symptoms even in advanced local disease. Rectal recurrence if at the site of the anastomosis of a low anterior resection or colo-anal resection can often be converted to an abdominoperineal resection. Localized pelvic side wall and presacral recurrences are harder to manage and attempted resection often causes profound morbidity. Further surgery and/or radiotherapy may provide palliation from distressing symptoms of pain or blood loss. Local surgical procedures such as repeated intrarectal resection may have a place in selected cases to provide palliation from distressing symptoms of recurrence such as tenesmus or bleeding. Decisions about the timing and extent of such treatments are difficult and are best done in close consultation between surgeon and oncologist.

All such problems of recurrence are easier to manage if discovered at an early stage and we advocate regular review by rectal examination, sigmoidoscopy with colonoscopy every 2–3 years; the place of CEA monitoring is currently the subject of an important large prospective randomized UKCCCR trial. The need to report symptomatology must be firmly established in the patient and regular clinic follow-up for examination is advocated 3 monthly initially before becoming twice yearly. Inspection of both the anastomosis and the remaining colonic mucosa are extremely important for detecting anastomotic recurrence and second primary tumours (which occur in 5–8% of cases).

42.9   FUTURE DIRECTIONS

The precise role of radiotherapy and adjuvant chemotherapy in both colon and rectal cancer needs to be established and proven in further well conducted large randomized clinical trials. The exact benefits in risk reduction need to be defined so that balancing the cost–benefit analysis becomes possible. Measures to assess not only quantity but also the quality of life of these patients must be studied as part of any therapeutic intervention. The need for novel active chemotherapeutic agents is apparent, as is the need to assess differing schedules of chemotherapy delivery.

Research into the genetics of colorectal cancer will be vital for both potential population screening and genetically mediated therapies. If high risk groups could be reliably detected, perhaps by genetic markers, then heightened surveillance and early intervention could possibly improve the outlook of colorectal cancers arising in such people immensely.

The role and extent of surgery in localized disease is established, but the exact place of laparoscopically assisted resection (if any) in the surgical treatment of colorectal cancer needs to be addressed urgently. The other main field of surgical research that remains in this area is investigating novel methods of dealing with isolated liver metastases. Laparoscopic or radiological approaches to the treatment of such metastases may be proven to be an advance over resection or for those with unresectable disease. The use of focused ultrasound or laser for hepatic resection tools is another exciting area of research aimed at improving the operative morbidity and mortality figures.

REFERENCES

Arbuck, S.G. (1989) Overview of clinical trials using 5FU and leucovorin for the treatment of colorectal cancer. *Cancer*, **63**, 1036–41.

Bodmer, W., Bailey, C., Bodmer, J. *et al.* (1987) Localisation of the gene for familial adenomatous polyposis on chromosome 5. *Nature*, **328**, 2–4.

Burkitt, D.P. (1971) Epidemiology of cancer of the colon and rectum. *Cancer*, **28**, 3–13.

Cady, B., Persson, A., Monson, D. *et al.* (1974) Changing patterns of colorectal cancer. *Cancer*, **33**, 433–6.

Cancer Research Campaign (1991) *Annual Report*, London.

Cummings, K., Michalek, A., Tidings, J. *et al.* (1986) Results of a public screening program for colorectal cancer. *New York State Journal of Medicine*, **86**, 68–72.

Dorudi, S., Wilson, N.M. and Heddle, R.M. (1990) Primary restorative colectomy in malignant left sided large bowel obstruction. *Annuals of Royal College of Surgery*, **72**, 393–5.

Dukes, C.E. (1932) The classification of cancer of the rectum. *Journal of Pathology and Bacteriology*, **35**, 323–32.

Dukes, C.E. and Bussey, H. (1958) The spread of rectal cancer and its effect on prognosis. *Cancer*, **12**, 309–20.

Ekbom, A., Helmick, C., Zack, M. *et al.* (1990) Ulcerative colitis and colorectal cancer. *New England Journal of Medicine*, **323**, 1228–33.

EORTC (1988) Preoperative radiotherapy as adjuvant therapy in rectal cancer. *Annals of Surgery*, **208**, 606–14.

Fearon, E.R. and Vogelstein, A. (1990) A genetic model for colorectal tumourgenesis. *Cell*, **61**, 759–67.

Gilbertsen, V.A., Williams, S., Schuman, L. *et al.* (1979) Colonoscopy in the detection of carcinoma of the intestine. *Surgery, Gynecology and Obstetrics*, **149**, 877–78.

GITSG (1986) Survival after postoperative combination therapy of rectal cancer. *New England Journal of Medicine*, **315**, 1294–5.

GITSG (1992) Radiation therapy and 5FU for the treatment of patients with carcinoma of the rectum. *Journal of Clinical Oncology*, **10**, 549–57.

Grage, T.B. and Moss S.E. (1981) Adjuvant chemotherapy in cancer of the colon and rectum. *Surgical Clinics of North America*, **61**, 1321–9.

Hardcastle, J.D., Thomas, W. Chainberlain J. *et al.* (1989) Randomised controlled trial of faecal occult blood screening for colorectal cancer. *Lancet*, **i**, 1160–1.

Heald, R. and Ryall, R. (1986) Recurrences and survival after total mesorectal excision for rectal cancer. *Lancet*, **i**, 1479–82.

Howe, G.R., Benito, E., Castelleto, R., Cornée, J. *et al.* (1992) Metanalysis of dietary fibre and colorectal cancer. *Journal of the National Cancer Institute*, **84**, 1887–96.

Hughes, K.S., Scheele, J. and Sugarbaker, P.H. (1989) Surgery for colorectal cancer metastatic to the liver. Optimising the results of treatment. *Surgical Clinics of North America*, **69**, 339–59.

Iwama, T. (1990) The Peutz Jeghers syndrome and malignant tumours, in *Hereditary Colorectal Cancer*, Springer Verlag, Berlin, pp. 337–42.

Iwatsuki, S., Esquivel, C.O., Gordon, R.D. and Starzl, T.E. *et al.* Liver resection for metastatic colorectal cancer. *Surgery*, **100**, 804–9.

Jass, J., Love, S. and Northover, J. (1987) A new prognostic classification of rectal cancer. *Lancet*, **i**, 1303–6.

Kane, M.J. (1991) Adjuvant sytemic treatment for carcinoma of the colon and rectum. *Seminars in Oncology*, **18**, 421–42.

Kirsner, J.B. (ed.) (1988) *Diseases of Colon, Rectum and Anal Canal*, Williams & Wilkins, Baltimore.

Kohne-Womper, C.H., Schmoll, H.J., Hastrick, A. *et al.* (1992) Chemotherapeutic stratagems in metastatic colorectal cancer. *Seminars in Oncology*, **19**, 105–25.

Lockhart-Mummery, H., Ritchie, J. and Hawley, P. (1976) Results of surgical treatment for carcinoma of the rectum at St Mark's Hospital from 1948–1972. *British Journal of Surgery*, **63**, 673–7.

Lorenz, H.P., Wilson, W., Leigh, B., Crombleholme, T. *et al.* (1991) Squamous cell carcinoma of the anus in HIV infection. *Diseases of the Colon and Rectum*, **34**, 336–8.

Lynch, H.T., Smyrck, T., Watson, P. *et al.* (1991) Hereditary colorectal cancer. *Seminars in Oncology*, **18**, 337–66.

McFarlane, J.K., Ryall, R. and Heald, R.T. (1993) Mesorectal excision for rectal cancer. *Lancet*, **341**, 457–60.

Midiri, G., Amanti, C., Consorti, F. *et al.* (1983) Usefulness of preoperative CEA levels in the assessment of colorectal cancer patient stage. *Journal of Surgical Oncology*, **22**, 257–60.

Morson, B.C. (1974) Evolution of cancer of the colon and rectum. *Cancer*, **34**, 845–9.

MRC (1984) Clinicopathological findings of prognostic significance in operable rectal cancer in 17 centres in the UK. *British Journal of Surgery*, **50**, 435–42.

NGTATG (1992) Expectancy or primary chemotherapy in patients with advanced asymptomatic colorectal cancer. *Journal of Clinical Oncology*, **10**, 904–11.

Office of Population Censuses and Surveys (1990) *Mortality Statistics* 1988. HMSO, London.

Rao, A., Kagan, A., Chan, P. *et al.* (1981) Patterns of recurrence following curative resection alone for adenocarcinoma of the rectum and sigmoid. *Cancer*, **48**, 1492–5.

Rifkin, M. and Marks, G. (1985) Transrectal ultrasound as an adjunct in the diagnosis of rectal and extrarectal tumours. *Radiology*, **157**, 499–502.

Scheithaeur, W., Rosen, H., Kornek, G.V. *et al.* (1993) Randomized comparison of combination chemotherapy in patients with metastatic colorectal cancer. *British Medical Journal*, **306**, 725–55.

Slater, G.I., Haber, R.H. and Aufses, J.H. (1984) Changing distribution of carcinoma of the colon and rectum. *Surgery, Gynaecology and Obstetrics*, **158**, 216–18.

Sontag, S., Durczak, C., Aranha, G. *et al.* (1983) Faecal occult blood screening for colorectal cancer in a Veteran's Administration hospital. *American Journal of Surgery*, **145**, 89–93.

Steele, G. and Ravikumar, T. (1989) Resection of hepatic metastases from colorectal cancer. *Annals of Surgery*, **210**, 127–38.

Weisburger, J.H. (1991) Causes, mechanisms and prevention of large bowel cancer. *Seminars in Oncology*, **18**, 316–36.

Whiston, R.J., Armitage, N.C., Wilcox, D. and Hardcastle, J.D. (1993) Hartmanns procedure: an appraisal. *Journal of the Royal Society of Medicine*, **86**, 205–8.

Winawer, S., Andrews, N., Flehinger, B. *et al.* (1980) Progress report on controlled trial of faecal occult blood testing for the detection of colorectal neoplasia. *Cancer*, **45**, 2959–64.

Winchester, D., Shull, J., Scanlon, E. *et al.* (1980) A mass screening program for colorectal cancer using chemical testing for occult blood in the stool. *Cancer*, **45**, 2955–8.

Vogelsten, B. (1990) The adenoma–carcinoma sequence. *Nature*, **348**, 681–2.

GASTRIC CANCER

Michael Findlay and David Cunningham

43.1 INTRODUCTION

Gastric cancer is the second most common tumour worldwide. Although there was a reduction in gastric cancer incidence during the early part of this century, in the last two decades this decline appears to have reached a plateau. The generally dismal outcome for the majority of patients with this disease underlines the need for a structured research based management programme. A comprehensive understanding of this disease enables rational planning of research in areas of greatest potential progress – in particular, prevention, screening and combined modality treatment. This chapter outlines the state of the art knowledge and the potential future directions in the management of this disease.

43.2 INCIDENCE

Wide variations exist in the incidence of gastric cancer in specific populations. In Japan the incidence is as high as 80 per 100 000 males while in most areas of Africa the overall incidence is approximately 5 per 100 000. Europe, the old USSR and parts of South America have incidence rates of 20–40 per 100 000 while North America, Australia and New Zealand have rates of approximately 10 per 100 000 (Parkin *et al.*, 1988). This wide range in incidence rates has made it possible to more accurately examine the aetiology of gastric cancer. Early this century gastric adenocarcinoma was the most common cause of cancer death both in the West

and in the underdeveloped countries. However, until recently there has been a decline in incidence of approximately 2.2% per year (Parkin *et al.*, 1988), such that it is now the second most common tumour globally. In the last two decades however the incidence of this tumour has remained static and is possibly increasing. There is also evidence that the proportion of patients having adenocarcinomas of the proximal stomach and gastro-oesophageal junction have increased while tumours of the distal stomach have reduced (Powell and McConkey, 1990). This is of potential prognostic importance as proximal tumours are more difficult to completely resect.

43.3 AETIOLOGY

The determination of various 'at risk' populations from epidemiological studies has given clues to the pathogenesis of this disease. Migrant studies of Japanese in North America and Europeans in Australia suggest environmental factors play a significant role in pathogenesis. Before adequate refrigeration of food was available meat was preserved using nitrite containing preservatives. These nitrites form N-nitroso compounds which are carcinogenic. The reduction in incidence of carcinoma of the stomach may be a result of widespread introduction of refrigeration and associated reduction in the use of such food preservatives. Similarly, dietary factors conferring an increased risk include pickled foods and those conferring a protective effect are allium vegetables (e.g. garlic), ascorbic acid, vitamin E and carotene, possibly through their antibacterial or anti-oxidant activity (You *et al.*, 1989). More recent interest has focused on the organism *Helicobacter pylori* which is a known causative factor in atrophic gastritis (Foreman *et al.*, 1991). Infections with this organism have been associated with a higher risk of developing gastric cancer. It is postulated that atrophic gastritis induced by this infection leads to a reduction in intraluminal acid secretion and a bacterial overgrowth which produces an increased nitrite formation. Although there is debate about the risk of subsequent gastric cancer in people with pernicious anaemia and previous distal gastrectomy, these conditions may be linked to tumour development by this mechanism.

The observation that patients with blood group A have higher relative risk of the diffuse type carcinoma of the stomach suggests a genetic predisposition to this disorder. There does appear to be a two–four fold increased risk of gastric cancer in first degree relatives; however, no specific pattern of inheritance has been identified. Barrett's oesophagus is the condition of the lower oesophagus where the squamous epithelium becomes columnar as a result of oesophago-gastric reflux and is associated with an increased risk of adenocarcinoma of the oesophago–gastric junction. Gastric cancer appears distinct from other upper aero-digestive tumours in that there is no evidence that it is associated with tobacco or alcohol consumption.

43.4 PATHOLOGY

Approximately 90% of gastric cancers are adenocarcinomas. The next most common types of pathology are lymphoma and leiomyosarcomas. It is therefore important to confirm the histology of gastric tumours as the management and outlook is quite different. Adenocarcinomas can be classified according to their differentiation or according to the Lauren system which divides the tumours into 'intestinal' and 'diffuse' (Lauren, 1965) Intestinal tumours are usually exophytic, often ulcerating and are associated with intestinal metaplasia of the stomach. Diffuse tumours are poorly differentiated infiltrating lesions which lead to thickening of the stomach (linitis plastica) while not necessarily penetrating the mucosa. Patients with diffuse type tumours appear to have a worse prognosis than those with intestinal type.

43.5 PRESENTATION

Patients presenting with gastric cancer often complain of symptoms that are non-specific. The vague nature of the symptoms may lead to delayed presentation on the part of the patient and delayed diagnosis on the part of the doctor who often makes a diagnosis of benign peptic ulcer disease. Weight loss and epigastric pain are the most common complaints while dysphagia, anorexia, nausea, vomiting and altered bowel habit occur less frequently. Haematemesis is not a common form of presentation for gastric adeno-carcinoma; however it is more frequently seen with leiomyosarcoma of the stomach.

With the increasing proportion of tumours occurring in the proximal stomach, the symptom of dysphagia may become a more prominent presenting feature of this disease. Although this should facilitate recognition of the diagnosis for the doctor, the fact remains that many patients will present with advanced disease with very little specific symptomatology. Knowledge of the common symptoms may help target populations for tumour screening in an attempt to diagnose early stage disease.

Clinical examination findings at presentation are frequently negative; however, a palpable epigastric mass is present in a third of patients. Metastatic spread may be clinically evident with supraclavicular and left axillary nodes, hepatomegaly or peritoneal disease with ascites, pelvic masses (Kruckenberg tumours), periumbilical nodules or a rectal mass (Blumer's shelf).

43.6 INVESTIGATION AND STAGING

After obtaining a full history and performing a physical examination the investigation most likely to yield the most diagnostic information is an endoscopy with biopsies. Endoscopy (Figure 43.1) should identify almost all intestinal type tumours as they are exophytic; however, diffuse (linitis plastica) tumours can be more problematical as there may be no obvious tumour visible on the mucosa and random biopsies may be negative. The only clue to the diagnosis may be a stomach that does not insufflate with air, generally appearing stiffened at endoscopy. It is important however to obtain a histological diagnosis because of the possibility of gastric lymphoma which would require a totally different management. This may necessitate a diagnostic laparotomy or laparoscopy.

Double contrast barium meal studies (Figure 43.2) have been widely used for screening gastric cancer in Japan (Kaneko

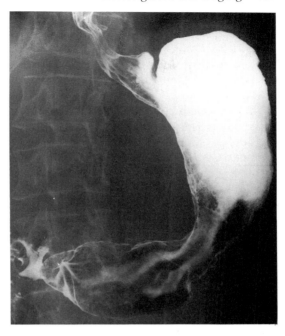

Figure 43.2 A barium study showing a tumour on the greater curve of the stomach. A central ulcer lies within the raised edges of the tumour.

et al., 1977) and appear to be only slightly less satisfactory than endoscopy for diagnostic

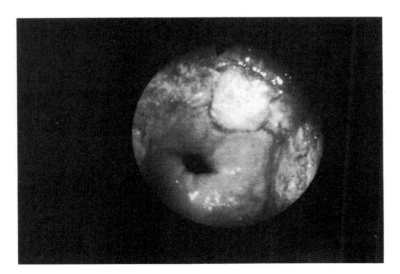

Figure 43.1 An endoscopic view of a carcinoma at the oesophago-gastric junction. (Courtesy of Mr N. Sacks, the Royal Marsden Hospital.)

purposes. Because a barium meal is less able to diagnose early gastric tumours and cannot provide histological information, the practice at this institution is to perform endoscopy with biopsy in the first instance.

In addition to identification of the tumour, its extent must be determined in order to direct treatment. CT (Figure 43.3) is the investigation of choice to establish the spread of tumour beyond the stomach. Distant metastases to liver, lung and ovary can usually reasonably be excluded using CT. Lymph node status is less accurately assessed on CT with sensitivity and specificity of 60–70%. The predictive value, however, can be improved when groups of nodes rather than isolated nodes are present. The definition of an abnormal node is based largely on size, which varies depending on the nodal group, but may also be differentiated by their contrast enhancing ability (normal nodes enhance with intravenous contrast). Other than the retrocrural nodes which should not exceed 0.5 cm in size, all other nodes should be 1.0 cm before being labelled pathological. The other area in which CT is of value is in determining the direct invasion of adjacent organs like pancreas, liver, colon, mesentery or spleen by the primary tumour. The sensitivity of this is often limited by the amount of intra-abdominal fat present which acts as a contrast between organs. Two areas in which CT is of less value are in diagnosis of peritoneal deposits and in estimation of depth of stomach wall invasion.

Endoluminal ultrasound is a newer technique which has shown promise in the accurate (80–90%) demonstration of tumour

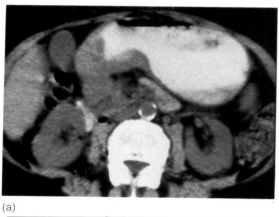

(a)

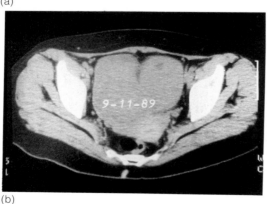

(b)

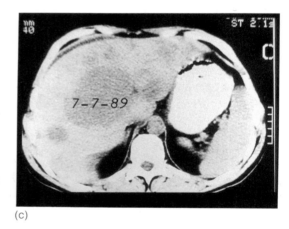

(c)

Figure 43.3 CT scans of patients with gastric cancer depicting: **(a)** a primary tumour in the distal stomach; **(b)** pelvic lymphadenopathy; **(c)** liver metastases.

penetration; however it is less satisfactory for lymph node evaluation (60–70% accurate). This technique is a very promising addition to the staging methods. However it is not yet widely available in clinical practice. Other than at laparotomy, peritoneal disease is best assessed using laparoscopy. However this technique is still being developed in the upper gastrointestinal area despite its extensive use in gynaecological disorders.

Ultimately, because of difficulties with the non-invasive methods of assessing disease, patients may need a diagnostic/therapeutic laparotomy, despite a comprehensive work-up. Unnecessary operations can however be avoided by correct patient investigation. Nevertheless, much of the information obtained with these investigations may prove more useful in investigating preoperative treatment strategies using chemotherapy or radiotherapy for patients with resectable tumours who are at high risk of relapse.

Using the internationally accepted TMN classification (American Joint Committee on Cancer Manual for Staging of Cancer, 1992), gastric cancer can be staged from I to IV (Table 43.1). Early gastric cancer according to the Japanese Research Society definition includes patients with T1 primary tumours with or without N1 nodes. This group of tumours has a very good prognosis with surgical resection. The survival of patients with different stages of disease at presentation is discussed in section 43.7.

43.7 PROGNOSTIC FACTORS

Indicators of prognosis in patients with gastric cancer may differ depending on the clinical setting in which they are used. Prognostic factors will be discussed in the context of outcome following primary surgery and for palliative treatment of advanced disease with chemotherapy.

The most important indicator of adverse outcome in this disease is the presence of an unresectable tumour. Survival at 12 months is poor (6%); however there appears to be some survival advantage in having a palliative resection, with a 21% 12 month and 7% 2 year survival. Resectability however is a function of the stage of the tumour (Allum *et al.*, 1989a). Survival according to stages devised using the TNM classification system is shown in Figure 43.4. Patients with stage I disease will have a 70% 5 year survival; however this is reduced to 60% with the presence of positive lymph nodes or penetration of the serosa by the tumour (20–40%). These high risk subgroups have been the subject of a variety of postoperative adjuvant studies. The histological classification of gastric cancer has some prognostic significance in that diffuse type tumours in the Lauren system have a poor survival after curative surgery, with less than 5% of patients surviving 5 years.

Within the large group of patients who either present with advanced tumours or relapse following surgery, a different set of prognostic factors may exist. Most patients considered for further active treatment will be offered chemotherapy with palliative intent. It is important therefore to identify patients who are unlikely to benefit from such treatment in order to minimize their exposure to cytotoxic side-effects. These factors will represent a function of the patient's general debility or tumour characteristics, or both. The most widely used predictor of outcome is the patient's pretreatment performance status. Few people who are bedbound and totally dependent for self-care (WHO grade 4 or Karnofsky < 30%) will benefit from chemotherapy. Tumour related factors such as previous weight loss and low serum albumin, the presence of measurable (large volume) disease and secretion of carcino-embryonic antigen predict poor outcome. However, tumour histology (diffuse vs intestinal) is a less clear predictor of outcome to chemotherapy although diffuse tumours more frequently have peritoneal metastases which are less likely to respond to treatment. In our experience the age of the patient is not

Table 43.1   TNM classification of gastric cancer

Definition of TNM
Primary Tumour (T)

TX	Primary tumour cannot be assessed
T0	No evidence of primary tumour
Tis	Carcinoma-*in-situ*: intraepithelial tumour without invasion of the lamina propria
T1	Tumour invades lamina propria or submucosa
T2	Tumour invades the muscularis propria or the subserosa
T3	Tumour penetrates the serosa (visceral peritoneum) without invasion of adjacent structures
T4	Tumour invades adjacent structures

Regional lymph nodes (N)

NX	Regional lymph node(s) cannot be assessed
N0	No regional lymph node metastases
N1	Metastasis in perigastric lymph node(s) within 3 cm of the edge of the primary tumour
N2	Metastasis in perigastric lymph node(s) more than 3 cm from the edge of the primary tumour, or in lymph nodes along the left gastric, common hepatic, splenic, or coeliac arteries

Distant Metastasis (M)

MX	Presence of distant metastasis cannot be assessed
M0	No distant metastasis
M1	Distant metastasis

STAGE GROUPING

Stage 0	Tis	N0	M0
Stage IA	T1	N0	M0
Stage IB	T1	N1	M0
	T2	N0	M0
Stage II	T1	N2	M0
	T2	N1	M0
	T3	N0	M0
Stage IIIA	T2	N2	M0
	T3	N1	M0
	T4	N0	M0
Stage IIIB	T3	N2	M0
	T4	N1	M0
Stage IV	T4	N2	M0
	Any T	Any N	M1

a significant predictor of outcome. The impact of these prognostic indicators on the survival of patients achieving response to chemotherapy however is minimal. Therefore if tumour response to treatment could be predicted within a short trial period of chemotherapy, the oncologist can provide better palliative management. Two non-invasive techniques have been used to predict response to 5-fluorouracil (5-FU) based treatment in gastrointestinal malignancy – magnetic resonance spectroscopy (MRS) and positron emission tomography (PET).

Identification of a 5-FU signal in a tumour using MRS, in our experience and that of others (Presant *et al.*, 1990; Findlay *et al.*, 1993a) predicts subsequent response to treatment. An advantage of this technique is that it can also identify changes in 5-FU metabolism at different stages of tumour treatment. PET scanning is a technique which from our own early experience (Findlay *et al.*, 1993b)

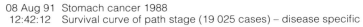

08 Aug 91 Stomach cancer 1988
12:42:12   Survival curve of path stage (19 025 cases) – disease specific

Graph of survival function
  Survival variable surv
    Grouped by npaths   path stage-group

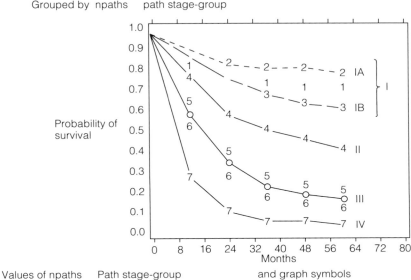

Values of npaths   Path stage-group   and graph symbols

Value	Graph Symbol	Value Label	Value	Graph Symbol	Value Label	Value	Graph Symbol	Value Label
1	1 – Stage 0		2	2 – Stage IA		3	3 – Stage IB	
4	4 – Stage II		5	5 – Stage IIIA		6	6 – Stage IIIB	
7	7 – Stage IV							

Figure 43.4 Survival of patients with gastric cancer according to tumour stage. (Reprinted from the *American Joint Committee on Cancer Manual for Staging Cancer*, 1992, with permission.)

appears to be predictive of response to chemotherapy when using the nonspecific marker of tumour metabolism – deoxyglucose labelled with [18]F (Chapter 7).

Development of new predictors of outcome remains an important aspect of the management of this disease, particularly as some chemotherapy regimens are not without significant toxicity. With the increasing interest in developing preoperative chemotherapy protocols, predictors of outcome may also help avoid inappropriate delay of curative surgery.

43.8 CURRENT MANAGEMENT

There are three major clinical entities in which this disease exists: resectable; unresectable; metastatic. Preoperative investigations may determine resectability of a tumour; however, the less than optimal predictive value of these techniques usually results in a laparotomy being performed. For this reason discussion of the current management of this disease will be based on is resectability and the presence of metastatic disease.

43.8.1 RESECTABLE GASTRIC CANCER

The type of operation required for gastric cancer depends on the site and extent of disease. Tumours of the distal stomach may be adequately treated with a partial gastrectomy while mid-stomach lesions usually require total or > 95% sub total gastrectomy –

Table 43.2 Adjuvant chemotherapy in gastric cancer

Chemotherapy	Tumour stage	No. patients	5 year survival %	Significance	Reference
Thio-TEPA i.p.+i.v. vs surgery alone	All curative resections	13 142	35 (3 years) 35	NS	Dixon et al., 1971
5-FU + FT-207 orally for 24–36 months vs surgery alone	'Suspected or definite invasion to serosa' (not T4)	57 78	45* 22	P < 0.005	Fujimoto et al., 1977
Mitomycin C twice weekly for 5 weeks vs surgery alone	II	89 99	78 42	'Highly significant'	Imanaga and Nakazato, 1977
Mitomycin C twice weekly for 5 weeks vs surgery alone	Involved serosa	136 135	49 22	P < 0.005	Nakajima et al., 1978
Mitomycin C 6 weekly × 4 vs surgery alone	All curative resections	33 37	76 (2 years) 30	P < 0.001	Alcobendas et al., 1983
Carbon absorbed mitomycin C i.p. ×1 vs control	T3–4	24 25	69 (3 years) 27	P < 0.005	Hagiwara et al., 1992
5-FU + methyl-CCNU (24 months) vs surgery alone	All curative resections	41 47	55* (4 years) 38	P = 0.03	Douglass et al., 1984 (GITSG)
5-FU + methyl-CCNU (2 years) vs surgery alone	All curative resections	66 68	38 (3.5 years) 39	NS	Higgins et al., 1983 (VASOG)
5-FU + methyl-CCNU (2 years) vs surgery alone	All curative resections	91 89	57 (2 years) 57	NS	Engstrom et al., 1985 (ECOG)
5-FU + mitomycin C vs 5-FU + mitomycin C + CMVF vs surgery alone	All curative resections	141 140 130	18* 10 18	NS	Allum et al., 1989 (BSCG)
5-FU + adriamycin + mitomycin C (12 months) vs surgery alone	Curative resections except T1 N0	133 148	46 35	P = 0.21	Coombes et al., 1990
5-FU + adriamycin + mitomycin C (12 months) vs surgery alone	IB,IC, II,III	83 93	Not stated	NS	Macdonald et al., 1992 (SWOG)

* Estimated from survival curve
CMVF, 5 day induction course of cyclophosphamide, methotrexate, vincristine + 5-FU.
NS, Not significant

the latter with the aim of leaving a small stump to which anastamoses are technically easier to attach. Proximal tumours and those extending to the oesophagus can be treated with oesophago-gastrectomy or a proximal gastrectomy.

Early gastric cancers, by virtue of their size, may be adequately treated with subtotal gastrectomy; nevertheless, proximal lesions may be more problematical due to a higher anastamotic leak rate. Distal partial gastrectomy however has less operative morbidity and mortality than total gastrectomy. The other issues in surgery of this disease are the need for extended radical lymph node dissection and splenectomy. Splenectomy has been performed largely to enable access for adequate lymph node dissection, but in distal tumours this is probably not necessary. Metastasis to the spleen from gastric cancer is very unusual. There is currently a study sponsored by the Medical Research Council in the United Kingdom where patients are randomized to receive a more limited (R1) or more extensive (R2) resection.

Patients found to have stage I disease on pathological review have a cure rate of at least 70% and are not likely to receive any major extra benefit from adjuvant treatment. More advanced tumours, however, particularly those which penetrate the serosa or have nodal involvement (T_2N_1, T_1N_2 or greater) have a much poorer outlook. There has been extensive investigation of postoperative adjuvant chemotherapy in these patients with mixed results.

(a) Adjuvant chemotherapy

Chemotherapy following successful complete resection of a primary gastric cancer is aimed at treating micrometastatic disease and local residual tumour. Earlier studies focused on the use of single agent drugs like thio-TEPA, 5-FU and mitomycin C. More recent studies have looked at the combination of 5-FU with methyl CCNU and at the FAM (5-FU, adriamycin and mitomycin C) regimen. In the 1960s, thio-TEPA, a drug not known for its activity in gastric cancer, was used intraperitoneally and intravenously postoperatively. No survival advantage was elicited in this large study (Dixon *et al.*, 1971). The early experience with fluoropyrimidines yielded mixed results. One study using fluorodeoxyuridine in all patients having had curative resection found there was no difference between treatment and control at 3 years. A Japanese study (Fujimoto *et al.*, 1977) treated patients with suspected serosal invasion using 5-FU and an analogue FT-207 2–3 years postoperatively. They found a significant difference in survival at 5 years. Four studies have examined single agent mitomycin C, three of them in patients whose tumours had serosal involvement. The results of these studies, three from Japan and one from Spain, all found a significant survival advantage with this treatment (Imanga and Nakazato, 1977; Nakajima *et al.*, 1978; Alcobendas *et al.*, 1983; Hagiwara *et al.*, 1992). The most recent study used a novel approach of administering mitomycin C absorbed to activated charcoal which was instilled at the time of surgical closure following primary resection (Hagiwara *et al.*, 1992). Four studies, three from the USA and one from Italy, have used 5-FU and methyl CCNU following curative resections (Gastrointestinal Tumor Study Group, 1982; Higgins *et al.*, 1983; Engstrom *et al.*, 1985; Italian Gastrointestinal Tumour Study Group, 1988). One of these studies found a difference in survival (Gastrxintestinal Tumour Study Group, 1982). One British study found giving 5-FU and mitomycin C following curative resection yielded no survival advantage, and in particular had problems with treatment related death due to the haemolytic uraemic syndrome – a known association with mitomycin C (Allum *et al.*, 1989b). Two groups have designed randomized controlled trials using the FAM regimen (Coombes *et al.*, 1990; Macdonald *et al.*, 1992). All patients with curative resections were included, except those with stage IA disease. Neither of these studies were able to demonstrate a survival benefit contradicting the earlier encouraging results using single agent mitomycin C.

Adjuvant chemotherapy currently does not have broad application in gastric cancer, and although in Japan it has now been accepted as standard treatment because of the results of the earlier Japanese single agent studies, its use should be limited to randomized clinical trials.

43.8.2   UNRESECTABLE GASTRIC CANCER

At laparotomy gastric cancer can be deemed unresectable for cure for various reasons – previously unknown metastatic disease in: liver; distant lymph nodes; and peritoneum may be recognized. The primary tumour however may be extensively adherent to adjacent structures precluding adequate resection with tumour free margins. If a palliative resection of the primary lesion can be achieved with minimum morbidity this then gives a better symptomatic result than a bypass procedure. If this is not possible, the options available for the symptomatic patient include intubation of the obstructing area of stomach or debulking of the tumour using laser endoscopy. Placement of tubes may often cause problems themselves with pain, dysphagia, reflux, aspiration pneumonia and tube migration. Repeated laser endoscopy in our view is a more satisfactory method of palliation, particularly in combination with chemotherapy (Harper *et al.*, 1992). The use of chemotherapy in unresectable tumours is discussed in a later section in this chapter (section 43.9).

43.8.3   METASTATIC GASTRIC CANCER

The aim of managing patients with metastatic gastric cancer is to optimize the quality of life, and if possible prolong survival. A randomized study of 41 patients with gastric cancer from Finland (Pyrhonen *et al.*, 1992) has demonstrated a 9 month median survival advantage (12 months vs 3 months) in patients given chemotherapy (5-FU, methotrexate and epirubicin) compared to those given best supportive care. The significant survival advantage found in this study makes it difficult to justify further trials of this type, particularly with an increasing patient perception that no treatment is a poor option. The most active drugs in gastric cancer appear to be 5-FU, mitomycin C, cisplatin and the anthracyclines, adriamycin and epirubicin. The first combination of cytotoxics to show major activity in this disease was 5-FU, adriamycin and mitomycin C (FAM) (Macdonald *et al.*, 1979). Two randomized studies have tested the activity of this combination: one showed an enhanced response rate compared to single agent 5-FU, but no survival advantage; the other showed both a response and survival advantage of FAM over 5-FU plus methyl-CCNU. A survival advantage in the former study may not have been detectable because of small patient numbers (Douglass *et al.*, 1984; Cullinan *et al.*, 1985).

The next most significant development was that of 5-FU, adriamycin and methotrexate (FAMTX) in combination. Following a Phase II study indicating activity of this regimen, it was examined in a Phase III study against the original FAM regimen (Wils *et al.*, 1991). It was found that the FAMTX regimen had a superior tumour response rate and patient survival when compared to the FAM regimen. The FAMTX regimen gave slightly more mucositis while the FAM regimen, due to the mitomycin C, gave more myelosuppression.

A German group developed a regimen using etoposide, adriamycin and cisplatin (EAP) (Preusser *et al.*, 1989). This regimen was based on preclinical studies suggesting synergy between cisplatin and etoposide, the latter being relatively inactive as a single agent. This regimen was found to have very high response rates initially, albeit with some

Table 43.3   Combination chemotherapy regimens used in gastric cancer

Combination	Number of responses/ number of patients	Percent response	Median survival (months)	Reference
FAM (5-FU, adriamycin, mitomycin)	151/453	33	5.5–7.2	Gohmann and Macdonald, 1989
FAMTX (5-FU, adriamycin, methotrexate)	22/67 (13% CR)	33	6	Wils *et al.*, 1991
EAP (etoposide, adriamycin, cisplatin)	95/181 (14% CR)	52	7.5–10	Wilke *et al.*, 1989 Lerner *et al.*, 1992
ELF (etoposide, leucovorin, 5-FU)	27/51 (12% CR)	53	11	Wilke *et al.*, 1990
ECF (epirubicin, cisplatin, protracted infusion 5-FU)	95/133 (11% CR)	71	8.2	Findlay *et al.*, 1993c

problems with myelosuppression. The EAP regimen has recently been compared to FAMTX in a randomized study (Kelsen *et al.*, 1992). The results of this trial show that despite the initial hope that this new regimen would be more active, it appears that its activity is little different to FAMTX, but more importantly its toxicity is substantially greater. The result of this study underlines the necessity to examine new combinations in randomized clinical trials. FAMTX currently remains the most appropriate standard treatment arm in a randomized study; however its mediocre overall impact in patients with this disease precludes it from being adopted as a standard treatment outside the context of a clinical trial. Newer more active, but less toxic chemotherapy combinations are required. The combination ELF (etoposide, leucovorin, 5-FU) was originally designed to be used on patients who were elderly or medically unfit for more intensive treatment (Wilke *et al.*, 1990). It has been shown to have reasonable activity against gastric cancer and is now the subject of a further Phase III study in comparison to FAMTX.

We have recently completed a Phase II study examining the role of epirubicin and cisplatin in combination with a protracted low dose infusion of 5-FU (Findlay *et al.*, 1993c). The rationale for this regimen is that the 5-FU as a continuous low dose infusion gives significantly less marrow toxicity than conventional bolus schedules. Epirubicin and cisplatin, both active in gastric cancer, were added to the infusion. Seventy-one per cent of patients had a response to this combination with 11% of patients achieving a complete response. Responses were seen at a variety of metastatic sites even in large volume disease. This high response rate was achieved with acceptable toxicity. This new regimen is now being studied in a multi centre randomized trial in the UK using FAMTX as the standard treatment arm.

43.9   FUTURE DIRECTIONS

43.9.1   SCREENING AND PREVENTION

Successful screening in any tumour relies on directing the screening at a suitably high risk population in which early stage tumours are detectable and, when upon detection, successful curative treatment can be instituted which ultimately changes the survival statistics for the at risk population. Such a screening and treatment programme also has to be economically feasible. In the UK approximately 80% of tumours of the stomach will, at presentation, be too far advanced for curative resection (Allum *et al.*, 1989a). There is therefore a good case for further investigating the role of screening for gastric cancer in this country. Screening has been successfully implemented in Japan using double-contrast barium meal and endoscopy (Kaneko *et al.*, 1977) with a resultant increase in the proportion of patients presenting with early gastric cancer (about 30–40%). One group in the UK designed a study to look at patients over 40 years of age presenting to their family practitioner with dyspepsia (Hallissey *et al.*, 1990). These patients were directly referred to a specialist endoscopy unit. Two per cent of all those referred were subsequently shown to have gastric cancer. One in every 117 patients studied had an early gastric cancer amenable to curative surgery. While these figures compare favourably with other screening programmes like breast mammography and cervical cancer screening, there is little information about the impact of a programme like this on survival in a UK population.

Another area of interest in populations bearing a high risk for gastric cancer is that of prevention. Studies are currently in progress in South America looking at the use of the anti-oxidant ascorbic acid and metronidazole which eradicates the *Helicobacter pylori* infection. However, until adequate screening or prevention programmes can be instituted the focus will be on the management of advanced disease.

43.9.2   SURGERY

While surgery remains the single most important therapeutic intervention in gastric cancer there are still purely surgical issues that can be clarified, e.g. the extent of nodal dissection required. We believe, however, the emphasis of further surgical studies will be on optimizing its timing with chemotherapy and radiation therapy.

43.9.3   RADIATION THERAPY

Radiation therapy is generally not considered a useful modality for gastric tumours; however, there has been little research in this area. Many of the randomized studies have used combination radiation/chemotherapy regimens from which no clear impact of radiation can be determined. Additionally, suboptimal radiation technique and dosing may have compromised results of otherwise well designed adjuvant studies (Allum *et al.*, 1989c).

We believe the future of radiation treatment in this tumour lies in either intraoperative or endoluminal treatment with or without radiosensitizing agents like 5-FU. Ultimately, the aim would be to investigate the application of systemic and local (pre- and postoperative) treatment using cytotoxins and radiation respectively.

43.9.4   CHEMOTHERAPY

While there have been improvements in chemotherapy for this disease there is still an urgent need for new anticancer agents based on classic or novel therapeutic targets. Two new compounds of interest in colon cancer offer hope of activity in gastric cancer. The campothecin analogue CPT-11 has shown significant activity in 5-FU resistant disease and the new thymidylate synthase inhibitor, D1694 undergoing Phase I/II development at the Royal Marsden Hospital and Institute of Cancer Research has to date shown encouraging activity. While awaiting new agents investigators must focus on specific problem areas in treatment failure, e.g. peritoneal metastases which may be better treated via

Table 43.4 Preoperative chemotherapy for locally advanced gastric cancer

Regimen	Timing of chemotherapy	Resectability	Number of evaluable patients	Complete responses (CR and PR)	Patients having surgery	Resection achieved	Pathological complete response
EAP (Wilke et al., 1989)	Pre	Unresectable	33	23/33 (70%)	19 + 1 NC	15/20 (75%)	5/20
EAP (Ajani et al., 1992)	Pre + post	Potentially resectable	48	15/48 (31%) 'major responses'	41	37/41 (90%)	0/41
FAMTX (Wils et al., 1991)	Pre	Unresectable	19	Not stated	7	3/7 (43%)	Not stated
FLC (Leichman and Berry, 1991)	Pre + post	Not stated	25	16/25 (64%) 'significant regression'	25	Not stated	0/25
EFP (Ajani et al., 1991)	Pre + post	Potentially resectable	25	6/25 (24%)	25	18/25 (72%)	0/25
CF (Lasser et al., 1991)	Pre	Clinically LAD	26	15/26 (58%)	15 + 11 NC + 1 NE	21/27 (78%)	Not stated
FLEP (Ishihara et al., 1991)	Pre	Unresectable	10	5/10 (50%)	5	5/5 (100%)	0/5
MF (Verschueren et al., 1988)	Pre	Unresectable (2 clinically LAD)	17	Not stated	13	7/13 (54%)	Not stated
ECF (Findlay et al., 1993c)	Pre	Unresectable or clinically LAD	35	28/35 (80%)	20	11/20 (55%)	4/20
ET (Roberts et al., 1991)	Pre + Post vs none	Potentially resectable T2–3 NOMO	92/2	Not stated	92/2	Not stated	Not stated (increased disease free survival with chemotherapy)

Abbreviations: CR – complete response; PR – partial response; NC – no change; EAP – etoposide, adriamycin, cisplatin; FLC – 5-FU, leucovorin, cisplatin; ECF – epirubicin, cisplatin, 5-FU; CF – cisplatin, 5-FU; ET – epirubicin, tegafur; FLEP – 5-FU, leucovorin, epirubicin, cisplatin; MP – methotrexate, 5-FU; FAMTX – 5-FU, adriamycin, methotrexate.

the intraperitoneal route with drugs that have had their pharmacokinetic features modified (e.g. mitomycin C absorbed to activated charcoal).

All these developments may be much better exploited by administering them where they exert the maximum biological effect, e.g. in the preoperative setting before resecting the tumour rather than after tumour resection. This approach however does provide some methodological difficulties. First, in order to determine the effect of a regimen on survival, randomized studies with a non-chemotherapy arm need to be performed in patients with advanced, but resectable disease. The difficulty with this is that patients with surgically curable non-advanced (stage I) disease are difficult to exclude by clinical staging. The risk to these patients in a surgery delaying preoperative chemotherapy programme, is that, unless the chemotherapy is 100% effective in preventing disease progression, there is a possibility of a surgically curable tumour becoming un-resectable. This obviously requires better methods of staging early gastric cancer and also necessitates very active chemotherapy regimens which not only have a high probability of inducing a response, but can also prevent frank progression of disease during the preoperative period.

The preliminary experience with pre-operative chemotherapy is outlined in Table 43.4. Some studies have used surgical criteria for operability while others have used clinical criteria (or both). The success of preoperative chemotherapy in gastric cancer can only be determined if these factors are standardized and prospectively evaluated in controlled studies.

43.10 CONCLUSIONS

Gastric cancer is a worldwide health care problem which despite a reduction in its incidence still continues to present several major problems. While targeting populations for screening and chemoprevention studies for this disease there are still many areas in which progress can be made in treating patients with gastric cancer.

REFERENCES

Ajani, J.A., Ota, D.M. and Jackson, D.E. (1991) Current strategies in the management of loco-regional and metastatic gastric carcinoma. *Cancer,* **57**, 260–5.

Ajani, J.A., Mayer, R.J., Ota, D.M. *et al.* (1992) Preoperative and postoperative chemotherapy for patients with potentially resectable gastric carcinoma. *Proceedings of the American Society of Clinical Oncology,* **11**, 165 (abstr. 475).

Alcobendas, F., Milla, A., Estape, J. *et al.* (1983) Mitomycin C as an adjuvant in resected gastric cancer. *Annals of Surgery,* **198**, 13–17.

Allum, W.H., Powell, D.J., McConkey, C.C. *et al.* (1989a) Gastric cancer: a 25-year review. *British Journal of Surgery,* **76**, 535–40.

Allum, W.H., Hallissey, M.T., Kelly, K.A. for the British Stomach Cancer Group. (1989b) Adjuvant chemotherapy in operable gastric cancer. *Lancet,* **I**, 571–4.

Allum, W.H., Hallissey, M.T., Ward, L.C. Hockey, M.S. for the British Stomach Cancer Group. (1989c) A controlled, prospective, randomised trial of adjuvant chemotherapy or radiotherapy in resectable gastric cancer: interim report. *British Journal of Cancer,* **60**, 739–44.

American Joint Committee on Cancer Manual for Staging of Cancer, 4th edn. Lippincott, Philadelphia, pp. 64–5.

Coombes, R.C., Schein, P.S., Chilvers, C.E.D. *et al.* for the International Collaborative Cancer Group (1990) A randomized trial comparing adjuvant fluorouracil, doxorubicin, and mitomycin with no treatment in operable gastric cancer. *Journal of Clinical Oncology,* **8**, 1362–9.

Cullinan, S.A., Moertel, C.G., Fleming, T.R. *et al.* for the North Central Cancer Treatment Group (1985) A comparison of three chemotherapeutic regimens in the treatment of advanced pancreatic and gastric carcinoma: fluorouracil vs fluorouracil and doxorubicin vs fluorouracil, doxorubicin, and mitomycin. *Journal of the American Medical Association,* **253**, 2061–7.

Dixon, W.J., Longmire, W.P. and Holden, W.D. (1971) Use of triethylenethiophosphoramide as an adjuvant to the surgical treatment of gastric and colorectal carcinoma: ten-year follow-up. *Annals of Surgery,* **173,** 26–37.

Douglass, H.O., Lavin, P.T., Goudsmit, A. *et al.* (1984) An Eastern Cooperative Oncology Group evaluation of combinations of methyl-CCNU, mitomycin C, adriamycin, and 5-fluorouracil in advanced measurable gastric cancer (EST 2277). *Journal of Clinical Oncology,* **2,** 1372–1381.

Engstrom, P.F., Lavin, P.T., Douglass, H.O. *et al.* (1985) Postoperative adjuvant 5-fluorouracil plus methyl-CCNU therapy for gastric cancer patients: eastern Cooperative Oncology Group Study (EST 3275). *Cancer,* **55,** 1868–73.

Findlay, M., Leach, M., Cunningham, D. *et al.* (1993a) Non-invasive monitoring of 5-fluorouracil modulation by Interferon alpha using 19F magnetic resonance spectroscopy in patients with colorectal cancer. *Annals of Oncology,* **4,** 597–602.

Findlay, M., Young, H., Hanrahan, A. *et al.* (1993b) Monitoring tumour response to infusional 5-fluorouracil in patients with colorectal cancer using positron emission tomography (PET) and 18F-deoxyglucose (FDG). *British Journal of Cancer,* **67,** (suppl. XX), 62 (abstr. p. 125).

Findlay, M., Cunningham, D., Norman, A. *et al.* (1993c) A Phase II study in advanced gastric cancer using epirubicin and cisplatin in combination with continuous infusion 5-fluorouracil (ECF). *Annals of Oncology,* in press.

Foreman, D., Newell, D.G., Fullerton, F. *et al.* (1991) Association between infection with *Helicobacter pylori* and risk of gastric cancer: evidence from a prospective investigation. *British Medical Journal,* **302,** 1302–5.

Fujimoto, S., Akao, T., Itoh, B. *et al.* (1977) Protracted oral chemotherapy with fluorinated pyrimidines as an adjuvant to surgical treatment for stomach cancer. *Annals of Surgery,* **85,** 462–6.

Gohmann, J.J. and Macdonald, J.S. (1989) Chemotherapy of gastric cancer. *Cancer Investigation,* **7,** 39–52.

Hagiwara, A., Takahashi, T., Kojima, O. *et al.* (1992) Prophylaxis with carbon-adsorbed mitomycin against peritoneal recurrence of gastric cancer. *Lancet,* **339,** 629–31.

Hallissey, M.T., Allum, W.H., Jewkes, A.J. *et al.* (1990) Early detection of gastric cancer. *British Medical Journal,* **301,** 513–15.

Harper, P., Highley, M., Houston, S. *et al.* (1992) Significant palliation of advanced gastric/oesophageal adenocarcinoma (G-O/C) with laser endoscopy and combination chemo-

therapy. *Proceedings of the American Society of Clinical Oncology,* **11,** 164 (abstr. 472).

Higgins, G.A., Amadeo, J.H., Smith, D.E. *et al.* (1989) A Veterans Administration Surgical Oncology Group Report. Efficacy of prolonged intermittent therapy with combined 5-FU and methyl-CCNU following resection for gastric carcinoma. *Cancer,* **52,** 1105–112.

Imanga, H. and Nakazato, H. (1977) Results of surgery for gastric cancer and effect of adjuvant mitomycin C on cancer recurrence. *World Journal of Surgery,* **1,** 213–21.

Ishihara, S., Nakajima, T., Ohta, K. *et al.* (1991) Evaluation of effective neo-adjuvant chemotherapy (FLEP therapy) in the treatment of advanced gastric cancer. *Gan-To-Kagakn-Ryoho,* **18,** 1748–52.

Kaneko, E., Nakamura, T. and Almeda, E. (1977) Outcome of gastric carcinoma detected by gastric mass survey in Japan. *Gut,* **18,** 6.

Kelsen, D., Atiq, O.T., Saltz, L. *et al.* (1992) FAMTX versus etoposide, doxorubicin, and cisplatin: a random assignment trial in gastric cancer. *Journal of Clinical Oncology,* **10,** 541–8.

Lasser, P.H., Rougier, P.H., Mahjoubi, M. *et al.* (1991) Neoadjuvant chemotherapy (NCT) in locally advanced gastric carcinoma (LAGC). *European Journal of Cancer,* **27,** S71, (suppl. 2)., (abstr. 396).

Lauren, P. (1965) The two histological main types of gastric carcinoma: diffuse and so-called intestinal type carcinoma. An attempt at a histo-clinical classification. *Acta Patrologica et Microbiologica Scandinavica,* **64,** 31–49.

Leichman, L. and Berry, B.T. (1991) Cisplatin therapy for adenocarcinoma of the stomach. *Seminars in Oncology,* **18,** (Suppl. 3), 25–33.

Lerner, A., Gonin, R., Steel Jr, G.D. and Mayer, R.J. (1992) Etoposide, doxorubicin, and cisplatin chemotherapy for advanced gastric adenocarcinoma: results of a Phase II trial. *Journal of Clinical Oncology,* **10,** 536–40.

Macdonald, J.S., Woolley, P.V., Smythe, T. *et al.* (1979) 5-Fluorouracil, adriamycin, and mitomycin-C (FAM) combination chemotherapy in the treatment of advanced gastric cancer. *Cancer,* **44,** 42–7.

Macdonald, J.S., Gagliano, R., Fleming, T., *et al.* (1992) Coordinated by the SWOG. A Phase III trial of FAM (5-fluorouracil, adriamycin, mitomycin-C) chemotherapy vs control as adjuvant treatment for resected gastric cancer (A Southwest Oncology Group Trial – SWOG 7804).

Proceedings of the American Society of Clinical Oncology, **11**, 168.

Nakajima, T., Fukami, A., Ohashi l, *et al.* (1978) Long-term follow-up study of gastric cancer patients treated with surgery and adjuvant chemotherapy with mitomycin C. *International Journal of Clinical Pharmacology*, **16**, 209–16.

Parkin, D.M., Laara, E. and Muir, C.S. (1980) Estimates of the worldwide frequency of sixteen major cancers in 1980. *International Journal of Cancer*, **41**, 184–97.

Powell, J. and McConkey, C.C. (1990) Increasing incidence of adenocarcinoma of the gastric cardia and adjacent sites. *British Journal of Cancer*, **62**, 440–3.

Preusser, P., Wilke, H., Achterrath, W. *et al.* (1989) Phase II study with the combination etoposide, doxorubicin and cisplatin in advanced measurable gastric cancer. *Journal of Clinical Oncology*, **7**, 1310–17.

Pyrhonen, S., Kuitunen, T. and Kouri, M. (1992) A randomised, Phase III trial comparing fluorouracil, epidoxorubicin and methotrexate (FEMTX) with best supportive care in non-resectable gastric cancer. *Annals of Oncology*, (1991) **3**, (suppl. 3) (abstr. 47).

Roberts, P.J., Antila, S., Alhava, E. *et al.* (1991) Results of peri-operative chemotherapy in patients with radically operated gastric cancer. *European Journal of Cancer*, **27**, S71 (suppl. 2). (Abstr. 398).

Gastrointestinal Tumor Study Group (1982) Controlled trial of adjuvant chemotherapy following curative resection for gastric cancer. *Cancer*, **49**, 1116–22.

Italian Gastrointestinal Tumor Study Group (1988) Adjuvant treatments following curative resection for gastric cancer. *British Journal of Surgery*, **75**, 1100–4.

Vershueren, R.J.C., Willemse, P.H.B, Sleijfer, D. Th. *et al.* (1988) Combined chemotherapeutic – surgical approach of locally advanced gastric cancer. *Proceedings of the American Society of Clinical Oncology*, **7**, 93, (abstr. 455).

Wilke, H., Preusser, P., Fink, U. *et al.* (1989) Preoperative chemotherapy in locally advanced and non-resectable gastric cancer: a phase II study with etoposide, doxorubicin and cisplatin. *Journal of Clinical Oncology*, **7**, 1318–26.

Wilke, H., Preusser, P., Fink, U. *et al.* (1990) *Journal of Clinical Oncology*, New developments in the treatment of gastric carcinoma. *Seminars in Oncology*, **17**, (suppl. 2) 61–70.

Wils, J.A., Klein, H.O., Wagener, D.J.T.H. *et al.* for the EORTC. (1991) Sequential high-dose methotrexate and fluorouracil combined with doxorubicin – a step ahead in the treatment of advanced gastric cancer: a trial of the European Organisation for Research and Treatment of Cancer Gastrointestinal Tract Cooperative Group. *Journal of Clinical Oncology*, **9**, 827–31.

You, W-C., Blot, W.J., Chang, Y-S., *et al.* (1989) Allium vegetables and reduced risk of stomach cancer. *Journal of the National Cancer Institute*, **81**, 162–4.

OESOPHAGEAL CANCER

44

S. Bal and Anthony G. Nash

Carcinoma of the oesophagus is a highly virulent tumour with an exceedingly poor prognosis. In spite of technical advances in surgery and radiation therapy there have been few improvements in outcome over the past 20 years and in most western countries the 5 year survival rates have been consistently under 10%. It is therefore fortunate that it is a relatively uncommon malignancy with a mean UK incidence of approximately 7.5 per 100 000 population; this translates into some 4000 deaths per annum. The significance of this malignancy lies in the major therapeutic challenge it poses, first from the magnitude of surgery required to excise the tumours and secondly the other techniques now available to relieve the patient's dysphagia.

44.1 EPIDEMIOLOGY

According to Schottenfeld (1984), the tumour is characterized by a large variation in its incidence in different parts of the world, among different ethnic groups and between males and females. It is a disease of the poor in most areas of the world. Among some populations major risk factors have been identified and the potential for prevention exists. The highest incidence in Europe occurs in the provinces of Normandy and Brittany. Higher incidences still occur in Transkei and East Africa, Northern China, and the highest reported incidence is in the Caspian littoral of Iran where the incidence reaches 260 per 100 000 population. In these areas of extremely high incidence, a 50 fold decrease in incidence occurs within a distance of a few hundred miles, suggesting the important role of environmental factors in aetiology.

44.2 AETIOLOGICAL FACTORS

44.2.1 RACE AND SEX

In multiracial areas, carcinoma of the oesophagus tends to be more common in blacks. In areas of high incidence in Northern China and Iran, the disease principally affects those of mongolian origin.

The malignancy is more common in males in most parts of the world. In high incidence areas, however, the incidence in females approaches or exceeds that in males. In Sweden, a higher proportion of oesophageal neoplasms in females were reported to occur in the upper third, a finding paralleled by Pearson's report from south-east Scotland. The female predominance and the geographical distribution of this unusual anatomical pattern was consistent with the concurrence of the Plummer–Vinson syndrome in these areas. In Mediterranean countries and those lying along the same latitude as India, a high oesophageal cancer incidence correlates significantly with high oral and pharyngeal cancer incidence suggesting a common aetiology.

44.2.2 ALCOHOL AND TOBACCO

No single environmental factor can account for the patterns of oesophageal cancer in all high incidence areas. In north America and western Europe, the major risk factors for oesophageal cancer are alcohol and tobacco which may account for about 80–90% of the cases each year. A dose–response relationship exists in that the relative risk increases with either the amount of alcohol consumed or tobacco smoked. Several prospective studies have noted that standardized mortality risk ratios for oesophageal cancer diminish after sustained smoking ceases.

44.2.3 DIET AND OTHER INGESTED SUBSTANCES

In many areas of high oesophageal cancer incidence such as Iran, soviet-central Asia and in parts of China, an aetiological role for a broad spectrum of nutritional deficiences has long been suspected (Watson, 1990). The association with dietary deficiency is consistent with the increased incidence of cancer of the oesophagus in low socio-economic groups.

The high incidence in certain parts of the world also reflects local habits and customs in relation to ingestion or inhalation of a wide variety of agents. In Iran and China where neither alcohol nor tobacco are relevant, opium smoking has been implicated, as are spices, bracken fern, betel nuts and cereals contaminated by the *Fusarium* species and fermented pickled vegetables. The last has been used to produce experimental oesophageal cancer in chicken.

The temperature of the ingested food also seems to be relevant in China, Singapore and Japan. In areas of highest incidence, the aetiology is probably multifactorial.

44.2.4 OTHER FACTORS

In Sweden, vulcanization workers have a ten fold increase in incidence of oesophageal cancer compared with matched controls.

There is little evidence of a strong genetic influence in the genesis of oesophageal cancer with the exception of sufferers from tylosis,

inherited and transmitted by an autosomal dominant gene.

44.3 PREMALIGNANT LESIONS

44.3.1 CORROSIVE STRICTURES

There have been several reports of squamous cell carcinoma developing many years after strictures caused by ingestion of caustic agents (Watson, 1990). These tend to occur 20–40 years after ingestion of the corrosive agent. It has been estimated that the presence of a corrosive stricture increases the likelihood of the development of a malignancy by 1000 fold. This is greater that any increased incidence reported due to other benign strictures causing stasis.

44.3.2 ACHALASIA

Chronic irritation due to stasis is considered the relevant aetiological factor for the development of carcinoma in this condition. The reported incidence varies between 2.8% and 4% (Watson, 1990). The tumours are squamous cell and can occur at all levels. Early treatment of achalasia has been advocated to prevent this although carcinomas have been known to occur after myotomy. Careful endoscopic surveillance of treated patients would therefore seem warranted. The co-existence of these two conditions may also occur by chance as they occur at a similar age and repeated biopsy may be necessary to eliminate malignancy in radiological cases of achalasia.

44.3.3 REFLUX STRICTURES

There is an increased incidence of oesophageal adenocarcinoma in patients with severe gastro-oesophageal reflux disease with, or without, reflux strictures (Moghissi, 1979), the likely mechanism being the presence of columnar metaplasia which is present in a large proportion of patients (Hill *et al.*,

1970). Surgical reflux control has been suggested as being protective (Watson, 1990), and if conservative management is opted for, regular surveillance and biopsy would seem indicated.

44.3.4 BARRETT'S OESOPHAGUS

Although originally described in 1950 as a congenitally short oesophagus, subsequent studies have clearly shown this condition to be acquired consequent to severe and long-standing gastro-oesophageal reflux (Bremner *et al.*, 1970). Barrett's oesophagus or more appropriately columnar epithelium lined oesophagus is associated with a high prevalence of oesophageal adenocarcinoma; the incidence is controversial and the risk has been estimated to vary from 1 in 56 per year of follow-up to 1 in 441 (Watson, 1990).

The controversy regarding the incidence of cancer has complicated the management and surveillance of this condition. In addition, there is no convincing evidence that regression occurs following successful antireflux treatment and development of adeno-carcinoma following successful antireflux treatment has been reported. Endoscopic surveillance following antireflux treatment has been recommended and evidence of dysplasia, particularly in male smokers, and columnar involvement of greater than 8 cm, should be taken as risk factors; high grade dysplasia is ominous and aneuploidy may be a sensitive indicator of malignant potential (Haggitt *et al.*, 1988). Prophylactic resection of the oesophagus has been recommended in patients with high grade dysplasia (Skinner, 1983). Many of these patients are found to have an adjacent focus of invasive carcinoma and the subsequent survival of such patients is significantly better than patients who are operated when symptomatic (Skinner, 1983).

In less florid cases, antireflux surgery and careful surveillance is recommended (Skinner, 1983).

44.4 PATHOLOGY

The oesophagus is only 20 cm in length from cricopharyngeal to oesophagogastric junction but is traditionally divided into thirds and the relative distribution of tumours within these segments of the oesophagus varies from series to series. Upper third lesions comprise 2–20% and remaining tumours are evenly distributed between the middle and lower thirds (Watson, 1990). The majority of tumours in the lower third are adenocarcinomas while tumours in the middle third are almost all squamous. Circumstantial evidence strongly suggests that long prodrome of mucosal epithelial alterations, i.e. dysplasia, atypical dysplasia and finally *in situ* carcinoma, precede the appearance of overt neoplasms (Mandard *et al.*, 1981; Fu Sheng *et al.*, 1982). In the high risk locales of China, where cytological screening is routinely performed, about half of the cases at the time of oesophagectomy are intra-epithelial neoplasms that occasionally show extension only to the submucosa, Foci of dysplasia are sometimes found at a distance from the cancerous lesion.

Morphologically, the tumours may appear as small grey mucosal plaques, but more often, they encircle the circumference of the oesophagus and simultaneously erode the submucosa. From this point, one of three gross morphological patterns emerges:

1. A fungating polypoid mass – 60%.
2. Ulcerating lesion that excavates into surrounding strictures – 25%.
3. A diffuse infiltrative tumour that causes thickening, rigidity and narrowing of the tumour with linear irregular ulcerations of the mucosa.

A large histological variety of primary oesophageal neoplasms has been reported:

1. Squamous cell carcinoma –
   Well differentiated
   Moderately differentiated
   Poorly differentiated

Spindle cell
Verrucous carcinoma
2. Adenocarcinoma
3. Adenoid cystic carcinoma
4. Mucoepidermoid carcinoma
5. Adenosquamous carcinoma
6. Carcinoid
7. Undifferentiated carcinoma
8. Small cell carcinoma
9. Basal cell carcinoma
10. Carcinoma (after Rosenberg *et al.*, 1985).

Ninety per cent of malignant oesophageal tumours are squamous cell carcinomas with varying degress of differentiation. The degree of differentiation has not been found to be of value in making a prognosis. Most of the remainder are adenocarcinomas beginning either in submucosal glands or in the metaplastic columnar epithelium of Barrett's oesophagus.

Oesophageal cancers are characterized by extensive local growth and lymph node involvement rather than early dissemination. Follow-up studies of early asymptomatic patients with *in situ* carcinoma have noted that it takes 3–4 years before advanced cancer develops (Guanrei *et al.*, 1982). The unique lymphatic drainage of the oesophagus and the long interval during which the tumour is asymptomatic account for extensive locoregional involvement. The absence of a serosal lining and the anatomical proximity to vital strictures are important contributors to non-resectability and poor prognosis.

Correlation exists between the length of the tumour and the extra-oesophageal spread and curability. When the tumour is smaller than 5 cm, 40% of specimens will demonstrate localized disease, 25% will be advanced locally and 35% will have distant spread or will be unresectable for cure. If the size exceeds 5 cm as determined by pathological examination, only 10% will be localized, 15% will be advanced locally and 75% will be beyond the limits of curative resection or will have distant disease.

Lymph node involvement carries a poor prognosis. A 5 year survival of 10–15% is reported following oesophagectomy when the lymph nodes are positive, and a survival two to three times these figures is obtained when these are not involved (Gunnlaugsson *et al.*, 1970).

44.5 CLINICAL PRESENTATION

The clinical presentation is usually with dysphagia but it must be stressed that difficulty in swallowing does not occur until the circumference of the oesophagus is narrowed to one-half to one-third the normal size. Pain radiating to the back on swallowing, dysphonia indicating laryngeal paralysis, diaphragmatic paralysis, evidence of tracheo-oesophageal fistula, the superior vena caval syndrome, palpable cervical lymph nodes in an intrathoracic growth and evidence of pleural effusion, ascites or bone pain are clinical indicators of unresectable disease.

Occasionally, a paraneoplastic syndrome is produced by an oesophageal tumour. Hypercalcaemia unrelated to bone involvement is the most common and gonadotropin and ACTH producing tumours have been described (Rosenberg *et al.*, 1985).

44.6 DIAGNOSIS

In a patient with advanced disease, the clinical presentation is unmistakable and diagnostic studies are confirmatory in nature. For earlier presentations the symptoms are minimal (Fu-Sheng *et al.*, 1982) and the level of suspicion should be high. Patients with symptoms related to the upper gastrointestinal tract, especially with onset of symptoms, in later life, need to be evaluated carefully. A plain chest radiograph is usually normal initially, and the initial diagnostic study of choice is the barium swallow; a double contrast study yields better results (Koehler *et al.*, 1976). Small carcinomas appear as sessile polyps or as focal areas of mucosal irregularities. The tumour tends to spread submucosally and if it encircles the entire wall, will present radiographically as a stricture with proximal dilatation. In the advanced stage it appears as an annular apple core lesion, a bulky mass, an irregular ulceration or an area of stricture that can have irregular or smooth margins (Dodds, 1988).

Endoscopy is performed for confirmation of diagnosis. Oesophageal cancer commonly infiltrates submucosally and the visual impression obtained at endoscopy may underestimate the true extent of the tumour. The mainstay of diagnosis remains the direct biopsy. Brushing for cytology is complementary and may increase the diagnostic yield. Because significant portions of the tumour may be submucosal, multiple biopsies should be taken and the endoscopist should be prepared to repeat the biopsy.

44.7   STAGING THE PATIENT

Before treating a patient with oesophageal carcinoma, several questions need to be answered: are metastases present; is the malignancy locally advanced so as to preclude resection; what is the status of the patient's cardiopulmonary function, and can the patient withstand an operation? Should radiotherapy be given as one attempt to cure, or as palliation with intubation, or combined with laser therapy?

As discussed the clinical features can provide important clues with respect to the local extent and metastatic involvement of a cancer of the oesophagus. Barium contrast studies are currently the best clinical method of determining the size of an oesophageal cancer and its extent of involvement, and may be complemented by CT. Attempts have been made to derive information from the oesophagogram with respect to resectability. The degree of deformity of the oesophagus produced by the tumour may be predictive of incurability (Akiyama, 1978). Between 75% and 80% of locally invasive tumours will have a deformed oesophageal axis with false-positive results in 10% of patients and false-negative results in 8% of locally invasive tumours (Akiyama, 1978).

CT is the best modality for staging but is not appropriate for screening. It can mistake a hiatus hernia for carcinoma and tends to underestimate the length of involvement of the oesophagus. It is also difficult to stage tumours located at the gastro-oesophageal junction.

The overall reported accuracy of staging by CT has varied from one study to another and ranges from 40% to more than 90%. In a critical review of literature, Halverson determined that CT was better in determining mediastinal invasion than in detecting lymph node metastasis. The sensitivity of detecting mediastinal invasion ranged form 88% to 94%, that of detecting involvement of the aorta, tracheobronchial tree and pericardium ranged from 94% to 97%. The sensitivity for detecting mediastinal adenopathy (48%) was less than that for abdominal nodes (61%). When a lymph node was enlarged, it had greater than 90% chance of being involved with metastatic tumour. CT can also diagnose liver (greater than 90%) and lung metastases. It is useful in planning if preoperative radiation with or without chemotherapy is being planned. It is certainly the method of choice for detecting local tumour recurrence and distant metastasis, post surgery.

Endoluminal ultrasound has assumed an important role in the staging of oesophageal tumours. the depth of invasion of the tumour and the presence of adenopathy may be elucidated transluminally. In a recent study by Tio *et al.* (1989), endosonography was able to identify the depth of penetration of the tumour correctly in 90% of 91 patients with oesophageal cancer. The study overstaged 6% and understaged 4% of these tumours, and was less successful in determining lymph node metastasis. Localized staging with endosonography is difficult after radiation therapy and may be impossible with stenotic lesions. It has been suggested that endo-luminal ultrasound is superior to CT scan-ning in the local staging of oesophageal carcinoma (Tio *et al.*, 1989).

The TNM and group staging criteria for oesophageal cancer were totally revised in 1987 (Gomes, 1992). The revised group staging scheme was based on a large Japanese study and separates regionally advanced from metastatic disease. The current staging system is close to that proposed by Skinner; the only two predictors of prognosis in this system were depth of wall (W) penetration and involvement of regional lymph nodes (N).

44.8   TREATMENT

Lack of progress in curative approaches has led to a great deal of pessimism and many oncologists emphasize palliation rather than cure. It is not necessary to separate objectives of management into palliation and cure; these two objectives can be integrated into a plan of management that may accomplish both. It is both futile and fruitless to attempt to define which therapeutic approach currently is most likely to result in cure. There are very few randomized comparisons of therapeutic approaches and comparison of published reports of a single institution's experience with one modality or another is hazardous and potentially misleading. Resection is con-sidered superior to radiation therapy in sur-gical literature (Oliver *et al.*, 1992). In the absence of prospective randomized trials to compare both modalities, this claim may not be valid. However, as the only treatment modality which has been repeatedly asso-ciated with prolonged survival in the litera-ture, albeit in a relatively small proportion of cases, resection is currently considered the treatment of choice in a fit patient with a rela-tively favourable tumour at least until the results of controlled clinical trials are known (Watson, 1990). In addition to allowing a small but definite cure rate, resection and

anastomosis usually mean permanent relief from dysphagia (Rosenberg *et al.*, 1985).

44.8.1   PREOPERATIVE CONSIDERATIONS

It is well recognized that eradication of the tumour is not the only problem facing the surgeon dealing with cancer of the oeso-phagus. In general terms surgery is a viable alternative provided the tumour is not too far advanced; obvious contraindications to use resection include distant metastasis or gross involvement of contiguous organs and extensive transmediastinal spread of tumour as determined by CT. The presence of enlarged nodes is not a contraindication to surgery (Watson, 1990) as these may not be metastatic, and there is no linear correlation between the presence of nodes and survival (Postlethwait, 1979).

In patients with operable tumours, Wong (1981) has shown the influence of age and intercurrent illness on operative mortality. Patients with significant cardiac and pul-monary insufficiency need to be excluded. It has also been shown that severe degrees of diabetes and impairment of renal and hepatic function are determinants of increased opera-tive mortality. Obviously each patient must be carefully evaluated. Statistics suggest that only about 30–40% of patients are selected for resection on the basis of this evaluation (Watson, 1990; Oliver *et al.*, 1992). While some patients unsuitable for surgery may be elig-ible for radical treatment using radio-therapy and/or chemotherapy, for the remaining majority, a palliative approach is appropriate; surgical heroism is undesirable as increases in resection rate are accompanied by a disproportionate increase in operative mortality (Ong *et al.*, 1978).

Most patients with oesophageal cancer are malnourished, anaemic and dehydrated. In an exhaustive review of the literature Chen *et al.*, (1991) documents the increase in protein synthesis and decrease in catabolism in these patients with nutritional support, all of which are biologically favourable to host viability. At this point, however, the data to support the premise that nutritional intervention in all patients with oesophageal cancer is clinically efficacious is lacking. However, if the patient has viable antineoplastic treatment options and has lost 10% of his pre-illness body weight and is hypoalbuminaemic, preoperative nutritional support needs to be seriously considered. The enteral route is preferable to total parenteral nutrition (TPN) because enteral nutrition has been shown to increase body weight and lead to positive nitrogen balance, and results of comparisons between TPN and enteral nutrition show marginal differences which do not lead to improved response rate and survival (Chen *et al.*, 1991).

The optimal duration of preoperative nutritional support is uncertain but most authorities would use it for a period of 7–10 days preoperatively. The nutritional support needs to be carried into the immediate postoperative period and can be conveniently given through the enteral route. Patients undergoing radiation and chemotherapy can also benefit from nutritional support when the appropriate patient population is selected (Chen *et al.*, 1991). Preoperative physiotherapy, prophylactic antibiotics, cessation of smoking and deep vein thrombosis prophylaxis are important adjuncts for successful outcome following surgery. The above measures, vigorously applied, account for the fact that at least 50% of patients with cancer of the oesophagus are presently considered operative candidates. While not all of these can be resected for cure (Oliver *et al.*, 1992), resection for cure or palliation may be possible in up to 90% (Rosenberg *et al.*, 1985).

44.8.2 SURGICAL THERAPY

Progress in anaesthesia, surgical care and operative techniques have led to a marked reduction in the rates of morbidity and mortality (Watson, 1990). Operative mortality rates of less than 5% are now commonly reported and rates less than 10% are the rule (Gomes, 1992). Controversy persists regarding the best surgical approach to this disease and strong arguments can be made for either transthoracic or extrathoracic oesophagectomies. The location and stage of the tumour are important factors in the choice of the surgical procedure and survival is probably determined by the stage of the tumour and its biological behaviour rather than the type of operation performed.

While the choice of operation is determined by the anatomical location of the tumour, the most important principle governing surgical therapy is determined by the unpredictable lymphatic drainage of the oesophagus (Gomes, 1992) and the pattern of submucosal spread of oesophageal cancer. Thus in one study of surgical specimens (Mandard *et al.*, 1981), 40% of oesophageal tumours in the upper third had metastasized to abdominal lymph nodes and 38% of tumours in the lower third had metastasized to cervical lymph nodes. This lymph node involvement can occur at some distance away from the site of the primary tumour and malignant cells can be found as far as 10 cm, from the primary tumour (Mandard *et al.*, 1981), thereby necessitating greater longitudinal clearance than normally practised in cancer surgery. It has only recently been suggested that this phenomenon of submucosal spread is primarily associated with distal oesophageal cancers (Wong, 1981). However, Watson *et al.* (1956) has adequately documented the case against segmental resection and Scanlon reported a 45% incidence of recurrence at the anastomotic site when segmental resection was performed. On the basis of available information, therefore, a resection that is less than subtotal may be inadequate and probably should not be attempted.

The other major consideration in determining operative approach and technique is the propensity of the intrathoracic anastomosis to leak because of the relatively poor blood supply of the oesophagus, the absence of a serous coat and high intraluminal pressures associated with swallowing. The complication of intrathoracic anastomotic leaks is devastating with a 50% or greater mortality and is the single greatest cause of mortality in many series (Ong *et al.*, 1978). This has led to the construction of the oesophagogastric anastomosis in the neck (Ong, 1969; McKeown, 1972) where the oesophageal blood supply is better and anastomotic leakage, although higher, is likely to be less serious. In addition, the procedure has the added advantage of achieving a wider longitudinal clearance. However, most of these benefits may be theoretical and the benefits may not be as great as we envisaged. Clinically significant anastomotic leakage from intrathoracic anastomosis is no longer a major problem (Watson, 1990); leaks from cervical anastomosis are well known to occur frequently into the mediastinum (Giuli *et al.*, 1986) and it has been shown that proximal clearance of 5–10 cm with an anastomosis at the apex of the mediastinum is accompanied by a very low rate of anastomotic recurrence (Watson, 1990).

A large number of operations have been described for oesophageal resection and excellent descriptions of operative techniques exist. These are described by Gomes (1992) and are briefly outlined below.

1. Ivor-Lewis (1946).
1a. Three stage oesophagectomy (McKeown, 1972).
2. Radical oesophagectomy (Skinner *et al.*, 1983).
3. Transhiatal oesophagectomy (Kirk, 1974; Orringer and Sloane, 1978).
4. Left thoracolaparotomy (Sweet, 1945).
5. Left sided subtotal oesophagectomy (Mathews and Steel, 1987).
6. Total pharyngolaryngectomy/total oesophagectomy for cervical, hypopharyngeal and upper third growths.

44.8.3 RECONSTRUCTION

Following oesophagectomy there are several options for restoration of gastrointestinal continuity, including the use of the entire stomach, a reversed or isoperistaltic gastric tube, colon or jejunal interposition. The subject has been brilliantly reviewed (Skinner, 1984) but the principal choice seems to lie between an isoperistaltic colonic segment or stomach for reconstruction. A jejunal segment is suitable for anastomosis below the aortic arch but spanning from the stomach to the base of the neck by the jejunum is difficult due to vascular anatomy, although this has been overcome by the use of microvascular anastomoses (Hester *et al.*, 1980).

The outcome of the anastomosis between the residual oesophagus and the replacement organ is a major factor in determining surgical morbidity and mortality. In reported series, leak rates of 15–30% are not uncommon (Skinner), although in recent years they have tended to be around 5%. The other important problem is the development of anastomotic strictures and these may be higher following use of mechanical stapling devices.

The results of surgical resection for oesophageal cancer are given in Table 44.1.

The parameters which have most attracted attention in the literature are the perioperative mortality and the 5 year survival (Beatty *et al.*, 1979). As already indicated, operative mortality varies greatly but Earlam and Cunha-Melo's review results cannot be taken to represent the outcome following surgery today (Earlam and Cunha-Melo, 1980a,b). Major British and American units with a special interest in oesophageal disease currently have a mortality of around 10% or less. It has been demonstrated (Belsey and Hiebert, 1974; Ong *et al.*, 1978) that operative mortality can exceed 40% when the majority of tumours are resected, emphasizing the importance of careful selection. Series from China (Huang, 1988) and Japan (Akiyama,

Table 44.1   Results of surgical resection for oesophageal cancer

Author	Year	Patients (no.)	Complication	Mortality	5 year survival (%)
Skinner	1983	80	52%	11%	18%
Orriger	1988	147	32%	6%	14%
Huang	1988	253 (Stage I)	NS	2.4%	89%
Wong	1988	189	NS	6%	30% at 3 yr
Shahian	1989	272	NS	4.6%	16%
Zhang	1986	973	NS	1.5%	19%
Lu	1987	1025	NS	4.9%	21%

After Games, 1992.

1978) with mortality of around 2% highlight the advantage of early detection. Long term survival in recent major western series vary between 10% and 20% at 5 years and are considerably less optimistic than the 96% 5 year survival reported in superficial lesions detected by screening (Huang, 1988). The major prognostic determinants are the depth of invasion and lymph node metastases. Adenocarcinoma have been thought to have an unfavourable prognosis but this may not be true (Hennessey, 1986).

44.8.4   RADIOTHERAPY

Radiation therapy of squamous cancers can be given with curative or palliative intent. While palliative treatment of adenocarcinoma is possible, curative radiotherapy should probably not be attempted for this tumour; combined modality approaches are discussed below.

A review of the literature (Hartar, 1992) suggests that using objective response data combined with symptomatic improvement, approximately 50% of patients will have relief of their dysphagia by radiotherapy lasting 2–6 months with little response in the other 50%.

For cervical and hypopharyngeal lesions curative irradiation is probably the treatment of choice. Radical surgical procedures in this region result in major functional impairment, with cure rates of 10–20%. Primary radiation

therapy series have produced similar results without the acute morbidity of surgery (Pearson, 1977; Lederman, 1966).

Recent literature confirming the results of irradiation alone is summarized in Table 44.2.

The modestly encouraging 20% 5 year survival reported by Pearson has not been duplicated and a paper updating the experience from Pearson's institution (Newaishy *et al.*, 1982) reveals substantial differences between the earlier and later series.

The theoretical advantage of radiotherapy in avoiding surgery is not borne out in literature. A 9% mortality has been reported (Cederquist *et al.*, 1978); continuing dysphagia is a problem needing dilatation or intubation and 20% are unable to complete treatment (Oliver *et al.*, 1992). Radiation toxicity and complications are substantial (Harter, 1992).

There are no direct comparisons between surgery and radiotherapy as far as survival is concerned. Since most patients with potentially operable disease do indeed undergo exploration, radiation series are probably heavily biased with poor risk patients. Data from Earlam and Cunha-Melo's (1981b) review would suggest that radiation may not be significantly worse than surgery as far as long term survival is concerned; palliation of dysphagia is probably not as good, although the recent development of intracavitary irradiation may overcome this problem (Rowland and Pagliero, 1985).

Table 44.2 Results of irradiation of oesophageal cancer (after Harter, 1992)

Author	Year	Patients (no.)	Dose (Gy)	5 year survival
Okawa	1989	288	6000–7000	T< 5 cm, 18% T 5–10 cm, 10% T > 10 cm, 3%
Steven and Stout	1988	108	6000– 6600	8%
Hyden	1988	33	5000 Ext. 2000 Brachy	Stage I/II, 12% Stage III/IV, 0%
Harrison	1988	99	6000–6600	6%

44.8.5 CHEMOTHERAPY

A number of single drugs and combinations have now been evaluated at least in preliminary fashion (Kelsen, 1984). It must be pointed out that almost all of these trials have been performed in patients with a Karnofsky performance status of 50 or better. Aggressive multidrug therapy is probably not indicated in severely ill patients.

Using multidrug treatment, cisplatin being the most common determinant, response rates of 40–50% have been achieved with reasonably well tolerated toxicities. The median duration of response (7 months), while still unsatisfactory, appears to be longer than that seen with most single agents. It should be emphasized that there are currently no randomized trials demonstrating the superiority of combination chemotherapy over single agents, nor is it clear whether one combination is superior to another. It is hoped that in future the role of combination chemotherapy as palliation for advanced disease, and as part of multimodality approaches, will be clarified. Until then, use of these agents should still be considered investigational.

44.8.6 CHEMOTHERAPY AND RADIATION WITHOUT SURGERY

A number of patients will either refuse surgery, will have medical contraindications or will have extensive locoregional disease considered unresectable on preoperative evaluation or occasionally at exploration (Kelsen, 1991). Attempts have been made to treat these patients with chemotherapy and radiotherapy. There are two current approaches. One involves chemotherapy followed by definitive radiotherapy. The second involves concurrent chemotherapy and radiotherapy (CT-RT). The ECOG study using the second approach has reported a survival advantage for the CT-RT arm as compared to radiotherapy alone. Similar results have been reported by the RTOG group. Morbidity was significant and treatment related death has been reported. Recently an intergroup prospective randomized trial comparing radiotherapy alone with concomitant radiotherapy and chemotherapy reported significant benefit from the combined modality approach. Radiotherapy was 64 Gy give in 2 Gy fractions over 6.5 weeks. The chemotherapy consisted of 4 courses of 5-fluorouracil (1 g/m^2 per day for 4 days) and cisplatin (75 mg/m^2 on first day); radiotherapy was given to a dose of 50 Gy in the combined modality arm. There was a significantly higher survival in patients treated with combined chemotherapy and radiotherapy, though the combined treatment arm was more toxic. An update reported 3/62 (5%) of patients on radiotherapy to be alive as compared to 20/61 (33%) of those treated with chemotherapy and radiotherapy. Contrary results have also been published showing little advantage over radiation alone (Kelsen, 1984).

There is little objective data for patients treated with chemotherapy followed by radiation. Most studies have not analysed failure patterns and median durations of survival are comparable to those seen with radiation therapy alone with occasional long term survival.

44.8.7 COMBINATION THERAPY (KELSEN, 1991)

The prognosis for patients treated with surgery or radiation therapy alone is poor and has led to the combination of various therapeutic modalities with an aim to improve success. There are several theoretical advantages including the down staging of tumour, thereby increasing resection rates, the control of micrometastases and the ablation of residual disease following resection for locally advanced tumours.

Autopsy studies indicate that in western patients oesophageal cancer is a disseminated disease at the time of diagnosis, systemic metastases are common and the local failure rate is high despite resection.

The most widely used combined modality technique has been preoperative radiation. The rationale for using this approach is that radiation may decrease tumour bulk, thereby increasing resection rates and can also treat peri-oesophageal disease. However, radiation therapy is a treatment of localized disease and does not address the risks of systemic failure.

Several preoperative radiation studies involving substantial number of patients have been performed (Kelsen, 1991). The majority of these trials are single arm, non-randomized studies using a historical control group. Three prospective randomized studies involving radiation therapy alone prior to operation have now been reported (Kelsen, 1991). There seem to be no differences in the percentage of patients who underwent exploration, resectability rate, operative mortality or survival. Although the uncontrolled trials have suggested a beneficial effect on resection rates and short term survival, this has not been confirmed by prospective studies and data to date suggest that preoperative radiation therapy should still be considered an investigational tool.

Postoperative radiation in the patient with resectable disease has not been systematically studied. Although small studies suggest a benefit, it is difficult to recommend the routine use of postoperative radiation for patients who are grossly free of disease at the end of the operative procedure. For residual tumour, the role of radiotherapy is again uncertain.

Phase II studies involving the use of chemotherapy alone prior to surgery have been reviewed in detail (Kelsen, 1991). A single phase III trial comparing surgery with adjuvant chemotherapy and surgery suggested that patients responding to preoperative chemotherapy had a substantial improvement in median survival (Kelsen, 1991). Further studies are needed, but since chemotherapy is efficacious for regression of localized disease as well as for systemic metastases, it seems logical to pursue chemotherapy in combined modality programmes. Preoperative chemotherapy and radiation prior to attempted resection has theoretical advantages, first in that drugs may act as radiation sensitizers and second that the chemotherapy will be effective against disease outside the radiated part. In the studies reported (Watson, 1990), although many patients had no residual tumour at the time of surgery, and operative mortality was low, no overall survival advantage could be claimed. There is evidence, however, that chemotherapy and radiation is superior to radiation alone (Kelsen, 1991). Certainly preoperative chemotherapy can be performed safely, is capable of inducing tumour regression in 50–60% of patients and does not increase morbidity or mortality. There are no data addressing the issue of purely postoperative adjuvant chemotherapy. A large scale intergroup trial is now underway to address the issue of pre- and postoperative chemotherapy for operable cancers, and more studies are urgently needed to resolve this issue.

44.8.8 PALLIATIVE THERAPY

The main aim of palliation for advanced oesophageal cancer is to restore nutritional function by relieving or bypassing the tumour, thereby improving malnutrition. Additional problems confronting the physician are chest pain and the development of broncho-oesophageal fistula. The role of chemotherapy and radiotherapy, both alone and in combination, has already been alluded to and will not be considered any further.

(a) Palliation

Until recently almost all discussions on the management of the disease have centred around maximizing survival time. As Oliver *et al.* (1992) has shown, this debate is irrelevant in the management of two-thirds of the patients. In the past decade, options for palliation have proliferated (Quinton and Lamouliatte, 1992).

A variety of intubation techniques have been used but the two most common procedures in the UK are intubation at laparotomy using a Celestin tube or the more popular fibre-optic endoscopic intubation. Procedure related mortality are similar for both techniques, as shown in the UK Thoracic Surgical Register, and both techniques should be available for continuity of care. The quality of palliation is reasonable (Watson, 1990). The intubation technique is also occasionally useful for patients with fistulas, with persistent dysphagia after radiotherapy and where local recurrence complicates surgical resection.

The increasing use of laser in palliating oesophageal carcinoma has been the subject of several reports (Quinton and Lamouliatte, 1992). The quality of palliation is good

although multiple treatments may be necessary and perforation is a risk. It is also expensive and its greatest role would appear to be in patients with failed or intubation tube blockage or proximal tumours which preclude intubation.

Surgical bypass although popular in the USA and the Far East has declined in popularity in the UK, following the development of intubation and laser techniques. Though surgical bypass gives a quality of palliation comparable to resection, it has a high operative mortality (Watson, 1990), and the only indication for it seems to be in patients found to be inoperable at exploration and in occasional patients with tracho-oesophageal fistulas. Intermittent endoscopic dilatation has been recommended as a palliative procedure, alone or combined with laser treatment. Recurrent dysphagia, however, occurs rapidly and the procedure needs to be repeated frequently, providing poor palliation. The patient with cancer pain may need to be treated in the setting of a pain clinic.

44.9 ADENOCARCINOMA

Much of the above discussion also applies to this histological variant which seems to be increasing in frequency (Oliver *et al.*, 1992). Surgically they are treated exactly as epidermoid tumours. Their response to radiation therapy has not been well established, although palliation may be possible. In the UK most surgeons do not use preoperative radiation therapy for adenocarcinoma. As the tumour often involves the upper third of the stomach, this organ is not available for reconstruction if a high resection is performed and will not thus allow a cervical anastomosis. The Ivor Lewis operation remains the basic operation for oesophagogastric adenocarcinoma (Faintuch *et al.*, 1984).

Although thought to have a poorer survival than the squamous cell variant, it probably has a survival similar to squamous cell carcinoma (Faintuch *et al.*, 1984; Hennessey, 1986).

44.10 SCREENING FOR OESOPHAGEAL CANCER

In geographical areas where there is a high risk of oesophageal cancer, analysis of cells obtained from the oesophagus has been used effectively to detect early lesions. This has been demonstrated on a large scale in studies from China. Using abrasive balloon cytology techniques (Fu-Sheng *et al.*, 1982), 75% of the cancers detected were early lesions with 5 year survivals exceeding 90%. Endoscopic follow-up indicates that dysplastic changes in the oesophageal mucosa are a common precursor of malignancy. This takes place over many years allowing a reasonable time for screening. Areas like the UK have a low incidence of disease and do not justify mass screening. However, there are smaller groups at risk where selective screening by cytology and endoscopic biopsy is recommended, usually every 1–3 years (Table 44.3, below).

In any of these groups where oesophageal biopsy reveals dysplasia, particularly graded severe, more frequent endoscopic surveillance is indicated. Careful inspection and systematic tissue sampling at 6 monthly intervals would seem most prudent with this finding, and persistence of severe dysphagia during the period of surveillance should warrant consideration of the use of surgical options.

REFERENCES

Akiyama, H.(1978) Surgery for carcinoma of the oesophagus. *Current Problems in Surgery*, **17**.

Beatty, J.D., DeBoer, G. and Rider, W.D. (1979) Carcinoma of the oesophagus: pretreatment assessment, correlation of radiation treatment parameters with survival, and identification and management of radiation treatment failure. *Cancer*, **43**, 2254–67.

Belsey, R. and Hiebert, C.A. (1974) An exclusive right thoracic approach for cancer of the middle third of the oesophagus. *Annals of Thoracic Surgery*, **18**, 1–15.

Bremner, C.G., Lynch, V.P. and Ellis, F.H. (1970) Barrett's oesophagus: Congenital or acquired; an experimental study of oesophageal mucosal regeneration in the dog. *Surgery*, **68**, 209–16.

Cederquist, C., Nielsen, J., Berthelsen A., *et al.* (1978) Cancer of the oesophagus II therapy and outcome. *Acta Chirurgica Scandinavica*, **144**, 233–40.

Chen, M.K., Souba, W.W. and Copeland, E.M. III (1991) Nutritional support of the surgical oncology patient. *Hematology/Oncology Clinics of North America*, **5**, 125–6.

Dodds, W.J. (1988) Radiology-oesophageal tumours, in *Alimentary Tract Radiology*, (eds A.R. Margulies and H.J. Burhenne), C.V. Mosby, St Louis, pp. 481–99.

Earlam, R. and Cunha-Melo, J.R., (1980a) Oesophageal squamous cell carcinoma I: A critical review of surgery. *British Journal of Surgery*, **67**, 381–90.

Earlam, R. and Cunha-Melo, J.R. (1980b) Oesophageal squamous cell carcinoma II: A critical review of radiotherapy. *British Journal of Surgery*, **67**, 457–61.

Faintuch, J., Shepard, K.V. and Levin, B. (1984) Adenocarcinoma and other unusual variants of oesophageal cancer. *Seminars in Oncology*, **11**, 196–202.

Fu Sheng, L., Ling Li and Song-Liang Qu (1982) Clinical and pathological characteristics of

Table 44.3 Screening of groups at risk from oesophageal cancer

Group	Risk (%)
Tylosis	95
Achalasia	1.7–8.2
Lye strictures	3.5–5.5
Plummer–Vinson syndrome	?
Coeliac disease	3
Head and neck cancer	2–4
Barrett's oesophagus	2–10

early oesophageal cancer. *Clinical Oncology*, **1**, 539–58.

Gomes, N.M. (1992) Oesophageal cancer: surgical approach, in *Gastro-intestinal Oncology*, (eds J.D. Ahlgren and J.S. Macdonald), J.B. Lippincott, Philadelphia, pp. 89–121.

Giuli, R. and Sancho-Garnier, H. (1986) Diagnostic, therapeutic and prognostic features of cancer of the oesophagus: results of the international prospective study conducted by the OESO group. *Surgery*, **99** (5), 614–22.

Guanrei, Y., He, H., Sunghong, Q and Yuning, C. (1982) Endoscopic diagnosis of 115 cases of early oesophageal carcinoma. *Endoscopy*, **14**, 157–61.

Gunlaugsson, G.H., Wychulis, A.R., Roland, C. and Ellis, F.H. (1970) Analysis of the record of 1675 patients with carcinoma of the oesophagus and cardia of the stomach. *Surgery, Gynecology and Obstetrics*, **130**, 997–1013.

Haggitt, R.C., Reid, B.J. and Rabinovitch P.S. (1988) Barrett's oesophagus: correlation between mucin histochemistry, flow cytometry, and histologic diagnosis for predicting increased cancer risk. *American Journal of Pathology*, **131**, 53–61.

Harter, W.K. (1992) Oesophageal cancer: management with radiation, in *Gastrointestinal Oncology*, (eds J.D. Ahlgren and J.S. Macdonald), J.B. Lippincott, Philadelphia, pp. 123–34.

Hennessey, T.P.J. (1986) Tumours of the oesophagus, in *Surgery of the Oesophagus*, (eds T.P.J. Hennessey and A. Cusehiere), Baillière-Tindall, London, pp. 307–57.

Hester, T., MConnel, F., Nahia, F, *et al*. (1980), Reconstruction of cervical oesophagus, hypopharynx and oral cavity using free jejunal transfer. *American Journal of Surgery*, **140**, 487–91.

Hill, L.D., Gelfard, M. and Bauermeister, D. (1970) Simplified management of reflux oesophagitis with stricture. *Annals of Surgery*, **172**, 638–46.

Huang, G.J. (1988) Recognition and treatment of the early lesion, in *International Trends in General Thoracic Surgery: oesophageal cancer*, Vol 4, (eds N.C. Delarue, E.W. Wilkins and C.J. Wang), C.V. Mosby, St Louis, pp. 146–66.

Kelsen, D. (1984) Chemotherapy of oesophageal cancer. *Seminars in Oncology*, **11**, 159–68.

Kelsen, D. (1991) Adjuvant therapy of upper gastro-intestinal tumours. *Seminars in Oncology*, **18**, 543–9.

Koehler, R.E., Moss, A.A. and Margulies, A.R. (1976) Early radiographic manifestations of carcinoma of the oesophagus. *Radiology*, **119**, 1–5.

Lederman, M. (1966) Carcinoma of the oesophagus, with special reference to the upper third: Part I, Clinical Considerations. *British Journal of Radiology*, **39**, 193–204.

Mandard, A.M., Chasle, J., Marnay, J. *et al*. (1981) Autopsy findings in 111 cases of oesophageal cancer. *Cancer*, **48**, 329–35.

Mathews, H.R. and Steel A. (1987) Left-sided subtotal oesophagecotomy for carcinoma. *British Journal of Surgery*, **79**, 1115–17.

McKeown, K.C. (1972) Trends in oesophageal resection for carcinoma. *Annals of the Royal College of Surgeons of England*, **57**, 213–38.

Moghissi, K. (1979) Conservative surgery in reflux stricture of the oesophagus associated with hiatus hernia. *British Journal of Surgery*, **76**, 221–5.

Newaishy, G.A., Read, G.A., Duncan, W. and Kerr, G.R. (1982) Results of radical radiotherapy of squamous cell carcinoma of the oesophagus. *Clinical Radiology*, **33**, 347–52.

Ong, G.B., Lam, K.H. and Wong, J. (1978) Factors influencing morbidity and mortality in oesophageal carcinoma. *Journal of Thoracic Cardiovascular Surgery*, **76**, 745–9.

Oliver, S.E., Robertson, C.S. and Logan, R.A.F.A. (1992) Oesophageal cancer: a population based study of survival after treatment. *British Journal of Surgery*, **79**, 1321–4.

Orringer, M.B. and Sloan, H. (1978) Oesophagectomy without thoracotomy. *Journal of Thoracic and Cardiovascular Surgery*, **76**, 643–51.

Pearson, J.G. (1977) The present status and future potential of radiotherapy in the management of oesophageal cancer. *Cancer*, **39**, 882–90.

Postlethwait, R.W. (1979) *Surgery of the Oesophagus*, Appleton-Century-Crofts, New York, pp. 341–414.

Quinton, A. and Lamouliatte, J. (1992) Laser applications in gastrointestinal cancer, in *Gastrointestinal Oncology*, (eds J.D. Ahlgren and J.S. Macdonald), J.B. Lippincott, Philadelphia, pp. 593–605.

Rosenberg, J.C., Roth, J.A. Lichter, A.S. and the oesophagus, in V.T. DeVita, (eds V.T. DeVita Jr, S. Hellman and S.A. Rosenberg), *Cancer Principles and Practice of Oncology*, J.B. Lippincott, Philadelphia, pp. 621–57.

Rowland, C.G. and Pagliero, K.M. (1985) Intracavitary irradiation in palliation of carcinoma of oesophagus and cardia. *Lancet*, **ii** 981–2.

Schottenfeld, D. (1984) Epidemiology of cancer of the oesophagus. *Seminars in Oncology*, **11**, 92–100.

Skinner, D.B. (1983) Enbloc resection for neoplasms of the oesophagus and cardia. *Journal of Thoracic and Cardiovascular Surgery*, **85**, 59–71.

Skinner, D.B. (1984) Surgical treatment for oesophageal carcinoma, *Seminars in Oncology*, **11**, 136–43.

Skinner, D.B. Walther, B.C. and Riddell, R.H. (1983) Barrett's oesophagus: comparison of benign and malignant cases. *Annals of Surgery*, **198**, 554–65.

Sweet, R.H. (1945) Transthoracic resection of the oesophagus and stomach for carcinoma: analysis of post-operative complications, causes of death and late results of operation. *Annals of Surgery*, **121**, 272–84.

Tio, T.L., Cohen, P., Coene, P.P. *et al.* (1989) Endosonography and computed tomography of oesophageal carcinoma: preoperative classification compared to the new (1987) T.N.M. system. *Gastroenterology*, **96**, 1478–86.

Watson, A. (1990) Carcinoma of the oesophagus, in *Surgical Oncology*, (eds C.S. McArdle), Butterworth, London, pp. 1–27.

Watson, W.L., Goodner, J.T., Miller, T.P. and Pack, G.T. (1956) Torek oesophagectomy: the case against segmental resection for oesophageal cancer, *Journal of Thoracic Surgery*, **32**, 347–57.

Wong, J. (1981) Management of carcinoma of the oesophagus: art or science? *Journal of the Royal College of Surgeons of Edinburgh*, **26**, 138–48.

PRIMARY LIVER AND BILE DUCT CANCER AND LIVER METASTASES

Dermot Burke and T.G. Allen-Mersh

45.1 PRIMARY LIVER CANCER (HEPATOCELLULAR CARCINOMA)

45.1.1 EPIDEMIOLOGY

Hepatocellular carcinoma is rare in Western Europe and the USA, the annual incidence being 1–2 per 100 000 population (Murray-Lyon, 1990). In Africa and South East Asia the incidence is about 20–30 times greater. In low incidence areas the disease is associated with cirrhosis in 80% of cases and is common in the 5th and 6th decades (Nagasue *et al.*, 1984). In high incidence areas the disease usually occurs two decades earlier and is associated with chronic liver disease secondary to Hepatitis B infection.

The natural carcinogen aflatoxin is also associated with hepatocellular carcinoma. This toxin is a product of the aspergillus fungus. The fungus thrives in hot, humid conditions and may commonly be seen as a white layer on the surface of stored rice. In Africa, the incidence of hepatocellular carcinoma correlates well with the data on aflatoxin contamination of food stuffs.

45.1.2 CLINICAL FEATURES

Presenting symptoms are usually abdominal pain and malaise. Unfortunately these symptoms are common in those with chronic liver disease. It is not until progressive jaundice or hepatomegaly occurs that the diagnosis is made. Thus, presentation occurs late in the course of the disease. The tumour presents as either a single mass or as multifocal nodules in the liver. Metastases are common. They present in the lung in 45% and in lymph nodes in 35% of cases (Liver Cancer Study Group of Japan, 1984). Untreated, it is rapidly fatal. Although survival to 14 months has been reported, the mean time from onset of symptoms to death in untreated cases is 4 months (Nagasue *et al.*, 1984).

45.1.3 SCREENING

As the disease is renowned for presenting at a late stage, attempts are now being made to screen high risk patients. If the tumours are detected while still small, then curative treatment should be possible. The following methods are used in screening.

(a) Alpha-fetoprotein (αFP)

In areas where hepatocellular carcinoma has a high incidence, attempts have been made to diagnose tumours at an earlier stage, by screening those at high risk. For patients with chronic active hepatitis screening using serum αFP levels and hepatic ultrasound is done every 3–6 months (Liaw *et al.*, 1986). Serum αFP is a relatively specific marker for hepatocellular carcinoma, but may be normal in up to 30% of those with tumours (Kubo *et al.*, 1978). For this reason it should not be used as the sole screening test. Despite diagnosing and treating tumours at an earlier stage, an increase in survival has not been seen using these methods.

The diagnosis is usually made clinically when a patient with chronic liver disease develops an abdominal mass or abdominal pain. For this reason, investigations are only used either to confirm clinical suspicions or to determine the extent of the disease.

45.1.4 INVESTIGATIONS

(a) Serum αFP

This helps to confirm the diagnosis in about 70% of cases. It may also be raised in testicular cancer.

(b) Ultrasound scan

Even if the liver is cirrhotic, this will show a space occupying lesion. In one series ultrasound detected over 80% of those lesions that were less than 3 cm in size (Nagasue *et al.*, 1987).

(c) Liver biopsy

This is not generally necessary as the diagnosis is usually obvious. It may be used in cases of doubt, but there is a risk that the procedure will spread malignant cells outside the liver capsule.

(a)

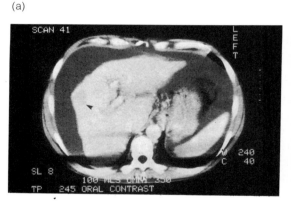

(b)

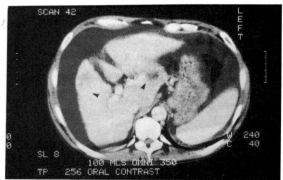

(c)

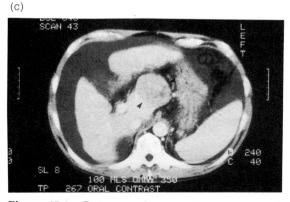

Figure 45.1 Contrast enhanced CT scan of a cirrhotic liver. A hepatoma is shown in the caudate lobe (**(a)**, **(b)**, arrowed). A satellite lesion is seen in the lateral aspect of the right lobe (**(c)**, arrowed). There is considerable ascites within the peritoneal cavity. (Courtesy of Dr J. Karani, King's College Hospital, London.)

Once the diagnosis is made, further investigation is necessary to determine whether or not the tumour is operable.

(d)   CT scan (Figure 45.1)

This will demonstrate the tumour's spread within the liver. Abdominal CT scan will reveal any intra-abdominal spread or diaphragmatic involvement. A CT scan of the thorax is necessary if pulmonary metastases are suspected.

(e)   Angiography (Figure 45.2)

This is the most useful and most accurate investigation in determining the resectability of the tumour. Selective angiography via the coeliac and superior mesenteric vessels reveals a hypervascular lesion in 90% of cases (Trede *et al.*, 1986). The venous phase of the angiogram is important because invasion of the portal vein will be seen as a filling defect. This will preclude surgery.

Small satellite tumours may be missed by these methods. It is unfortunate if these remain undiscovered until laparotomy, as they may make the tumour inoperable. Arteriography with ultrafluid Lipiodol injection, followed by CT scan 10–15 days later, is said to be a very sensitive method for detecting these small tumours (Belghiti, 1991).

45.1.4   CURATIVE TREATMENT

The only curative treatment is complete resection of all malignant tissue. No other treatment has yet demonstrated a survival benefit.

Unfortunately, most tumours are too advanced to be considered operable. Between 10% and 20% are thought to be operable before surgery (Ong and Chaw, 1976; Murray-Lyon, 1990). Despite thorough preoperative investigation, many of these tumours are actually more extensive at operation. In one series only 40% of tumours resected had a disease free margin (Bismuth *et al.*, 1992). As much information as possible should be gained before surgery. Recently, intra-operative ultrasound scan has become available. It can detect nodules as small as 0.5 cm in size and so is invaluable in detecting lesions that my otherwise be missed.

Resectability depends on:

1. The extent of tumour growth.
2. The functional capacity of the diseased liver.
3. The patient's general condition.

(a)   Tumour growth

The following are indications for surgery (Lin *et al.*, 1987; Bismuth *et al.*, 1992):

1. No evidence of distal metastases.
2. No involvement of the hepatic artery or portal vein.
3. Unilobar distribution of tumour.
4. Tumour less than 5 cm in size.
5. Three or fewer separate tumours.

(b)   Hepatic function

Up to four segments of an otherwise healthy liver may be resected and compensatory regrowth will occur (Okamoto *et al.*, 1984).

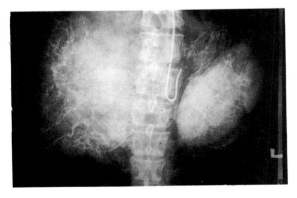

Figure 45.2   Angiogram of a hepatoma. Contrast agent is seen throughout the tumour, demonstrating its vascular nature.

However a cirrhotic liver is less capable of re-generation and, following resection, hepatic failure may occur. Therefore it is important to assess hepatic function preoperatively.

In cirrhotic patients, liver function is tradi-tionally assessed by Child's classification. However, if surgery is contemplated, it is useful to have a more exact measure of hepatic functional capacity. One such measure is the indocyanine green retention time (ICG R_{15}) (Okamoto *et al.*, 1984). The urea-nitrogen synthesis rate (UUN) may also be used (Paquet *et al.*, 1991). Postoperative morbidity and mortality are reduced in the following circumstances:

1. Child's classification B or C
2. No jaundice
3. No ascites
4. ICG R_{15} less than 10%
5. UUN at least 6 g/day.

(c)   Patient's general condition

The patient's performance status at pre-sentation is a good indicator of likely outcome (Falkson *et al.*, 1978). Those with a poor performance status have a bad prog-nosis. Any concurrent illnesses, e.g. diabetes, ischaemic heart disease, lessen the chances of a successful outcome.

(d)   Morbidity and mortality

Complications of surgery include: hepatic failure, biliary leaks, jaundice, ascites and oedema. The latter three are more common in cirrhotic patients (Lin *et al.*, 1987).

Reported mortality rates vary, but should now be reduced to below 5% (Lin *et al.*, 1987). Careful patient selection can reduce mortality to 0% (Ikeda *et al.*, 1993). Postoperative death is due to hepatic failure, gastrointestinal haemor-rhage or tumour cachexia (Liver Cancer Study Group of Japan, 1984; Lin *et al.*, 1987).

(e)   Follow-up after surgery

Regular monitoring with serum αFP and hepatic ultrasound should be employed.

Reported recurrence rates vary from 70% to 100% (Lin *et al.*, 1987; Belghiti, 1991). It is un-certain whether the recurrence is due to growth of residual disease or growth of a new tumour. The former is thought more proba-ble.

(f)   Transplantation

This is controversial. However, there is a definite benefit to the patient when a tumour is discovered incidentally in a diseased liver that is being transplanted for a non-malignant con-dition (Iwatsuki *et al.*, 1985). If transplantation is used to enable a large, otherwise un-resectable tumour, to be resected, then no benefit is seen. In this latter case, the operative mortality rate is 30%. If the patient survives the operation, recurrence occurs in 74%.

45.1.5   PALLIATIVE TREATMENT

Palliative treatment is the only treatment possible in 80–90% of cases. It is used if the tumour is unresectable, or the patient is too ill for surgery. There are now a wide variety of techniques available.

(a)   Surgery

This may be used to provide pain relief or to debulk the tumour. With the introduction of less invasive techniques, it is used less frequently.

(b) Chemotherapy

This has had little success. The following agents have all been used:

5-Fluorouracil (5-FU
Methotrexate   } in combination (Choi
                        et al., 1984)

Cyclophosphamide
Vincristine

                       } alone and in
Streptozotocin   combination with
Methyl-CCNU   5-FU (Falkson *et al.*,
                       1978)

Cisplatin   (Epstein *et al.*, 1991)
Adriamycin   (Sciarrino *et al.*, 1985)

The most successful approach has been with adriamycin as sole agent. It is given at a dose of 60 mg/m^2 intravenously every 3 weeks. The maximum cumulative dose is 450 mg/m^2, as it is cardiotoxic (Sciarrino *et al.*, 1985). It stimulated appetite and stabilized weight in 18% of patients in this series. Unfortunately, alopecia occurs in most patients. Other side-effects include: nausea, vomiting, mucositis and leukopenia. More recently it has been given in combination with the carrier Lipiodol via the hepatic artery (Katagari *et al.*, 1989). This technique is currently being evaluated. If, after 3 doses, there is no response to adriamycin, then further doses should not be give. A response is unlikely and toxic effects will occur (Sciarrino *et al.*, 1985).

(c) Radiotherapy

Hepatocytes are radiosensitive. Thus external beam irradiation of the liver is dose-limited. The healthy liver can tolerate 20–35 Gy, but this will cause hepatic failure in the cirrhotic liver (Novell *et al.*, 1991). Thus internal irradiation, which reduces the dose delivered to non-malignant hepatocytes, is used.

Iridium-192 wires can be implanted in the tumour either at laparotomy or transhepatically (Novell *et al.*, 1991). Yttrium-90 has been combined with microspheres for regional infusion. Unfortunately, yttrium accumulates in bone marrow, to which it is toxic. Iodine-131 incorporated into Lipiodol, which is selectively retained by hepatic tumours, has been shown to reduce symptoms (Bretagne *et al.*, 1988).

(d) Percutaneous ethanol injection therapy

Using ultrasound guidance, ethanol can be injected into and around the tumour. It can destroy tumours less than 3 cm in size (Shiina *et al.*, 1990). It is relatively non-invasive, but

causes pain and an elevation of liver enzymes due to tumour necrosis.

(e) Embolization

Particles can be injected via the hepatic artery. Microspheres, and gelatin sponge particles have been used. The latter have been combined with adriamycin to produce a partial response rate of 72% (Ikeda *et al.*, 1991). Side-effects, due to hepatic ischaemia, include nausea, vomiting and abdominal pain.

(f) Laser hyperthermia

Using ultrasound guidance and the Nd : YAG laser, small tumours can be destroyed. As laparotomy is not needed, the technique is relatively non-invasive (Masters *et al.*, 1991).

(g) Cryotherapy

This involves liquid nitrogen at –196°C. It requires a laparotomy.

45.2 PRIMARY BILE DUCT CANCER (CHOLANGIOCARCINOMA)

Epidemiology

Carcinoma of the bile duct is rare, with an incidence of 0.01–0.46% at post-mortem (Sako *et al.*, 1957). It has a peak incidence in the seventh and eighth decades and is equally common in the sexes. It is classified into intra- and extrahepatic lesions.

45.2.1 INTRAHEPATIC LESIONS

These present with abdominal pain, jaundice and hepatomegaly. They are locally invasive. They are managed in the same way as hepatocellular carcinoma except that the patients do not have chronic liver disease. They have a poor prognosis, with a survival time of 3–6 months from diagnosis.

45.2.2   EXTRAHEPATIC LESIONS

(a)   Clinical features

Cholangiocarcinoma presents with obstructive jaundice in 90% of patients. This is frequently associated with abdominal pain and hepatomegaly (Gibby *et al.*, 1985). It is locally invasive and rarely metastasizes. However, as it invades the liver, portal vein and hepatic arteries at an early stage, it is rarely curable.

(b)   Investigations

Serology

Bilirubin, alkaline phosphatase and aspartate transferase are raised. Serum albumin is usually normal.

Ultrasound scan

This is the first investigation in jaundiced patients. It shows biliary duct dilatation, the level of which indicates the level of the obstruction. The latter has therapeutic implications. It may show a mass.

CT scan

This is complementary to ultrasound. It may provide more accurate information about tumour extent. CT scan of the abdomen and thorax is useful in demonstrating metastases. The proximal extent of the tumour has important implications for therapy. Investigations should therefore be continued until the full extent of the tumour is known.

Percutaneous transhepatic cholangiography (PTC) (Figure 45.3)

This is the investigation of choice for evaluating the growth of high bile duct tumours. It shows characteristic signs of malignancy in 100% of cases (Gibby *et al.*, 1985).

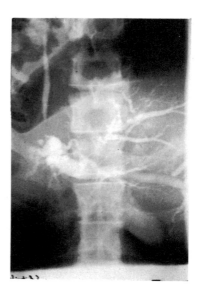

Figure 45.3 Percutaneous transhepatic cholangiogram showing a cholangiocarcinoma obstructing the common bile duct. The right hepatic duct is grossly dilated above the tumour, but contrast can still be seen in the common hepatic duct.

Endoscopic retrograde cholangiopancreatography (ERCP)

This is useful for low tumours. A biopsy may be taken or cells taken for cytology. This will distinguish a carcinoma of the ampulla of Vater from a cholangiocarcinoma (Stain *et al.*, 1992). If there is a complete obstruction of the bile duct, ERCP may not demonstrate the proximal extent of the tumour and PTC will be necessary.

Arteriography

This must be performed if surgery is contemplated. The late phase of a selective arteriogram will give an indirect portogram. Involvement of the portal vein or the hepatic arteries indicates an unresectable tumour. Arteriography will not, however, demonstrate the inferior vena cava and caudate lobe particularly well (Voyles *et al.*, 1983).

(c) Curative treatment

The only curative treatment is surgery. Unfortunately, only about 30% are thought suitable for surgery. Of these, at best two-thirds have a curative resection (Evander *et al.*, 1980; Voyles *et al.*, 1983).

Site of the tumour

The tumour prognosis and the type of operation are dependent on the site of the tumour. The bile duct may be divided into thirds as described below.

Upper third These have the worst prognosis. They are frequently unresectable. If the tumour is at the bifurcation of the hepatic duct, it is known as Klatskin's tumour. If the tumour invades the liver, a partial hepatectomy may be necessary. In these cases a hepaticojejunostomy is performed.

Middle third These have a relatively good prognosis if resectable. A choledochojejunostomy is performed. This has a low operative mortality rate.

Lower third If these are resected, a Whipple's procedure is necessary. This has an operative mortality rate of about 20% (Tompkins *et al.*, 1981).

Preoperative drainage of jaundice

There is an increased risk of coagulation disorders and postoperative renal failure after surgery in the jaundiced patient. It was thought, therefore, that preoperative decompression of jaundice would benefit these patients and improve operative mortality (Denning *et al.*, 1981). However, two randomized, controlled trials comparing laparotomy alone to preoperative percutaneous transhepatic biliary drainage (PTBD) for at least 18 days followed by laparotomy, showed no difference in either morbidity or mortality

between the two groups (Benjamin *et al.*, 1984; Gibby *et al.*, 1985)

Indications for surgery are:

1. No evidence of distant metastases.
2. No evidence of lymph node metastases beyond the hepatic pedicle.
3. No involvement of the hepatic artery or portal vein.
4. Liver disease limited to one lobe (Bismuth *et al.*, 1992).

Morbidity The main complications are biliary fistulas, anastomotic failure and renal failure (Evander *et al.*, 1980).

Mortality This depends on the site of the tumour and on careful patient selection. Rates vary between 23% and 0 (Tompkins *et al.*, 1981; Bismuth *et al.*, 1992). Causes of death include hepatic failure, tumour growth and gastrointestinal haemorrhage.

Recurrence rates These depends on the completeness of resection. If the resection is complete, then a 50% 3 year survival rate, without recurrence, is possible. If there is evidence of residual microscopic disease after resection, the recurrence rate may reach 90% (Bismuth *et al.*, 1992).

(d) Palliative treatment

Surgery

If unresectable disease is found at laparotomy, then a bypass procedure, e.g. cholecystojejunostomy, should be performed (Benjamin, 1989). Operative insertion of a 'U'-tube was popular in the early 1970s (Terblanche *et al.*, 1972). This had an arm which was exteriorized and which increased the risk of sepsis.

Since the late 1970s, however, it has been possible to bypass tumours without recourse to laparotomy (Nakayama *et al.*, 1978). Stents can be inserted via PTC or ERCP. If the tumour is known to be unresectable, it is reasonable to use these methods to bypass the obstruction before resorting to laparotomy (Stain *et al.*, 1992). Bypassing the obstruction will relieve symptoms and improve quality of life. It may increase survival to about 6 months (Evander *et al.*, 1980).

Radiotherapy

External beam radiotherapy at doses of 10–60 Gy, in fractions of 2 Gy/day, may be given (Hashikawa *et al.*, 1983). It relieves jaundice, but causes nausea, vomiting and anorexia. Implanted iridium-192 wires have been tried, but made little difference.

Chemotherapy

Mitomycin, 5-FU and adriamycin have been given systemically, with a 20% response rate, and regionally, with a 40% response rate. There has been no demonstrated increase in survival (Liver Cancer Study Group of Japan, 1984; Oberfield and Ross, 1988).

45.3 LIVER METASTASES

Liver metastases occur in approximately 25% of all patients with cancer (Bengmark, 1989). They can arise from any primary, but are particularly common in cancers of the gastrointestinal tract, of the breast and of melanocytes. Due to their frequency, most attention has been focused on liver metastases from colorectal cancer.

45.3.1 CLINICAL FEATURES

Most hepatic metastases are asymptomatic. Our experience suggests that up to 30% of the liver can be replaced before symptoms occur. At this stage, curative treatment is unlikely. Abdominal pain or mass, weight loss and anorexia are features of advanced metastatic disease. Jaundice is uncommon unless the bile ducts are blocked by diseased hilar lymph nodes. For curative treatment to be possible, metastases need to be found while they are small and asymptomatic.

45.3.2 INVESTIGATIONS

(a) Serology

Bilirubin, alkaline phosphatase (ALP) and lactic dehydrogenase (LDH) levels are raised only when the disease is very advanced. Serum carcinoembryonic antigen (CEA) levels greater than 5 ng/ml are a sensitive indicator of colorectal malignancy (Wanebo *et al.*, 1978) and should be performed monthly in the follow-up period (Neville, 1986; Wiggers *et al.*, 1988).

The best method of screening for hepatic metastases is to combine measurement of serum CEA, ALP and LDH levels with one imaging technique (Kemeny *et al.*, 1986). Once they have been detected though, a more accurate assessment of their extent is necessary, in order to provide appropriate treatment. Radiological imaging techniques are the best method of assessment.

(b) Ultrasound scan

This is probably the most commonly used method due to its availability, speed, low cost and non-invasive nature. It has good specificity for metastases, but is unlikely to detect those less than 1 cm in size (Gunven *et al.*, 1985). Unfortunately, results depend largely on the experience of the sonographer, and up to 20% of scans may be technically inadequate (Bernardino and Lewis, 1982) due to the position of the liver or due to intestinal gas.

(c) CT scan (Figure 45.4)

This is less operator dependent than ultrasound. It is a sensitive investigation, detecting some lesions < 1 cm in size (Bernardino and Lewis, 1982). A significant advantage is that it can be combined with either intra-arterial or intravenous injection of contrast material to increase its sensitivity. False-positive results

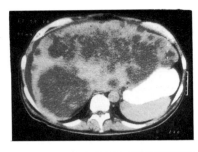

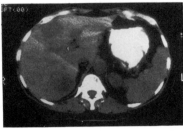

Figure 45.4 Contrast enhanced CT scan of colorectal liver metastases. The contrast opacifies normal hepatic parenchyma, but the metastases, being avascular, do not opacify and are seen as defects. Oral contrast agent is also seen in the stomach.

include lesions such as haemangiomas and adenomas. Unfortunately, like ultrasound, it is not good at detecting extrahepatic disease, e.g. hepatic lymph nodes, and may miss lesions in the left lateral lobe (Clarke *et al.*, 1989).

From examination of the CT images it is possible to calculate the percentage hepatic replacement (PHR) of the liver by tumour. This correlates well with the actual tumour volume and is an objective measurement which is useful in determining the effects of treatment (Hunt *et al.*, 1989).

(d) CT portography

This is an extremely sensitive investigation which will detect small hepatic lesions (Soyer *et al.*, 1992). It is invasive and is only used when surgery is contemplated. A contrast medium is injected via a catheter whose tip lies in the superior mesenteric artery. The liver is scanned when the contrast appears in the portal vein.

(e) Angiography

Visualization of the hepatic vasculature may be obtained by injection of contrast via a catheter in the hepatic artery. This is not useful in detecting metastases as they are hypovascular (Bernardino and Lewis, 1982), but is useful in determining the hepatic vasculature prior to either hepatic resection or insertion of a hepatic artery catheter for local chemotherapy infusion.

(f) Intraoperative ultrasound scan

This is a recent development which may be more accurate than CT (Clarke *et al.*, 1989). It can detect up to 40% more lesions than can be detected by palpation or visualization at operation. It is only useful when hepatic surgery is being performed as the liver must be fully mobilized to use the scanner. Thus it is not used to screen for metastases at the time of primary colonic surgery.

(g) Radionuclide scintigraphy/assessment at operation

These have been superseded by the above methods. They are not very sensitive and are only useful for detecting widespread disease (Bernardino and Lewis, 1982; Finlay *et al.*, 1982)

45.3.3 TREATMENT OF LIVER METASTASES

The only curative treatment for liver metastases is surgery. Chemotherapeutic treatment is under evaluation, but responses are limited. Radiotherapy has no role to play at present.

(a) Surgery

Of those who develop liver metastases, only 20–25% will be suitable for tumour resection (August *et al.*, 1984). Of these, only 20–25% will survive 5 years (Attiyeh and Stearns, 1981). Thus the proportion that can be said to be cured by surgery is small, but none the less significant. Hepatic resection should only be performed by appropriately experienced surgeons. Patients with the following features should be considered for surgery:

1. Less then four metastases (Ekbert *et al.*, 1986).
2. A unilobar distribution (Attiyeh and Stearns, 1981).
3. No extrahepatic disease (extrahepatic disease is associated with a poor prognosis) (Wagner *et al.*, 1984).
4. A PHR < 25%.

Contraindications include: more than four metastases, moderate/severe cirrhosis, unresectable extrahepatic disease, involved hepatic lymph nodes. The following are not contraindications: Duke's stage C, a high preoperative CEA level (Ekberg *et al.*, 1986; Petrelli *et al.*, 1991).

Morbidity is due to sepsis, e.g. wound infection, subphrenic abscess, pneumonia, and occurs in about 30% of patients (Petrelli *et al.*, 1991). It increases with age, extent of resection and preoperative systemic disease.

Mortality should be less than 5% (Vetto *et al.*, 1990). It is due to haemorrhage, overwhelming sepsis and liver failure.

(b)   Operative details

The understanding of the liver's segmental blood supply has led to better and safer hepatic surgery (McPherson *et al.*, 1984). The liver can be divided into eight segments by the hepatic veins and branches of the portal vein. This means that localized resection is possible with much less blood loss than previously. Right and left hepatectomy, single segmentectomies and bisegmentectomies are now associated with low morbidity and mortality (Bismuth, 1986).

(c)   Recurrence after liver resection

Recurrence occurs in 60–80% (Ekberg *et al.*, 1986). Of these, approximately 33% will have disease confined to the liver, the rest will have either extrahepatic disease only, or both extrahepatic and liver disease. Those with disease confined to the liver may be suitable for further surgery, the rest are not.

(d)   Chemotherapy

In view of the limited number of patients with liver metastases that can be helped by surgery, attempts have been made to reduce tumour burden with chemotherapy. The agent which has been most widely used for colorectal metastases is 5-FU (Chapter 42) either systemically (Kemeny, 1983) or intra-arterially, when fluorodeoxyuridine has a higher first pass take up (Van de Velde *et al.*, 1988). Death usually occurs due to progression of disease outside the liver (Kemeny, 1992).

(e)   Lipiodol

As mentioned previously, this has been used in primary liver tumours. It may be combined with iodine-131.

It is selectively taken up by tumour cells. Unfortunately, as liver metastases are hypovascular, it seems to effect only those cells at the periphery of the metastasis (Bretagne *et al.*, 1988).

(f)   Embolization

This is a non-selective method of attacking malignant cells. Inoperable liver metastases tend to be multifocal. Therefore widespread ischaemic damage to normal hepatocytes may result from embolization. Although microspheres and gel foam may reduce tumour size, an increase in survival has not been demonstrated (Bengmark, 1989).

REFERENCES

Attiyeh, F.F. and Stearns, M.W. (1981) Second look laparotomy based on CEA elevations in colorectal cancer. *Cancer*, **47**, 2119–25.

August, D.A., Ottow, R.T. and Sugarbaker, P.H. (1984) Clinical perspective of human colorectal cancer metastases. *Cancer Metastasis Reviews*, **3**, 303–24.

Belghiti, J. (1991) Resection of hepatocellular carcinoma complicating cirrhosis. *British Journal of Surgery*, **78**, 257–8.

Bengmark, S. (1989) Palliative treatment of hepatic tumours. *British Journal of Surgery*, **76**, 771–3.

Benjamin, I.S. (1989) Progress in liver resection. *Cancer Topics*, **7**, 54–6.

Bismuth, H. (1986) Surgical Anatomy of the Liver in Recent Results in Cancer Research, in *Therapeutic Strategies in Primary and Metastatic Liver Cancer* (eds Ch. Herfath, P. Schlag and P. Hohenberg), Springer-Verlag, Berlin, pp. 170–84.

Bismuth, H., Nakache, R. and Diamond, T. (1992) Management strategies in resection of hilar cholangiocarcinoma. *Annals of Surgery*, **215**, 31–8.

Bretagne, J., Raoul, J., Bourget, P. *et al.* (1988) Hepatic artery injection of I-131 labelled Lipiodol part II.: preliminary results of therapeutic use in patients with hepatocellular carcinoma and liver metastases. *Radiology*, **168**, 547–50.

Choi, T.K., Nim, W.L. and Wong, J. (1984) Chemotherapy for advanced hepatocellular carcinoma. Adriamycin versus quadruple chemotherapy. *Cancer*, **53**, 401–5.

Clarke, M.P., Kane, RA., Steele, G. Jr *et al.* (1989) Prospective comparison of preoperative imaging and intraoperative ultrasonography (IOUS) in the detection of liver tumours. *British Journal of Surgery*, **76**, 1323–9.

Denning, D. A., Ellison, E.C. and Carey, L.C. (1981) Preoperative percutaneous transhepatic biliary decompression lowers operative morbidity in patients with obstructive jaundice. *American Journal of Surgery*, **141**, 61–5.

Ekberg, H., Tranberg, K-G., Anderson, R. *et al.* (1986) Determinants of survival in liver resection for colorectal secondaries. *British Journal of Surgery*, **73**, 727–31.

Epstein, B., Ettinger, D., Leuchner, P.K. and Order, S.E. (1991) Multimodality cisplatin treatment in non-resectable alpha-fetoprotein positive hepatoma. *Cancer*, **67**, 896–900.

Evander, A., Freudland, P., Hoevels, J. *et al.* (1980) Evaluation of aggressive surgery in carcinoma of the extrahepatic bile ducts. *Annals of Surgery*, **191**, 23.

Falkson, G., Moertal, C.G., Lavin, P. *et al.* (1978) Chemotherapy studies in primary liver cancer. A prospective randomised clinical trial. *Cancer*, **42**, 2149–56.

Finlay, I.G., Meek, D.R., Gray, H.W. *et al.* (1982) Incidence and detection of occult hepatic metastases in colorectal carcinoma. *British Medical Journal*, **284**, 803–5.

Gibby, D.G., Hanks, J.B., Wanebo, H.J. *et al.* (1985) Bile duct carcinoma: diagnosis and treatment. *Annals of Surgery*, **202**, 139–44.

Gunven, P., Makuuchi, M., Takayasu, K. *et al.* (1985) Preoperative imaging of liver metastases. Comparison of angiography, CT scan and ultrasonography. *Annals of Surgery*, **202**, 537–9.

Hashikawa, Y., Shimada, T., Miura, T. and Imajyo, Y. (1983) Radiation therapy of carcinoma of the extrahepatic bile ducts. *Radiology*, **146**, 787–9.

Hunt, T.M., Flowerdew, A.D.S., Taylor, I. *et al.* (1989) A comparison of methods to measure the Percentage Hepatic Replacement in colorectal liver metastases. *Annals of the Royal College of Surgeons of England*, **71**, 11–13.

Ikeda, K., Kumada, H., Saitoh, S. *et al.* (1991) Effect of repeated transcatheter arterial embolisation on the survival time in patients with hepatocellular carcinoma: an analysis by Cox proportional hazard model. *Cancer*, **68**, 2150–4.

Ikeda, K., Saitoh, S., Tsubota, A. (1993) Risk factors for tumour recurrence and prognosis after curative resection of hepatocellular carcinoma. *Cancer*, **71**, 19–25.

Iwatsuki, S., Gordon, R.D., Shaw, B.W. and Starzl, T.E. (1985) Role of liver transplantation in cancer therapy. *Annals of Surgery*, **202**, 401–7.

Katagari, Y., Mabuchi, K., Itakura, T. *et al.* (1989) Adriamycin-Lipiodol suspension for i.a. chemotherapy of hepatocellular carcinoma. *Cancer Chemotherapy and Pharmacology*, **23**, 238–42.

Kemeny, N. (1983) The systemic chemotherapy of hepatic metastases. *Seminars in Oncology*, **10**, 148–58.

Kemeny, N. (1992) Review of regional therapy of liver metastases in colorectal cancer. *Seminars in Oncology*, **19**, (Suppl. 3), 155–62.

Kemeny, M.M., Ganteaume, L., Goldberg, D.A. *et al.* (1986) Preoperative staging with Computed Axial Tomography and biochemical laboratory tests in patients with hepatic metastases. *Annals of Surgery*, **203**, 169–72.

Kubo, Y., Okuda, K., Musha, H. and Nakashima, T. (1978) Detection of hepatocellular carcinoma during a clinical follow-up of chronic liver disease. Observations in 31 patients. *Gastroenterology*, **74**, 578–82.

Liaw, J.F., Tai, D.I., Chu, C.M. *et al.* (1986) Early detection of hepatocellular carcinoma in patients with chronic type B hepatitis. A prospective study. *Gastroenterology*, **90**, 263–7.

Lin, T.Y., Lee, C.S., Chan, K.M. and Chen, C.C. (1987) Role of surgery in the treatment of primary carcinoma of the liver: a 31 year experience. *British Journal of Surgery*, **74**, 839–42.

Liver Cancer Study Group of Japan (1984) Primary liver cancer in Japan. *Cancer*, **54**, 1747–55.

Masters, A., Steger, A.C. and Bown, S.G. (1991) Role of interstitial therapy in the treatment of liver cancer. *British Journal of Surgery*, **78**, 518–23.

McPherson, G.A.D., Benjamin, I.S., Hodgson, H.J.F. et al. (1984) Preoperative percutaneous transhepatic biliary drainage. The results of a controlled trial. *British Journal of Surgery*, **71**, 371–5.

Murray-Lyon, I.M. (1990) Liver tumours, in *Oxford Textbook of Medicine 1990*, 2nd edn, (eds D.J. Weatherall, J.G.G., Ledingham and D.A. Warrell), Oxford University Press, Oxford, pp. 12.256–9.

Nagasue, N., Yukaya, H., Chang, Y.C. et al. (1987) Appraisal of hepatic resection in the treatment of minute hepatocellular carcinoma associated with liver cirrhosis. *British Journal of Surgery*, **74**, 836–8.

Nagasue, N., Yukaya, H., Hamada, T. et al. (1984) The natural history of hepatocellular carcinoma. A study of 100 untreated cases. *Cancer*, **54**, 1461–5.

Nakayama, T., Ikeda, A. and Okuda, K. (1978) Percutaneous transhepatic drainage of the biliary tract. *Gastroenterology*, **74**, 554.

Neville, A.M. (1986) International Union against Cancer Report. Workshop on Immunodiagnosis. *Cancer Research*, **46**, 3744–6.

Novell, J.R., Hilson, A. and Hobbs, K.E.F. (1991) Therapeutic aspects of radio-isotopes in hepatobiliary malignancy. *British Journal of Surgery*, **78**, 901–6.

Oberfield, R.A. and Ross, R.N. (1988) The role of chemotherapy in the treatment of bile duct cancer. *World Journal of Surgery*, **12**, 771–3.

Okamoto, E., Kyo, A., Yamanaka, N. et al. (1984) Prediction of the safe limits of hepatectomy by combined volumetric and functional measurements in patients with impaired hepatic function. *Surgery*, **95**, 586–92.

Ong, G.B. and Chaw, P.R.W. (1976) Primary carcinoma of the liver. *Surgery, Gynecology and Obstetrics*, **143**, 31–8.

Paquet, K.J., Koussouris, P., Mercado, M.A. et al. (1991) Limited hepatic resection for selected cirrhotic patients with hepatocellular or cholangiocellular carcinoma: a prospective study. *British Journal of Surgery*, **78**, 459–62.

Petrelli, N., Gupta, B., Piedmonte, M. and Herrera, L. (1991) Morbidity and survival of liver resection for colorectal carcinoma. *Diseases of the Colon and Rectum*, **34**, 899–904.

Sako, K., Seitzinger, G.L. and Garside, E. (1957) Carcinoma of the extrahepatic bile ducts: review of the literature and report of six cases. *Surgery*, **41**, 416.

Sciarrino, E., Simaretti, R.G., Le Moli, S. and Pagliaro, L. (1985) Adriamycin treatment for hepatocellular carcinoma. Experience with 109 patients. *Cancer*, **56**, 2751–5.

Shiina, S., Tagawa, K., Unuma, T. et al. (1990) Percutaneous ethanol injection therapy of hepatocellular carcinoma: analysis of 77 patients. *American Journal of Roentgenology*, **155**, 1221–6.

Soyer, P., Levesque, M., Elias, D. et al. (1992) Preoperative assessment of resectability of hepatic metastases from colonic carcinoma: CT portography vs sonography and dynamic CT. *American Journal of Roentgenology*, **159**, 741–4.

Stain, S.C., Baer, H.U., Dennison, A.R. and Blumgart, H. L. (1992) Current management of hilar cholangiocarcinoma. *Surgery, Gynecology and Obstetrics*, **175**, 579–88.

Terblanche, J., Saunders, S.J. and Louw, H.J. (1972) Prolonged palliation in carcinoma of the main hepatic duct junction. *Surgery*, **71**, 720.

Tompkins, R.K., Thomas, D., Wile, A. and Longmire, W.P. Jr (1981) Prognosis factors in bile duct carcinoma: analysis of 96 cases. *Annals of Surgery*, **194**, 447–57.

Trede, M. and Raute, M. (1986) Surgical therapy of primary liver tumours, in *Recent Results in Cancer Research. Therapeutic Strategies in Primary and Metastatic Liver Cancer*, (eds Ch. Herfath, P. Schlag and P. Hohenberger), Springer-Verlag, Berlin, pp. 197–211.

Van de Velde, C.J.H., Maurits de Brau, L., Sugarbaker, P.H. and Tranberg, K-G. (1988) Hepatic artery infusion chemotherapy: rationale, results, credits and debits. *Regional Cancer Treatment*, **1**, 93–101.

Vetto, J.T., Hughes, K.S., Rosenstein, R. and Sugarbaker, P.H. (1990) Morbidity and mortality of hepatic resection for metastatic colorectal carcinoma. *Diseases of the Colon and Rectum*, **33**, 408–13.

Voyles, C.R., Bowley, N. J., Allison, D J. et al. (1983) Carcinoma of the proximal extrahepatic biliary tree: radiological assessment and therapeutic alternatives. *Annals of Surgery*, **197**, 188–93.

Wagner, J.S., Adson, M.A., Van Heerden, J.A. et al. (1984) The natural history of colorectal metastases from colorectal cancer. A comparison with resective treatment. *Annals of Surgery*, **199**, 502–8.

Wanebo, H., Bhaskar, R., Pinsky, C.M. et al. (1978) Preoperative carcinoembryonic attention level as a prognostic indicator in colorectal cancer. *New England Journal of Medicine*, **299**, 443–51.

Wiggers, T., Arendo, J.W. and Volovics, A. (1988) Regression analysis of prognosis factors in colorectal cancer after curative resections. *Diseases of the Colon and Rectum*, **31**, 33–41.

EXOCRINE PANCREATIC CARCINOMA 46

J-C. Gazet

46.1 INCIDENCE

It is now considered that cancer is responsible for a third of all deaths in the UK and the lifetime risk for males was 33.73 and for females 32.03 as calculated in 1985. Total deaths from cancer in 1986 were 158 770, of which pancreatic cancer accounted for 3300 in males (4%) and 3480 in females (5%).

The incidence in the UK in 1984 was 121 per million, ranked 8th in males with 3330, and 110 per million ranked 10th in women with 3184 reported cases. The incidence was similar in 1988 with a lifetime risk of 0.94 in males and 0.92 in females. Examining the EC cancer statistics, it did not rank in the first 10 for 1978–82. The 5 year survival is approximately 4.5% and the lowest for any gastrointestinal tumour. This suggests that the reported incidence and known mortality are virtually the same.

It is interesting to note that the incidence of pancreatic carcinoma, where recorded, is twice as high in developed countries as in underdeveloped countries.

The incidence varies with age, sex and race. It is rare under 30; the incidence rises steeply and progressively after 50, so that in males aged 75 or over, the tumour occurs eight to ten times more commonly than in the general population. Whereas it is more common in males than females in the UK (1.2 to 1), this rises for example to 4 to 1 amongst the Chinese in Singapore. The factors underlying racial differences are not obvious but there are gross differences between the black population in the USA compared with Nigeria, suggesting environmental causes which though related to socio-economic status are confirmed by studies on migrant populations.

46.2 AETIOLOGY

The aetiology of pancreatic carcinoma is unknown. The environmental factors which have been involved include tobacco, diet and alcohol. Host factors include diabetes mellitus, genetic factors, chronic pancreatitis and biliary tract disease. None of these factors stand up to critical statistical analysis as few series include sufficient cases to allow the data to be evaluated. This is due in part to the low incidence in the general population which prevents successful screening for early diseases in which epidemiological studies could be performed (Howat and Sarles, 1979).

46.3 PATHOLOGY

The histological classification of pancreatic cancer has received little attention in the past. This was due in part to the known clinical poor prognosis, and a genuine doubt as to the effect, if any, such a classification might have on the management of the patient.

The recognition of endocrine tumours of the gastrointestinal tract and the development of sophisticated immunocytochemical technique has allowed a complete re-appraisal of the situation. Whereas it had been generally accepted that 90% of pancreatic carcinomas were adenocarcinomas of ductal origin, the realization that some patients did not follow the anticipated course of such tumours has led to two fundamental changes.

The first is that the only way to confirm the diagnosis of a pancreatic carcinoma is by histological examination (Rode, 1990). The corollary is that it is not only necessary to differentiate between endocrine and exocrine tumours of the pancreas as their prognosis and treatment are completely different, but within each group to classify the tumour present by cell type.

Thus the first rule must be to accept that it is mandatory to diagnose and classify pancreatic tumours on histological grounds. Most classifications accept that cancer of the pancreas is basically an epithelial tumour of ductal or acinar cell type. Subgroups due to metaplasia, solid/cystic lesions and connective tissue tumours complete the picture. To this must be added the endocrine tumours which are usually non-functional. This classification is a synthesis of many: non-exhaustive and arguable (Table 46.1). The commonest site for an adenocarcinoma of the pancreas is the head (75%); the body (15%) and the tail (10%) account for the rest. The average size at presentation of a cancer of the head is 5 cm and the body and tail somewhat larger (5–7 cm). This in part is related to the development of obstructive jaundice with lesions in the head, whereas the presenting problem is pain with tumours of the body and tail. Resected tumours are usually considerably smaller (< 3.5 cm).

A pancreatic cancer is macroscopically hard, often fixed to the posterior abdominal wall with tell-tale invasion of the root of the mesentery.

Table 46.1   Primary tumours of the pancreas

EXOCRINE

	Benign	Malignant
Acinar cells	Adenoma	Acinar cell carcinoma
Ductal cells	Adenoma	Solid adenocarcinoma
	Cystadenoma	Cyst adenocarcinoma
Metaplastic cells		Adenosquamous carcinoma
		Adenoacanthoma
Solid/cystic		Giant cell carcinoma
		Mixed cell carcinoma
		Osteoblastic type carcinoma
Connective tissue	Lipoma	Sarcomas
	Fibroma	
	Haemangioma	
	Lymphangioma	

ENDOCRINE

Tumours with no perceptible hormone secretion (benign or malignant), e.g.

Islet cell tumour
Carcinoid
Hormone secretory tumours (benign or malignant)
Insulinoma (ZE syndrome)
Gastrinoma
Vipoma
Glucagonmona
Somatostatinoma
Carcinoid

The typical carcinoma elicits a marked desmoplastic reaction which accounts for its consistency and compounds the diagnosis with chronic pancreatitis. Differentiation between poorly and moderately differentiated adenocarcinoma is probably of little value. Of great significance is vascular, lymphatic and perineural invasion as evidence of spread and poor prognosis. The lymphatic drainage and node distribution is complex but basically nodal involvement carries a poor prognosis in patients undergoing pancreatectomy.

46.4 PRESENTATION

The clinical manifestations of pancreatic carcinoma are vague and ill defined. Abdominal pain is the most common symptom often associated with backache. Weight loss and anorexia complete the triad which often suggests a dyspeptic disorder. During the interval of 6 months between the onset of symptoms and a definitive diagnosis, the disease progresses inexorably and spreads. Obstructive jaundice is the most striking sudden and arresting symptom, present in over 50% of patients, but occurs late in the disease. Liver enlargement is common but is not diagnostic of liver involvement, rather of biliary obstruction.

The pain of cancer of the head of the pancreas is predominently in the epigastrium and radiates to the right hypochondrium.

Lesions of the body and tail produce pain in the left hypochondrium radiating to the ribs and back. The pain is severe, unremitting and dull. It can mimic that of peptic ulceration and the actual presence of duodenal ulcer does not exclude a pancreatic neoplasm which may encroach and invade the duodenum. Back pain is a symptom of cancer of the body but is also present in tumours of the head.

Loss of weight is a constant unvarying symptom of pancreatic cancer and cannot be precisely explained by anorexia or nausea which are not features of the early disease.

Dyspepsia has already been mentioned, but change in bowel habit, flatulence and intolerance to fatty foods occurs. Neuropsychiatric symptoms are common with emotional disturbance, depression and anxiety. The relation of this to pain, weight loss and anorexia are hard to define.

Migratory thrombophlebitis first described by Trousseau in 1877 in association with pancreatic cancer is well known but not associated with either invasion or compression of veins by tumour. Hypoglycaemia has been reported as has pancreatitis, with both commonly being present together.

Dark urine, skin irritation and frank jaundice are late symptoms all too familiar in the diagnosis of cancer of the pancreas.

The physical signs may be few and indistinct. An enlarged liver, a palpable gallbladder and obstructive jaundice are obvious signs of a tumour in the head of the pancreas. Courvoisier in 1890 simply stated that in the presence of jaundice if the gallbladder was palpable, the cause (of the jaundice) was unlikely to be due to stones. This implied that with cholelithiasis, it was uncommon not to have a degree of cholecystitis with associated fibrosis of the gallbladder.

A palpable mass in the epigastrium associated with vomiting is a sign of advanced disease. A pancreatic cancer is rarely palpable at the stage at which it is operable. Similarly, the presence of ascites and palpable skin nodules are signs of impending dissolution not pancreatic cancer.

It has been said many times that the diagnosis of pancreatic cancer is made when the diagnosis is thought of. Several series of patients with symptoms referrable to the gastrointestinal system have shown that once the diagnosis of pancreatic cancer was entertained, the diagnosis were made in 17–25% of patients where preliminary investigations excluded other upper gastrointestinal disease.

46.5 INVESTIGATIONS

There are no reliable specific diagnostic tumour markers for pancreatic carcinoma. Furthermore, specific tests of pancreatic function such as glucose tolerance or pancreatic secretory test are usually of little help. Serological tests have been criticized because they fail to detect pancreatic carcinoma at a treatable stage and tend to be less reliable in the presence of jaundice. Thus such a test should be effective in a symptomatic non-jaundiced patient with small tumours. Due to the rarity of the tumour (say 20 per 10^5 population in the western countries), a screening test would have to be 100% sensitive and 99.95% specific to be effective. If it were 100% sensitive and only 99% specific there would be 1020 positive test with only 20 true positive and 1000 false positive requiring further exhaustive investigations (Rhodes and Ching, 1990).

The monoclonal antibodies raised against colorectal tumours, Ca 19.9 and Ca 50 are sensitive to 68–93% and 60–81% respectively for pancreatic tumours. DU-PAN-2 raised against pancreatic cancer is only 36–68% sensitive. Oncofetal pancreatic antigen like carcinoembryonic antigen both raised against fetal tumour are too unreliable.

These tests have all been shown to be of greater value in assessing progress and recurrence of the tumour itself and metastases. Nothing has changed in the last decade.

Having considered the diagnosis, then the first valuable investigation is abdominal ultrasonography. This can demonstrate an abnormality of the pancreas, be it a distinct mass or general enlargement. It is possible to detect bile duct and common bile duct dilatation in the absence of obstructive jaundice. Furthermore, vascular abnormalities such as portal vein or superior mesenteric vein obstruction can be shown, apart from metastatic lesion in the liver and ascites in the peritoneal cavity.

Where ultrasound investigation is indeterminate or further evaluation is required, a CT scan is of great value. Both these investigations allow safe image-guided percutaneous pancreatic core biopsy. Rode (1990) has pointed out the value of this technique when, using a spring-loaded device (Biopsy Gun) and a suitable needle, a core measuring 1.7 × 1.2 mm can be obtained for histological measurement. The speed of the device in obtaining the specimen and size of the needle prevents haemorrhage and fistula formation. Using this technique 602 biopsies were performed in 241 patients investigated for biliary obstruction or pancreatic pain where a mass was found by ultrasound in the pancreatic area. One hundred and seventy neoplasms in 241 patients were diagnosed (70.5%).

In the presence of jaundice it is possible to proceed to percutaneous transhepatic cholangiography which not only allows the biliary tree to be delineated but sites the position of the obstruction. It allows aspiration biopsy and the insertion of a stent to overcome the obstruction by internal drainage, or if this is not possible by external drainage. Alternatively, it is possible by endoscopic examination of the duodenum to perform endoscopic retrograde cholangio-pancreatography (ERCP) which will outline the biliary and/or pancreatic ducts, insert a stent, obtain a biopsy and exclude an ampullary lesion.

Thus the nature of the lesion in the pancreas can be histologically proven, the size delineated by ultrasound or CT scan. Finally vascular involvement of the portal vein and superior mesenteric vein can be excluded or confirmed by digital subtraction angiography using the Seldinger percutaneous trans-femoral approach. This will also delineate the arterial blood supply, highlighting any vascular abnormalities seen including those found with metastases.

The sequential investigation of the patient allows for a proper assessment as to whether the primary lesion is resectable and allows by a staging algorithm to decide on appropriate therapy.

46.6 STAGING

The classification and staging of pancreatic carcinoma is a recent development and has been controversial. The UICC (1987) and American Joint Committee on Cancer (1983) have agreed a classification based on the TNM classification of malignant tumours. This has effectively been a compromise of a variety of proposed stages (Gazet, 1986) and is different from the staging classification of pancreatic carcinoma proposed by the Japanese Pancreatic Society (1982).

Enough data from composite groups has been collected and published to justify the use of comparable staging and allow refinements to develop in the future for results from single institutes to be collated. For example, it has become crystal clear that tumour size (T) is critical in exocrine carcinoma of the pancreas. Tsuchiya *et al.* (1986) reported a 96.7% resectability for tumours less than 2 cm (T1) falling to 18.3% in those with tumour greater than 6 cm (T4). The overall cumulative survival after operation for T1 tumours was 26.6% at 8 years compared with 6.6% for T4 tumours. However, only 240/4406 (5.4%) were T1 and comprised 232/2097 (11.1%) of all resections. Thus the Japanese classification is based on T1 tumours < 2 cm, T2 2.1–4 cm, T3 4.1–6 cm and T4 > 6 cm. The American staging takes no account of size, but considers stage on involvement of adjacent structures. The UICC TNM classification is a compromise accepting the importance of 2 cm as the earliest stage (Table 46.2). The Japanese take into account lymph node involvement as: N1, primary nodes immediately draining the tumour; N2, involvement of the secondary group of lymph nodes draining the whole pancreas; N3, involvement of lymph nodes beyond the local regional lymphatics. Both the UICC and American Joint Committee on Cancer consider only whether regional lymph nodes are involved or not.

Similarly over the question of involvement of the pancreatic capsule (S), retroperitoneal structures (Rp) and portal vein (V), the Japanese classification distinguishes between: S1 Rp1 V1, suspected invasion; S2 Rp2 and V2, minimal invasion, S3 Rp3 and V3, marked tumour invasion. This is only discussed as distant metastases M1 in the UICC and AJCC classifications.

Whereas, it can be accepted that overcomplicated staging details may be counterproductive in their collection and collation, if minimal data only is assessed then significant trends will not be noted. It follows therefore that in a disease which at present defies cure in a reasonable proportion of cases, data collection must still play a major role in assessing the strategies employed in managing the problem. Recently Bakkevold and Kambestad (1993) have reviewed the Norwegian experience in staging and have shown using the UICC, TNM classification that survival is strictly related to stage with a median survival of 342 days for Stage I, 229 for Stage II, 169 for Stage III and 79 for Stage IV. Where the stage could not be identified the median survival was 135 days.

46.7 PROGNOSTIC FACTORS

There is strong evidence from the literature over the last decade to confirm that tumour site, TNM stage, vascular invasion, lymph node metastases and distant metastases are all independant prognostic factors in survival.

Age, sex, patient status (Karnofsky index), histological grade and capsular invasion are more contentious. Radical surgery is an independent valid prognostic indicator which is enhanced by small tumour size (T1). The exception is with endocrine tumours where size is not important.

The three most significant factors in operative risk in pancreatic resection are the presence of jaundice, the age of the patient and the ability of the surgeon (Jeekel, 1992). An

Table 46.2   Stages of exocrine pancreatic carcinoma

STAGE	JAPANESE	UICC	ACC
I	T1 (< 2 cm) NO	T1 limited to pancreas	T1 limited to pancreas
	S0	T1A (< 2 cm)	
	RpO	T1B (> 2 cm)	
	V0	T2 Extension duodenum, bile duct, pancreatic tissue	
		N0 M0	N0 M0
II	T2 (2.1–4 cm)	T3 Extension stomach, spleen, colon, large vessels	
	N1 (Primary nodes)	N0	Not resectable
	SI	M0	N0 M0
	Rp1		
	V1		
III	T3 (4.1–6 cm)	T1–3	T1–3
	N2 (Secondary nodes)	N1 (Regional lymph nodes)	N1 (Regional lymph nodes)
	S2	M0	M0
	Rp2		
	V2		
IV	T4 (> 6.1 cm)	T1–3	T1–3
	N3	N0–1	N0–1
	S3	M1	M1
	Rp3		
	V3		

operative mortality or greater than 5% for a radical resection of the pancreas is no longer acceptable. The Johns Hopkins group concluded that the improvment in surgical end results is due to fewer surgeons performing more radical pancreatectomies in less time and less blood loss. This view highlights reports of current mortality rates exceeding 20% in the hands of surgeons with occasional experience. These facts strengthen the case for regionalization of this type of surgery (Warshaw and Swanson, 1988).

It had been suggested that preoperative decompression of the biliary tract by external drainage in jaundiced patients reduced the operative mortality. Sadly, controlled clinical trials did not confirm this; however it stimulated the search for effective drainage which has resulted in endoscopic stenting. This procedure is less invasive, allows evaluation of the patient and planned treatment and has been shown to be highly effective in relieving the acute symptoms of obstructive jaundice.

It was traditionally considered that patients aged 70 and over were not candidates for radical surgery. Most experienced surgeons set no age limit, but rather base their decision on the general assessment of the patient including renal function, cardiopulmonary status and mental state.

Thus the first and most important prognostic factor is whether the patient is treated in a dedicated pancreaticobiliary unit. However, generally speaking improved resection rate with lowered mortality, although now the expected standard, has not led to a dramatic increase in 5 year survivors. This is directly related to the stage at which the disease is detected.

It is therefore necessary to look at the ability of radiotherapy and chemotherapy to improve the general results of radical surgery. Thus the second important prognostic factor is whether the patient has access to a multidisciplinary unit comprising surgeon, radiotherapist and physician with a special expertise in the management of cancer.

46.8   CURRENT MANAGEMENT

The current management depends upon the extent of the disease on full staging.

46.8.1   SURGERY

If the patient has evidence of distant metastases (M1), surgery is not indicated except for relief of obstruction. Biliary obstruction is best dealt with by stenting either introduced by PTC or ERCP. In spite of a high failure rate from obstruction with biliary sludge, stents usually can be easily replaced by an experienced interventionalist radiologist or gastroenterologist. Gastric obstruction will occur in 10% of patients and is best dealt with by gastrojejunostomy. If this becomes necessary it is possible at the same operation to perform a triple bypass (gastrojejunostomy, choledocho loop jejunostomy and jejunojejunostomy).

When staging has suggested that the tumour is resectable then laparotomy should be performed with the intent of performing radical surgery. On this basis between 1982 and 1989 Jeekel (1992) performed 206 laparotomies achieving 108 radical pancreaticoduodenectomies with a 2% mortality.

Three procedures are currently performed, namely a radical pancreaticoduodenectomy (classical Whipple's operation), total pancreaticoduodenectomy and pylorus preserving pancreaticoduodenectomy (PPP – a variation on the classical Whipple's operation). Each of these operations can be associated with either a radical lymphadenectomy of the surrounding lymph nodal drainage area including skeletonization of the porta hepatis vessels (R1) or an extended radical pancreaticoduodenectomy (R2) which can remove en bloc the pancreas, regional lymph nodes, duodenum, gastric antrum and intrapancreatic portal vein.

One of the major problems with all operations for ductal carcinoma of the pancreas is the complication rate. A radical pancreaticoduodenectomy removes the head of the pancreas, gastric antrum and duodenal loop. Pancreatic fistula will occur in 10% of patients at the anastomosis of the pancreatic duct and body of the pancreas to the jejunum. Gastric retention is a well documented complication especially after pyloric preserving pancreaticoduodenectomy. Biliary fistulas usually heal spontaneously, though a late stricture with jaundice can be a serious problem. Total pancreatectomy eliminates pancreatic fistulas, which have a mortality, but at the price of diabetes which can be brittle and difficult to treat.

Haemorrhage is the most feared complication often associated with infection and a potent cause of death unless dealt with promptly by re-operation. Large volumes of blood can be rapidly lost.

Late complications of all these procedures include as already stated jaundice from stricture of the choledochojejunostomy, gastric ulceration, diabetes mellitus even in subtotal pancreatic resection (25%), steatorrhoea and finally recurrent disease.

Despite the complications experienced even by an expert surgeon, the results in the last decade are encouraging with a range of 30–78% 1 year survival down to 0–37% 5 year survival. These results are directly related to the experience of the surgeon and number of procedures performed.

However, there is little evidence to suggest the more radical procedure (extended pancreaticoduodenectomy – R2) produces better results except in the most specialized units. Thus morbidity and mortality outweigh theoretical gain (Hiraoka *et al.* 1990).

46.8.2 RADIOTHERAPY

There is ample evidence that preoperative, introperative (IORT) or postoperative radiotherapy improves survival. Furthermore, preoperative radiotherapy will improve the resectability rate.

Jeekel (1992) has proposed that where a primary tumour with no visible metastases (M0) is not resectable, the patient should be treated with radiotherapy and 5-FU with a second look procedure at 6 months. In six cases following postlaparotomy radiation, a Whipple's procedure was possible with survival at 10, 10, 36 and 80 months. In a personal series of similar cases, we have noted a 50% resection rate after radiotherapy at second look surgery, confirming observations by others that preoperative radiotherapy is effective in downstaging pancreatic surgery. Thus preoperative radiotherapy increases the overall resectability rate and can have a positive effect on patient survival.

Hiraoka *et al.* (1990) have combined extended radical pancreaticoduodenectomy (R2) with IORT with a projected 5 year survival of 33%. Ozaki *et al.* (1990) combined extended surgery (R2) and 30 Gy IORT with intraoperative hepatic artery or portal vein mitomycin C and postoperative systemic

mitomycin C. Sixteen patients so treated had a 88% 1 year survival and 53% 3 year survival. Despite the quite dramatic increase in survival in patients receiving postoperative radiotherapy and 5-FU as shown by the Gastrointestinal Tumour Group (GITSG) in 1985 (Kalser and Ellenberg, 1985) and in 1987 (Douglas), this therapy has failed to be used routinely in clinical practice. It is difficult to understand the reasons for this. It is accepted that in 1993 it is as yet not possible to give IORT in the UK but it is standard practice in some EC countries. Preoperative radiotherapy does require a dedicated assessment of the patient presurgery. However, postoperative radiotherapy is freely available. Evidence has been presented that local control of pancreas can be achieved with interstitial implantation of radioactive isotopes such as iodine-125. It will boost the effect of postoperative radiotherapy and appears to offer consistent improved local control, particularly after resection (Shipley *et al.*, 1980; Perez *et al.*, 1989). This has been our experience even with radioactive gold ([198]AU) in improving the median survival following palliative resection.

46.8.3 CHEMOTHERAPY

Chemotherapy has been used for 30 years in advanced pancreatic carcinoma. Its development has been slow, mainly because of all the agents tested only 5-FU has been the most consistently effective drug. Partial response seen with single agents is usually short lived. It is now considered that the most effective drug combinations for pancreatic carcinoma include 5-FU, mitomycin C, epirubicin, cisplatinum and streptozotocin. Current studies are examining the value of ECF (epirubicin, 5-FU and cisplatinum) with or without streptozotocin (ECFS) against conventional regimens, as epirubicin is less cardiotoxic than doxorubicin and is being used in combination with 5-FU and mitomycin C (FEM). The two most favoured regimens have been FAM (5-FU doxorubicin and mitomycin C) and SFM (streptozotocin, mitomycin C and 5-FU). S-FAM has been our usual combination therapy in advanced disease. Combination treatment such as radiotherapy and 5-FU followed by SMF has shown a significant increased survival rate over patients treated by standard therapy (SMF) only. However, with all therapies of this type, an account must be taken of possible additional toxicity.

It can be said that postoperative radiotherapy with 5-FU should be standard adjuvant therapy for patients undergoing a curative resection of a pancreatic carcinoma.

If the tumour, at explorative surgery, is found to be unresectable, then the ideal treatment is immediate IORT or insertion of iodine-125 granules. If this is not possible, postoperative radiotherapy with chemotherapy (epirubicin, 5-FU and cisplatinum). The patient should be reassessed with CT scanning and where apparent downstaging has occurred then re-exploration within 6 months in an attempt to remove residual tumour should be the rule. When at surgery the tumour is not only found to be unresectable but also undetected metastases are found precluding subsequent surgery, IORT and postoperative chemotherapy is of value. However, a triple bypass should be performed.

Patients with tumours involving portal vein or superior mesenteric vessels will benefit in many cases from radiotherapy which may subsequently, by downstaging the tumour, allow an exploratory laparotomy.

46.9   CURRENT CLINICAL RESEARCH

Current clinical research has three aims. The primary aim is to standardize optimal treatment for patients with resectable cancer of the pancreas.

Ultrasonography is already an established technique in primary diagnosis, but endoscopic ultrasonography with endoprobes as small as 3 mm in diameter has opened up a new field of diagnostic assessment. The latest equipment can pick up tumours with 100% accuracy less than 20 mm in size, and with a working channel provide the possibility for improved accuracy of biopsy under endoscopic guidance. The overall accuracy of staging is quoted as 80–90%, with positive lymph node detection of about 75%.

Radioimmunolocalization of tumours is another fascinating and rapidly progressive field. At present CEA CA 19-9 TAG 72 (tumour associated antigen) and BW494 (an antigenic epitope present in pancreatic cancer cells recognized by murine monoclonal antibody BW 494) all show promise more for the diagnosis of recurrent disease than primary diagnosis.

The second aim has been to study the molecular biology of pancreatic exocrine tumours and their relationship to endocrine tumours. Insulin and IGF-I are mitogenic for pancreatic epithelial cells. Structural and functional abnormalities have been noted in growth factors such as EGF receptor and in oncogenes such as C-*erb*B-2, Ki-*ras* and the tumour suppressor gene p53. All studies show an increasing and complex relationship which requires extended *in vitro* and *in vivo* studies before the neoplastic phenotype is defined.

Finally, it is essential that multicentre randomized clinical trials of Phase II and Phase III drugs and their combinations continue in a new environment of multidisciplinary management of the primary tumour.

The management and results of treatment of endocrine tumours particularly the stent or non-secretory types with cure must stimulate further study of the exocrine lesion.

46.10   SYMPTOMATIC TREATMENT

Pancreatic cancer is a usually fatal painful debilitating disease. Too much stress cannot be applied to the palliative care, be it to relieve biliary and gastric obstruction or pain. Relief of pain and improvement of the quality of life is a major consideration. It is now well documented that IORT is highly effective in relieving pain and is more effective than either pre- or postoperative radiotherapy.

Paravertebral and coeliac plexus block with 100% absolute alcohol is equally effective either intraoperatively or postoperatively. Pain relief with drug therapy though effective can produce unacceptable side-effects of nausea, constipation, drowsiness and general sensation of loss of control. General medication, maintenance of body weight, relief of anorexia, nausea and control of diarrhoea or steatorrhoea are equally important. The help of a dedicated dietician is invaluable.

46.11 CONCLUSIONS

A nihilistic approach to pancreatic cancer must be avoided. The fatalistic approach has given way to a realistic and optimistic approach which can only be engendered by a deeply committed physician dedicated to the management of this form of cancer. Ralph Riddall Dobelbower Jr (1992) has summarized it best:

> Pancreatic carcinoma
> Many physicians advocate only supportive care for most patients with cancer of the pancreas. Such a philosophy ensures that most of the patients will die of cancer and that new treatment regimens will not be evaluated, thus creating a self-fulfilling prophecy. Similar philosophies have been promulgated in the past for Hodgkin's disease, advanced testicular cancer, and childhood leukaemia, all of which are now curable.
>
> Ralph Riddall Dobelbower, Jr (1992)
> Medical College of Ohio, USA.

REFERENCES

American Joint Committee on Cancer (1983) in *Manual for Staging of Cancer*, 2nd edn, (eds O.H. Beahrs and M.H. Myer), J.B. Lippincott, Philadelphia.

Bakkevold, K.E. and Kambestad, B. (1993) Long-term survival following radical and palliative treatment of patients with carcinoma of the pancreas and papilla of vater – the prognostic factors influencing the long-term results. A prospective multicentre study. *European Journal of Surgical Oncology*, **19**, 147–61.

Gazet, J-C. (1986) Surgeons as philatelists: collectors and classifiers. Part I. The problem in pancreatic cancer: Staging. *European Journal of Surgical Oncology*, **12**, 325–33.

Hiraoka, T. Uchino, R., Kanemitsu, K. *et al.* (1990) Combination of intraoperative radiation with resection of cancer of the pancreas. *International Journal of Pancreatology*, **7**, 201–7.

Howat H.T. and Sarles H. (eds) (1979). *The Exocrine Pancreas*, W.B. Saunders, Philadelphia.

Japanese Pancreatic Society (1982) *General rules for Surgical and Pathological Studies on Cancer of the Pancreas*, 2nd edn, Kanehara Publishing, Tokyo (in Japanese).

Jeekel, J. (1992) Radical surgery in pancreatic cancer, Lecture, ESSO, Helsinki.

Kalser, M.H. and Ellenberg, S.S. (1985) Pancreatic cancer. Adjuvant combined radiation and chemotherapy following curative resection. *Archives of Surgery*, **120**, 899–903.

Ozaki, H., Kinoshita, T., Kosuge, T. *et al.* (1990) Effectiveness of multimodality treatment for resectable pancreatic cancer. *International Journal of Pancreatology*, **7**, 195–200.

Peretz, T., Nori, D., Hilaris, B. *et al.* (1989) Treatment of primary unresectable carcinoma of the pancreas with I[125] implantation. *International Journal of Radiation Oncology, Biology, Physics*, 1989, **17**, 931–5.

Rhodes, J.M. and Ching, C.K. (1990) Serum diagnostic tests for pancreatic cancer. *Clinical Gastroenterology*, **4.4**, 833–52.

Rode, J. (1990) The pathology of pancreatic cancer. *Clinical Gastroenterology*, **4.1**, 793–813.

Shipley, W., Nardi, G.G., Cohen, A.M. and Ling, C.C. (1980) Iodine[125] implant and external beam irradiation in patients with localised pancreatic carcinoma. A comparison study to surgical resection. *Cancer*, **45**, 709–14.

UICC (1987) *TNM Classification of Malignant Tumours*, 4th edn, (eds P. Hermanek and L.H., Sobin), Springer-Verlag, Berlin.

Tsuchiya, R., Noda, T., Harada, N. *et al.* (1986) Collective review of small carcinomas of the pancreas. *Annals of Surgery*, **203**, 77–81.

Warshaw, A.L. and Swanson, R. (1988) Pancreatic cancer in 1988. Possibilities and probabilities. *Annals of Surgery*, **208**, 541–52.

INDEX